AF567002

Reoperative Gynecologic and Obstetric Surgery

Second Edition

A wise and experienced surgeon has said, "The second most difficult decision to make in surgery is when to operate. The most difficult decision is when to reoperate." The truth of this aphorism is readily apparent to most clinical surgeons.

Ronald K. Tompkins, M.D., 1988

Reoperative Gynecologic and Obstetric Surgery

Edited by
David H. Nichols, M.D.

Visiting Professor of Obstetrics, Gynecology, and Reproductive Biology
Harvard Medical School
Boston, Massachusetts

Past-Professor and Chairman of Obstetrics and Gynecology
Brown University School of Medicine
Providence, Rhode Island

Lecturer in Obstetrics and Gynecology
Tufts University School of Medicine
Boston, Massachusetts

Past-Professor of Gynecology and Obstetrics
State University of New York at Buffalo
Buffalo, New York

Second Edition
With 336 illustrations and 8 color plates

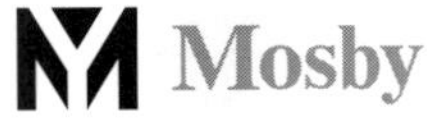

St. Louis Baltimore Boston Carlsbad Chicago Naples New York Philadelphia Portland
London Madrid Mexico City Singapore Sydney Tokyo Toronto Wiesbaden

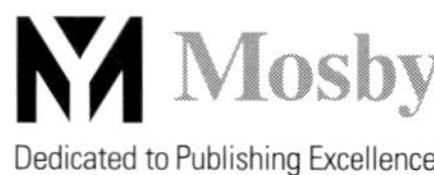

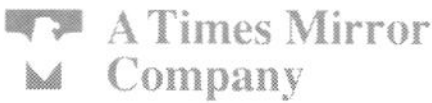

Vice President and Publisher: Anne S. Patterson
Editor: Susie Baxter
Developmental Editor: Anne Gunter
Project Manager: John Rogers
Project Specialist: Kathy Teal
Senior Production Editor: Helen Hudlin
Designer: Yael Kats
Manufacturing Supervisor: Don Carlisle

Second Edition

Printed in the United States of America
Composition by Graphic World, Inc.
Color film by Color Dot Graphics, Inc.
Lithography by Color Dot Litho, Inc.
Printing/binding by Maple-Vail Book Manufacturing Group

Mosby–Year Book, Inc.
11830 Westline Industrial Drive
St. Louis, Missouri 63146

ISBN 0-8151-6452-1

97 98 99 00 01 / 9 8 7 6 5 4 3 2 1

Contributors

Shahriar Alikhani, M.D.
Chief Resident
Department of Anesthesia
Massachusetts General Hospital
Boston, Massachusetts

Michael Bailin, M.D.
Instructor
Department of Anesthesia
Harvard Medical School
Associate Anesthetist
Massachusetts General Hospital
Boston, Massachusetts

David I. Barclay, M.D.
Professor
Department of Obstetrics and Gynecology
University of Arkansas for Medical Sciences
Little Rock, Arkansas

James L. Breen, M.D.
Clinical Professor
Department of Obstetrics and Gynecology
Jefferson Medical College
Philadelphia, Pennsylvenia
Chairman
Department of Obstetrics and Gynecology
Saint Barnabas Medical Center
Livingston, New Jersey

Jennifer Y. Choe, M.D.
Fellow in Urogynecology
Department of Obstetrics and Gynecology
Harbour—University of California at Los Angeles Medical Center
Torrance, California

John O.L. DeLancey, M.D.
Associate Professor
Director, Division of Gynecology
Department of Obstetrics and Gynecology
University of Michigan Medical School
Ann Arbor, Michigan

Philip J. DiSaia, M.D.
The Dorothy J. Marsh Chair in Reproductive Biology and
Professor, Department of Obstetrics and Gynecology
Division of Gynecologic Oncology
University of California College of Medicine—Irvine
University of California Irvine Medical Center
Orange, California

James H. Dorsey, M.D.
Assistant Professor
Gynecology and Obstetrics
Johns Hopkins School of Medicine
Johns Hopkins University
Chairman
Department of Obstetrics and Gynecology
Greater Baltimore Medical Center
Baltimore, Maryland

Bruce H. Drukker, M.D.
Professor
Department of Obstetrics, Gynecology, and Reproductive Biology
Michigan State University
East Lansing, Michigan

Thomas E. Elkins, M.D.
Abe Mickal Professor
Department of Obstetrics and Gynecology
Louisiana State University School of Medicine
New Orleans, Louisiana

Celso-Ramón Garcia, M.D.
Professor Emeritus
University of Pennsylvania Medical Center
Philadelphia, Pennsylvania

Rene R. Genadry, M.D.
Associate Professor of Obstetrics and Gynecology
Johns Hopkins School of Medicine
Johns Hopkins University
Baltimore, Maryland

David L. Hemsell, m.d.
Professor and Director
Division of Gynecology
Department of Obstetrics and Gynecology
University of Texas Southwestern Medical Center
Chief of Gynecology
Parkland Memorial Hospital
Dallas, Texas

Jaroslav F. Hulka, m.d.
Professor Emeritus
Obstetrics and Gynecology and Maternal and Child Health
University of North Carolina School of Medicine
Chapel Hill, North Carolina

W. Glenn Hurt, m.d.
Professor
Department of Obstetrics and Gynecology
Medical College of Virginia
Richmond, Virginia

Keith B. Isaacson, m.d.
Assistant Professor
Department of Obstetrics and Gynecology
Harvard Medical School
Chief, Vincent Memorial Reproductive Endocrinology and Infertility Division
Vincent Memorial Gynecology Service
Massachusetts General Hospital
Boston, Massachusetts

Louise Lapensee, m.d.
Fellow
Vincent Memorial Gynecology Service
Massachusetts General Hospital
Boston, Massachusetts

Saul Lerner, m.d.
Professor
Department of Obstetrics and Gynecology
University of Massachusetts Medical School
Worcester, Massachusetts

L. Russell Malinak, m.d.
Professor and Vice Chairman for Clinical Affairs
Director, Residency Training Program
Department of Obstetrics and Gynecology
Baylor College of Medicine
Houston, Texas

Douglas J. Marchant, m.d.
Adjunct Professor
Department of Obstetrics and Gynecology
Brown University School of Medicine
Director, Breast Health Center
Women & Infants Hospital of Rhode Island
Providence, Rhode Island

George B. McClure, m.d.
Instructor in Obstetrics, Gynecology, and Reproductive Biology
Harvard Medical School
Fellow in Reconstructive Pelvic Surgery and Urogynecology
Department of Obstetrics and Gynecology
Massachusetts General Hospital
Boston, Massachusetts

Harold Michlewitz, m.d.
Director
Vulvar Clinic
Vincent Memorial Gynecology Service
Massachusetts General Hospital
Boston, Massachusetts

George W. Mitchell, m.d.
Clinical Professor
Department of Obstetrics and Gynecology
University of Texas Health Science Center
San Antonio, Texas

Bradley J. Monk, m.d.
Assistant Professor and Director of Gynecologic Oncology
Department of Obstetrics and Gynecology
Texas Tech University Health Sciences Center
Lubbock, Texas

David H. Nichols, m.d.
Visiting Professor of Obstetrics, Gynecology, and Reproductive Biology
Harvard Medical School
Chief of Pelvic Surgery
Vincent Memorial Gynecology Service
Massachusetts General Hospital
Boston, Massachusetts

Samantha M. Pfeifer, m.d.
Assistant Professor
Division of Human Reproduction
Department of Obstetrics and Gynecology
University of Pennsylvania School of Medicine
Philadelphia, Pennsylvania

Howard T. Sharp, m.d.
Assistant Professor
University of Utah Medical Center
Salt Lake City, Utah

John D. Thompson, m.d.
Professor Emeritus of Gynecology and Obstetrics
Emory University School of Medicine
Atlanta, Georgia

Marc R. Toglia, m.d.
Clinical Assistant Professor of Obstetrics and Gynecology
Hahnemann University School of Medicine
Department of Obstetrics and Gynecology
Graduate Hospital
Philadelphia, Pennsylvania

Dionysios K. Veronikis, m.d.
Instructor in Obstetrics, Gynecology, and Reproductive Biology
Harvard Medical School
Fellow in Reconstructive Pelvic Surgery and Urogynecology
Department of Obstetrics and Gynecology
Massachusetts General Hospital
Boston, Massachusetts

Paul J. Wendel, m.d.
Assistant Professor
Department of Obstetrics and Gynecology
Division of Maternal-Fetal Medicine
University of Arkansas for Medical Sciences
Little Rock, Arkansas

Clifford R. Wheeless, Jr., m.d.
Director
The Institute of Special Pelvic Surgery
Sinai Hospital of Baltimore
Baltimore, Maryland

Anne Wiskind, m.d.
Urogynecology
Piedmont Hospital
Atlanta, Georgia

Lynda J. Wolf, m.d.
Assistant Professor of Obstetrics and Gynecology
Medical College of Ohio
Toledo, Ohio

To Robert, Amanda, Landel, David Andrew, Brynne, and David Reeves, to carry on further the surgical traditions and principles in which their grandfather has so firmly believed.

Preface

In this era of cost containment and an environment of managed care, our society cannot afford the frequent investment of resources expended by reoperation for the relief of the symptoms of the original condition, to say nothing of the pain, suffering, and risk imposed on the patient. Knowing how to stay out of trouble is more important than knowing how to get out of trouble. This new edition emphasizes both.

Reoperation is often the consequence of an inappropriate choice of the original operative procedure, inexpert surgical performance, some failure to recognize and treat all of the symptom-producing elements that were present, or failure to recognize and treat coincident pathologic weaknesses.

Surgeons who train themselves to choose and correctly perform the most effective procedures the first time around will in the future be busier than their peers and will earn the undying gratitude of their patients and their patients' loved ones. New techniques of diagnosis and surgery are constantly evolving as are appropriate remedies to restore and enhance a patient's quality of life.

Experienced and authoritative national teachers have carefully revised and updated each of the chapters of this new edition, and new and important chapters have been added to provide information of value well into the next century.

David H. Nichols

Acknowledgments

The editor acknowledges with pleasure the skilled contributions and illustrations of Melvin Diedrich, Allison Boisselle, and Lori Vaskalis. The editorial skills and patience of Susie Baxter and Anne Gunter of Mosby–Year Book have been invaluable and I sincerely appreciate them. The patience and forebearance of my coworkers at Harvard University and at the Massachusetts General Hospital have been an indulgence without parallel. My skillful secretaries, Sara Mallari and Maureen Melanson, have ably borne the burden of typing and retyping the manuscript and their help and suggestions have been invaluable.

David H. Nichols

Contents

Surgery being an art, the description of methods of operation will always be colored subjectively, the various schools and operators deviating from each other in technical details. Each intervention expresses the individuality of the concerned surgeon and the best surgical textbook will not transform a bungler into an artist. For purpose of instruction, the special characteristics of technique and the methods of various schools are by no means the most important. . . . What is of decisive importance pertains to the proper anatomic place when the ligation and section is executed.

Heinrich Martius, Göttingen, November 1936

A surgeon should have the eye of an eagle, the heart of a lion, and the touch of a woman. Your mission in life is to relieve not to cause suffering and pain.

George E. Goodfellow

I

General Considerations

DAVID H. NICHOLS

The goals of reoperative gynecologic surgery are the same as those of primary gynecologic surgery: the relief of symptoms, the restoration of useful function, and the reestablishment of anatomic relationships. A decision for reoperation requires some assumptions concerning the causes of failure of the original surgery. Understanding of the etiology of the failure may evolve from the surgeon's consideration of the following issues: Is it clear that the original surgery was the best solution to relieve the patient's symptoms? If so, was the best of several possible operations selected for this particular patient? Was the procedure performed expertly by an experienced surgeon? Was the quality of postoperative care appropriate to the needs of this particular patient?

Some introspective soul-searching is required if the original operation was performed by the surgeon who is considering reoperation. All gynecologic surgeons should develop the habit of reviewing objectively their personal record of success and noting the long-term results after prolonged longitudinal postoperative follow-up of their patients.

For effectiveness the holistic approach to surgery requires not only an anatomically correct end result and a restoration of normal function, but also relief of the patient's symptoms. Patient gratitude and surgical effectiveness are lacking when troublesome pelvic symptoms persist or are magnified or new and usually unexpected symptoms arise postoperatively.

Failure to achieve surgical success should be rare, but such unhappy patients, though small in number, constitute a proportion of those seen in surgical consultation. Before considering the possibility of reoperation, the surgeon must thoughtfully study the patient and her personality and draw conclusions that have been tempered by personal experience as well as that of others. This is not an easy task, but an essential one if the patient is to be comfortable. Suspicions of maladjustment are not just intuitive. The surgeon must analyze the patient's delineation of her pelvic expectations, her home structure, and the possibility that she had significant misperceptions at the time of the previous, usually surgical, treatment. It is well worth investing in this process to develop an appropriate solution.

Any operative exercise must have realistic goals to be achieved. The surgeon must faithfully determine postoperatively whether or not these expectations have been realized and, if not, why not. If the results are less than ideal, the surgeon must develop a plan to prevent these problems among future patients.

The surgeon should take a detailed history from the patient, once again emphasizing subtle clues concerning the onset and progression of the patient's disability or of its persistence since the previous surgery. It is helpful to ask and understand the patient's perception of her problem.

Copies of previous surgical dictations, pathology reports, and discharge summaries should be obtained, whenever possible, and studied. The surgeon should ask the patient's permission to contact the original surgeon when this might seem likely to produce candid answers not evident in the signed dictations.

Having considered what steps have already been taken to relieve her suffering, the surgeon should note whether they were even partially effective.

A careful and unhurried physical examination seeking mechanical clues that might explain the operative failure should be performed. The surgeon should endeavor to correlate the patient's symptoms with positive findings, and these observations should be promptly recorded. For those suspected conditions likely made worse by the pull of gravity, pelvic examination should be conducted with the patient in the standing as well as lithotomy position, first while she is at rest and then while she is bearing down.

Positive findings relevant to the patient's problem must be summarized.

A firm and definitive preoperative diagnosis should be made and recorded. There must be careful correlation between symptoms and findings with realistic assessment of both patient and physician expectations of the results of surgery. Before developing and offering a new surgical plan, the surgeon must be convinced that it is likely, though not guaranteed, to provide relief for the patient. If there is any doubt as to the appropriateness of a surgical remedy, the counsel and consultation of a more experienced colleague should be obtained.

All of these findings and conclusions should be reviewed to refresh the surgeon's memory immediately before reoperation.

Unproved or novel procedures should be considered only with great caution, especially in the patient for whom reoperation is a consideration; however, when there are no obvious surgical alternatives, the patient must be clearly informed of the risks involved and the likelihood of success of the procedure. If the surgeon's optimism is unsubstantiated by a record of success, corroboration by consultation with a more experienced colleague should be sought, particularly if there is any doubt in the surgeon's mind about the efficacy of the surgical plan. Nevertheless, as Zollinger says, "There must be only one 'captain of the ship,' and one surgeon alone must coordinate all diagnostic procedures, consultations, and treatments. There is no place for fragmentation of responsibility in any part of the preoperative, operative, or postoperative care of the patient who requires reoperative surgery."[1]

PREOPERATIVE CARE

A recommendation and decision for reoperation should be implemented only after meticulous assessment of the patient's history and correlation with the objective findings of physical examination. The surgeon should be familiar with all recent relevant surgical advances and described techniques that are likely to be applicable to this particular clinical problem.

There should be careful psychologic assessment of the patient's expectation of the results of the surgery, balanced with those of the surgeon. It is imperative that the surgeon's expectations be based on fact and experience and not on wishful thinking.

When indicated, appropriate preoperative recognition, evaluation, and treatment of coincident medical disorders that are likely to affect the risk and outcome of surgery should be undertaken. The patient's status with respect to problems such as heart disease, pulmonary disease, obesity, diabetes, and hypoestrogenism should be thoughtfully considered before the final presentation to the patient of the problem and its proposed solution. All necessary or desirable laboratory work should be completed and evaluated. When medical consultation will effectively provide an unprejudiced risk-benefit assessment, it should be obtained, recorded, and followed. The proposed length of hospitalization and the need and place for appropriate postoperative convalescence should be carefully outlined. Necessary alterations in lifestyle should be discussed with the patient.

The timing of reoperative surgery should be optimized. It is important that physiologic homeostasis after the previous surgery has been obtained and that edema and wound healing have stabilized. An operative time is selected that will provide unhurried surgical intervention in the patient's condition. The surgeon should be unencumbered by pressures of surgical overcommitment or by the patient's unresolved physiologic or psychologic adjustment. The usual skills needed to drive a car or use a computer do not require a detailed knowledge of the mechanisms of the equipment's assembly and how it works. Surgical effectiveness, in contrast, is diametrically opposed to this situation—optimal effectiveness requires a detailed knowledge of anatomy, developmental anatomy, the extremes of individual variation, and both normal and abnormal physiology, tempered by the effects of aging, parity, lifestyle, and heredity.

Survival in and of our discipline requires a detailed and individualized application of all of these considerations to each patient.

Intraoperative Care

Morning surgery, when the minds and bodies of the surgeon and surgical team are alert and unfatigued, is best for reoperation. The surgeon should arrange for the best qualified assistants with whose skills the surgeon is both familiar and comfortable.[2] An adequate length of time for surgery is booked. An appropriate anesthetic is planned following preoperative evaluation by a skilled anesthetist.

Thoughtful consideration is given to patient positioning, choice of incision, choice of suture material, and availability of special instruments that may be required. Confirmation of previous findings should be obtained by examination under anesthesia, provision having been made in the informed consent to allow last-minute changes in the planned surgical techniques. Antibiotics do not replace adequate surgical asepsis, and drains do not replace adequate and effective hemostasis. The surgeon should dictate the operative report promptly and thoroughly while the details are still fresh in mind.

Postoperative Care

Postoperative care begins the minute the patient leaves the operating room and enters the recovery room. The patient's loved ones should be promptly informed of the details of surgery and told when it is likely that they may see the patient and what they may expect.

The surgeon should make daily unhurried postoperative hospital visits to the patient with assessment of her responses to healing and therapy. Recognizing and responding to her psychologic concerns are important. With the implementation of discharge planning, the patient must be given information as to the surgeon's availability postoperatively for advice, counsel, and concern. She must be told in detail of changes such as unexpected pain, bleeding, or fever that should be brought to the surgeon's attention. Her convalescence should be outlined, questions solicited, and a plan made for postoperative examination. Verbal instructions are so often misinterpreted or forgotten that brief written instructions are desirable and valuable.

Each surgeon should develop a plan for long-term follow-up and analysis of patients both as individuals and within series of cases so that the end results and effectiveness in reaching the surgical goals may be correlated with the techniques performed and the passage of time. Thus the need for future modifications in technique and care will become obvious and can be implemented, underlining the dynamic and evolutionary character of our surgical discipline.

Hospitalization is expensive, and becoming more so, imposing a predictable burden upon the patient's and the public's purse. Necessity and duration of hospitalization must be carefully monitored within set limits to avoid waste if hospital care is to remain affordable and therefore available. Better yet, a detailed analysis of need, an accurate diagnosis, and an appropriate choice of remedy, skillfully performed, should be determined at the time of the initial hospitalization. This would lessen the suffering, risk, and expense of reoperative surgery.

References

1. Zollinger RM, editor: Some principles of reoperative surgery. In Tompkins RK: Reoperative surgery, Philadelphia, 1988, JB Lippincott.
2. Nichols DH, editor: The role of the surgical assistant, Gynecologic and obstetric surgery, St Louis, 1993, Mosby.

2

Anesthetic Considerations for the Reoperated Patient with Associated Disease

MICHAEL BAILIN
SHAHRIAR ALIKHANI

Anesthetic considerations for reoperative surgery after initial gynecologic or obstetric procedures are similar to those for other surgical procedures. Patients presenting for reoperative surgery may have serious coronary, chronic pulmonary, and other associated diseases. This chapter focuses on reoperation in patients who have additional nonsurgical conditions. Preoperative assessment should identify abnormalities that may become significant if unrecognized. Even in emergency situations, the anesthesiologist should make every attempt to understand the current surgical requirements, associated medical conditions, present therapies, and overall health of the patient.

Anesthetic care is designed to render the patient insensible to pain during surgical procedures, to ensure an adequate circulating blood volume, and to maintain appropriate ventilation and oxygenation. The specific therapies and interventions used by anesthesiologists include airway management techniques, volume assessment, fluid resuscitation maneuvers, and specific drugs to control or stabilize blood pressure. Attention to individual organ systems, in concert with consideration of all the issues involving reoperated patients, allows the anesthesia care team to provide optimal and safe treatment.

Experience dictates that we make every attempt to review all of the available and necessary data *before* surgical intervention, especially in patients requiring emergent reoperative surgery. A summary of preoperative concerns are listed in Table 2.1. Depressed hematocrit level or platelet count may necessitate specific orders to the blood bank, whereas a recent abnormal electrocardiogram (ECG) may indicate need for consultation and arrangement for postoperative intensive care. If significant questions about the etiology, diagnosis, or treatment of a particular abnormality remain, further review is indicated. Examples of previously unrecognized but potentially significant problems include the patient with unexplained thrombocytopenia or new-onset dyspnea or chest pain. Medical advice is particularly effective when the consultant addresses a set of specific questions. Comprehensive assessment will emphasize the following: (1) the need for further diagnostic evaluation (Is the work-up complete?); (2) the need for further medical optimization (Is the patient in optimal condition?); and (3) risk assessment (What is the likelihood of complications?). Patients with long-standing illnesses or those with acute or uncharacterized disease may benefit from evaluation by an internist when unfamiliar problems arise.

The following case illustrates this process. A 74-year-old woman 1 week after total abdominal hysterectomy required laparotomy for peritonitis. On the morning of surgery she had an episode of angina and a cardiologist was asked to see her. The cardiologist's note concludes: "Given the urgency of the clinical situation, further cardiac work-up will not be performed at this time. The patient clearly has myocardium at risk but no evidence of ventricular dysfunction. I have increased her antianginal program and encourage meticulous intraoperative control of blood pressure and heart rate. She is at greater-than-average risk for a perioperative ischemic event. I will follow

Table 2.1 Preoperative issues

- Chart review
  - General record
  - Anesthetic record
  - Intensive care unit (ICU)/postanesthesia care unit (PACU) hemodynamic record
- Patient assessment
  - Review of systems
  - History and physical
  - Medications/infusions
  - Allergies
- Laboratory assessment (if indicated)
  - Hematocrit level
  - Coagulation studies
  - Electrolyte levels
  - ECG
  - Arterial blood gas concentration
  - Chest x-ray examination
- Volume and hemodynamic assessment
  - Jugular venous distension
  - Invasive monitoring
    - Central venous monitoring
    - Pulmonary artery pressures
- Blood and blood products
  - Ensure presence of sample in blood bank
  - Ensure availability of blood
- Establish sufficient intravenous access
  - Central access
  - Peripheral access
- Understand surgical requirements
- Notification of appropriate personnel
  - Personnel taking care of patient (ICU, PACU, ward)
  - Notification of operating room personnel
- Contact consultants as necessary
- Obtain informed consent
- Devise anesthetic and monitoring plan
- Arrange for postoperative care
  - ICU
  - PACU
- Notify family

with you postop." In the case cited, the cardiologist addressed each element of assessment and concluded that surgery should not be delayed despite the potential for cardiac ischemia.

The issues of timing and urgency of reoperation must be addressed concurrent with the overall patient assessment. Concerns surrounding the "fresh" postoperative patient still in the recovery room differ significantly from those regarding the patient who was operated on several days previously. Immediately following surgery patients may experience such routine anesthetic complications as hypotension, the need for airway support, or nausea and vomiting.[1] Several days postoperatively more serious complications may arise, including hemorrhage, sepsis, thromboembolism, or wound dehiscence.[2-6] We will consider several organ systems within the context of both the immediate postoperative period and the delayed postoperative period (postoperative day 1 and beyond).

General Considerations

Of utmost importance to this discussion is communication. The decision whether to bring a patient back to the operating room (OR) or not is ultimately that of the primary obstetrician or gynecologist. Once the decision to reoperate has been made, however, this conclusion must be promptly and clearly communicated to the entire patient care team. Alerting the anesthesiologist allows preanesthetic evaluation of the patient to be initiated. The OR personnel should be notified to ensure the availability of appropriate nursing staff, sterile surgical equipment, and the OR. Notifying the care providers on the floor, in the recovery room, or in the intensive care unit (ICU) will expedite preparation of the patient. Such preparation may include performing or confirming laboratory studies, checking the availability of a sample in the blood bank, or simply requesting and reviewing the patient record.

Classification of the reoperative procedure is an important communication issue for every member of the team. The decision to schedule a procedure as "emergent" should not be a precipitous one. In pressing situations, thoroughness is sometimes compromised in the name of speed. Frequently it may behoove the perioperative team to proceed expeditiously, but not emergently, to ensure thorough preparation. We believe successful communication provides the basis for safe and optimal patient care. Since the etiology and pathophysiology of urgent or emergent surgical diseases are so diverse, careful and complete assessment of the patient's status by the anesthesiologist is imperative. Reoperation for life-threatening complications (e.g., hemorrhagic hypovolemia) cannot be delayed while attempts are made to improve the patient's condition if there is a reasonable expectation for surgical correction. Immediate reexploration with simultaneous resuscitative care can be best performed in the OR.

As reoperation per se may increase the surgical level of difficulty, the anesthesia team may face challenges created by prior interventions. Line placement may be restricted by scarring, hematoma, thrombosis, or hypovolemia. Anemia, volume abnormalities, and edema are not unexpected prior to reoperation, especially if the primary operation was performed within a few days preceding the reoperation.

There is no preferred anesthetic technique or drug for the patient undergoing reoperative surgery since any suitable agent may be used to achieve satisfactory anesthesia. Induction of general anesthesia usually begins with single or multiple injections of intravenous (IV) agents listed in Table 2.2. Neuromuscular blockers are used to facilitate endotracheal intubation or to maintain muscle relaxation. Maintenance of anesthesia with intravenous or inhalational agents is routinely practiced. Administration of nitrous oxide may be curtailed when there is potential or real evidence of bowel obstruction or air embolus. Most anesthesiologists tend to control the airway with endotracheal intubation and mechanical ventilation during urgent conditions. Although specific anesthetic considerations are derived from the clinical presentation, the medical status, and the current surgical requirements, certain commonalities exist. These include assessment of volume status, the potential for a full stomach, and an estimation of cardiovascular and pulmonary function.

Although there is little evidence of improved postoperative outcomes for combined epidural and general anesthesia (CEGA) in gynecologic surgery, many anesthesiologists employ CEGA in their attempt to combine the advantages of general and regional anesthesia (Table 2.3). At the Massachusetts General Hospital, CEGA is the standard technique for primary or reoperative major vascular and noncardiac thoracic surgery. We routinely insert epidural catheters preoperatively in patients scheduled for postoperative intensive care. The decision to induce complete epidural sensory and motor blockade prior to incision or to defer epidural injection until the postoperative period is made on an individual basis. Determining factors for practicing CEGA in reoperative gynecologic surgery include the clinician's familiarity with the technique, the surgical urgency, the medical contraindications, and the patient's understanding and consent.

Table 2.2 Anesthetic agents

Agent	Use	Route
Barbiturates (thiopental)	Induction	IV
Benzodiazepines	Induction	IV
Ketamine	Induction	IV
Etomidate	Induction	IV
Propofol	Induction/ maintenance	IV
Inhalational agents	Induction/ maintenance	Inhaled
Opioids	Induction/ maintenance	IV

Airway Considerations

Airway management is one of the main responsibilities of the anesthesiologist. Patients may require airway management or control for any of the following:

Table 2.3 General anesthesia versus regional anesthesia

Advantages	Disadvantages
General anesthesia	
Reliability	Potential cardiac depression
Controllability	Loss of temperature control
Speed of induction	
Early airway protection	
Regional anesthesia	
Awake patient	Uncontrolled airway
Postoperative pain control	Awake patient
Potential decreased blood loss	Hypotension from vasodilation
Decreased incidence of thromboembolism	Intraoperative nausea or vomiting
Earlier ambulation	May conceal diagnostic pain

1. Acute or chronic respiratory insufficiency
2. Loss of airway reflexes
3. As an adjunct to general anesthesia
4. Oversedation causing respiratory distress

During a procedure, airway management ranges from minimal assistance (with respect to positioning of the head and mouth) in a spontaneously breathing patient, to mask ventilation and intubation in the unconscious patient. Examination of the airway prior to instrumentation is very important. The most common airway classification is that described by Mallampatti in 1983[7] (Table 2.4). The Mallampatti classification, combined with poor neck extension (decreased mobility at the atlanto-occipital joint) and the presence of a retracted mandible, among other factors, may predict a difficult intubation.

In the immediate postoperative period, airway obstruction is commonly due to upper airway problems.[1] In the pharynx, posterior tongue displacement or soft tissue collapse or edema may obstruct the airway, whereas in the larynx, foreign body, laryngeal edema, or laryngospasm may be responsible for obstruction. Pharyngeal and laryngeal edema may make endotracheal reintubation more difficult. Airway edema may occur in operations during which the patient has been in the Trendelenberg position for prolonged periods, in lengthy pelvic or abdominal procedures, or in cases where significant volume replacement has occurred. Partial airway obstruction may also derive from tracheal compression secondary to hematoma formation. Hematoma may result from attempts at central venous cannulation or from surgery or trauma to the neck.

In instances of potential loss of the airway, immediate assistance is essential. Both mask ventilation and intubation may be challenging. The airway must be clear of vomitus or foreign bodies and should be maintained with simple maneuvers, including administering oxygen, providing jaw lift (mandibular elevation), placing an oropharyngeal or nasopharyngeal airway, or lateral positioning. An expanding neck hematoma must be relieved immediately. In any situation involving obstruction of the airway, seeking timely assistance from an experienced anesthesiologist or surgeon capable of providing invasive airway support may mean the difference between a routine complication and a crisis secondary to respiratory arrest.

In the early postoperative period, patients may be under the influence of residual IV or inhalational anesthetics, narcotics, or muscle relaxants. These agents may compromise airway and respiratory management. Patients must be examined to determine the residual activity of previously administered anesthetics. Anesthesiologists must carefully review the preceding anesthetic record and the nursing record in the postanesthesia care unit (PACU) for information pertinent to medical management during surgery. Decreasing subsequent doses of sedatives or hypnotics may be indicated in patients demonstrating excessive drowsiness, sedation, hypoventilation, or hypoxemia in the PACU.

Reoperation mandates airway reevaluation just prior to the induction of anesthesia. The anesthesiologist cannot rely on a history of "easy" mask ventilation or intubation as a guide to airway management—even if the anesthetic management was uncomplicated only hours earlier. A determination that pharyngeal or laryngeal edema or swelling is present should change the anesthesia care plan. A patient with airway edema should be presumed to be at high risk for airway complications, occasionally necessitating an awake or fiberoptic intubation. These procedures are vital to the administration of anesthesia and are thoroughly reviewed by Roberts.[8]

Patients with esophageal reflux, gastroparesis, ileus, or bowel obstruction may aspirate stomach contents on induction of general

Table 2.4 Mallampati classification

Class I: Ability to visualize the posterior pharynx, pharyngeal pillars, and uvula on preoperative examination
Class II: Partial visualization of the posterior pharynx, pharyngeal pillars, and uvula
Class III: Minimal visualization of posterior pharynx; inability to visualize the uvula or pharyngeal pillars
Class IV: Inability to visualize the posterior pharynx, pharyngeal pillars, or the uvula

anesthesia since airway reflexes are eliminated. In addition, parturients, the morbidly obese, and adults with recent ingestion of solids (less than 8 hours before surgery) or liquids (less than 4 hours before surgery) are at increased risk for pulmonary aspiration of stomach contents when laryngeal competence is impaired. In these high-risk patients, we frequently use rapid-sequence induction. Rapid-sequence induction involves preoxygenation, application of cricoid pressure, rapid administration of a predetermined dose of IV anesthetic and muscle relaxant, avoidance of insufflating the stomach with gas, and timely endotracheal intubation with a cuffed endotracheal tube. Prompt protection of the airway decreases the likelihood of aspiration in the aforementioned high-risk groups.

Patients who required rapid-sequence induction for a prior surgery may or may not be treated similarly for reoperation in the postoperative period. Factors affecting the decision to employ rapid-sequence induction include choice of anesthesia, recent medical course, and associated medical conditions. Since there is no guarantee that the airway can be easily secured, suspending the patient's ability to breathe with muscle relaxants may be hazardous. Gastric motility is decreased in the postoperative period, especially in patients treated with opioids. The reality of a "full stomach" with increased gastric pressure and acidity still accounts for major morbidity in the peripartum cohort.[9-11] The parturient should be considered at increased risk for aspiration from the twelfth week of gestation until 6 weeks after delivery, when the physiologic changes associated with pregnancy normalize.[12] We medicate parturients, postparturients, patients with esophageal reflux, some diabetics, and morbidly obese patients with nonparticulate antacids (sodium citrate, 30 mg administered orally [po])[13] and histamine H_2 blockers (cimetidine, 300 mg IV, or ranitidine, 150 mg IV) in order to decrease gastric acidity[14] and metoclopramide (10 mg IV) to increase gastric motility[15] prior to airway manipulation.

PULMONARY CONSIDERATIONS

Effective alveolar ventilation may be impaired in both the immediate and delayed postoperative period and should be closely monitored, especially in patients with pulmonary disease. Anesthetic agents, analgesics, or muscle relaxants may delay the return of effective spontaneous ventilation. Sudden respiratory insufficiency may result from aspiration, mucus plugging, or administration of an opioid overdose in the postoperative period. Careful attention to the respiratory system is essential for appropriate management of the surgical population.

Perioperative pulmonary problems may be divided into three categories: (1) iatrogenic, (2) anatomic, and (3) pathophysiologic. Evaluation of the postoperative patient for reoperation requires careful consideration within each category.

Iatrogenic effects include the consequences of residual IV or inhalational anesthetics and account for the blunting of ventilatory response to hypoxia and hypercarbia. Careful review of the anesthetic record and the nursing record should include the doses, times, and routes of administration of all analgesics and sedatives. The onset of hypoventilation and hypercarbia often begins during transfer to the OR after premedication is given. Similarly, respiratory depressants administered en route to the PACU will have their peak effect in the recovery room. Epidural or spinal morphine may cause respiratory depression up to 24 hours after administration.[16] Peridural opiates may cause patients to suffer from decreased respiratory drive and diminished pulmonary reserves, and they may be more likely to experience hypoxemia and respiratory acidosis during reoperation.

Anatomic factors may also affect ventilation and gas exchange. Pneumothoraces may first present in the postoperative period. Causes include spontaneous occurrence, lung perforation secondary to central venous catheter placement, or barotrauma from mechanical ventilation.[17] Thoracentesis or other invasive thoracic procedures for staging of gynecologic tumors may cause pneumothorax, diaphragmatic dysfunction, or impairment of the chest wall bellows.[18] Jugular venous distension, contralateral tracheal deviation, ipsilateral hyperresonance to chest percussion, or a sudden increase in central venous pressure (CVP) or peak inspiratory pressure in a mechanically ventilated patient may suggest the diagnosis of a pneumothorax.

Small pneumothoraces, less than 10% of the lung volume, frequently go undetected based on clinical signs, and they may resolve spontaneously. Chest radiographs, routinely obtained after central venous cannulation and thoracic and laparoscopic procedures, will help with diagnosis and management of patients with pneumothoraces.[19] Definitive treatment of a pneumothorax with a thoracostomy tube in an unstable patient should not be delayed while awaiting the chest film. Positive pressure ventilation in a patient with a tension pneumothorax may result in profound hypotension secondary to decreased venous return to the heart. If reoperation is planned in a patient with pneumothorax, we recommend considering thoracostomy tube placement prior to induction of anesthesia, or as soon thereafter as possible.

Pathophysiologic factors in the patient requiring reoperation may include atelectasis, bronchospasm, pneumonia, bronchitis, pleural effusion, or respiratory insufficiency secondary to aspiration of gastric contents. Mucus plugging and adult respiratory distress syndrome may worsen underlying lung disease. Patients in the early postoperative period are at increased risk for atelectasis, pulmonary infection, and fluid shifting into alveolar spaces.[20] If careful attention to the lung examination in the perioperative patient suggests any abnormalities, then serial chest films, frequent vital signs, and meticulous recording of fluid intake and output are advised. If time permits, the patient's pulmonary disease should be optimized prior to reoperation. This may include initiating antibiotic treatment, aggressive chest physical therapy, incentive spirometry, administration of bronchodilators, and occasionally steroid therapy.

The choice of regional anesthetic techniques includes epidural, spinal, or nerve block anesthesia. Selecting regional anesthesia and minimizing airway manipulation in patients with compromised pulmonary reserves should be balanced against selecting a general anesthetic designed to protect and support pulmonary function.[21,22] There are many considerations in providing anesthesia for reoperation to the patient with respiratory disease. The choice of anesthetic should be at the discretion of the anesthesiologist. This decision is ideally based on the patient's specific needs and the skills of the anesthesiologist. Of importance is the optimal medical management of patients with pulmonary disease prior to any anesthetic or surgical manipulation.

Cardiovascular Considerations

A detailed history of cardiovascular problems should be obtained from all patients prior to any surgical intervention. Cardiovascular complications in the postoperative period may range from benign electrocardiographic changes to myocardial ischemia or ventricular dysfunction leading to cardiovascular collapse. Knowledge of previous and current cardiac pathologic conditions helps guide therapy in these patients.

Myocardial infarction (MI) may occur at any time in the perioperative period, but it is statistically more likely to occur after the first postoperative day. Signs and symptoms such as atypical chest pain, upper abdominal pain, or abnormal enzyme profiles may confuse the diagnosis. Clinical evidence of chest pain, changes in the ECG (e.g., ST segment elevation or Q waves), together with a previous history of heart disease, should raise the index of suspicion for myocardial ischemia or infarction. The most striking risk factors for a perioperative ischemic event are unstable angina or recent MI.[23-25] Patients exhibiting signs consistent with infarction should be managed with continuous multilead electrocardiographic monitoring to detect cardiac arrhythmias and ischemia. Supplemental oxygen, pain medications, and nitroglycerin should be used when appropriate. Once stable, the patient may be transferred to a cardiac unit for further monitoring and care. The decision whether to administer heparin or not should be evaluated on a case-by-case basis, weighing the risks of potential surgical bleeding against the benefits of anticoagulation. Cardiology consultation will assist in the consideration of coronary angiography, coronary angioplasty, or surgical revascularization.

Patients with a recent MI can be divided into three groups: (1) those for whom reoperation is lifesaving and emergent, (2) those for whom surgery is elective and may be delayed, and (3) those for whom surgery is not absolutely emergent but cannot be postponed indefinitely.

Cardiology consultation may be beneficial for surgical patients with recent MI. Some references suggest that during the 3 to 6 months following an MI, the cardiac muscle heals and the patient returns to a normal risk class.[26] However, others suggest that coronary artery disease (CAD) can be expected to progress in 6 months and thereby increase the risk of perioperative reinfarction.[27] Patients who have completed an infarction and demonstrate no further "myocardium at risk," through radionuclide scintigraphy or by "passing" a stress test, are in a lower risk class than patients experiencing postinfarction angina or congestive failure.

Preoperative evaluation assessing exercise tolerance, ventricular function, and ischemic potential should be performed on patients with uncharacterized heart disease or those with recent cardiac decompensation. Optimizing antianginal therapy and rehabilitation activity will improve overall cardiovascular function. The surgeon, the anesthesiologist, and the medical consultant can then counsel the patient on the risks of proceeding with surgery compared with that of facing a worsening surgical condition. For each group of patients, the competing risks of the cardiac pathologic condition must be weighed against delaying surgical intervention.[23,28]

Although abnormalities of cardiac rhythm occur in one third of general anesthetics,[29] dysrhythmias causing hemodynamic compromise are rare. Benign dysrhythmias are also common in the immediate as well as the late postoperative period. Patients with a history of perioperative cardiac rhythm disturbance should be thoroughly evaluated by electrocardiographic analysis prior to reoperation. Secondary causes of dysrhythmia, such as electrolyte abnormalities, hypoxemia, hypercarbia, or drug effects, should be ruled out. Myocardial ischemia may either precipitate or result from dysrhythmia. Patients with benign supraventricular or junctional rhythms or those with infrequent ventricular ectopic beats may be safely anesthetized for reoperation after appropriate evaluation. Certain sympathomimetic medications such as epinephrine can predispose patients to dysrhythmia and should probably be avoided. Frequent ventricular dysrhythmias or hemodynamically significant rhythm disturbances should be controlled prior to surgery.

Congestive heart failure (CHF) may present postoperatively with shortness of breath, tachypnea, chest pain, and tachycardia. It is most likely to occur in the setting of fluid overload in a patient with a serious intrinsic cardiac disorder. Crackles on lung auscultation, decreased urine output, distension of neck veins, and edema of the lower extremities may indicate biventricular CHF. Treatment consists of restricting IV fluids, inducing diuresis, morphine in small amounts, and supplemental oxygen. Management of surgical pain should not be overlooked during evaluation and treatment of pulmonary edema. The anesthesiologist should identify and treat cardiac symptomatology in order to avoid complications such as ischemia or infarction prior to reoperation. Specific considerations, such as the extent of hemodynamic monitoring and the choice of anesthetic technique, should be up to the discretion of the attending anesthesiologist. The patient's cardiac condition should be optimized prior to proceeding with any surgical or anesthetic intervention. Arrangements for a monitored bed with close nursing supervision in the postoperative period should be made.

Renal Considerations

Patients with renal disease are more likely to have electrolyte and acid-base disturbances and abnormal volume status. An increased volume of distribution, which affects drug distribution, may be seen in patients with renal dysfunction. Aberrant drug disposition may result in heightened or diminished physiologic responses to a drug that would otherwise have predictable consequences. Renal failure patients are at increased risk for hypervolemia and fluid overload as impairment of water or solute excretion leads to fluid retention. In the absence of some mechanism for removing excess volume (urine output, dialysis, or filtration), hypervolemia will usually progress to hypertension, edema, and congestive failure. In some cases, overly aggressive fluid restriction can lead to hypovolemia, especially in patients sustained by dialysis. Unrecognized or underestimated volume deficits may lead to profound hypotension particularly evident during induction of anesthesia. Anesthetic management will have to account for these possible changes in volume status and the presence of acidosis or hypoproteinemia. The anesthesiologist should pay careful attention to blood loss, blood pressure, serum electrolyte levels, and blood pH. Central venous or pulmonary artery catheters may help guide fluid management. Knowledge of cardiac filling pressures and stroke volume can differentiate hypovolemic hypotension from low systemic vascular resistance.

Hyperkalemia is common in renal failure patients secondary to hemolysis and limitations in excretion of solutes. As the serum potassium level approaches and goes beyond 7 mEq/L, hypotension, weakness, and electrocardiographic abnormalities may appear. Cardiac arrest from ventricular fibrillation will occur unless pharmacologic management is instituted. Kayexalate with sorbitol enema or dialysis will lower the potassium load. Calcium chloride or calcium gluconate injections are indicated when there is progression of electrocardiographic evidence of hyperkalemia. Metabolic acidosis commonly accompanies renal insufficiency and may worsen the hyperkalemic state, inducing further myocardial irritability.

Hypokalemia usually results from potassium deficits secondary to vomiting, diarrhea, or diuretics. Our practice does not discriminate against asymptomatic chronic hypokalemia. We treat patients with 10 mEq of potassium chloride per hour when the serum potassium level is less than 2.5 mEq/L, and we generally do not administer potassium when values are greater than 3 mEq/L. Rapid potassium repletion may cause life-threatening arrhythmias.

Acute decompensation of renal function may occur in the perioperative period, especially in patients with preexisting renal disease, such as renal artery stenosis, diabetic nephropathy, or long-standing hypertension.[30] Additional factors responsible for the development of perioperative renal injury include fluid restriction, dehydration, nephrotoxic antibiotics, IV contrast agents, and ischemia from low flow states. Renal function may abruptly cease when renal plasma flow decreases below a threshold level.

Table 2.5 Anesthetic considerations in the patient with renal insufficiency
Blood volume abnormalities
Dialysis schedule
Oliguria or anuria
Hypoalbuminemia
Anemia
Platelet abnormalities
Abnormalities of potassium, calcium, magnesium, and phosphate
Associated disease (e.g., diabetes)
Metabolic acidosis
Altered pharmacodynamics and pharmacokinetics

Renal decompensation may be more likely in reoperated patients who have subclinical or overt hypovolemia with impending renal injury. The role of osmotic or loop diuretics in conferring renal "protection" in at-risk patients has not been elucidated. Patients with renal failure requiring reoperation are at risk for complete renal shutdown. The anesthesiologist should search for anemia, metabolic acidosis, and coagulation and platelet abnormalities (Table 2.5). The causes of renal disease must also be taken into account, since the presence of atherosclerotic renovascular disease, diabetic nephropathy, or polycystic kidney disease may have important ramifications for other organ systems. Patients with uremia, especially those undergoing hemodialysis, may have an acquired platelet dysfunction, which may be partially reversed with intravenous arginine desmopressin (DDAVP).[31]

Hematologic Considerations

The presence of coexisting coagulation disorders may complicate the course of some surgical patients. The potential for abnormal or excessive bleeding may be acquired or congenital. Clinical considerations in treating nonsurgical bleeding depend on the appropriate investigations into the cause of the bleeding. Hypovolemia is to be expected when bleeding necessitates reoperation. With unstaunched and continued hemorrhage, hypotension, tachycardia, and anemia may make a dramatic appearance, requiring immediate volume and red blood cell (RBC) resuscitation to avoid cardiovascular collapse. Although current transfusion practices are quite restrictive, and clear guidelines exist for allogeneic RBC replacement,[32-34] there are occasions when it is necessary to proceed with transfusion before laboratory tests return. For example, it is reasonable to administer blood to an elderly patient with baseline anemia and CAD facing reoperation for hemorrhage. Myocardial ischemia may also occur in this setting, and the benefit of increasing RBC mass probably outweighs the infectious risks. The risks of transmitting blood-borne infections through transfusion of blood products are low, such that further safety of the blood supply would be difficult to prove in a clinical study.[35,36] We emphasize that a thoughtful rationale should accompany the administration of any colloid (e.g., packed cells, fresh frozen plasma or albumin). Anesthetic management is predicated on careful hemodynamic assessment and monitoring combined with the maintenance of normovolemia through appropriate volume resuscitation. Although consideration is given to the bleeding patient in Chapter 19, we will briefly review three specific causes of hemorrhage: hemophilia, von Willebrand's disease, and acquired factor VIII antibody.

The two most common bleeding disorders are a deficiency of factor VIII (hemophilia A) and von Willebrand's disease (VWD).[37,38] Patients with low levels of factor VIII have a normal prothrombin time (PT) and a prolonged partial thromboplastin time (PTT), indicating a defect in the intrinsic limb of the coagulation cascade. Females rarely exhibit hemophilia A since the factor VIII gene resides on the X chromosome. These individuals may carry one defective gene and as heterozygotes, do not display a bleeding tendency. A deficiency of factor VIII function is more likely to be caused by an acquired factor disorder, usually a circulating anticoagulant.[39] Although hemophilia A may present as postsurgical bleeding requiring reexploration, a congenital deficiency would not only be rare, but there would typically be a family history of bleeding as well.

Although there are several clinical presentations of VWD, the diagnosis is often made in patients suffering from menorrhagia, epistaxis, and mucosal or gastrointestinal (GI) bleeding. Bleeding after surgery or dental extractions may be the first clue, prompting hematologic evaluation. VWD may occur either as a quantitative or qualitative deficiency of the von Willebrand (VW) factor, and there are more than a dozen genetic subtypes.[40] The VW factor forms an essential complex with factor VIII and serves as the factor VIII carrier. The VW factor also plays a vital role linking platelets to the endothelium. Clinical presentation ranges from mild bleeding, effectively treated with DDAVP, to severe hemorrhage requiring large doses of cryoprecipitate.[31] Bleeding times may not be useful in the diagnosis or treatment of this disease. Consultation and follow-through with a hematologist are recommended for patients suspected of having this condition.

There are many causes of exceptional perioperative bleeding that are neither congenital nor surgical. Patients who sustain significant intraoperative blood loss may present with perioperative coagulopathy. This coagulopathy may manifest as generalized oozing, together with various coagulation disorders The anesthesiologist must be able to diagnose and treat the major causes of abnormal, nonsurgical bleeding, namely, platelet and coagulation factor disorders. Normal hemostasis depends on an intact vasculature and the presence of sufficient quantities of coagulation factors and functional platelets. Spontaneous or excessive bleeding therefore stems from a defect in one or more of these areas and may require treatment with packed red blood cells, fresh frozen plasma, platelet concentrates, cryoprecipitate, and/or antifibrinolytic agents.

An illustrative case is that of a 72-year-old woman with adult-onset diabetes mellitus and stable angina who underwent a lengthy and complicated total abdominal hysterectomy (TAH)/bilateral salpingo-oophorectomy (BSO) under general anesthesia. Blood loss was estimated at 1500 ml, and fluid replacement comprised 2 units of packed red blood cells and 7000 ml of crystalloid. After the first hour in the PACU, she exhibited pallor, hypotension, and nausea. Samples were drawn for blood gas analysis and determination of hematocrit and glucose levels. An ECG was performed, and a second IV line was initiated. Warm Ringer's lactate solution was infused rapidly, and the OR was notified of a potential emergent laparotomy. Insufficient blood was crossmatched for this patient, necessitating a crossmatch waiver. Laparotomy demonstrated 1 L of free blood without much evidence of clot.

The differential diagnosis of bleeding in this scenario includes several nonsurgical etiologies, such as factor deficiency (including hemophilia), platelet disorders (including VWD), circulating anticoagulants, and disseminated intravascular coagulation (DIC). Hematologic testing revealed a normal PT and an abnormal PTT, suggesting deficiency in factor VIII, IX, XI, or XII. Acquired bleeding disorders are frequently secondary to circulating inhibitors, which are immunoglobulins and are commonly anti–factor VIII.[39,41] Although these antibodies may occur spontaneously in normal individuals, they often manifest in the postpartum period, in cancer patients, following certain medications, and in patients with systemic lupus erythematosis (SLE). Treatment in this case required fresh frozen plasma, factor VIII concentrate, cryoprecipitate, platelets, and packed red blood cells. The factor VIII antibody was ultimately controlled with prednisone therapy. In the example just given, fibrin degradation products were not elevated, suggesting no intravascular fibrinolysis, although consultation with a hematologist was crucial for diagnosis and treatment.

When surgical bleeding must be controlled, transportation to the OR should not be delayed. The advantages of performing volume resuscitation in the OR are realized when the personnel, blood warming equipment, and monitoring devices are readily available. Induction of general anesthesia with endotracheal intubation is preferably done in the OR as well, with the absolute control of the airway being a vital adjunct in the patient with an unstable or uncertain cardiovascular status.

Infectious Considerations (Shock)

Sepsis usually results from bacterial infection; however, it also may be a direct consequence of viremia or fungemia. The surgical patient with wound infection, abscess, peritonitis, or sepsis must be managed with early and appropriate antimicrobial therapy to prevent progression to septic shock. The antibiotic therapy may be empirical or specific, and in either case, it should be based on clinical presentation and/or culture data. Occasionally antibacterial therapy may be delayed until appropriate tissue samples (wound, peritoneal fluid, or blood) are obtained for culture. However, deliberate omissions of therapy should be reviewed with the surgeon and other care providers. Early recognition and treatment of sepsis are crucial, since the concomitants of this condition, which include hypovolemia, vasodilation, and myocardial depression, may cause cardiovascular collapse.

In the initial stages of sepsis syndrome, fever, tachycardia, and increased cardiac output are apparent. An early sign of sepsis is reduced systemic vascular resistance, which may result in increased skin perfusion, diaphoresis, and flushing. As shock progresses, vascular resistance increases and cardiac output falls, resulting in skin hypoperfusion and multiorgan ischemia. Tachycardia is generally present in early and late sepsis, but isolated heart rate increases do not reliably indicate shock, especially in anesthetized patients.

Making the distinction between hypovolemic and septic shock may be challenging because they share some common signs and symptoms. Such signs include tachycardia, hypotension, decreased cardiac stroke volume, oliguria, and mental status changes. Skin hypoperfusion and impairment of oxygen delivery and utilization may also be present during both septic and hypovolemic shock and may result from cardiovascular decompensation. Pulmonary edema, hypovolemia, and considerable third-space losses may be seen as a result of transudation of intravascular volume secondary to impaired capillary integrity.

In the clinical setting both hypovolemic and septic shock are generally treated with administration of Ringer's lactate or normal saline solution, which increases intravascular volume and normalizes blood pressure. Bolus infusions of 10 to 20 ml/kg body weight are used, and several multiples of this therapy may be necessary to support the circulation. Invasive monitoring is used to help guide fluid therapy in patients exhibiting cardiovascular instability. Direct arterial access enables frequent blood sampling to monitor hematocrit and electrolyte levels and acid-base disturbances. Central venous and pulmonary artery catheters are necessary to estimate preload and cardiac output, permitting assessment of cardiovascular function and intravascular volume. Central venous cannulation also allows infusion of vasoactive drugs directly into the superior vena cava, which is particularly important during periods of diminished cardiac output.

Comprehensive therapy of patients who display signs of septic shock and must return to the OR should include the diagnosis of the likely origin of the infection, collection of the pertinent cultures, and the rapid institution of broad-spectrum or targeted antibiotic coverage. When appropriate, debridement, drainage of infection, and removal of packing are essential in the overall management of such patients. In addition, indwelling catheters may need to be replaced to prevent contamination. The administration of IV vasoactive agents, such as phenylephrine, epinephrine, and norepinephrine, may be indicated when stabilization or maintenance of blood pressure cannot be achieved using volume resuscitation.

DIC may be a dire consequence of sepsis syndrome and is optimally treated by correcting the underlying disease process. Laboratory tests of the coagulation and fibrinolytic systems should be obtained. These tests include PT, PTT, platelet count, fibrinogen levels, fibrinogen degradation products, and D-dimers. When a coagulopathy is suspected, a simple but effective "bedside" test may be performed that involves adding 10 ml of the patient's blood to a glass test tube. Blood that does not form a solid coagulum within a few minutes indicates a coagulation abnormality. A clot may form but readily dissolve; this is an indication of fibrinolysis and may indicate further testing and antifibrinolytic therapy. If bleeding is significant, replacement of coagulation factors and platelets may be needed. Successful management of sepsis-induced DIC requires treatment of the infectious cause with appropriate antibiotics and surgical intervention.

Hepatic Considerations

Patients with hepatocellular insufficiency may be asymptomatic or severely incapacitated with ascites, encephalopathy, jaundice, coagulopathy, and hepatorenal syndrome. Several studies suggest that the presence of acute hepatitis or advanced cirrhosis is an independent risk factor increasing surgical morbidity of laparotomy.[42,43] However, patients with asymptomatic liver disease probably have normal surgical risk, since well-compensated cirrhosis and mild hepatitis do not seem to add to perioperative morbidity.[44]

When reoperation is elective, the anesthesiologist should consider three important issues in the preoperative evaluation of the patient with abnormal liver function: diagnosis, prognosis, and functional capacity of the liver. If the diagnosis is unknown, a history of drug or alcohol abuse, past history of hepatitis or jaundice, and history of blood transfusions may be revealing. The two most common forms of liver disease are hepatitis (acute or chronic) and cirrhosis. Acute hepatitis is typically caused by viral infection or alcohol hepatotoxicity. Clinical presentation ranges from mild right upper quadrant discomfort to fulminant hepatic failure. Elective surgery is usually delayed until liver function tests have normalized.

Cirrhosis may be secondary to any type of liver disease causing hepatocyte death with resultant fibrosis. Progressive end-stage fibrosis is termed cirrhosis. Anesthetic considerations in cirrhosis reflect the degree of hepatic functional impairment. Severe hepatic impairment leads to fluid and electrolyte abnormalities, specifically hyponatremia and decreased intravascular volume. Patients taking diuretics to control ascites are likely to experience hypotension on the induction of anesthesia since the combination of fluid restriction, hypovolemia, and vasodilation caused by anesthetic agents may markedly diminish venous return. Phenylephrine, an effective vasoconstrictor, may be used to support systemic vascular tone and arterial blood pressure.

In advanced forms of liver disease, the reduction in hepatic protein synthesis results in hypoalbuminemia and decreased production of coagulation factors. As protein binding of anesthetic drugs to albumin is decreased, the free drug fraction will increase. This may cause exaggerated responses to medications, such as excessive sedation and hypotension. A coagulopathic state caused by liver disease may be multifactorial. Since the liver synthesizes most of the coagulation proteins and it is also responsible for the absorption of vitamin K, an abnormal coagulation profile may follow hepatic disease. Additionally, portal hypertension may lead to platelet sequestration with resultant thrombocytopenia. The anesthesiologist must be prepared to administer vitamin K, fresh frozen plasma, and platelets to control intraoperative hemorrhage.

Oliguria, hypoxemia, and hypoglycemia may also occur in surgical patients with liver disease. Diuretic dependence and renal hypoperfusion may account for specific cases of decreased urine output. Intrapulmonary shunting, pulmonary effusions, and atelectasis may accompany advanced liver disease, and each can induce arterial hypoxemia. The anesthesiologist should be prepared to support respiration with endotracheal intubation and mechanical ventilation in patients with hepatopulmonary syndrome. A summary of anesthetic concerns is found in Table 2.6. If there are doubts as to the type and extent of liver disease, medical consultation should be obtained and a liver biopsy may be necessary for diagnosis.

Table 2.6 Manifestations of liver disease of importance to the anesthesiologist

Coagulopathy
Thrombocytopenia
Hypoxemia
Ascites
Varices
Encephalopathy
Altered pharmacokinetics
Hypoalbuminemia
Fluid and electrolyte abnormalities
Oliguria

Summary

The potential for increased complexity and greater variability exists during a return to the OR. Medical management "answers" may not be as important as asking the right questions. What is the patient's volume status? Is it changing? What are the particular surgical requirements? How will the airway be secured? What are the anesthetic choices? Are medical consultations necessary to improve the patient's medical status and to better define risk stratification? The response to many of these questions is sometimes a function of uncertain physiologic and clinical presentation.

The ability to identify options and consider relative risks and benefits is of vital importance to the anesthesiologist faced with any complicated surgery. Certain challenges arise even in straightforward reoperative procedures. The administration of an appropriate anesthetic should include careful questioning and examination of the patient, a search for associated diseases, the development and communication of the anesthesia plan, and careful intraoperative and postoperative vigilance.

References

1. Hines R and others: Complications occurring in the postanesthesia care unit: A survey, Anesth Analg 74(4):503, 1992.
2. Clagett GP: Prevention of postoperative venous thromboembolism: An update, Am J Surg 168(6):515, 1994.
3. Crandon AJ, and Koutts J: Incidence of postoperative deep venous thrombosis in gynecologic oncology, Aust N Z Obstet Gynaecol 23:216, 1983.
4. Kadivar TF and Nahhas WA: Nongynecologic surgical procedures performed on a gynecologic oncology service, Gynecol Oncol 35(1):78, 1989.
5. Kearon C and Hirsh J: Starting prophylaxis for venous thromboembolism postoperatively, Arch Intern Med 155(4):366, 1995.
6. Kendrick JH and others: The complicated septic abdominal wound, Arch Surg 117:464, 1982.
7. Mallampatti SR: Clinical signs to predict difficult tracheal intubation, Can Anaesth Soc J 30:316, 1983.

8. Roberts JT, editor: Clinical management of the airway, Philadelphia, 1994, WB Saunders Co.
9. Baggish MS and Hooper S: Aspiration as a cause of maternal death, Obstet Gynecol 43(3):327, 1974.
10. Dick W: Maternal risk from general anaesthesia and regional anaesthesia, Anaesthesist 29(5):219, 1980.
11. Mendelson CL: The aspiration of stomach contents into the lungs during obstetric anesthesia, Am J Obstet Gynecol 52:191, 1946.
12. Barash PG, Cullen BF, and Stoelting RK, editors: Clinical Anesthesia, ed 2, Philadelphia, 1992, JB Lippincott Co.
13. Gibbs CP and others: Antacid pulmonary aspiration in the dog, Anesthesiology 51:380, 1979.
14. McCaughey W and others: Cimetidine in elective caesarean section: Effect on gastric acidity, Anaesth 36(2):167, 1981.
15. Howard FA, and Sharp DS: Effect of metoclopramide on gastric emptying during labour, Br Med J 1:446, 1973.
16. Baroka A, Noveihid R, and Hajj S: Intrathecal injection of morphine for obstetric analgesia, Anesthesiology 54:136, 1981.
17. Jayr C and others: Preoperative and intraoperative factors associated with prolonged mechanical ventilation: A study in patients following major abdominal vascular surgery, Chest 103(4):1231, 1993.
18. Farn J, Hammerman AM, and Brunt LM: Intraoperative pneumothorax during laparoscopic cholecystectomy: A complication of prior transdiaphragmatic surgery, Surg Laparosc Endosc 3(3):219, 1993.
19. Barlow DW, Weymuller EA, and Wood DE: Tracheotomy and the role of postoperative chest radiography in adult patients, Ann Otol Rhinol Laryngol 103(9):665, 1994.
20. Sleszynski SL and Kelso AF: Comparison of thoracic manipulation with incentive spirometry in preventing postoperative atelectasis, J Am Osteopath Assoc 93(8):834, 1993.
21. Rivers SP and others: Epidural versus general anesthesia for infrainguinal arterial reconstruction, J Vasc Surg 14(6):764, 1991.
22. Shir Y, and others: Postoperative morbidity is similar in patients anesthetized with epidural and general anesthesia for radical prostatectomy, Urology 44(2):232, 1994.
23. Goldman L: Cardiac risk in noncardiac surgery: An update, Anesth Analg 80:810, 1995.
24. Larsen SF and others: Prediction of cardiac risk in non-cardiac surgery, Eur Heart J 8:179, 1987.
25. Steen P, Tinker J, and Tarhan S: Myocardial infarction after anesthesia and surgery, JAMA 239:2566, 1978.
26. Rao TLK, Jacobs KH, and El-Etr AA: Reinfarction following anesthesia in patients with myocardial infarction, Anesthesiology 59:499, 1983.
27. Shah KB and others: Reevaluation of perioperative myocardial infarction in patients with prior myocardial infarction undergoing noncardiac operations, Anesth Analg 71:231, 1990.
28. Fleisher LA and Barash PG: Preoperative cardiac evaluation for noncardiac surgery: A functional approach, Anesth Analg 74:586, 1992.
29. O'Kelly B and others: Study of Perioperative Ischemia Research Group: Ventricular arrhythmias in patients undergoing noncardiac surgery, JAMA 268:217, 1992.
30. Wilkes BM and Mailloux LU: Acute renal failure: Pathogenesis and prevention, Am J Med 80:1129, 1986.
31. Rodeghiero F, Castaman G, and Mannucci PM: Clinical indications for desmopressin (DDAVP) in congenital and acquired von Willebrand disease, Blood Rev 5(3):155, 1991.
32. Metz J and others: Appropriateness of transfusions of red cells, platelets and fresh frozen plasma: An audit in a tertiary care teaching hospital, Med J Aust 162(11):572, 1995.
33. Soumerai SB and others: A controlled trial of educational outreach to improve blood transfusion practice, JAMA 270(8):961, 1993.
34. Stehling L and others: Guidelines for blood utilization review, Transfusion 34(5):438, 1994.
35. Heymann SJ and Brewer TF: The infectious risks of transfusions in the United States A decision-analytic approach, Am J Infect Control 21(4):174, 1993.
36. Sloand EM, Pitt E, and Klein HG: Safety of the blood supply, JAMA 274(17):1368, 1995.
37. Bell B, Canty D, and Audet M: Hemophilia: An updated review, Pediatr Rev 16(8):290, 1995.

38. Ruggeri ZM and Zimmerman TS: Von Willebrand factor and von Willebrand disease, Blood 70(4):895, 1987.

39. Hauser I, Schneider B, and Lechner K: Postpartum factor VIII inhibitors: A review of the literature with special reference to the value of steroid and immunosuppressive treatment, Thromb Haemost 73(1):1, 1995.

40. Bona RD: Von Willebrand factor and von Willebrand's disease: A complex protein and a complex disease, Ann Clin Lab Sci 19(3):184, 1989.

41. Neidhardt B, Bartels O, and Hahn B: Postpartum hemophilia A with factor VIII inhibitor, Deutsche Medizinische Wochenschrift 110(20):799, 1985.

42. Friedman LS and Maddrey WC: Surgery in the patient with liver disease, Med Clin North Am 71(3):453, 1987.

43. Gholson CF, Provenza JM, and Bacon BR: Hepatologic considerations in patients with parenchymal liver disease undergoing surgery, Am J Gastroenterol 85(5):487, 1990.

44. Conn M: Preoperative evaluation of the patient with liver disease, Mt Sinai J Med 58(1):75, 1991.

3

Evisceration

CLIFFORD R. WHEELESS, JR.

Evisceration may be vaginal or abdominal. Fortunately this complication is rare. Both vaginal and abdominal evisceration are preceded by disruption of the vaginal or abdominal wound. Would disruption, or dehiscence, generally refers to a separation of the abdominal wound involving the anterior fascia sheath and peritoneum. Vaginal evisceration has been reported with or without a history of pelvic surgery following the spontaneous rupture of a large enterocele without previous hysterectomy.

Both vaginal and abdominal evisceration are associated with high mortality. Although one recent series reported a mortality of 34% in patients who had operative closure of an abdominal wound evisceration, most authorities report that operative mortality has been reduced to less than 1% in recent years. Few operative complications in modern gynecology have this range of mortality associated with a surgical procedure.

ABDOMINAL EVISCERATION

The frequency of abdominal wound disruption averages 2.6% when all abdominal operations are considered collectively, but the literature ranges from 0.5% to 3%. The etiology of this phenomenon is secondary to systemic as well as local factors.

Systemic factors associated with wound separation and evisceration include age, obesity, atelectasis, coughing, retching, hiccuping, cancer, jaundice, malnutrition, corticosteroids, and immunosuppressive drugs. The most common systemic factors associated with wound separation are those pathophysiologic phenomena associated with increased intraabdominal pressure such as atelectasis with its associated coughing, nausea, and vomiting, all of which increase the intraabdominal pressure and put a strain on the suture line in the abdominal wall. Systemic factors that are associated with decreased properties of wound healing play roles in the reduction and alteration of collagen synthesis, collagen reorganization, and influence the effectiveness of the phases of wound healing, such as inflammation, contraction, and epithelization.

Local Risk Factors

The most important local factors predisposing to wound separation and evisceration are inadequate closure, inadequate suture material, hemorrhage, and wound infection. The most frequent local factor in wound dehiscence and evisceration is inadequacy of surgical technique. Occasionally the first sign of wound dehiscence becomes manifest when the skin sutures are removed and evisceration of intraperitoneal contents, either intestinal or omental, occurs (Figure 3.1). Closing the midline abdominal wall incision in layers with fine absorbable suture approximating the peritoneum and the edges of the fascia with permanent suture material has generally been replaced with the mass closure technique. Mass closure techniques involve placing sutures 3 cm from the fascia edge and including all layers of the abdominal wall, fascia, muscle, and peritoneum. It was generally thought that interrupted mass closure sutures would have a greater success rate than running mass closure sutures. A recent multicenter prospective randomized trial compared continuous versus interrupted sutures in midline abdominal incisions. The overall dehiscence rate was 1.6% in patients with continuous sutures versus 2% in patients with interrupted sutures.

Many have thought that the design of the abdominal incision contributes to the inci-

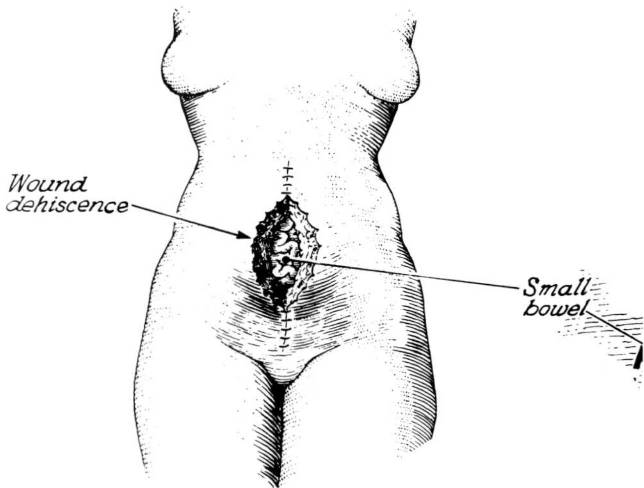

FIGURE 3.1 Abdominal wound separation with dehiscence of small bowel through the wound. (From Wheeless CR Jr: Abdominal wound dehiscence. In Wheeless CR Jr, editor: Atlas of pelvic surgery, ed 2, Philadelphia, 1988, Lea & Febiger.)

dence of dehiscence and evisceration. With the exception of long paramedian incisions that denervate much of the rectoabdominal wall, there is no evidence that the kind of incision is related to the incidence or frequency of wound dehiscence or evisceration. The exteriorization of drains or stomas through the midline incision rather than exteriorization through separate stab wound incisions is another factor that may contribute to wound disruption and evisceration.

Wound infection, particularly if catgut sutures have been used, can be associated with a higher incidence of wound disruption and evisceration. Catgut sutures use the process of phagocytosis for absorption in wounds. Phagocytosis reduces suture tensile strength. The role of catgut sutures in modern gynecologic surgery is limited, and they should be replaced with modern synthetic absorbable, delayed absorbable, or permanent sutures.

The dehiscence rate in interrupted suture lines is significantly higher than in continuous suture lines when wounds are contaminated. Several well-controlled series have shown no significant differences in the type of synthetic absorbable used, for example, polyglycolic acid versus polyglactin 910 or polyglactide L lactide. Currently the single knot suture line using the size "O" loop PDS (Polydioxanone) may be the procedure of choice for closing long midline incisions in cancer patients. Most of the studies on the subject show that the weakest point in a suture line is the knot: one knot equals one weak point, two knots equal two weak points, etc.

Diagnosis and Management

The drainage of serosanguineous fluid after 24 hours from an abdominal incision is virtually pathognomonic of wound separation of some degree and raises the possibility of evisceration. The patient often describes a popping sensation associated with severe coughing or retching.

The mortality associated with wound disruption and evisceration can be dramatically influenced by modern surgical techniques. The patient should immediately be returned to bed, the abdominal viscera covered in moist, sterile towels, and the patient taken to the OR. The cough reflex should be immediately suppressed by the IV or intramuscular (IM) injection of opiates such as codeine that block the cough center. After general anesthesia, the abdominal contents should be copiously washed with saline or Ringer's lactate solution. All necrotic tissue needs to be excised and all sutures removed (Figure 3.2). The intestines

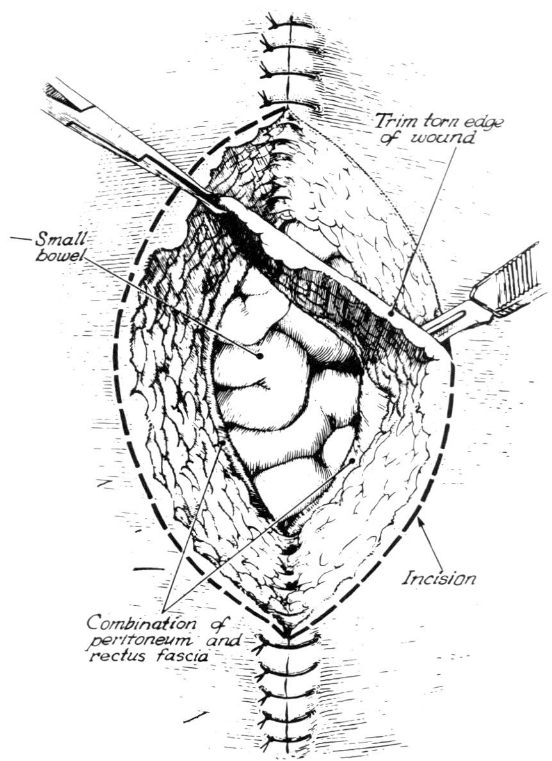

FIGURE 3.2 All necrotic tissue, including skin, rectus fascia muscle, and peritoneum, should be excised. Necrotic sutures should be removed. (From Wheeless CR Jr: Abdominal wound dehiscence. In Wheeless CR Jr, editor: Atlas of pelvic surgery, ed 2, Philadelphia, 1988, Lea & Febiger.)

should be thoroughly inspected from the ligament of Treitz to the rectosigmoid colon. Any devitalized intestine should be resected and reanastomosis performed (see Figure 3.9). The wound should be closed in a mass closure technique utilizing the running Smead-Jones far-near-near-far technique (Figure 3.3) or the mass closure single knot loop suture running technique (Figure 3.4). This should be performed with large synthetic permanent suture (such as Prolene or nylon). Through-and-through sutures of the entire abdominal wall from the skin to the peritoneum using large-gauge wire have generally been replaced with synthetic permanent sutures such as nylon or prolene. If the wound is not infected or if it is infected and there has been adequate surgical debridement of necrotic tissue (see Figure 3.2), an alternative to open or delayed wound closure may be considered; the skin and subcutaneous tissue are closed, and a closed suction drain is placed over the fascia and under the skin and subcutaneous tissue (Figure 3.5). Intravenous antibiotics, while initially used in most cases, can be tailored according to cultures taken at the time of operation and the patient's postoperative clinical course. In obese patients the use of a surgical binder may relieve stress on the wound from the large fat pad and panniculus.

Recurrence of evisceration after reclosure of a dehisced wound is rare, although incisional hernias are later found in approximately 20% of such patients, usually in those with wound infection in addition to dehiscence.

VAGINAL EVISCERATION

Fortunately, vaginal evisceration of the intestine is rare (Figure 3.6). The literature consists

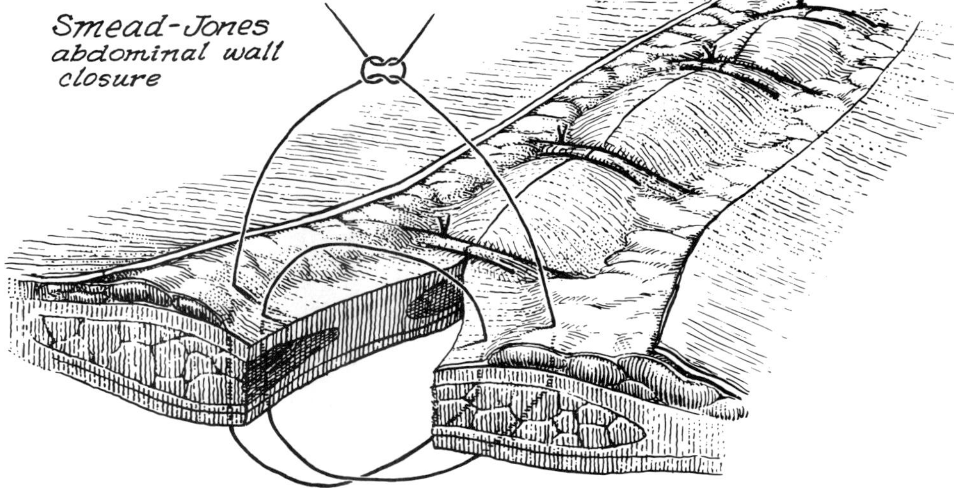

FIGURE 3.3 Smead-Jones abdominal wall closure using far-near-near-far sutures.

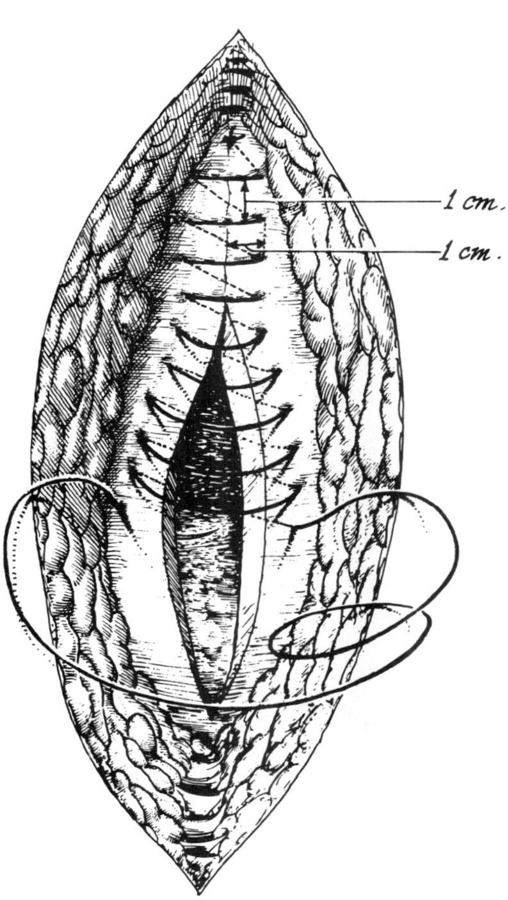

FIGURE 3.4 Through-and-through technique of mass closure with running technique placing sutures 1 cm apart.

of individual case presentations with an occasional review article; fewer than 62± cases have been reported.

Evisceration occasionally follows vaginal hysterectomy, usually within the immediate postoperative period. However, there are cases reported years later. It has been reported after abdominal hysterectomy and as a spontaneous sequela of ruptures of large enteroceles with and without previous hysterectomy.

A contemporary source of vaginal eviscerations has been suction curettage for termination of pregnancy during which the small intestine is sucked into the eye of a vacuum curette that has perforated the uterine wall and the small intestine is pulled through the perforation in the uterus and out into the vagina (Figures 3.7 and 3.8).

The etiology of vaginal evisceration, except for that associated with suction termination of pregnancy, is confusing. There has been no specific pattern of events that can be related in a cause-and-effect manner.

The anatomy of the small bowel and its mesentery should make vaginal evisceration difficult. Most anatomists describe the mesentery of the small bowel as being from 15 to 20 cm in length. Obviously this distance is insufficient to allow the terminal ileum and/or jejunum to exit the peritoneal cavity through the vaginal cuff or a uterine perforation and eviscerate. There appear to be two possibilities: first, certain individuals could have a longer mesentery than the 15-to-20 cm average; sec-

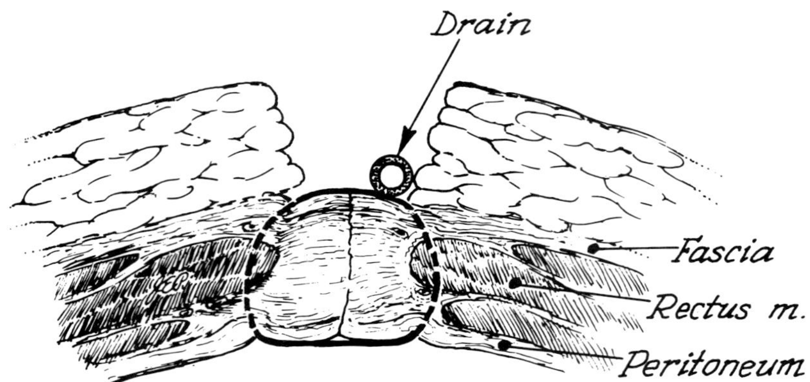

Figure 3.5 Cross section of the mass closure, including all layers, fascia, muscle, and peritoneum. If the subcutaneous tissue and skin are to be closed, a closed suction drain is placed over the fascia and brought out through a separate stab wound.

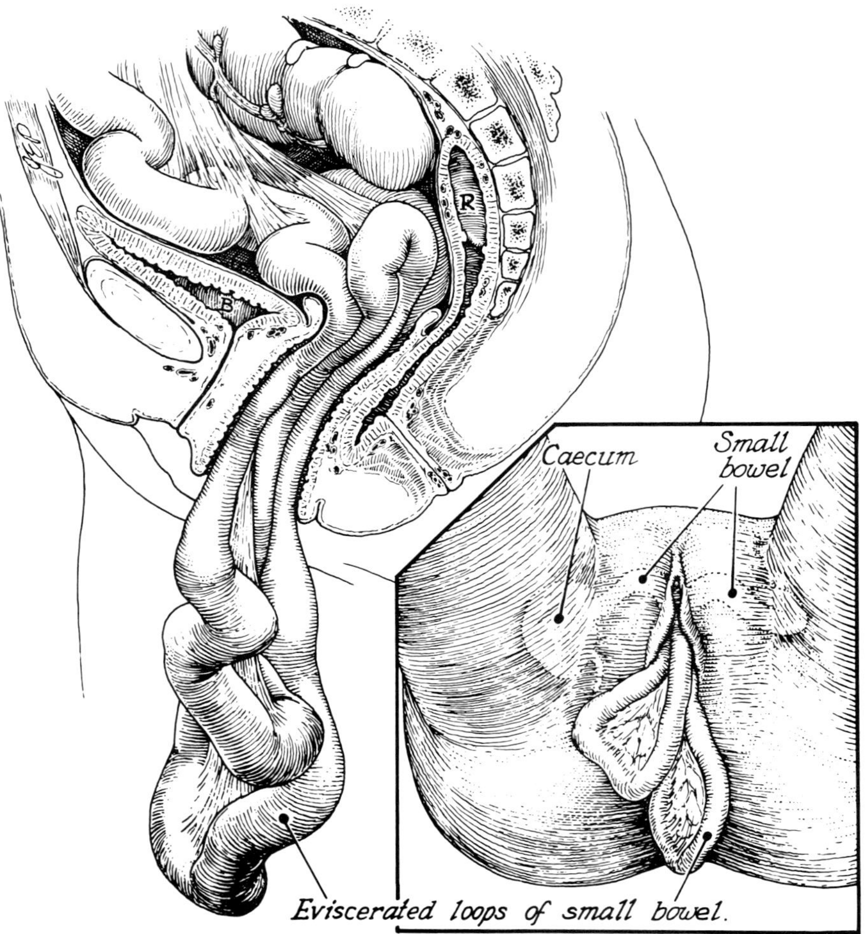

Figure 3.6 Sagittal view of the lower abdomen and pelvis plus a perineal view *(inset)* with the patient in the lithotomy position show the vaginal evisceration. The sagittal view in particular emphasizes the point that, for complete vaginal evisceration to occur, there must be some technique of mobilization of the small bowel mesentery. Otherwise, the length of small bowel mesentery is generally insufficient for the evisceration to occur. (Redrawn from Wheeless CR Jr: Vaginal evisceration following pelvic surgery. In Nichols DH, editor: Clinical problems, injuries, and complications of gynecologic surgery, ed 2, Baltimore, 1988, Williams & Wilkins.)

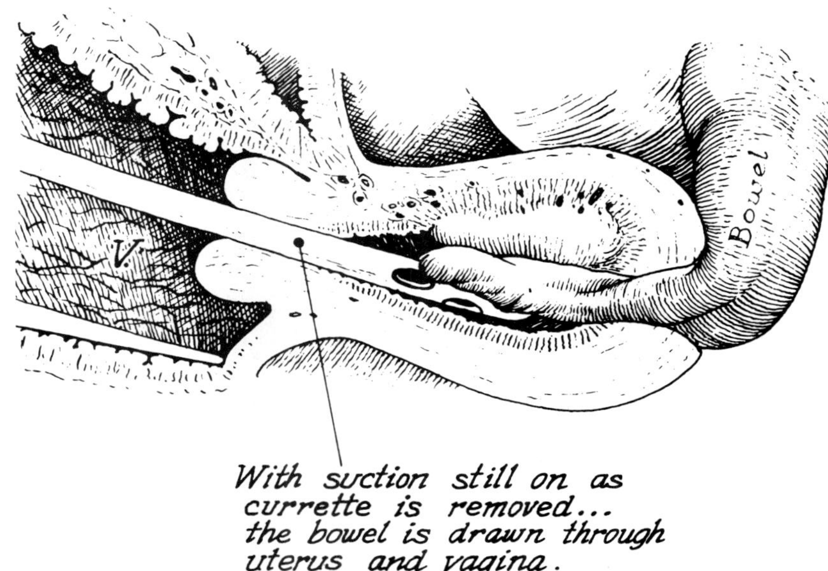

FIGURE 3.7 Sagittal view showing the suction curette with attached bowel being pulled through the perforated uterus during a termination of pregnancy. The gestational contents have not been removed. *V,* vagina. (From Wheeless CR Jr: Vaginal evisceration following pelvic surgery. In Nichols DH, editor: Clinical problems, injuries, and complications of gynecologic surgery, ed 2, Baltimore, 1988, Williams & Wilkins.)

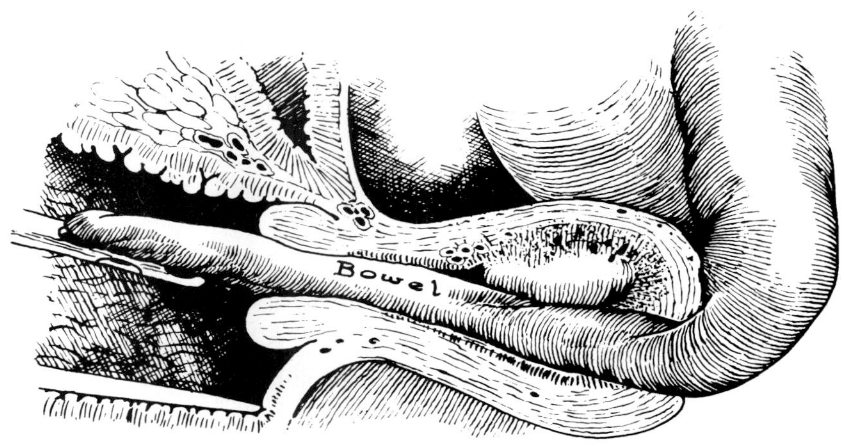

FIGURE 3.8 The intestine is eviscerated through the cervix out into the vagina. It is at this point that the intestine is most likely to be injured by confusing it with fetal parts. (From Wheeless CR Jr: Vaginal evisceration following pelvic surgery. In Nichols DH, editor: Clinical problems, injuries, and complications of gynecologic surgery, ed 2, Baltimore, 1988, Williams & Wilkins.)

ond, the process involved in evisceration may lengthen the small intestine mesentery by mobilizing it secondary to lacerations in the mesentery at the root of its origin (Figure 3.9, *A*). It is likely that both phenomena occur. Laceration of the small bowel mesentery threatens the continuity of the blood supply to the intestine. However, the laceration could occur in such a location as to spare specific vascular arcades within the small bowel mes-

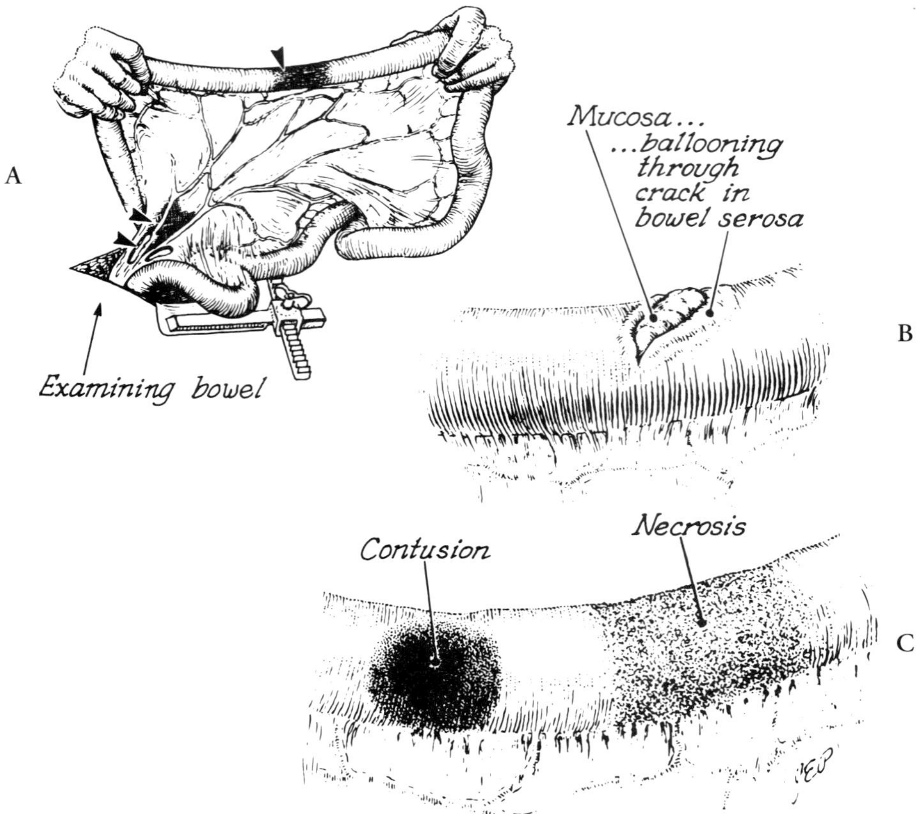

Figure 3.9 A, This drawing demonstrates the need for complete examination of the intestine from the ligament of Treitz to the cecum. Specific areas of laceration within the mesentery should be searched for and the relationship between the laceration and the vascular integrity of the bowel should be confirmed. B, Intestinal enterotomies or tears should be searched for and appropriately repaired. C, Areas of contusion and necrosis should be identified. (From Wheeless CR Jr: Vaginal evisceration following pelvic surgery. In Nichols DH, editor: Clinical problems, injuries, and complications of gynecologic surgery, ed 2, Baltimore, 1988, Williams & Wilkins.)

entery. This may explain why there are successful reports of simply replacing the small bowel into the peritoneal cavity via the vaginal route without performing a laparotomy and the patient recovering without incident. However, a procedure such as replacement of the intestine through the vaginal opening without laparotomy could be perilous. The overall mortality from vaginal evisceration has been reported at approximately 10%. From a review of the literature, it appears that much of this mortality is secondary to peritonitis, possibly related to intestinal necrosis. On the other hand, the morbidity from laparotomy in a modern hospital is minimal. Via laparotomy the intestine can be thoroughly inspected and suspicious areas of compromised intestine resected with primary reanastomosis (Figures 3.9, *B* and *C*, and 3.10).

Prevention

Prevention of vaginal evisceration following hysterectomy has several possibilities. A collective series of a significant number of patients for statistically valid results is unavailable. Therefore the precise cause of this problem in most cases remains unknown, except for those cases that occurred during termination of pregnancy in which the intestine was pulled through a perforation in the uterine wall. Possibilities for prevention that require discus-

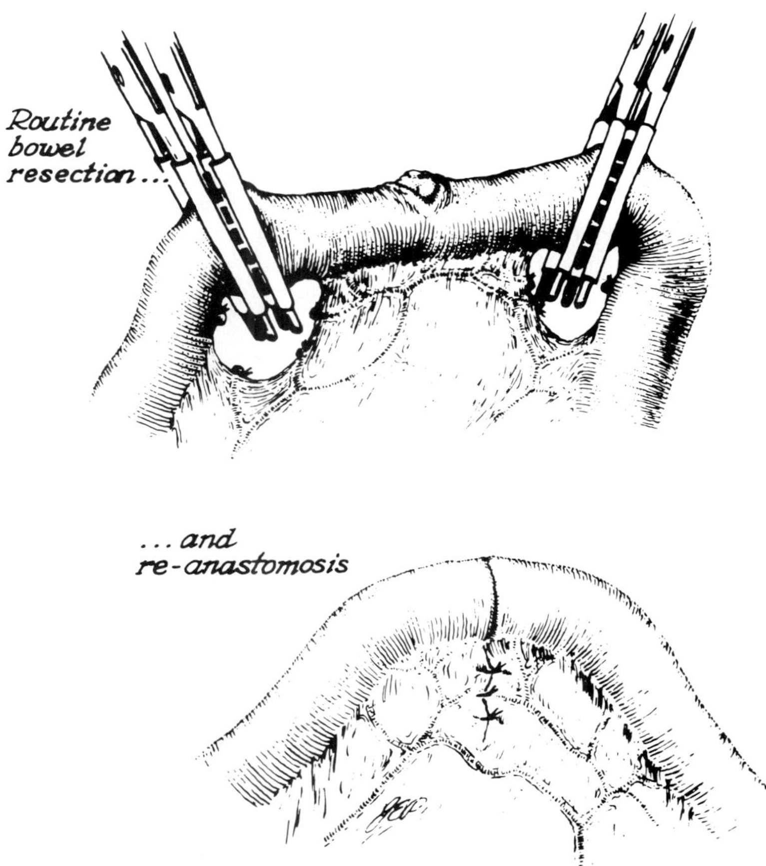

FIGURE 3.10 Areas of severe intestinal damage and vascular necrosis should be surgically resected and reanastomosis performed. (From Wheeless CR Jr: Vaginal evisceration following pelvic surgery. In Nichols DH, editor: Clinical problems, injuries, and complications of gynecologic surgery, ed 2, Baltimore, 1988, Williams & Wilkins.)

sion include the following: (1) the repair of an enterocele or cystocele present at the time of hysterectomy; (2) the pros and cons of leaving the vaginal vault open at the time of hysterectomy; (3) the choice and size of suture material used in closure of the vaginal vault and particularly the technique of anastomosis of the stumps of the supporting ligaments of the pelvis to the angles of the vagina.

Although vaginal eviscerations have occurred in a variety of clinical and anatomic situations, the majority of eviscerations have occurred in association with poor support of the vaginal cuff, posterior fornix, and cul-de-sac after vaginal hysterectomy.

The open vaginal vault is an attractive and tempting possibility for the cause of vaginal evisceration. However, the open vaginal vault is the technique of many gynecologists, and thousands of hysterectomies have been performed leaving the vaginal vault open without the rare event of postoperative vaginal evisceration. When the vaginal vault is left open, its edge is usually sutured with a running locked synthetic absorbable suture, referred to as "reefing" the margin of the vaginal cuff. At the vaginal angles this "reefing suture" usually includes the stumps of the uterosacral and cardinal ligaments and anastomoses them to the angle of the vagina for additional support. In addition, most surgeons (but not all) peritonealize the pelvis by approximating the anterior and posterior peritoneal surfaces. This covers the open vaginal cuff. However, if one returns to the classic anatomic situation where the average length of the mesentery of the small bowel is 15 to 20 cm, evisceration would be virtually impossible unless an additional event occurred to excessively mobilize the intestine, producing sufficient length to push it through an opening in the vaginal cuff. Therefore open vaginal cuffs alone are generally insufficient to be the cause of all vaginal eviscerations. In addition, most vaginal eviscerations reported have occurred after the vaginal cuff has been surgically closed with interrupted sutures.

The choice of suture material may be a factor involved in the occurrence of vaginal evisceration, but, like the open vaginal cuff, an additional factor is usually required to mobilize sufficient intestine to eviscerate out the vagina. If fine synthetic absorbable suture material is used (size 3-0 or less), there is the attractive thesis that the anastomosis of the stumps of the cardinal and uterosacral ligaments could break down and set up the anatomic situation for evisceration. In addition, if enough pressure were acutely exerted on the mesentery of the small bowel via a large Valsalva maneuver to lacerate the mesentery and thereby mobilize the intestine, evisceration could occur. However, insufficient evidence exists to state that the cause of vaginal evisceration is the choice of suture material. We believe synthetic absorbable suture in sizes of 2-0 to zero represents the ideal suture material for management of the vaginal cuff and reanastomosis of the stumps of the uterosacral and cardinal ligaments to the angle of the vaginal cuff. Permanent suture used in this area would not eliminate eviscerations but would add morbidity from suture abscesses.

The method of closure of the vagina could also represent a potential threat for vaginal evisceration. All too often the vaginal cuff is closed with figure-of-eight sutures. A figure-of-eight suture, especially if tied tightly, promotes necrosis and healing by second intention. This is not the purpose of the suture in the vaginal cuff. Single sutures of synthetic absorbable material tied gently enough to approximate the tissue and prevent hemostasis without strangulation and necrosis are sufficient.

In addition, it is important to plicate the uterosacral ligaments behind the vaginal vault to reduce the cul-de-sac and reduce the tendency toward enterocele formation. We do not believe that the complete classic McCall's plication of the uterosacral ligament is necessary in all hysterectomies, and in fact it represents a threat of suture ligation of the ureter if the uterosacral ligaments are plicated for a distance of more than 4 cm.

Although the factors discussed may play a role in this problem, we are impressed that most vaginal eviscerations are associated predominantly with large Valsalva maneuvers, namely, vomiting, coughing, and lifting heavy objects. Severe vomiting and coughing have been reported in most cases in which evisceration has occurred after hysterectomy. Therefore prevention must include moderating these factors by eliminating overzealous oral feeding and excessive induction of postoperative coughing. Prevention of evisceration at suction abortion must include the safe utilization of techniques for performing the operation, that is, careful dilation of the cervix and repeated sounding of the uterine cavity.

Early Recognition

The key to reduction of severe morbidity and mortality associated with evisceration must be early recognition. Most eviscerations through the vagina are associated with lacerations of the mesentery of the small bowel, and the vascular integrity of the small bowel is at stake (see Figure 3.9). When evisceration is caused by suction abortion, the additional factor of trauma by the suction curette to the wall of the bowel makes early recognition extremely important (see Figure 3.8). Early recognition allows surgical intervention before intestinal necrosis and leakage of intestinal contents into the peritoneal cavity.

Appropriate Treatment

Treatment of evisceration through the vagina should start with pelvic laparotomy. Initial first aid upon discovering the evisceration should be the physiologic protection of the eviscerated loop of intestine by wrapping it in sterile saline–soaked gauze or a sterile moist towel. An exploratory laparotomy through a midline incision should be performed immediately. We emphasize a midline incision; we do not think that the mesentery of the intestine can be inspected adequately through a Pfannenstiel's incision. The intestine is carefully

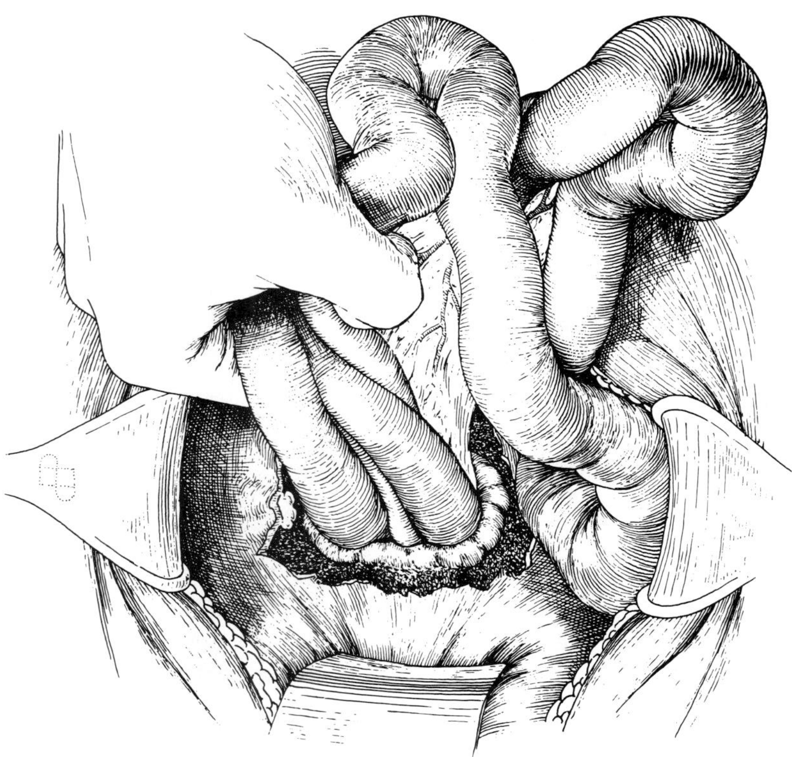

FIGURE 3.11 Pelvic laparotomy showing the replacement of the intestine back into the peritoneal cavity through the ruptured vaginal cuff surrounded by the torn peritoneal margins. (From Wheeless CR Jr: Vaginal evisceration following pelvic surgery. In Nichols DH, editor: Clinical problems, injuries, and complications of gynecologic surgery, ed 2, Baltimore, 1988, Williams & Wilkins.)

withdrawn through the defect whether it is the perforated uterus or the vaginal cuff (Figure 3.11). A complete inspection of the entire intestine and its mesentery from the ligament of Treitz to the cecum is indicated (see Figure 3.9). The mesentery is carefully inspected for lacerations and vascular injuries and hemostasis. Suspicious areas of intestine are resected and reanastomosis performed (see Figure 3-10). We believe there is no role for transvaginal or transuterine replacement of the intestine into the abdominal cavity without laparotomy because of the possibility of lacerations in the mesentery and undetected injury to the small bowel. This is especially true when evisceration has occurred through the perforated uterus during the performance of a suction abortion. The suction curette could have damaged several pieces of small intestine other than the piece eviscerated through the uterine perforation. When the intestine has been appropriately replaced into the abdominal cavity and inspected carefully, and damaged areas have been resected, the entire peritoneal cavity is copiously lavaged with normal saline. A nasogastric gastrostomy tube is inserted into the stomach and left in place until the patient has resumed intestinal function. All patients who have sustained vaginal evisceration should be covered with broad-spectrum antibiotics. Antimicrobial therapy should be guided by appropriate cultures taken at the time of laparotomy, but therapy should be directed toward the gram-negative anaerobic group D *Enterococcus* organisms.

In those cases of evisceration associated with termination of pregnancy, it is vital to complete the termination as part of the repair procedure. All too often in the panic of this unexpected and severe complication, attention is directed toward the intestinal problem and away from the potential severe complica-

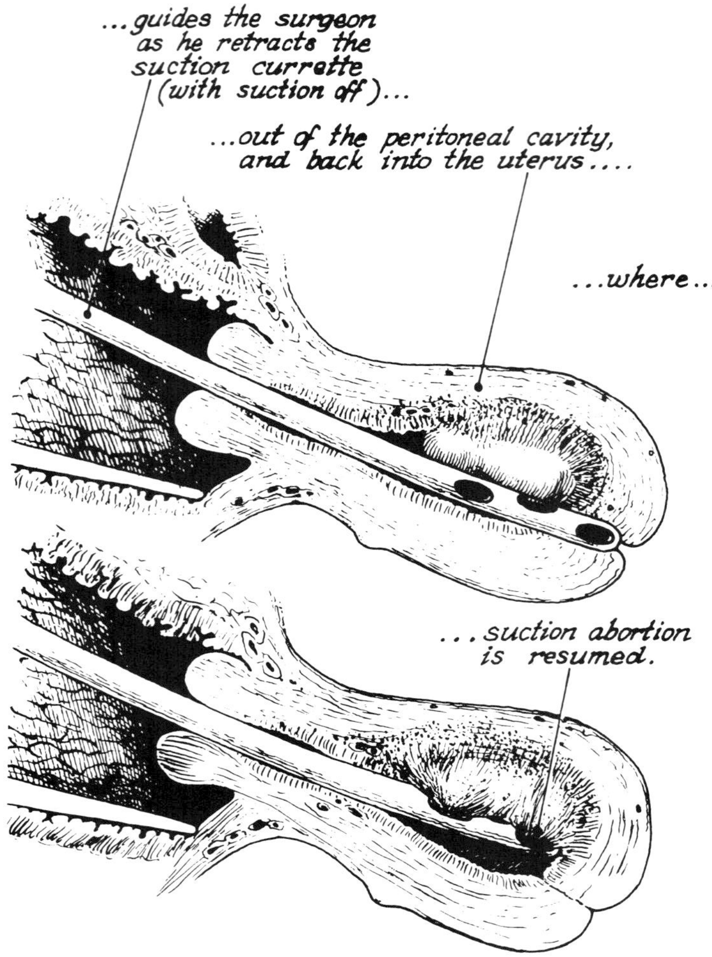

Figure 3.12 Sagittal drawing showing suction cannula withdrawn into endometrial cavity. (From Wheeless CR Jr: Vaginal evisceration following pelvic surgery. In Nichols DH, editor: Clinical problems, injuries, and complications of gynecologic surgery, ed 2, Baltimore, 1988, Williams & Wilkins.)

tion of incomplete septic abortion with retained gestational contents. One solution is to have a second surgeon immediately perform a laparotomy and guide the withdrawal of the bowel out of the uterus and the suction cannula out of the peritoneal cavity and back into the endometrial cavity, where the suction can be resumed and the termination of pregnancy completed. The bowel can be inspected and repaired if needed (Figure 3-12). Failure to do this leaves products of gestation within the endometrial cavity and creates the potential for the sequelae of incomplete septic abortion.

Repair of the ruptured vagina or perforated uterus differs. The perforation site in the uterus can be closed with simple through-and-through sutures of absorbable material. However, in the case of the ruptured vagina, careful closure with a well-designed plan of ligament suspension and obliteration of the cul-de-sac should be made (Figure 3.13). The suture material should be absorbable and care taken to reduce areas of necrosis to a minimum. The opening in the vagina should be excised back to fresh, healthy tissue. Closure with interrupted absorbable sutures is preferable. A separate step to locate and suture the stumps of the uterosacral and cardinal ligaments to the angles of the vagina should be made (see Figure 3.13, *A*). In addition, the anterior surface of the

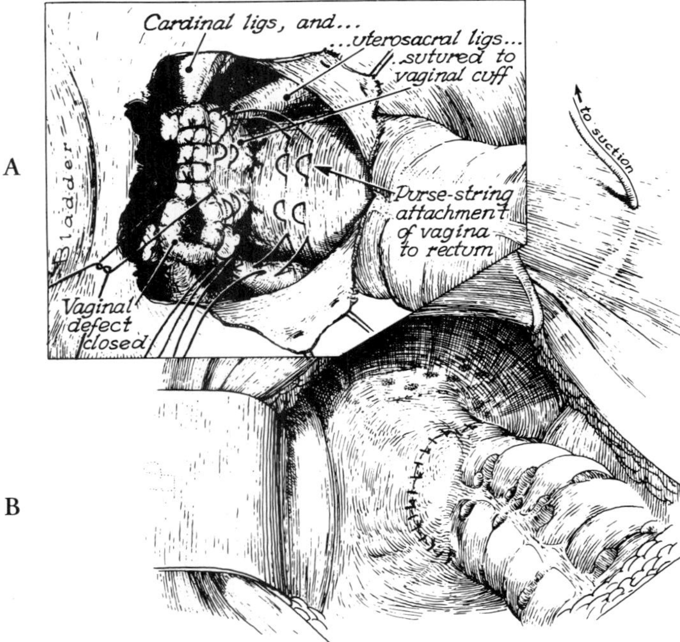

FIGURE 3.13 **A,** Repair of ruptured vagina and suture of rectosigmoid colon to posterior vaginal cuff. **B,** Reperitonealization of pelvis. (From Wheeless CR Jr: Vaginal evisceration following pelvic surgery. In Nichols DH, editor: Clinical problems, injuries, and complications of gynecologic surgery, ed 2, Baltimore, 1988, Williams & Wilkins.)

rectosigmoid colon is sutured to the posterior vaginal cuff to eliminate the cul-de-sac (see Figure 3.13, *B*). Complete resection of all necrotic tissue along the vaginal cuff and stumps of the supporting ligaments is necessary. This is a particularly important step if fecal material has spilled into the peritoneal cavity. The surgeon should not be surprised at the development of a postoperative pelvic abscess if necrotic tissue that has been bathed in the intestinal contents is left within the pelvis postoperatively. Antibiotic therapy will not be sufficient to override this breach in surgical technique. We advocate intermittent pneumonic pressure cuffs to the legs for 5 days for all of these patients. Those patients who do not have return of intestinal function within 3 to 4 days postoperatively should be given intravenous hyperalimentation (total parenteral nutrition, 30 calories/kg). In many of the series reported in the literature, prolonged ileus has followed vaginal evisceration. If the entire intestine has been completely explored and the surgeon is comfortable as to the vascular integrity of the intestine, prolonged ileus should be treated conservatively with nasogastric or gastrostomy drainage and IV hyperalimentation. However, if the intestine has been replaced vaginally and it has been inadequately explored, the question of vascular integrity and necrosis of the bowel must be considered. Repeat, or second-look, laparotomy should be considered, and the vascular integrity of the bowel ensured.

Although evisceration of the small intestine through the vagina is an extremely serious event, patients have an excellent chance for recovery if intestinal necrosis and peritonitis have not occurred. Moreover, if proper closure of the vaginal vault with elimination of the cul-de-sac and careful approximation of the supporting ligaments to the angles of the vagina is made during the repair process, the likelihood of recurrence is small.

A gynecologist could practice for a lifetime and never encounter a case of vaginal evisceration. Because of its rarity, it has been difficult for any one clinic to gain a large volume of experience in treating this phenomenon. Nevertheless it seems logical to treat vaginal evisceration as one would treat abdominal evisceration following dehiscence of a postoperative abdominal incision. In treating evisceration of the abdominal wall, the surgeon would never consider replacing the intestine through the traumatic abdominal opening or dehiscent wound without a thorough inspection of the peritoneal cavity. This same principle should be carried out in vaginal evisceration.

BIBLIOGRAPHY

Alexander HC and Prudden J: The causes of abdominal wound dehisced disruption, Surg Gynecol Obstet 122:1223, 1966.

Banerjee SR and others: Abdominal wound evisceration, Current Surg 40:432, 1983.

Fagniez JL and others: Abdominal midline incision closure, Arch Surg 120:1351, 1985.

Farrell SA and others: Massive evisceration: A complication following sacrospinous vaginal vault fixation, Obstet Gynecol 78:560, 1991.

Fox PF and Kowalczyk AS: Ruptured enterocele, Am J Obstet Gynecol 111:592, 1971.

Fox WP: Vaginal evisceration, Obstet Gynecol 50:223, 1977.

Gammelgaard N, and Jensen J: Wound complications after closure of abdominal incisions with Dexon or Vicryl, Acta Chir Scanda 149:505, 1983.

Goligher JC and others: A controlled clinical trial of three methods of closure of laparotomy wounds, Br J Surg 62:823, 1975.

Goss CM: The digestive system. In Gray H, editor: Anatomy of the human body, ed 28, Philadelphia, 1973, Lea & Febiger.

Greenburg AG, Saik RP, and Peskin GW: Wound dehiscence, Arch Surg 114:143, 1979.

Halasz NA: Dehiscence of laparotomy wounds, Am J Surg 116:210, 1968.

Hall BS and others: Vaginal evisceration during coitus, Am J Obstet Gynecol 131:115, 1978.

Hunt TK: Disorders of repair and their management. In Hunt TK, and Dumphy JE, editors: Fundamentals of wound management, New York, 1979, Appleton-Century-Crofts.

Karam JA, Wengert PA, and Kerstein MD: Vaginal evisceration, South Med J 88:355, 1995.

McNellis D, Torkelson L, and McElin TW: Late postoperative vaginal vault disruption, Am J Obstet Gynecol 94:543, 1966.

Nichols DH and Randall CL: Complications of vaginal surgery. In Nichols DH and Randall CL: Vaginal surgery, ed 2, Baltimore, 1996, Williams & Wilkins.

Pemberton LA and Manax WG: Complications after vertical and transverse incisions for cholecystectomy, Surg Gynecol Obstet 132:892, 1971.

Penninck FM and others: Abdominal wound dehiscence in gastroenterological surgery, Ann Surg 189:342, 1979.

Powell JL: Vaginal evisceration following vaginal hysterectomy, Am J Obstet Gynecol 115:276, 1973.

Powell JL: Transvaginal evisceration after hysterectomy, Am J Obstet Gynecol 172:1656, 1995.

Rollinson D and others: Transvaginal small-bowel evisceration: A case report, Mt Sinai J Med 62:235, 1995.

Rolf BB: Vaginal evisceration, Am J Obst Gyn 107:369, 1970.

Sanders RJ and DiClementi D: Principles of abdominal wound closure: Prevention of wound dehiscence, Arch Surg 112:118, 1977.

Somkuti SG and others: Transvaginal evisceration after hysterectomy in premenopausal women: A presentation of three cases, Am J Obstet Gynecol 171:567, 1994.

Wax JR, Segna RA, and Vandersloot JA: Magnesium toxicity and resuscitation: An unusual cause of postcesarean evisceration, Int J Gynaecol Obstet 48:213, 1995.

Wheeless CR Jr: Abdominal wound dehiscence. In Wheeless CR Jr, editor: Atlas of pelvic surgery, ed 2, Philadelphia, 1988, Lea & Febiger.

4

Incisional Hernia

George W. Mitchell

Predisposing Factors

If all gynecologic operations were performed on young healthy individuals, there would be few incisional, or ventral, hernias, but this is not the group most liable to surgery and its consequences. Factors predisposing to the development of ventral hernia are listed in Table 4.1. In life-threatening situations requiring surgical intervention, all of these factors must be ignored, but in the decision to perform elective surgery, herniation is one of the possible complications that must be taken into account. Adverse predisposing factors of a general systemic type are for the most part self-evident, but even in a healthy person a well-healed wound leaves the abdominal wall weaker than it was before, and additional incisions through the same site weaken it still further.

Incisions

The surgeon has some control over operative factors, but this control is not absolute. For instance, if the same area must be reentered a few hours or even a few weeks after a preceding operation, the surgeon is well advised to reopen the original incision, since a new parallel or perpendicular incision may further compromise the regenerating blood and nerve supply of the area. The most commonly used incisions for gynecologic operations are shown in Figure 4.1; of these, the lower midline is certainly the most popular. For cesarean section, the transverse modified Pfannenstiel incision is replacing the vertical incision, probably because of the marked diastasis of the rectus muscles produced by pregnancy and the easy access to the lower uterine segment. Transverse muscle-cutting incisions, the Maylard (Figure 4.2) and the Czerny (Figure 4.3), provide excellent exposure for retropubic operations, such as those performed by gynecologic urologists, and for the resection of the lymph nodes of the lateral pelvic walls. Transverse skin incisions leave a cosmetic scar and are more in demand by patients. Some statistics suggest that transverse incisions undergo fewer dehiscences than vertical incisions and give rise to fewer postoperative hernias, but the tension on both types of incision is equal, as is the quality of the tissue, and it is possible that the reported differences may be due to other variables such as the suture material used and the type of closure. Transverse incisions can be an embarrassment if the focus of the operation proves to be higher in the abdomen.

Rather than seriously damage the rectus muscle in a frustrating attempt to find the midline after previous surgery, it is sometimes advisable to do a muscle-splitting incision directly through the sheath of the rectus itself. This incision offers exposure just as good as a midline incision and can be extended above the umbilicus without difficulty, but it has the disadvantage that more bleeding may be encountered as a result of vessels perforating the sheath from the inferior epigastric artery. Incisions close to or along the semilunar line at the junction of the transversalis and oblique muscles (pararectus) are sometimes used for retroperitoneal operations involving the ureter, pelvic lymph nodes, or localized infections, but the resulting scar is relatively weak. The healing process is also affected by the length of the incision despite the much quoted apocryphal statement that incisions heal from side to side and not from top to bottom. The tension on the closure of a midline incision is proportional to the square of the length of the incision, which means that the longer the incision, the more likely it is to pull apart.

TABLE 4.1 Factors predisposing to wound disruption

Preoperative
Age
Systemic disease
Diabetes, cancer, anemia, pulmonary disability
Nutrition
Obesity, hypoproteinemia
Previous surgery
Irradiation
Drugs
Chemotherapy, steroids
Operative
Type and length of incision
Length of operation
Poor hemostasis
Necrotic tissue
Type of closure
Suture material
Postoperative
Wound infection
Hematomas, seromas
Distention
Ileus, ascites
Exertion
Coughing, vomiting, hiccups

Closure of Incisions

Hemostasis should be 100% complete when the incision is closed. Seromas and hematomas accumulating in the subcutaneous space or deep to the fascia give rise to infection and may even burst open the incision by the pressure of their accumulation. The cautery is a valuable tool in this process, since it is both effective and expeditious, but the overuse of the cautery causes necrosis and gives rise to infection. When the subcutaneous tissues have been widely undercut during the closure or there is likely to be a considerable dead space left behind, drainage is desirable, and this should be done by suction drains brought out through a stab wound at least 5 cm away from the incision. In operations involving gross infection or fecal contamination, the skin should be left open and closed several days later.

Wound dehiscence through one or more layers of the abdominal wall is a complication of gynecologic surgery that occurs in between 0.3% and 3% of cases. When only the skin opens in isolated areas postoperatively, it is of no great significance, but the more common separation of the skin and subcutaneous tissues down to the fascia, usually caused by infection, prolongs hospitalization and requires either

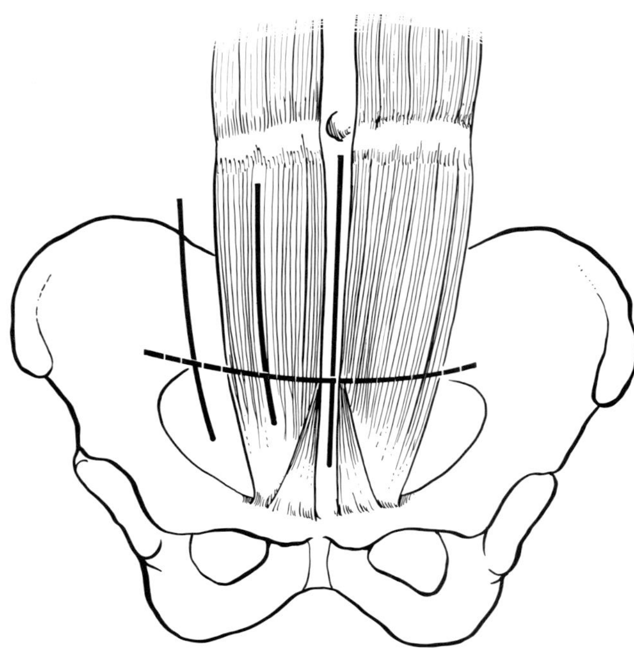

FIGURE 4.1 Placement of midline, muscle-splitting, pararectal, and low transverse incisions.

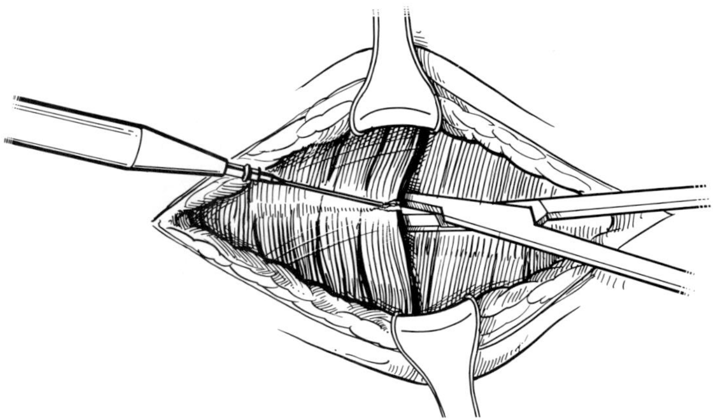

Figure 4.2 Maylard incision. A long Kelly's clamp is thrust under the rectus muscle, and the muscle is transsected with the Bovie cautery, taking care not to damage the inferior epigastric vessels.

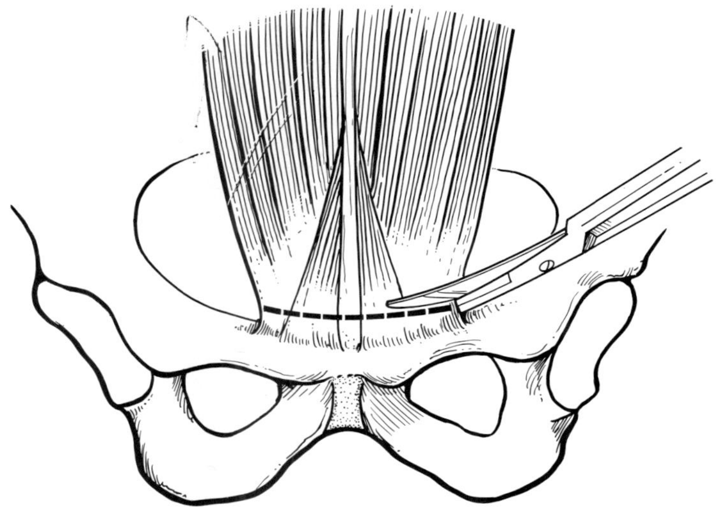

Figure 4.3 Czerny incision. The tendinous insertion of the rectus muscles and the origin of the pyramidial muscles are cut away from the pubis and reflected upward.

reclosure after the wound is clean and granulating or a protracted period of healing by second intention. If the fascia is involved in the infection or gives way as a result of tension, the situation is more serious and subsequent herniation more likely. Complete dehiscence, for which the term *evisceration* is frequently used, implies the extrusion of abdominal contents through the incision and requires immediate surgical intervention. The mortality rate from the complication remains high, and in those who survive, the possiblity of hernia formation is great.

Suture Materials. All experts agree that the type of closure of the incision has an important bearing on the likelihood of dehiscence and the possibility of the future development of the hernia, but there is little agreement regarding what the exact nature of that closure should be. There is a similar lack of consensus regarding appropriate suture material. From the beginning of the twentieth century, general surgeons preferred to close their patients' wounds in layers with nonabsorbable suture material, usually silk, although cotton and linen were also used. Metallic sutures have been available for more than 100 years, and monofilament steel wire remains to this day the preference in some quarters. Gynecologists often followed suit, but with the development of the chromicized catgut in the 1920s, most turned to that type of suture material. During this era, statistics were adduced to show that closures with catgut were as strong as those with nonabsorbable material and that the incidence of dehiscence and herniation was not increased.

The development of longer-lasting synthetic absorbable suture material and relatively inert nonabsorbable suture material in the 1960s again radically altered the pattern of usage. The commercial market for products of this kind is active, and as each new product comes on the market, it quickly develops a coterie of adherents. Nevertheless, those who were trained with the more old-fashioned materials may continue to adhere doggedly to them and claim their superiority. The wide range of choices is shown in Tables 4.2 and 4.3. Even though the surgeon's preference has a major role in determining what is to be used, the following objective points can be made:

1. Nonabsorbable sutures are strong and last for months, but they are foreign bodies that may serve as niduses for infection.
2. Silk is facile to use but reactive in tissue, cotton is obsolescent, and linen is obsolete.
3. Wire is relatively inert but hard to handle.
4. Nylon and polyester are more flexible than wire but require five throws per knot.
5. Braided sutures are more likely to promote infection than monofilament sutures.
6. The tensile strength of absorbable sutures lasts from 10 (catgut) to 40 days (synthetic).
7. Synthetic nonabsorbable sutures are stiff, tend to come untied, and require five throws per knot.
8. Catgut sutures are more difficult to standardize for quality and give way early but require only three throws per knot.
9. Synthetic absorbable suture material lasts long enough for complete wound healing.

A sensible middle-of-the-road position based on the facts would suggest that silk and catgut should not be used as the principal suture in fascial closure, that long-lasting synthetic absorbable sutures are satisfactory in most instances, and that relatively inert synthetic nonabsorbable material is advantageous in difficult cases, for single running sutures, and in hernia repair.

Suturing Techniques. As has been noted, a variety of different techniques of closure have evolved that have been shown by various authors to be successful in reducing the incidence of postoperative dehiscence. The only conclusion to be reached is that there is no universal method that can be acclaimed supremely successful. One important variable other than the technique may explain the discrepancy in statistics: in many centers that accumulate large volumes of cases, the incisions are closed by personnel low on the hierarchical totem pole, often without supervision. This is particularly true of cæsarean sections, and the results of these closures are bound to reflect the inexperience. On the other hand, future authors interested in compiling data to support their particular method are more likely to remain in attendance and either perform or supervise the closure.

The peritoneum is usually closed with a running absorbable suture. Since this mesothelial layer ordinarily regenerates spontaneously within 24 hours, some surgeons believe that it is unnecessary to close it, but common sense suggests that an additional layer might be helpful in some instances in preventing total extrusion of the intestines after fascial separation. The fascia may be closed with straight interrupted sutures (see Figure 4.12), with figure-of-eight sutures (Figure 4.4), or with a running suture (Figure 4.5). The first takes more time but has the advantage that if one goes, all of them do not go. The second is less likely to pull out but bunches up tissue, making it more likely to undergo necrosis. The third is faster and probably satisfactory if the suture material can be depended on. Possibly influenced by tradition, my preference is for the first. Important principles in all of these techniques are white fascia to white fascia apposition, the placement of sutures at least 1 cm from the fascial edge, the ability to tie securely but not to maximum constriction, and closure without tension. The anesthesi-

Table 4.2 Nonabsorbable sutures

Type	Generic Name	Ethicon, Inc.* Trade Name	Davis & Geck† Trade Name	Deknatel, Inc.‡ Trade Name
Synthetic braided	Uncoated polyester	Mersilene	Dacron	Cottony Dacron
	Polybutilate-coated polyester	Ethibond		
	Silicone-coated polyester		Ti-cron	
	Polytetrafluoro-ethylene-coated polyester			Polydek
	Polytetrafluoro-ethylene-coated polyester			Tevdek
	Uncoated nylon	Nurolon		
	Uncoated nylon with tubing fluid	Pliabilized Nylon		Braided Nylon
	Nylon-coated with silicone		Surgilon	
Synthetic monofilament	Monofilament nylon	Ethilon	Dermalon	Monofilament Nylon
	Monofilament nylon with tubing fluid	Pliabilized Nylon		
	Polybutester		Novafil	
	Polyethylene		Dermalene	
	Polypropylene	Prolene	Surgilene	Deklene
Metallic	Stainless steel (316L)			
	Monofilament	Monofilament Stainless Steel	Monofilament Stainless Steel	Monofilament Stainless Steel
	Twisted	Twisted Stainless Steel	Flexon	
	Braided	Braided Stainless Steel		
Natural fiber	Uncoated twisted silk	Virgin Silk	Virgin Silk	
	Twisted silk coated with silicone		Twisted Silk Coated with Silicone	
	Uncoated braided silk	Perma-Hand		
	Braided silk coated with silicone	Perma-Hand	Braided Silk Coated with Silicone	
	Twisted cotton	Surgical Cotton	Surgical Cotton	

From Edlich RF, Rodeheaver GT, and Thacker JG: J Urol 137:373, 1987.
*Somerville, NJ.
†Danbury, Conn.
‡Queens Village, NY.

ologist can be of great help in the latter respect. Closure of transverse incisions is very similar except at the lateral margins, where the fascia of the internal oblique must be united with that of the external oblique on each side of the incision. An attempt should be made to incorporate the rectus muscle in the fascial suture in the midportion of the incision when a Maylard incision (see Figure 4.4) has been made or to pull the tendons of

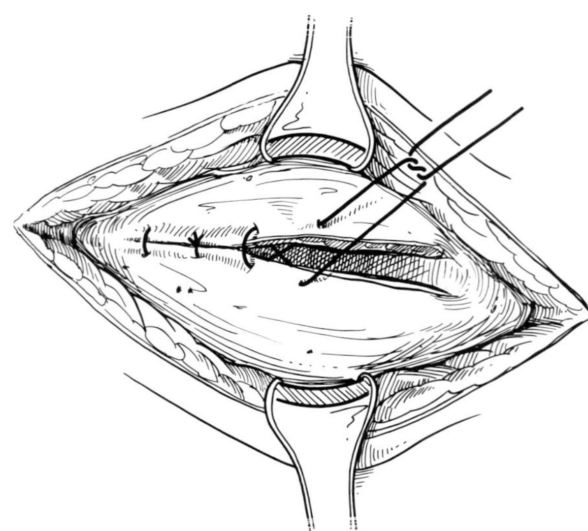

Figure 4.4 Closure of the Maylard incision with interrupted figure-of-eight sutures incorporating the severed ends of the rectus muscles.

Table 4.3 Absorbable sutures

Type	Generic Name	Ethicon, Inc. Trade Name	Davis & Geck Trade Name	Deknatel, Inc. Trade Name
Synthetic braided	Coated polyglactin 910	Vicryl		
	Uncoated polyglycolic acid		Dexon "S"	
	Coated polyglycolic acid		Dexon Plus	
Synthetic monofilament	Polyglyconate		Maxon	
	Polydioxanone	PDS		
Natural fiber	Plain gut with tubing fluid	Plain Gut	Plain Gut	Plain Gut
	Chromic gut with tubing fluid	Chromic Gut	Chromic Gut	Chromic Gut
	Plain gut impregnated with glycerin		Soft Gut	
	Chromic gut impregnated with glycerin		Soft Gut	
	Reconstituted plain collagen	Plain Collagen		
	Reconstituted chromic collagen	Chromic Collagen		

From Edlich RF, Rodeheaver GT, and Thacker TG: J Urol 137:373, 1987.

the rectus muscle under the distal fascial edge in the case of the Czerny incision (Figure 4.6). Failure to do so does not necessarily initiate hernia formation but may cause an unsightly subfascial muscle bulge that subsequently can be seen and felt by the patient.

The Smead-Jones closure, far-near-near-far, and its modification (Figure 4.7) have

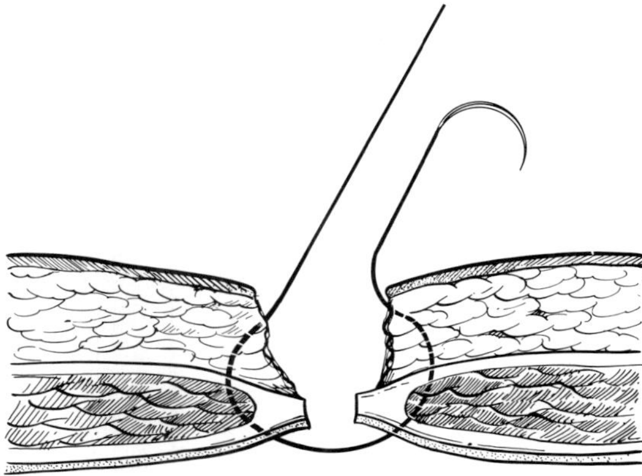

FIGURE 4.5 The continuous closure with nonabsorbable suture includes all layers.

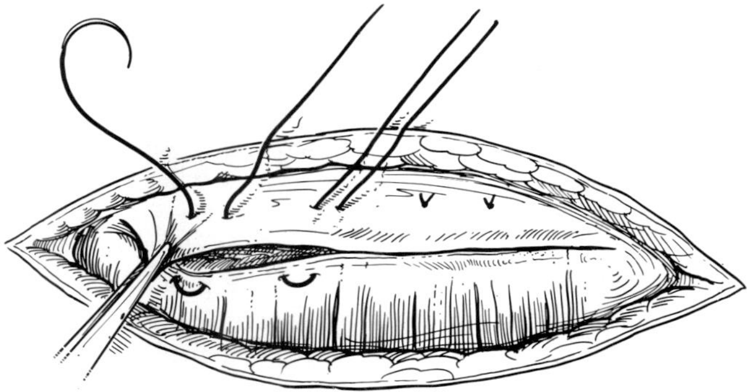

FIGURE 4.6 Closure of the Czerny incision using interrupted pulley sutures to draw the tendinous insertions of the rectus muscles beneath the distal fascia.

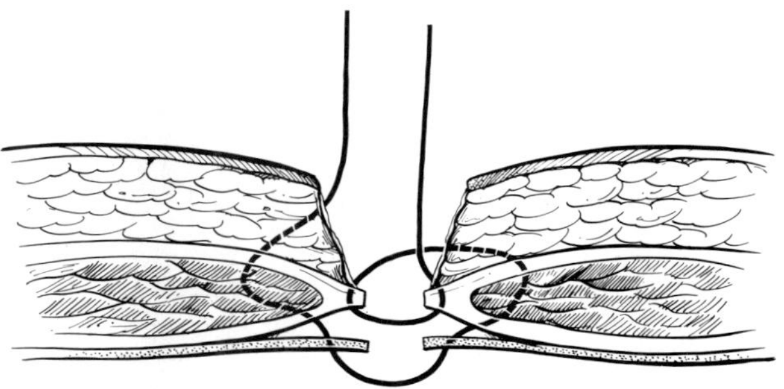

FIGURE 4.7 The modified Smead-Jones far-far-near-near closure includes all layers except the skin.

achieved great popularity in recent years and are often used in what the surgeon believes to be difficult cases. I have always believed that what is good for difficult cases might also be appropriate for simple cases, but this philosophy does not seem to be widespread. The data indicate that this is an excellent type of closure in that dehiscences are rare.

Even more recently, many general surgeons have adopted a form of mass closure using a nonabsorbable running suture to unite all layers of the abdominal wall except the skin (see Figure 4.5). This has been advocated by Gallup et al. for gynecologic surgery, including prolonged difficult oncologic operations. The apparent effectiveness of this method makes it another option for those seeking a rapid simple technique with which to conclude surgery. The results match those of other types of closure.

The use of through-and-through stay sutures, either of wire, nylon, or polyester, to add support to layer-for-layer closures has been advocated for many years. Like adding a belt to suspenders to hold up the trousers, this double harness would seem to be superior to either method alone, but statistics on dehiscence do not support that concept.

HERNIAS

Incisional hernias occur when the fascial margins and adjacent muscles separate, leaving a defect through which peritoneal pouches containing abdominal contents protrude. More often than not the poor protoplasm of the patient is responsible, but additional factors include infection, defective suture material, and tension on the closure from abdominal distension or any type of unusual exertion (see Table 4.1). In a lower abdominal vertical incision, this is more likely to happen in the lower pole of the incision because of the weakness of the posterior sheath of the rectus muscle below the semicircular line, where only the transversalis fascia is present. The rate of occurrence of ventral hernias varies according to the population at risk, but it is reported to occur following approximately 1% of all gynecologic surgery. The incidence increases after superficial wound infection and even more drastically after dehiscence and reclosure. The size of the fascial defect may have no bearing on the volume of the hernia, since escaping loops of bowel and omentum may quickly undermine the superficial subcutaneous tissues and skin and spread out over much of the abdominal wall. Of course, the smaller the fascial defect, the greater the likelihood of incarceration of the intestine with possible constriction of blood supply and infarction. The fascial ring is usually quite large in ventral hernias, however, and vascular impairment of the bowel is rare compared with inguinal hernias.

The development of hernias following laparoscopy is so uncommon that it is sometimes not included in large series of cases listing complications, but isolated cases are reported often enough to justify a word of warning regarding the possibility. The most important preventive measures are the evacuation of all intraperitoneal gas before withdrawal of the scope and palpation of the under fascial edges of the trocar site to prevent protrusions of viscera or omentum.

If a large trocar has been used, leaving a defect of 1 cm or more, it is generally agreed that the fascia should be closed with an appropriate number of interrupted sutures. Placing these sutures through the small skin incision in obese patients without incorporating intestine can be difficult. Various techniques have been recommended, including placing the sutures under direct vision with the laparoscope, elevating the fascial edges with Allis' clips and inserting a Foley catheter, which, when the balloon is inflated and raised, keeps intestinal contents away from the suture site and can be deflated and withdrawn before the sutures are tied. The prolonged operating time of some laparoscopic procedures and the perceived need to shorten it should not obviate the necessity to protect the patient against this rare complication by closing the large holes.

The actual occurrence of postlaparoscopy hernias may become manifest acutely, when intestinal vasculature is compromised, or chronically, when it may be confused with postoperative ileus. In either case, physical examination of the operative site usually solves the problem. Bowel resection is seldom necessary; replacement of protruding viscera and suture of the defect are all that is required.

Diagnosis

The diagnosis of incisional hernia is usually made by the patient, who feels lower abdominal pressure and discomfort and occasionally can observe peristalsis of the intestine beneath the skin. She may also note that the lump becomes worse with straining, coughing, or even standing and recedes when she lies down. Occasionally she will have the impression that something is giving away and will note that the hernia becomes larger over a period of time, especially when her lifestyle requires considerable exertion. The patient's story is not absolutely pathognomonic of the presence of hernia but is very close to being so; objective evidence is provided by palpation of the edge of the fascial ring, sometimes very difficult in the obese patient. Additional evidence often can be obtained by ultrasound cuts through the abdominal wall, which, in the hands of an expert, can demonstrate even very small protrusions. Mistakes are also made with this technique. Of the triad of history, physical examination, and ultrasonography, it is well to have at least two of the three positive before proceeding with surgical treatment.

Some hernias are extremely large, making it seem as if the entire abdominal contents are within the hernia sac, and some such patients are very old, very sick, or morbidly obese. The likelihood of failure of surgical correction under these circumstances is high, and, since the operation is always lengthy, the patient may die as a result of anesthesia or postoperative complications. The failure rate also increases with the number of previous unsuccessful attempts at repair. Under any of these circumstances, decision analysis requires the careful balancing of the pros and cons of surgery with the possibility of managing the patient with abdominal binders and an adjusted lifestyle. Large hernias of long standing may be well tolerated by some individuals, and medical supply houses offer a variety of adjustable garments that can be made to fit almost any abdominal distortion.

Surgical Repair

Once surgery has been elected, a well-planned preoperative regimen should be initiated (Table 4.4).

TABLE 4.4 Treatment before hernia surgery

1. Shave, shower, and cleanse abdomen not more than 1 hr before
2. Nasogastric tube
3. Foley catheter
4. Bowel prep
   - Cathartics, enemas
   - Neomycin, 1 gm 4 times in 24 hr
   - Erythromycin, 1 gm 4 times in 24 hr
5. Prophylactic antibiotics IV at time of incision

The patient should be admitted in time to permit appropriate measures to cleanse the bowel and reduce the bacterial content. These measures are necessary because the bowel is frequently adherent in the peritoneal sac, and dissection of adhesions may cause bowel perforation at a time when it is least expected. Proper preoperative preparation reduces the morbidity following such an accident. A nasogastric tube should be placed so that the intestine can be completely decompressed, and the skin should be cleansed well before the patient's call to the OR. Shaving is usually unnecessary for vertical incisions and should be kept to a minimum for all types because of increased bacterial contamination of the skin. If it is necessary, it should be done close to the time of surgery.

The basic principles of hernia repair have been sacred since the days of Halsted: dissection and excision of the peritoneal sac, high ligation of the peritoneal defect, fascia to fascia closure without tension, and absolute hemostasis. In addition, it is desirable to excise excess skin and subcutaneous tissue in amounts appropriate for a cosmetic superficial closure. A broad-spectrum antibiotic should be given IV before the skin incision is made.

The previous scar is resected along with a margin of normal skin (Figure 4.8), and the

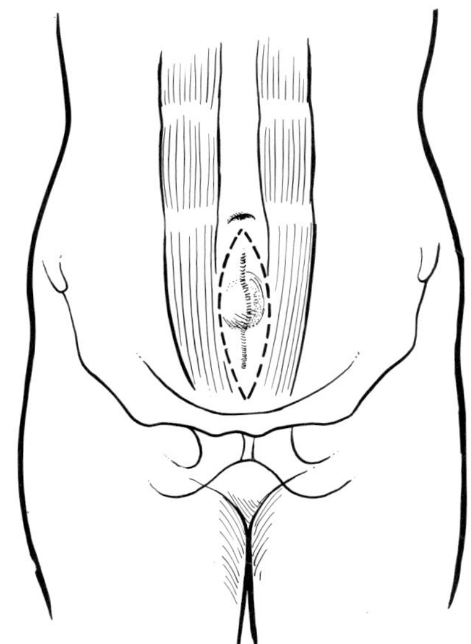

FIGURE 4.8 Elliptical incision to excise previous scar and redundant skin over the hernia.

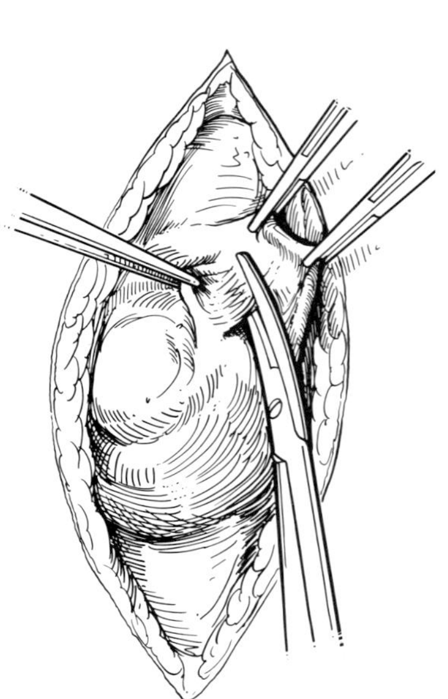

FIGURE 4.9 While traction is maintained on the fascial edge, the peritoneal covering of the hernial sac is cut away from its undersurface.

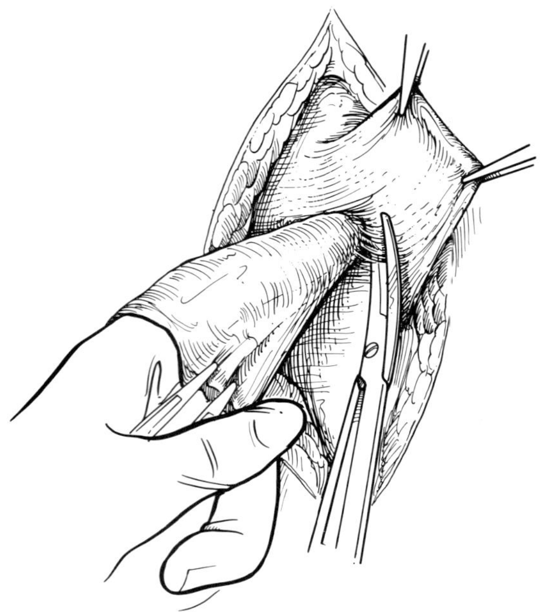

FIGURE 4.10 The hernial sac is opened and kept on traction while a finger inside guides the dissection downward to the origin of the hernia.

subcutaneous tissues are sharply dissected from the surface of the hernial sac (Figure 4.9). When the sac is exposed, I prefer to open it, being careful not to injure adherent underlying structures, and with a finger inside as a guide, to continue the dissection of subcutaneous tissue and muscles down to the point of protrusion above the fascia (Figure 4.10). The sac may now be more fully opened and its edges grasped with Kocher's clamps to provide countertraction while the surgeon mobilizes bowel and omentum away from the peritoneal surface by cutting adhesions (Figure 4.11). Metzenbaum's scissors are ideal for this purpose, and the dissection continues until all abdominal contents are free of the sac and returned to the abdominal cavity. Before the omentum and intestines are abandoned, a sharp search for possible bleeding points is imperative. The redundant peritoneum is then excised; often at the fasical level the peritoneum and rectus sheath are fused, and the fascial edges are attenuated and ragged. When this is the case, it is essential to resect the combined fascia and peritoneum ruthlessly, mobilizing the rectus muscles as necessary in the process, until a level where the fascia is healthy and strong is reached. Attempts to retain and use fascia of obviously poor quality in the repair are certain to increase the likelihood of failure.

Before the repair is begun, each fascial edge is grasped with an Allis' clamp, and the two edges are drawn together to see whether there will be tension on the closure. In the event that there is no tension and the underlying peritoneum is not fused to the fascia, the peritoneum is closed separately with a running suture, and the fascia is closed with interrupted synthetic monofilament nonabsorbable material, placing the sutures at least 1 cm from the edge and 1 cm apart (Figure 4.12). The overlapping double-layer imbrication of the fascia has not been shown to have any advantage over a simple side-to-side technique.

When traction on the fascial edges indicates that the incision cannot be closed without undue tension, the problem may be solved by extensive mobilization of the anterior rectus fascia, cutting back the subcutaneous tissue from the surface as far as is necessary to permit the fascial edge to be pulled to the midline (Figure 4.13). It is usually also necessary to separate the rectus muscle from its fascial

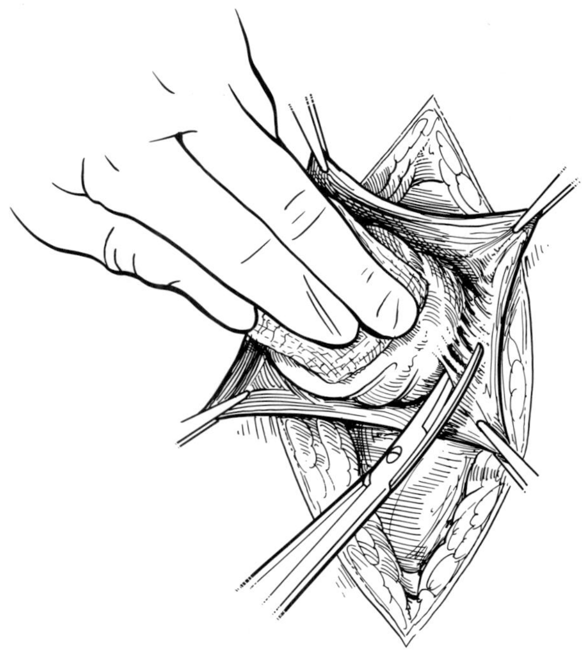

Figure 4.11 Traction is maintained on the peritoneum and countertraction on the contents of the hernia while internal adhesions are lysed to permit return of the intestines and omentum to the general abdominal cavity.

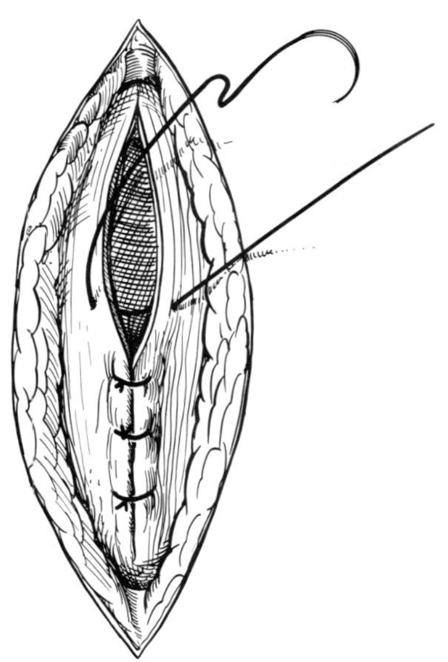

Figure 4.12 The fascia is being closed over the mesh with interrupted nonabsorbable sutures.

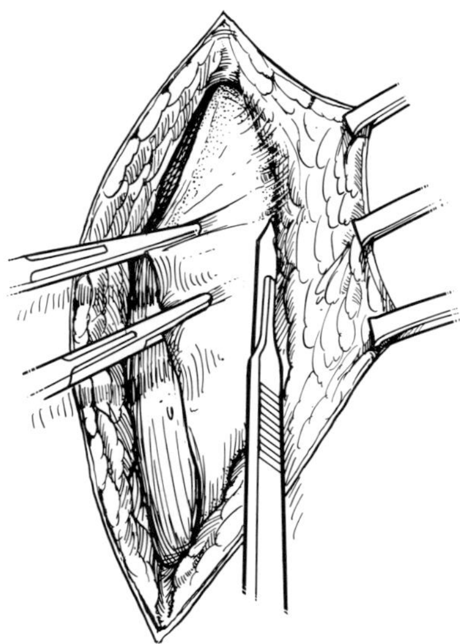

Figure 4.13 The subcutaneous tissues are mobilized from the superior surface of the fascia so that it can be resected as necessary and closed without tension.

attachments and to mobilize the posterior sheath as well. This maneuver is often successful in allowing closure without tension, and since the peritoneum is often fused with the fascia, as previously noted, both layers may be united at the same time with interrupted sutures. Further mobilization of the rectus fascia also can be achieved by relaxing incisions close to the semilunar line, where the transversalis muscle joins the oblique musculature, but this weakens the abdominal wall in that area and has been superseded by the use of prostheses.

When a large amount of fascia has been resected to obtain a substantial layer for closure or the hernia defect is unsusually wide, it may be impossible to bring the fascial edges together. This absolute tissue deficiency may be compensated by the use of prostheses, a bewildering variety of which have been promoted over the past 100 years. In the nineteenth century, animal tendons, skin, and fascia, and metal filigrees, particularly silver, were tried with little success. Early in this century the patient's own transplanted fascia and skin were used with some successes but a high morbidity. In the 1920s, preserved ox fascia seemed to hold promise because of its successful use in dogs, but it was not well tolerated in humans. During the following decade, tantalum mesh was introduced and was not only well tolerated but could be placed directly in contact with the underlying intestine without causing complications. Over the years it underwent work fracture, but by then the mesh was extensively replaced by the ingrowth of connective tissue. Although tantalum and steel mesh are still available for this purpose, more flexible and durable synthetic materials have been developed, of which polyethylene and polypropylene are the most frequently selected. These are inserted in the wound in the form of a fine, gauzelike mesh. When the peritoneum and fascial edges cannot be approximated, the mesh is tailored with scissors to the size of the defect and sutured to the retracted fascial margins around its perimeter (Figure 4.14). The edge of the mesh is doubled over for about 1 cm so that the sutures can be placed through a double layer to avoid their pulling out. The mesh thus lies directly over and in contact with the intestine, and the subcutaneous tissues and skin are closed over it.

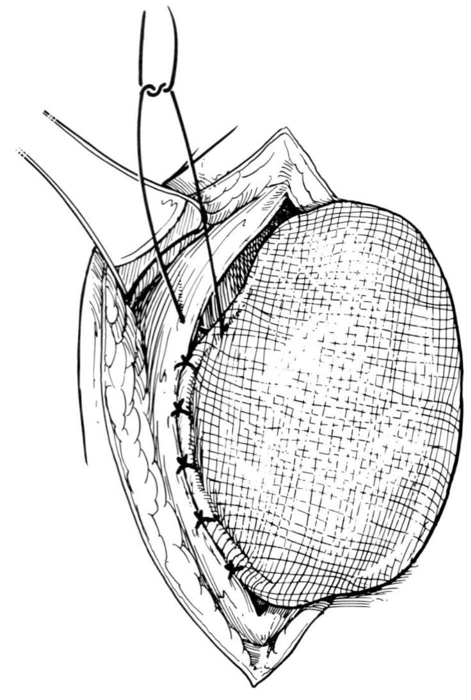

Figure 4.14 Because of an absolute deficiency of fascia and peritoneum, the folded edge of the mesh is sutured to the retracted fascial edge. It lies in contact with the intestines below and the subcutaneous tissues above.

When all of the fascia is unduly attenuated and the closure is considered insecure, the repair can be reinforced with mesh placed either beneath or above the fascial closure. It is technically easier to place it above the fascia, but in this position it is more likely to give rise to infection in the subcutaneous tissues, since the mesh is a major foreign body lying in a large dead space where fluid collection is certain. The mesh is in a relatively protected position below the facial closure, but it is more difficult and time consuming to suture it in this location (Figure 4.15). Nonabsorbable sutures are desirable. When the repair is successful, the mesh is eventually completely replaced by connective tissue.

The essential feature of hernia repair is the fascial closure, with or without the addition of a prosthesis, but careful attention must be paid to the subcutaneous tissues and the skin. Because they often have been extensively undercut, these structures must be examined for bleeding points, however minute, and

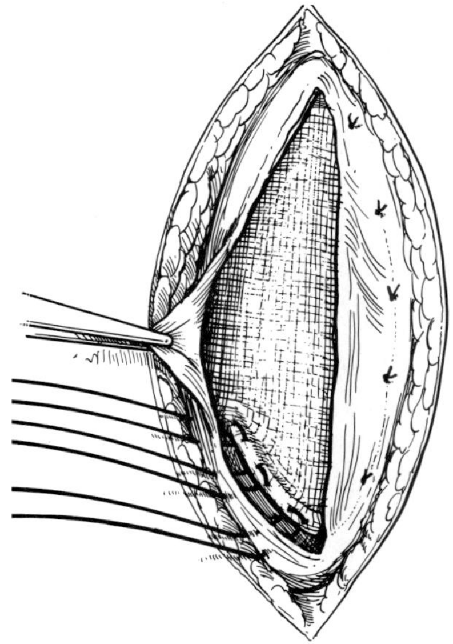

Figure 4.15 The synthetic mesh has been tailored and placed beneath the fascia to support the closure. The folded edge of the mesh is being drawn beneath the fascia with pulley sutures placed well back from the edge.

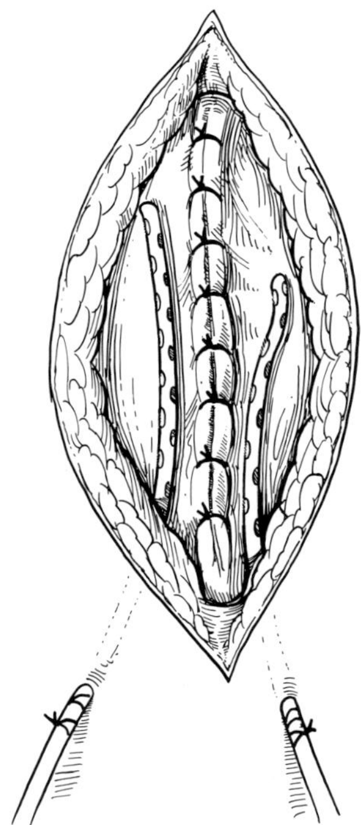

Figure 4.16 Suction drains are inserted through separate stab wounds in the dead space left by undercutting the subcutaneous tissues and are sutured at the skin level.

patches of redundant fat likely to become necrotic must be excised. The skin that has been mobilized by undercutting should be resected enough to provide a firm but not taut closure and joined by clips or sutures according to the surgeon's preference. Before the skin is closed, one or two suction drains, depending on the amount of dead space beneath the skin, are inserted through separate stab wounds and sutured at the skin level (Figure 4.16). A tight dressing is applied for 24 hours, and the patient is taken to the recovery room.

Postoperative Care

Postoperatively the patient's nasogastric tube is kept in place until she begins to pass gas per rectum. Until that time, she is fed IV, beginning a liquid diet at the onset of bowel function and progressing to a soft and then regular diet. Early removal of the tube and oral feeding are likely to cause abdominal distension that may jeopardize the repair. Early ambulation is advisable, supporting the abdominal wall with some type of soft binder. Prophylactic antibiotics are not continued for more than 24 hours. Smoking is discouraged, and every attempt is made to alleviate coughing, vomiting, and hiccups. The dressing is removed in 24 hours and the wound inspected. After that a light dressing may be applied or the would left open to the air, and inspections are carried out at least once daily. The drain or drains are removed within 48 hours unless the volume of drainage remains high (100 ml or more daily). At the time of discharge, the patient is instructed to reduce physical activities for a least 1 month and cautioned about the possibility of superficial fluid collection, especially when a prosthesis has been used. When such collections occur, they must be either aspirated, or, if chronic, again placed on constant suction drainage. Infections are treated as in any other wound, but occasionally removal of a prosthesis may be necessary for healing. Since no hernias are alike, success rates are difficult to determine.

Bibliography

Amid PK and others: Biomaterials for abdominal wall hernia surgery and principles of their applications, Langenbecks Arch Chir 379(3):168, 1994.

Baggish MS and Lee WK: Abdominal wound disruption, Obstet Gynecol 46:530, 1975.

Bucknall TE, Teare L, and Ellis H: The choice of a suture to close abdominal incisions, Eur Surg Res 15:59, 1983.

Chan STF and Esufali ST: Extended indications for polypropylene mesh closure of the abdominal wall, Br J Surg 73:3, 1986.

Edlich RF, Hodeheaver GT, and Thacker JG: Considerations in the choice of sutures for wound closure of the genitourinary tract, J Urol 137:373, 1987.

Gallup DG, Talledo OE, and King LA: Primary mass closure of midline incisions with a continuous running monofilament suture in gynecologic patients, Obstet Gynecol 73:675, 1989.

George CD and Ellis H: The results of incisional hernia repair: a twelve year review, Ann R Coll Surg Engl 68:185, 1986.

Gilsdorf RB and Shea MM: Repair of massive septic abdominal wall defects with Marlex mesh, Am J Surg 130:634, 1975.

Halevy A, Oland Y, and Adam YG: Stainless steel wire for closure of abdominal operative wounds, Am Surg 44:342, 1978.

Helmkamp BF: Abdominal wound dehiscence, Am J Obstet Gynecol 128:803, 1977.

Howard FM and Sweeney TR: Omental herniation after operative laparoscopy, J Reprod Med 39(5):415, 1994.

Israelsson LA and Jonsson T: Suture length to wound length ratio and healing of midline laparotomy incisions, Br J Surg 80 (10):1284, 1993

Jager RM: Safe repair of umbilical fascial wounds after laparoscopy, J Laparoendoscopic Surg 4(3):199, 1994.

Jenkins SD, Klamer TW, and Parteka JJ: A comparison of prosthetic materials used to repair abdominal wall defects, Surgery 94:392, 1983.

Kadar N and others: Incisional hernias after major laparoscopic gynecologic procedures, Am J Obstet Gynecol 168:1493, 1993.

Katz S, Izhar M, and Mirelman D: Bacterial adherence to surgical sutures: a possible factor in suture induced infection, Ann Surg 194:35, 1981.

Kenady DE: Management of abdominal wounds, Surg Clin North Am 64:803, 1984.

Kon ND and others: Abdominal wound closure: a comparison of polydioxanone, polypropylene, and Teflon-coated Dacron sutures, Am Surg 50:549, 1984.

Koontz, AR: Preliminary report on the use of tantalum mesh in the repair of ventral hernias, Ann Surg 127:1079, 1948.

Koontz AR and Shackelford RT: Tissue reaction to ribbon catgut and preserved ox fascia lata strips, Ann Surg 115:1186, 1942.

Kurtz BR, Daniell JF, and Sparo AT: Incarcerated incisional hernia after laparoscopy, J Reprod Med 38(8):643, 1993.

Lewis RT: Knitted polypropylene (Marlex) mesh in the repair of incisional hernias, Can J Surg 27:155, 1984.

Mead PB and others: Decreasing the incidence of surgical wound infections, Arch Surg 121:458, 1986.

Murray DW Jr and Blaisdell FW: Use of synthetic absorbable sutures for abdominal and chest wound closure, Arch Surg 113:477, 1978.

Nehme AE: Repair of large incisional hernias with Marlex mesh, Int Surg 67:398, 1982.

Nichols RE: Postoperative wound infection, N Engl J Med 307:1701, 1982.

Osther PJ and others: Randomized comparison of polyglycolic acid and polygluconate sutures for abdominal fascial closure after laparotomy in patients with suspected impaired wound healing, Br J Surg 82(8):1080, 1995.

Rock JR and Thompson JD: TeLinde's operative gynecology, ed 8, Philadelphia, 1996, JB Lippincott Co.

Rubin LK and Maplesden DC: Suturing with stainless steel wire, Vet Med p 1431, September 1977.

Rubio PA: New technique for repairing large ventral incisional hernias with Marlex mesh, Surg Gynecol Obstet 162:275, 1986.

Skandalakis JE and others: Hernia: surgical anatomy and technique, New York, 1989, McGraw-Hill Book Co.

Sloop RD: Running synthetic absorbable suture in abdominal wound closure, Am J Surg 141:572, 1981.

Sowa DE and others: Effects of thermal knives on wound healing, Obstet Gynecol 66:436, 1985.

Stillman RM, Marino CA, and Seligman SJ: Skin staples in potentially contaminated wounds, Arch Surg 119:821, 1984.

Varma S and others: Tissue reaction to suture materials in infected surgical wounds: a histopathologic evaluation, Am J Vet Res 42:563, 1981.

Wallace D and others: Prevention of abdominal wound disruption utilizing the Smead-Jones closure technique, Obstet Gynecol 45:226, 1980.

5

"Recurrent" Stress Urinary Incontinence

W. Glenn Hurt

Stress urinary incontinence (SUI) is the involuntary loss of urine that occurs as a direct result of sudden, stress-induced increases in intraabdominal pressure. Characteristically, the loss of urine occurs coincident with the acme of the stress. Stress urinary incontinence becomes clinically significant when it is an embarrassing social and hygienic problem.

"Recurrent" SUI is used in the generic sense to refer to all cases of SUI, both persistent and recurrent, that may follow an operation undertaken to cure the condition. It is necessary to consider other types of urinary incontinence in the diagnosis and management of patients with "recurrent" SUI.

Incidence

Urinary continence in women is not always absolute. At least 50% of young adult nulliparous women admit to some leakage of urine when coughing or sneezing or as a result of some other forms of physical exertion. Usually their leakage is not so severe or so frequent as to be a social or hygienic problem and is of little clinical consequence.

It is estimated that at least 10% of women 20 to 60 years of age and 30% of women more than 60 years of age have significant urinary incontinence.[1] The majority of these women have SUI. One half of all women with SUI have "pure" SUI; the other half have SUI in combination with some other cause of urinary incontinence, usually detrusor instability.

More than 150 surgical procedures have been recommended for the treatment of SUI. This large number of procedures attests to the fact that no one operation can cure all patients. Patient, diagnostic, operative, and assessment variables make it difficult to review the surgical literature and predict the cure rates of various surgical procedures. Studies that have attempted the objective assessment of the results of SUI surgery report anterior vaginal repair cure rates of 36% to 60% and abdominal retropubic colpopexy (i.e., Burch) cure rates of 80% to 90%.[2,3] Following primary surgical procedures, 15% to 20% of the patients will have recurrent SUI, and an additional 15% to 20% will have urge incontinence or some other type of lower urinary tract dysfunction that causes them to be dissatisfied with the results of their surgical procedure. All such cases are, in a sense, therapeutic failures.

It is important that every effort be made to ensure the success of the first operative procedure undertaken as treatment of SUI. This is especially true since it is the first operative procedure that is most likely to cure a patient's SUI. Subsequent procedures have failure rates that increase in proportion to their number.

To improve the chances for cure, I will review the preoperative, operative, and postoperative factors that are thought to contribute to surgical failure. I will discuss the evaluation of patients with recurrent SUI and will make recommendations regarding the treatment of patients with recurrent SUI.

Preoperative Factors

There are many different causes of urinary incontinence (Table 5.1). The treatment of each is vastly different. Therefore it is the physician's responsibility to evaluate each patient in a manner that will precisely diagnose the cause of her urinary incontinence. Preoperative diagnostic errors can result in failure to

Table 5.1 Causes of urinary incontinence
Stress urinary incontinence
Urge incontinence
Detrusor instability
Irritative conditions
Neuropathic incontinence
Overflow incontinence
Psychogenic incontinence
Miscellaneous causes
Urethral diverticulum
Drug induced
Congenital incontinence
Urethral hypospadias
Ectopic ureter
Bladder exstrophy
Genitourinary fistula
Ureteral
Vesical
Urethral

recognize the cause or causes of a patient's urinary incontinence and therefore be a major contributor to the failure of the operation.

Many patients have had surgery for SUI when their preoperative diagnosis was based solely on their history of urine leakage. Although the clinical history is valuable in documenting urinary symptomatology and its onset and severity, it cannot be depended on to accurately diagnose the specific cause of a patient's urinary incontinence. One study undertaken to determine the ability of the urologic history to predict urodynamically proved SUI concluded that the symptom of stress incontinence is highly sensitive (93%) with respect to the final diagnosis, but when taken alone, it has such low specificity (19%) that it is of little diagnostic value.[4]

The physical examination should be used to evaluate the patient's mental attitude, her overall state of health, and the current status of all medical conditions that might be related to her urinary incontinence. Chronic respiratory diseases, neurologic disorders, and hormonal deficiencies should receive special attention. They may cause or contribute to a patient's urinary incontinence.

The pelvic examination of patients who complain of urinary incontinence should be more than an attempt to demonstrate pelvic organ prolapse. It is a common mistake for clinicians to use evidence of anterior vaginal prolapse to confirm the diagnosis of SUI. The two should not be equated. SUI is frequently seen in patients with little or no pelvic organ prolapse. At the other extreme, some patients with marked degrees of pelvic organ prolapse will find themselves unable to pass urine unless they manually reduce the prolapse. When the symptom of stress incontinence is combined with evidence of anterior vaginal prolapse in an effort to predict urodynamically proved genuine SUI, the positive predictive value of pure SUI is 60% and the false positive diagnosis rate is 40%.[4]

The pelvic examination should be used not only to look for weaknesses within the pelvic support system but also to determine the condition of all pelvic tissues and to demonstrate the patient's urinary incontinence. Stress testing is the most reliable method of diagnosing SUI. It has the highest predictive values, both positive and negative, of all tests. Unfortunately, it cannot be used to distinguish pure SUI from those mixed forms of incontinence of which SUI may be only one component. Stress testing should be performed when the patient has a full bladder. If stressful maneuvers do not demonstrate a patient's incontinence when she is in the lithotomy position, she should be allowed to assume the erect position for additional attempts at demonstrating her incontinence. The diagnosis of urinary incontinence should not be made unless the incontinence is objectively demonstrable. A patient whose SUI cannot be demonstrated should not be considered a candidate for SUI surgery.

Patients who complain of urinary incontinence should have their urine tested to rule out the possibility of a urinary tract infection (UTI). Such infections can cause lower urinary tract dysfunction and result in urinary incontinence. The eradication of a UTI will often relieve the patient's symptoms and preclude the need for further diagnostic procedures. Sterile urine should be a prerequisite for urodynamic testing. Invasive testing in patients with infected urine places them at risk for developing an acute UTI and casts doubt on the reliability of all urodynamic studies.

No urinary incontinence evaluation is complete unless cystometry has been performed. It is used to determine bladder capacity and neurologic control of the micturition reflex. Cystometry is the primary method of detecting detrusor instability, which is the cause of at least 10% to 15% of all female urinary incontinence. Detrusor instability is also a frequent finding in those patients who have mixed forms of urinary incontinence. One third to one half of all patients with SUI have some evidence of detrusor instability. The treatment of detrusor instability is primarily medical; the treatment of SUI is primarily surgical. Patients who have SUI and detrusor instability should be told of the significance of the coexistence of the two types of urinary incontinence. Detrusor instability should be aggressively treated before any attempt is made to surgically correct SUI. If a patient's preoperative detrusor instability cannot be corrected and persists after surgery, or if it occurs for the first time after surgery, it may be a cause of urgency, frequency, and urge incontinence. The patient with postoperative urinary incontinence due to detrusor instability will consider surgery undertaken to correct her condition a failure, even though she may have been cured of her coexistent SUI.

In the treatment of SUI, surgical failure predisposes the patient to subsequent surgical failure. This fact emphasizes the need for the careful selection and performance of each continence procedure. Historically, anterior vaginal repairs have been considered the operation of choice for all cases of SUI. There is a dictum, "Do the first operation from below, and if it fails, then go above." This dictum has been cited as the reason for many cases of recurrent SUI. It is now apparent, by objective assessment, that the cure rates of SUI treated by a retropubic procedure are consistently better than the cure rates of SUI treated by an anterior vaginal repair.[3] Consequently, it makes little sense to routinely perform an anterior vaginal repair as treatment for SUI. The routine anterior vaginal repair, as performed by most surgeons, is not a procedure designed primarily for the cure of SUI. It is an operation designed for the correction of anterior vaginal wall prolapse; it is limited in the extent to which it can elevate and stabilize the urethrovesical junction. Even its most ardent proponents do not recommend it for the treatment of patients with recurrent SUI.

OPERATIVE FACTORS

From a surgical standpoint there are two types of SUI. One type of SUI is due to hypermobility of the urethrovesical junction in the presence of an otherwise normal urethral sphincter mechanism. It is often referred to as "anatomic SUI." A second type of SUI is due to a damaged urethral sphincter mechanism. It is referred to as "intrinsic sphincter deficiency" (ISD). Anatomic SUI is much more common than SUI due to ISD.

The primary aim of the surgical treatment of anatomic SUI is to elevate the urethrovesical junction to a retropubic position within the abdominal zone of pressure and to maintain its position during sudden increases in intraabdominal pressure. To be most effective, the operation must preserve posterior rotational descent of the trigone and base of the bladder, the compressibility of the urethra, and the integrity of the urethral sphincter mechanism.

The primary aim of the surgical treatment of urinary incontinence due to ISD is coaptation of the proximal urethral lumen or partial obstruction of the bladder neck. The patient typically has what is referred to as a fixed, functionless, "drain-pipe" urethra. Damage to the urethral sphincter mechanism may have been the result of previous surgery that has resulted in fibrosis and fixation of the pelvic tissues. Such scarring can adversely affect the continence mechanism by distorting the anatomic relationship between the urethra and bladder that favors continence, by interfering with posterior rotational descent of the bladder during stress; and by damaging the urethra's internal and external sphincteric mechanisms and its overall compressibility, or both. All pelvic operations should avoid direct and indirect injuries to the urethra. Laceration, devascularization, or denervation of the urethra may cause it to lose its sphincteric capability and become a functionless conduit. It also may cause urinary incontinence as a result of lower urinary tract dysfunction or the formation of a genitourinary fistula.

Failure to accomplish the goals of a particular SUI procedure may be due to lack of knowledge of the technical aspects of the procedure or to lack of experience in performing it. Unfortunately, training programs are limited in the experience that they can provide in the performance and follow-up of procedures to correct incontinence. As a result, the gynecologic surgeon who does not become proficient in several different types of SUI procedures will be limited in the ability to successfully perform surgery for incontinence when different types of SUI are diagnosed and when intraoperative findings dictate the need for modification of an operative procedure.

The results of incontinence procedures depend on the integrity of the tissues that are used to support the urethrovesical junction. Since injury, attenuation, and atrophy of the tissues that normally support the proximal urethra and the urethrovesical junction contribute to the development of SUI, it is important to prepare all pelvic tissues for surgery and to use the tissues to provide permanent support for the proximal urethra and the urethrovesical junction. When the patient's tissues are inadequate for this purpose, it may be necessary to consider the use of fascial or synthetic straps for a more durable repair.

Suture material and suture placement are critical to the success of continence surgery. Catgut is a poor choice for repair and suspension operations. It causes an intense inflammatory response, promotes fibrosis, has poor tensile strength, and is rapidly absorbed. The newer delayed absorbable and permanent suture materials are recommended because of their low reactivity, their higher tensile strength, and their slower rate of absorption. The critical sutures in needle retropubic and abdominal colposuspension procedures are the ones that are placed in tissues on either side of the urethrovesical junction. These sutures are used to elevate and maintain the urethrovesical junction within the retropubic space (of Retzius). It is recommended that permanent suture be used for such suspensions and that it be tied in a manner that will not result in necrosis or release. Furthermore, it is important that the primary suspending sutures be placed on either side of the urethrovesical junction, which is normally about 4 cm from the external urethral meatus. If these sutures are placed below the urethrovesical junction, they fail to restore it to its normal retropubic position. If they are placed above the urethrovesical junction, they tend to "urethralize" the trigone and interfere with the posterior rotational descent of the trigone and base of the bladder.

It is important in incontinence surgery to detect and correct all weaknesses within the pelvic support system. To concentrate on the elevation and stabilization of the urethrovesical junction and to neglect other evidence of pelvic organ prolapse predisposes the operation to failure. The function of the urinary continence mechanism depends on the relationship of the urethra and bladder, but this relationship can be influenced by the presence of a cystocele, enterocele, rectocele, or prolapsed uterus. Suspension of the urethrovesical junction and failure to correct other evidence of pelvic organ prolapse are likely to accentuate weaknesses within the pelvic support system and require the patient to have additional surgery.

Postoperative Factors

During the immediate postoperative period, hematomas, infections, and overdistension of the bladder can cause recurrent incontinence through damage to the suspending sutures and tissues, the bladder, or the urethra. It is recommended that all patients who have operations for pelvic support defects avoid constipation and observe a period of physical restraint to permit adequate healing. Patients should be advised that excessive coughing, straining, or lifting during the healing phase can cause recurrent incontinence and pelvic organ prolapse. An increasing number of patients are involved in strenuous occupational and recreational activities. If such activities are likely to contribute to recurrent incontinence or prolapse, they should be reduced or eliminated.

Estrogen prevents weakening and atrophy of the pelvic support system, enhances the function of the internal urethral sphincter mechanism, and preserves the pliability of the soft tissues of the pelvis. Menopausal patients need long-term estrogen replacement therapy. If they quit taking estrogen, they may see a gradual deterioration in the efficiency of their continence mechanism.

Chronic respiratory diseases that cause sudden increases in intraabdominal pressure may contribute to the failure of surgery for incontinence. The repetitive stress of a chronic cough may be more than tissues can bear. Smokers who undergo incontinence surgery should be advised to quit smoking or risk the return of urinary incontinence.

A number of postoperative complications may result from incontinence surgery and cause urinary leakage. Detrusor and urethral instability may cause urge incontinence, bladder neck obstruction may cause overflow incontinence, and genitourinary fistula may cause continuous leakage.

EVALUATION

Patients who have "recurrent" SUI should have a complete urogynecologic evaluation with urodynamic studies (Table 5.2). Every effort should be made to determine the reason for the failure of the operative procedure or procedures; the anatomic, physiologic, and pathologic changes that are present; and the current cause or causes of urinary incontinence.

The patient should be asked to keep a urinary diary for at least 3 consecutive days as she goes about her daily routine. She should record the time and amount of fluid intake and urinary output. Also, she should record all episodes of urgency and incontinence and make some comment regarding the circumstances associated with each. The urinary diary provides objective evidence of the patient's symptomatology. It is also a valuable means of assessing the results of therapy.

The patient's general history should be supplemented by an incisive urologic history that documents the urinary symptoms and their onset and severity. Incontinence questionnaires have proved helpful in assuring completeness of the urologic history. It is also useful for the questionnaire to include a space for the patient to list significant medical illnesses, previous surgical procedures, allergies, and all recent and current medications.

The general physical examination should detail the patient's body habitus, the condition of her respiratory system, and any findings that are the result of chronic illnesses or previous surgery. The neurologic examination should be focused to detect central, spinal, and peripheral nervous system disorders that might affect the lower urinary tract. Attention should be given to the evaluation of sacral nerves 2, 3, and 4 that provide the principal motor supply for the detrusor and for the periurethral striated muscle. A detailed pelvic examination should be performed to ascertain the condition of the tissues, to determine the size, shape, position, and mobility of the pelvic organs, and to detect all weaknesses within the pelvic organ support system.

Every effort should be made to demonstrate the patient's urinary incontinence. If the patient comes to the examining room with a full bladder, she may be asked to cough while in the lithotomy and erect positions, to heel bounce, and to listen to the flow of running water to see if leakage will occur. After the patient has emptied her bladder, she should be catheterized for measurement of residual urine. The specimen should be tested for evidence of a UTI or sent for bacteriologic culture. At this time, a Q-tip test may be performed to quantify the mobility of the urethrovesical junction. If the patient did not demonstrate her incontinence when previously stress tested, a straight catheter should be used to slowly fill the bladder with sterile room temperature saline. An effort is made to determine the bladder volume when she feels the

TABLE 5.2 Evaluation of patients with recurrent SUI
Urinary diary
History and physical examination
Q-tip quantification of urethral mobility
Urinary residual measurement
Urine culture
Stress testing to demonstrate incontinence
Uroflowmetry
Multichannel urethrocystometry
Urethral pressure profilometry
Valsalva leak point pressure
Voiding cystourethrography
Periurethral electromyography
Urethrocystoscopy
Optional studies
Bead chain urethrocystocolpography
Voiding cystourethrography
Intravenous urography
Videocystourethrography
Consultation

first urge to void and when she is at maximum capacity. When the bladder is full, the catheter is removed and stress testing is repeated with the patient in the erect position. It is important to actually observe the patient's leakage in an effort to determine its timing in relationship to stress and to document the characteristics of urine leakage.

Uroflowmetry may be performed following initial stress testing, before instrumentation of the lower urinary tract, when the patient is asked to empty her bladder. It is a study that should be repeated to verify its results.

Cystometry should be performed in all patients who are being evaluated for urinary incontinence. It is the primary method of assessing detrusor activity, bladder sensation, and bladder capacity. Multichannel urethrocystometry is recommended for those with recurrent SUI. It should simultaneously measure bladder, urethral, and abdominal (vaginal or rectal) pressure. Subtracted measurements may be used to calculate detrusor pressure and urethral closure pressure. During the filling of the bladder, it is important to note the first sensation of filling, the first desire to void, and the maximum cystometric capacity. Passive and dynamic urethral pressure profilometry may be performed as part of the urethrocystometric examination. This provides a urethral pressure profile and permits calculation of the maximum urethral closure pressure, the functional profile length, and pressure transmission ratios. When the bladder is full, the patient should be stress tested in the erect position to detect detrusor instability and to demonstrate urinary incontinence. Valsalva leak point pressure determination is helpful in the diagnosis of ISD. Voiding cystometry may be performed to evaluate the contractile function of the detrusor. Electromyography of the periurethral striated muscle is useful in detecting vesicourethral sphincter dyssynergia.

Urethrocystoscopy is performed to detect mucosal lesions, growths, diverticula, and so on within the bladder and urethra. It is important to observe the reaction of the detrusor and urethra during filling and to observe the base of the bladder, the urethrovesical junction, and the proximal urethra when the patient is asked to squeeze as if voluntarily interrupting her urinary stream and to bear down as if she were trying to have a bowel movement. Dynamic urethrocystoscopy is used to confirm the findings of the Q-tip test in determining the mobility of the urethrovesical junction and of the pelvic examination in determining the presence or absence of a cystocele or cystourethrocele.

A number of imaging techniques are available for documenting the anatomic relationships of the pelvic organs, for detecting urethral diverticulum, and for visualizing the function of the lower urinary tract. Bead chain urethrocystocolpography is useful in documenting the anatomic relationships of the urethra, bladder, and vagina and the location of each with respect to recognizable bony landmarks within the pelvis. It is recognized as the gold standard for determining the anatomic changes wrought by surgical procedures. Intravenous urography, voiding cystourethrograms, and other tests may be indicated to determine the condition of the urinary tract, to detect genitourinary fistulas, to demonstrate a diverticulum, and so forth. Such tests should be freely utilized.

Many urologic laboratories use ultrasound and videocystourethrography in diagnosing lower urinary tract disorders. The latter, combined with urethrocystometry, gives a comprehensive evaluation of the anatomic and physiologic functions of the lower urinary tract.

In the evaluation of a patient with recurrent SUI it is important to know when consultation or referral is in order. Urodynamic testing and surgery for recurrent SUI is most beneficial when undertaken by physicians who have a special interest in urogynecology.

Therapy

Detrusor instability can be a cause of urgency, frequency, nocturnal enuresis, and urge incontinence in persons who have had continence surgery. It is helpful to know if this problem was a preoperative finding that persists, if it developed for the first time during the immediate postoperative period, or if it was a delayed complication. Detrusor instability that develops during the immediate postoperative period is often due to a lower urinary tract infection or to bladder trauma. It usually resolves promptly following the eradication of the infection and completion of the healing process.

Preoperative detrusor instability that persists into the postoperative period or that occurs as a delayed complication of incontinence surgery is much more refractory to bladder retraining and pharmacologic therapy.

As a result of a suspension procedure, patients with a weak detrusor may have their postoperative course complicated by voiding dysfunction or urinary retention. They may benefit from pressure-flow studies and electromyography of their periurethral striated muscle to define the status of their voiding mechanism. Some will learn to void efficiently using alternative voiding techniques. Pharmacologic therapy may be used to reduce outlet resistance. Intermittent self-catheterization is recommended to prevent overdistention of the bladder.

Bladder neck obstruction may cause detrusor instability or retention and overflow incontinence. If there is significant obstruction of the bladder neck, release of the suspending sutures may be necessary. Before reoperation to release the suspending sutures, it is important to define the patient's detrusor function because she may decide that self-catheterization is preferable to urinary incontinence.

Therapy for recurrent SUI will, of course, be dictated by the patient's current type of incontinence, its severity, and her physical condition and findings. Mild recurrent SUI may be managed by perineal pads, pelvic muscle exercises, pharmacologic therapy, or insertion of a pessary. Estrogen augments the internal urethral sphincter mechanism by its action on the mucosa, the vascular plexus, the connective tissue, and the smooth muscle. It also contributes to the pliability of the pelvic tissues and the integrity of the pelvic support system. α-Adrenergic agonist therapy, such as imipramine, may be used to strengthen the internal urethral sphincter mechanism.

After a complete evaluation of their condition, patients with moderate or severe recurrent SUI should be considered candidates for repeat continence surgery. There is general agreement that surgery for recurrent anatomic SUI should consist of some type of retropubic urethral suspension. The standard anterior colporrhaphy has no place in the treatment of recurrent SUI.

The procedures that I currently recommend as treatment for recurrent SUI and indications for each are listed in Table 5.3. Most recurrent anatomic SUI can be cured by an abdominal retropubic colposuspension. Recurrent SUI due to ISD may be treated by an abdominal retropubic colposuspension or by the placement of a suburethral sling if there is hypermobility of the urethrovesical junction. If there is IDS, no hypermobility of the urethrovesical junction, and no significant pelvic organ prolapse or detrusor instability, surgical options include periurethral bulk injections, the placement of a suburethral sling, or the placement of an artificial sphincter. The three procedures that will be described are abdominal retropubic colposuspension, suburethral fascial sling urethropexy, and periurethral bulk injections. The artificial sphincter is recommended only for patients with intractable incontinence. At this time, I believe that the placement of an artificial sphincter should remain in the hands of those with special expertise in its insertion and use.

Retropubic (Modified Burch) Colposuspension

The patient is placed on the operating table, and anesthesia is administered. The patient's heels are strapped in stirrups (Allen Universal), and she is placed in a modified lithotomy position with hips slightly flexed and the lower extremities slightly abducted. The foot of the operating table is dropped from under the lower extremities. The abdomen, inner thighs, perineum, and vagina are prepared and draped

Table 5.3 Recurrent SUI: procedures and their indications

Procedure / Indication
Retropubic colposuspension
Adequate vagina with mobile walls
Bladder neck descent
Depressed pressure transmission
Suburethral sling urethropexy
Inadequate vagina with immobile walls
Open bladder neck
Low urethral closure pressure
Periurethral bulk injections
Good anatomic relationships
Low urethral closure pressure
Low Valsalva leak point pressure
Artificial sphincter
Intractable incontinence

to allow simultaneous abdominal and vaginal access. A sterile Foley catheter is placed transurethrally into the bladder and connected to straight drainage.

A lower abdominal incision is made into the peritoneal cavity. If a hysterectomy or salpingo-oophorectomy is indicated, it is performed, and the pelvis is reperitonealized. A Moschcowitz or Halban closure of the cul-de-sac (of Douglas) is completed using permanent suture. The anterior parietal peritoneum is approximated.

The patient is placed in a slight reverse Trendelenburg's position. A small retractor (Balfour) is used to retract the lower medial margins of the rectus muscles. Moist small laparotomy packs are used to dissect the retropubic space (of Retzius). If the patient has had a previous retropubic procedure, an extraperitoneal cystotomy may be performed and the bladder separated from the pubis and pubic symphysis under direct vision using sharp dissection. Once the depths of the retropubic space have been dissected bilaterally, the operating surgeon should place a sterile sleeve and glove onto the nondominant arm and hand. Approximately 50 ml of indigo carmine–colored sterile saline is instilled into the bladder via the Foley catheter's drainage system, and the catheter is clamped to prevent the escape of the colored solution from the bladder.

The first and second fingers of the surgeon's nondominant hand are placed into the vagina so the tips of the fingers will straddle the urethrovesical junction as identified by the Foley balloon. The urethrovesical junction should be about 4 cm from the external urethral meatus. The tip of one of the vaginal fingers is used to elevate the vaginal wall that overlies it into the retropubic space. A sponge stick or Kelly dissector is used to move the lateral aspect of the urethrovesical junction from over the elevated vaginal wall. When the overlying tissues have been removed, the fibromuscular wall of the vagina appears glistening white, and on palpation, the vaginal wall will be all that is felt between the tips of the vaginal and abdominal fingers.

A no. 0 or 00 permanent suture is threaded onto a needle (Mayo, no. 5) and passed twice through the entire thickness of the anterior vaginal wall at a point 1.5 to 2 cm lateral to the urethrovesical junction. A second suture of similar material is placed in a similar manner 1 to 1.5 cm lateral and superior to the first (Figure 5.1). The long arms of both sutures are clamped with different small clamps so as to distinguish the medial from the lateral suture. The vaginal wall on the opposite side of the urethrovesical junction is elevated, and the overlying tissues are moved medially. Identical suture placement is undertaken, and the long arms of each suture are clamped with the same small clamp sequence to differentiate the medial from the lateral suture. The sutures are elevated to judge their potential for suspending the urethrovesical junction. If it is satisfactory, a needle is threaded sequentially onto one arm of each suture, and that arm of the suture is passed through Cooper's ligament at a point above its location in the anterior vaginal wall. One arm of each suture is placed before any of the suspending sutures are tied (Figure 5.2).

The elevation of the urethrovesical junction may be determined by elevation of the tips of the surgeon's vaginal fingers, observation of the urethrovesical junction via a cystoscope, Q-tip deflection of approximately −20 degrees with respect to the horizontal, or observation of the bladder neck via the suprapubic cystostomy. The extent of elevation of the urethrovesical junction is determined more by experience than by scientific measurement. Once the surgeon feels that the urethrovesical junction is in proper position, the suspending sutures are tied to elevate and maintain the urethrovesical junction within the retropubic space (Figure 5.3). Care should be taken to be sure that the urethra is not compressed against the symphysis pubis or otherwise unduly obstructed. If there has been excessive bleeding within the retropubic space, suction drains (Jackson-Pratt) may be placed and brought out through separate stab incisions in the lower abdomen.

The medial margins of the rectus muscles are loosely approximated along the midline to prevent ventral herniation of the dome of the bladder. The anterior abdominal incision is closed in the routine manner. A suprapubic catheter is preferred for postoperative bladder drainage. Following its placement, the transurethral Foley catheter is removed, and the patient is sent to the recovery room.

The suprapubic catheter is clamped on the third or fourth postoperative day to permit

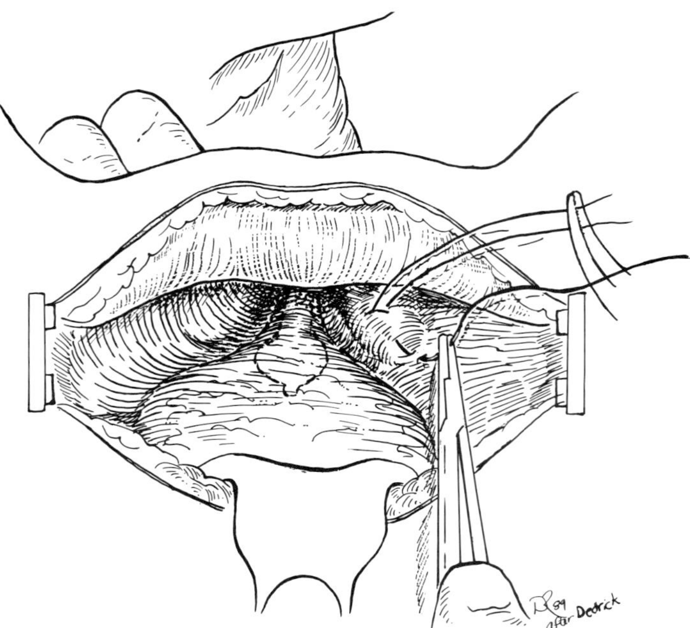

Figure 5.1 Retropubic colposuspension. A vaginal finger elevates the anterior vaginal wall into the retropubic space for placement of the second suture to the right of the urethrovesical junction.

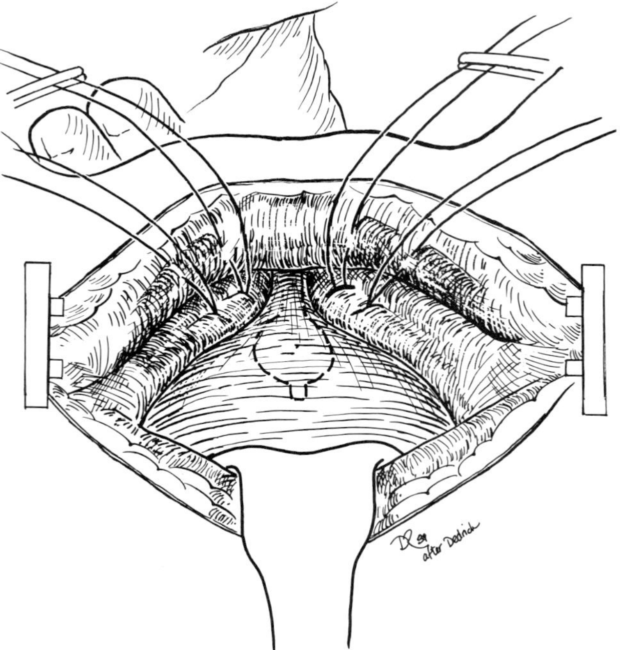

Figure 5.2 Retropubic colposuspension. The four suspending sutures have been placed through Cooper's ligament.

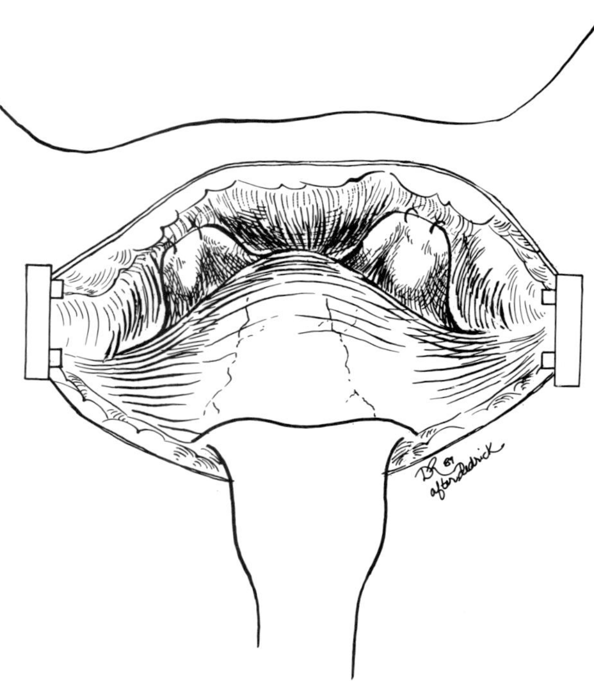

Figure 5.3 Retropubic colposuspension. The four suspending sutures have been tied.

voiding trials. It is not removed until the postvoid residual urine is consistently less than 80 to 90 ml.

The most frequent complications of a retropubic colposuspension are delayed voiding, UTI, pyrexia, lower urinary tract injury, and wound infection. The expected cure rate of recurrent SUI with a retropubic colposuspension should be 85% to 90%.

Suburethral Sling Urethropexy

The patient is placed on the operating table and anesthesia is administered. If a strip of the patient's fascia lata is to be used for the sling, the patient is placed on her side, with thighs and legs parallel, slightly flexed, and with a pillow between them. The upper part of the thigh is prepared and draped. A transverse 4-cm incision is made through the skin above the inferior condyle and just above the superior margin of the patella. The subcutaneous tissues are retracted to expose the fascia lata. Two parallel incisions are made 1.5 to 2 cm apart and in line with the fibers of the fascia lata. Another incision in the fascia joins the distal ends of the two parallel incisions. The flap of fascia lata is lifted and threaded into a fascial stripper (Masson or Wilson) (Figure 5.4). The fascia lata is stripped for a distance of at least 18 cm. The strip is removed by cutting the superior end of the fascial strip. The exposed fascial incisions are approximated with delayed absorbable or permanent suture, the skin incision is closed, and bandages are applied. This fascia is laid aside in a moistened sterile towel until it is needed.

The patient's heels are strapped in stirrups (Allen Universal), and she is placed in a modified lithotomy position with hips moderately flexed and the lower extremities slightly abducted. The foot of the operating table is dropped from under the lower extremities. The abdomen, inner thighs, perineum, and vagina are prepared and draped to allow simultaneous abdominal and vaginal surgery, preferably by two surgical teams. A sterile Foley catheter is placed transurethrally into the bladder and connected to straight drainage. Indigo carmine–colored saline is instilled into the bladder, and the Foley catheter clamped so as to retain the colored saline within the bladder.

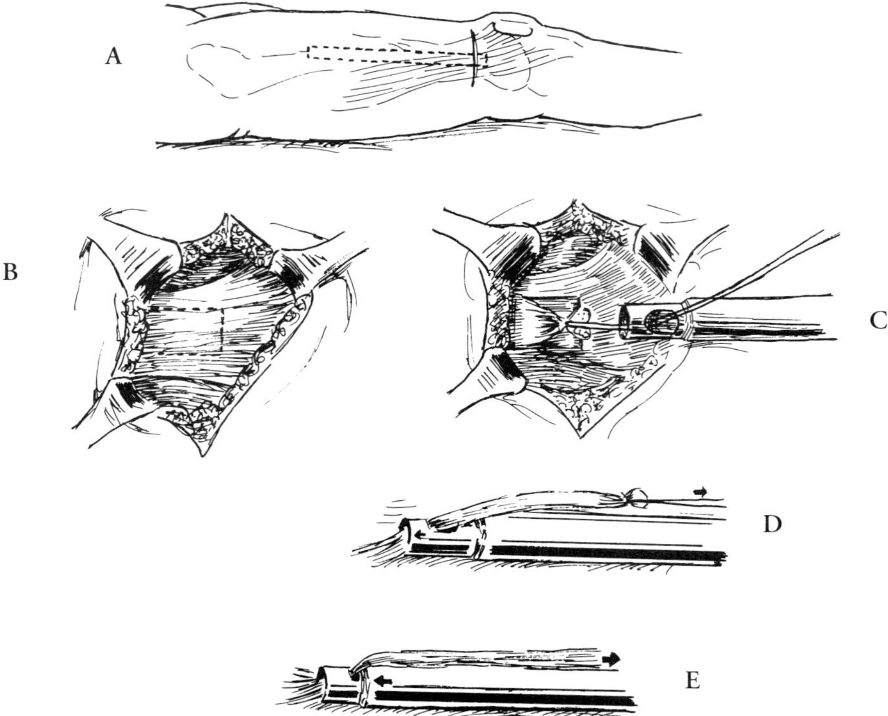

FIGURE 5.4 Suburethral sling urethropexy. **A,** The thigh has been prepared and draped, and the incisions have been made for obtaining the fascia lata strap. **B,** The fascia is incised as indicated by the *dashed line.* The incised fascia is threaded into the fascia stripper (**C**), and the stripper advanced subcutaneously (**D**) as far as it will go, while traction to the free end of the strip is maintained in the opposite direction, as shown by the *small arrow.* When the stripper can be advanced no further, the outer sleeve is unscrewed and slid distally as a guillotine over the opening in the central barrel (**E**), transecting the fascia. The fascial strap and the stripper are removed, and the visible fascial defect closed with a few interrupted sutures, as in the skin incision. (Redrawn from Nichols DH: The sling operation. In Cantor EB, editor: Female urinary stress incontinence, Springfield, Ill, 1979, Charles C Thomas.)

Subsequent leakage of the blue dye into the operative field should alert the surgeons to the possibility of bladder injury.

The abdominal surgical team makes a transverse curvilinear 8- to 10-cm incision in the lower abdomen approximately 3 cm above the symphysis and exposes the anterior abdominal aponeurosis. The vaginal surgical team incises the full thickness of the anterior vaginal wall in the midline from within 1 cm of the external urethral meatus to the vaginal apex. The vesicovaginal space is widely dissected bilaterally to the pubic rami. The vaginal surgeon uses the index finger to pierce the endopelvic fascia laterally and dissect the retropubic space (of Retzius) the full depth of the symphysis on either side of the urethrovesical junction. The pubocervical fascia is plicated beneath the urethrovesical junction. This fascia will act as a cushion between the urethra and the fascial sling.

The abdominal surgical team should make bilateral 2-cm incisions through the abdominal aponeurosis at the lateral margins of the rectus muscles or 3 to 4 cm from the midline. A long uterine packing forcep or a suture ligature carrier (Pereyra type) is passed through one incision in the anterior abdominal aponeurosis into the retropubic space so that it comes into direct contact with the

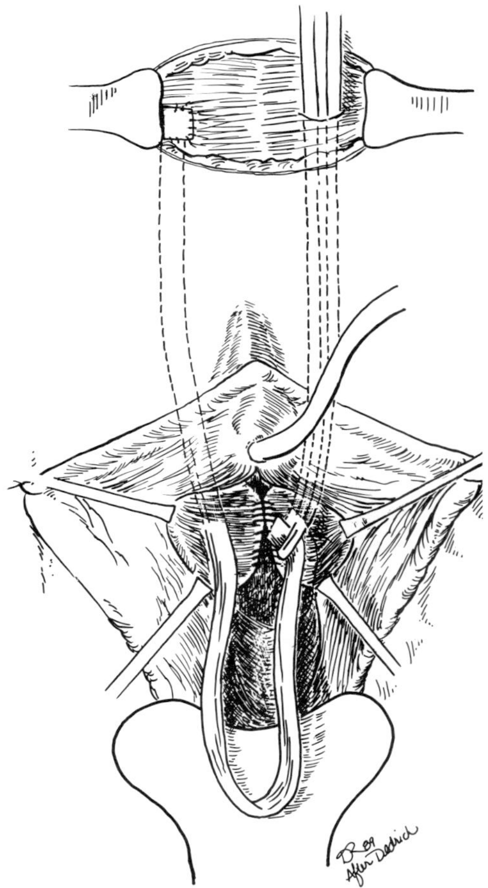

Figure 5.5 Suburethral sling urethropexy. The fascia lata strap is in place on the right side of the urethra and is being retrieved on the left side of the urethra.

vaginal surgeon's index finger. The forcep or ligature carrier is guided down through the retropubic space and out of the vaginal port on the corresponding side of the urethra. The end of the fascial or synthetic strap is picked up by the uterine packing forcep, or sutures in the end of the strap are threaded into the ligature carrier. The retrieving instrument is drawn up through the retropubic space bringing the end of the strap through the incision in the abdominal aponeurosis. The same procedure for the retrieval of the opposite end of the strap is performed on the opposite side (Figure 5.5). Care is taken to keep the strap flat throughout its course.

One end of the strap is sewn to the superior surface of the anterior abdominal aponeurosis with permanent suture in a manner that will secure it and at the same time close the fascial defect within the aponeurosis. The opposite end of the strap is then drawn up through the anterior abdominal aponeurosis so that the suburethral portion of the strap barely supports the urethrovesical junction. Interrupted permanent sutures are used to attach the suburethral portion of the strap to those tissues on either side of the urethrovesical junction to help hold the strap in place. The unsecured end of the strap is then sewn to the superior surface of the anterior abdominal aponeurosis with permanent suture in a manner that will secure it and also close the fascial defect. The medial edges of the anterior vaginal wall are trimmed and approximated with interrupted delayed absorbable suture. The anterior abdominal wall is closed in a routine manner. A suprapubic catheter is preferred for postoperative bladder drainage. After it is placed, the transurethral Foley catheter is removed.

When voiding trials are to be undertaken, the suprapubic catheter is clamped. The suprapubic catheter is not removed until the postvoid residual urine is consistently less than 90 ml.

The most frequent complications of the suburethral sling procedures include delayed voiding, UTI, pyrexia, hematuria, seroma, lower urinary tract injury, wound infection, and urinary fistula. Parker and others[5] report a cure rate of 84%, and Beck and others[6] report a cure rate of 98% when a suburethral fascia lata sling is used as treatment for recurrent SUI.

Periurethral Bulk Injections

Women who are to have periurethral bulk injections must be collagen-sensitivity tested by the intradermal injection of 0.1 ml of purified bovine dermal collagen at least 4 weeks prior to their periurethral injection session. The collagen supplied for skin testing is a non–cross-linked collagen preparation, which is more likely to provoke a sensitivity reaction than is the purified bovine dermal glutaraldehyde cross-linked collagen used for periurethral bulking. Patients with a positive skin test (approximately 3% of patients tested) are not candidates for periurethral bulk injections using bovine dermal cross-linked collagen.

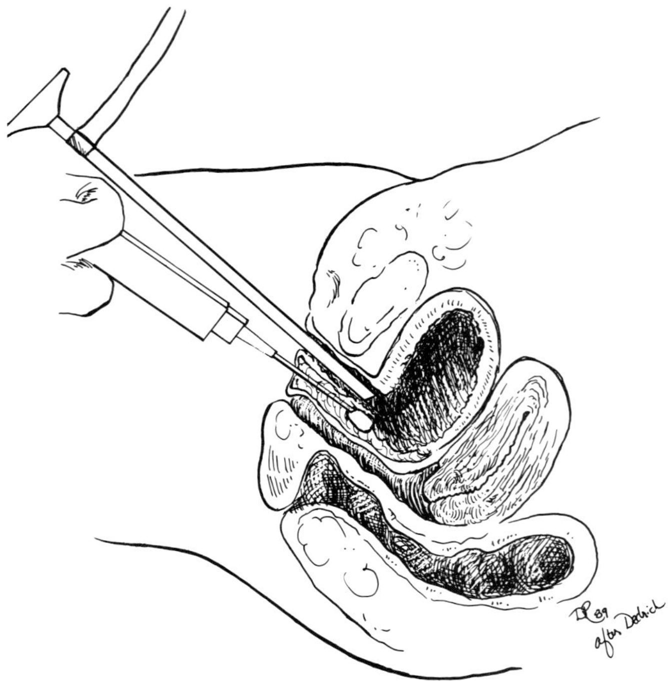

FIGURE 5.6 Collagen is being injected about the proximal urethra.

In preparation for periurethral bulk injections, the patient is asked to void. She is then placed on the examining table in the lithotomy position. The periurethral skin is prepared with an antiseptic solution, and a topical anesthetic gel is applied to the periurethral skin. A sterile Q-tip is used to apply 2% lidocaine gel throughout the urethra. Using a sterile 30-gauge hypodermic needle, 2 to 4 ml of local anesthetic (1% Xylocaine without epinephrine) is injected into the tissues adjacent to the external urethral meatus at the 4 and 8 o'clock positions. The bladder is drained, and videourethroscopy is performed. A 22-gauge sterile spinal needle is inserted next to the external urethral meatus at the 4 o'clock position and advanced the length of the urethra to position its beveled tip just beneath the urethral mucosa and within the submucosa of the most proximal portion of the urethra (Figure 5.6). A sufficient amount of GAX cross-linked bovine collagen is injected to cause the urethral mucosa to bulge into the lumen of the urethra. The same procedure is performed on the opposite side of the urethra following insertion of the spinal needle at the 8 o'clock position next to the external urethral meatus. The goal is to inject that amount of GAX cross-linked collagen necessary to increase outflow resistance by causing coaptation of the mucosal surfaces of the proximal urethra. Reinjection sessions should be at least 1 month apart.

Complications of periurethral bulk injections include transient urinary retention, which may be treated by intermittent clean self-catheterization; lower urinary tract infection; and rare collagen-sensitivity reactions.

Approximately 50% of women with mild or moderate degrees of SUI due to ISD and with no detrusor instability incontinence or significant pelvic organ prolapse can be cured of their incontinence by periurethral bulk injections. Another 20% will be improved, and 30% will fail treatment. It is difficult to predict which women will experience maximum benefit.[7]

REFERENCES

1. Urinary incontinence in adults, Natl Inst Health Consensus Dev Conf Statement 7:1, 1988.

2. Hilton P: Urinary incontinence in women, Br Med J (Clin Res) 195:426, 1987.

3. Elia G and Bergman A: Prospective randomized comparison of three surgical procedures for stress urinary incontinence: Five year follow-up, Neurourol Urodyn 13:498, 1994.

4. Walters MD and Shields LE: The diagnostic value of history, physical examination, and the Q-tip cotton swab test in women with urinary incontinence, Am J Obstet Gynecol 159:145, 1988.

5. Parker RT, Addison WA, and Wilson CJ: Fascia lata urethrovesical suspension for recurrent stress urinary incontinence, Am J Obstet Gynecol 135:843, 1979.

6. Beck RP, McCormick S, and Nordstrom L: The fascia lata sling procedure for treating recurrent genuine stress incontinence of urine, Obstet Gynecol 72:699, 1988.

7. Appell RA: Collagen injection for urinary incontinence, Urol Clin North Am 21:177, 1994.

Bibliography

Appell RA: Artificial sphincter and periurethral injections. In Benson JT, editor: Female pelvic floor disorders, New York, 1992, WW Norton & Co, Inc.

Burch JC: Urethrovaginal fixation to Cooper's ligament for correction of stress incontinence, cystocele, and prolapse, Am J Obstet Gynecol 81:281, 1961.

Burch JC: Cooper's ligament urethrovesical suspension for stress incontinence, Am J Obstet Gynecol 100:764, 1968.

Webster GD and others: Management of type III stress urinary incontinence using artificial urinary sphincter, Urology 39:399, 1992.

6

Eversion of the Vagina

David H. Nichols

Recurrent massive eversion of the vagina is not uncommon. It may be of various degree, with or without recurrence of the other forms of genital prolapse such as enterocele, cystocele, and rectocele. It involves a significant redescent of the vaginal vault, at first a partial eversion (Figure 6.1), which, if unattended, proceeds to a complete eversion of the vagina (with the uterus, if it is present). Descent of the uterus is a passive accompaniment of the vaginal vault prolapse and is therefore the result and not the cause of genital prolapse. Hysterectomy, though usually desirable, is but one feature of surgical pelvic reconstruction. The essential steps toward successful pelvic reconstruction lie within a recognition of all of the sites of pelvic damage and its probable etiology, the choice of appropriate corrective procedure, the techniques of the repair itself, and the precision and proficiency of the surgeon.

Posthysterectomy vaginal vault prolapse is preventable in most instances by definitive attaching of the transected cardinal uterosacral ligaments to the vault of the vagina at the time of hysterectomy[1] if they are strong, by the McCall cul-de-plasty if they are strong and elongated,[2,3] or by some coincident colpopexy if they are weak.

Usually there is a history of preceding hysterectomy, either transabdominal or transvaginal. Often there was a particular weakness in the support of the vaginal vault, which may or may not have been recognized and effectively addressed by the initial surgeon (Figure 6.2). The onset of recurrent massive eversion of the vagina is sometimes insidious. At other times it follows directly some sudden increase in intraabdominal pressure as from a fit of coughing or vomiting or having lifted something heavy, such as a piece of furniture. The patient, often older and frequently dehydrated, may be given to a chronic habit of straining at stool. She may become aware of a sudden sensation of something having given way within the pelvis, with an accompanying backache and feeling of fullness, which is worse in the erect position. An obvious and externally visible bulge in the vagina may become evident. It enlarges over a period of time but invariably recedes when the patient lies down, when gravity pulls her genital parts in another direction.

The sole exception to this situation is the patient with an incarcerated procidentia, in which the amount of tissue edema becomes so severe that spontaneous or induced manual reduction within the pelvis is no longer possible (Figure 6.3). Such incarceration constitutes a surgical emergency, because ureteral obstruction, necrosis, and gangrene of the tissues may supervene if the condition is not relieved. For the patient with an incarcerated prolapse, the immediate treatment is strict bed rest. The prolapsed parts should be wrapped in soaks of hypertonic saline to reduce the edema. Manual reposition within the pelvis may be tried two or three times daily as the edema subsides, the tenderness abates, and reduction once again becomes possible. The reposited prolapse should be held in place with an intravaginal pessary until appropriate reconstructive surgery can be performed. If irreducible after 2 or 3 days of therapy, surgery should not be delayed.

The patient often describes the bulge of recurrent prolapse as a "bubble" involving the bladder. When it begins to interfere with the wearing of her clothing or the comfort of sitting down, she will request relief. There is a surprising lack of initial urinary symptoms or incontinence, although later digital elevation of the bladder may be required for urination. Half of urinary-incontinent women with vagi-

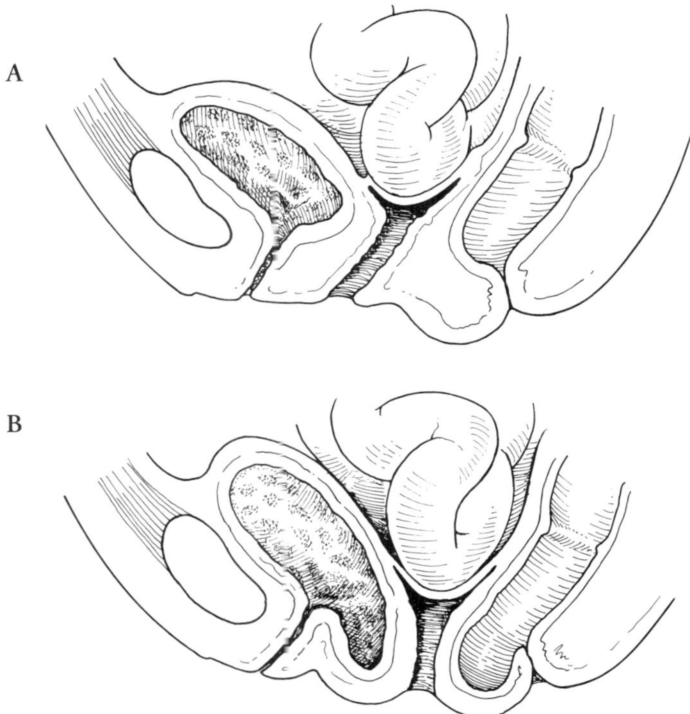

FIGURE 6.1 **A,** Partial posthysterectomy eversion of the vagina without cystocele and rectocele. **B,** Partial posthysterectomy eversion of the vaginal vault with obvious cystocele and rectocele. (Redrawn from Nichols DH and Randall CL: Vaginal surgery, ed 4, Baltimore, 1996, Williams & Wilkins.)

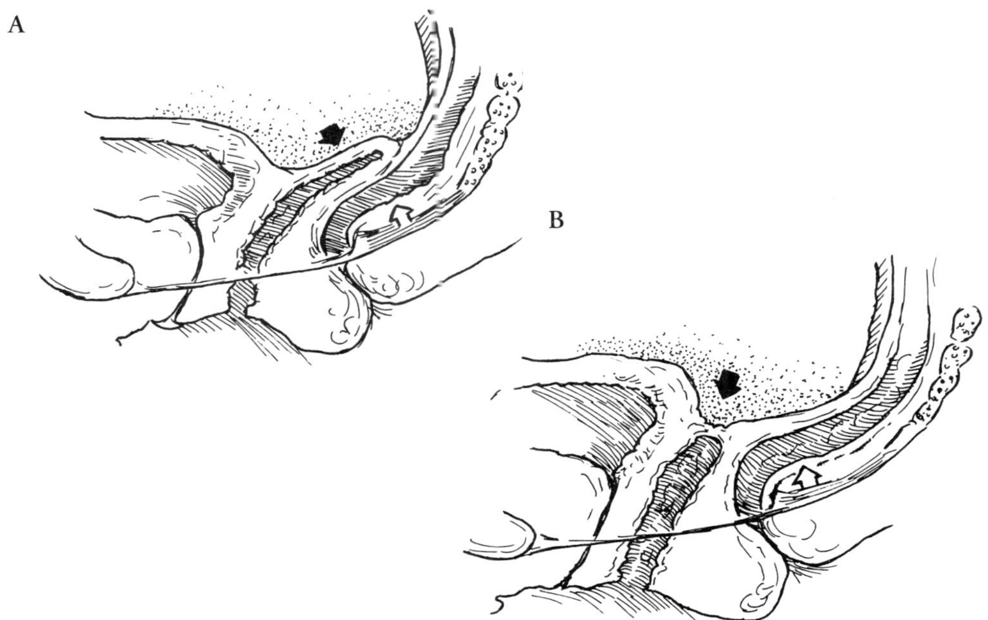

FIGURE 6.2 **A,** The long posthysterectomy vagina in which the vaginal vault is supported above the intact levator plate *(white arrow)* and posterior to its anterior margin. Increases in intraabdominal pressure *(black arrow)* tend to squeeze the vagina against the intact levator plate. In **B,** however, the vault of a shorter posthysterectomy vagina ends anterior to the intact levator plate *(white arrow),* and increases in intraabdominal pressure *(black arrow)* are exerted in the axis of the vagina, tending to cause it to telescope and to become even shorter. (Redrawn from Amreich J: Wien Klin Wochenschr 63:74, 1951.)

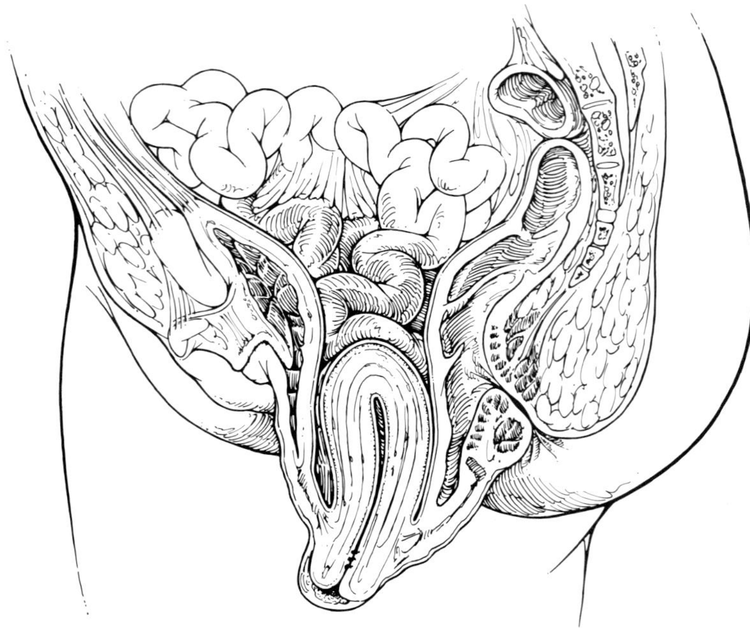

FIGURE 6.3 Massive eversion of the vagina and the organs to which it is attached are shown in sagittal section. (From Nichols DH, editor: Gynecologic and obstetric surgery, St Louis, 1993, Mosby.)

nal vault prolapse will demonstrate urinary incontinence once the prolapse has been reduced.[4] This risk can be uncovered during preoperative testing[5] while the prolapse has been reduced (pessary or vaginal packing). If incontinence is seen, appropriate steps must be undertaken to establish a preoperative confirmatory diagnosis, and a proper surgical remedy applied to the anterior vaginal wall. Symptoms of rectal dysfunction or pain are uncommon. Rectal prolapse may coexist (Figure 6.4) and should be repaired separately.

The patient with recurrent massive eversion of the vagina is usually, though not invariably, postmenopausal and parous. There may be a family history of severe genital prolapse. Recent weight loss may precipitate aggravation of the prolapse by removing ischiorectal fat from its supporting position beneath the pelvic diaphragm (Figure 6.5). The presence of wide abdominal striae strongly suggests an underlying elastic tissue defect.

PATHOGENESIS

Initially there is eversion of a poorly supported vaginal vault, with coexistent enterocele in 60% to 70% (Figure 6.6) of patients. At first the surgeon may note only a small displacement type of cystocele, which will often disappear with replacement of the vault. There is usually an abnormally inclined, vertically oriented vaginal axis,[6] signifying some disturbance in the integrity of the levator plate. When this is severe, there may be some flattening of the anorectal angle. Upon questioning, the patient may admit a minor degree of loss of confidence in her rectal continence.

As the vault descends further, it brings with it more of the bladder as a larger cystocele. Later the lower supports of the vagina are compromised. As the urogenital diaphragm becomes stretched, there is a degree of rotational descent of the bladder neck. Since the posterior portion of the bladder has come

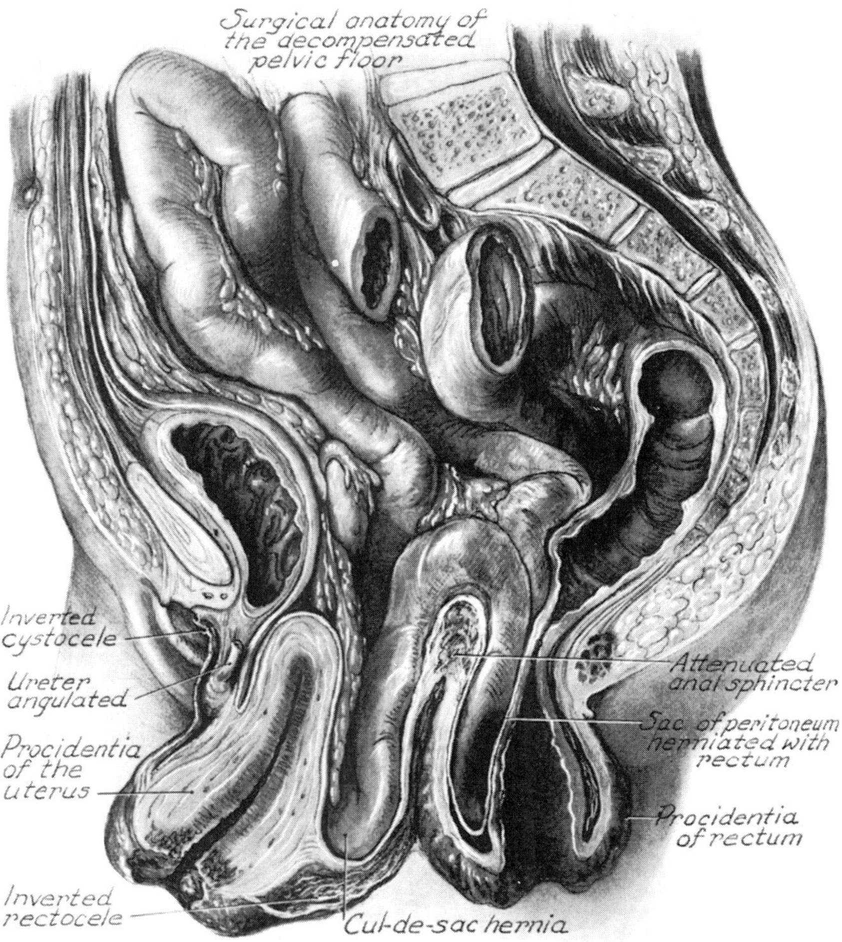

Figure 6.4 Simultaneous genital prolapse and rectal prolapse are shown in sagittal section. Because they are each of entirely different cause, each must be repaired separately. (From Ball TL: Gynecologic surgery and urology, ed 2, St Louis, 1963, Mosby.)

down first, there is usually with its unimpeded descent some expected persistence and even increase in the cystourethral angle with preservation or return of urinary continence. As the prolapse progresses to total vaginal eversion, the dilating wedgelike effect of the prolapse on the levator ani increases the width of the genital hiatus and accentuates the defect in the integrity of the pelvic diaphragm and then of the perineal body. Coincident full-length rectocele and perineal body defect become evident.

If the surgeon is seeing the patient for the first time at this stage of her disease, it may be difficult to establish the site of primary damage. Sending for and reviewing the surgical dictation of the patient's past records may be, but is not invariably, helpful. However, determining the location of the major initial defect with reasonable certainty is important so that Bonney's precept of overrepair of the primary site can be accomplished to lessen the chance of recurrence.[7] Examining the unanesthetized patient in a lithotomy position and gently

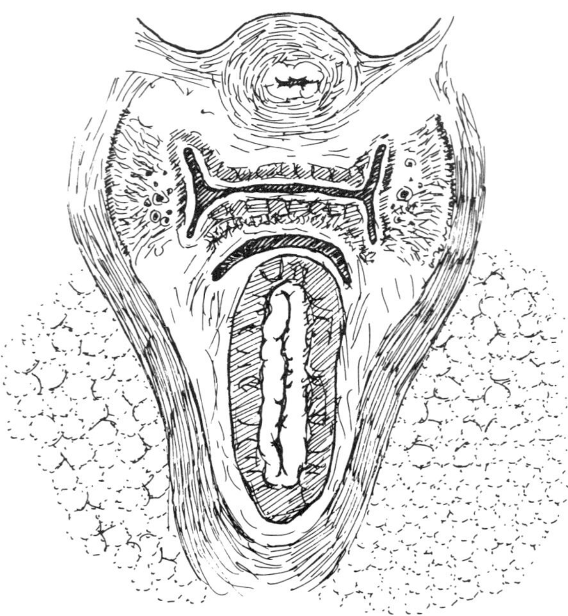

FIGURE 6.5 A cross-section through the lower midportion of the pelvis is shown. Notice the fibers of Luschka that attach the lateral walls of the vagina to the fascia of the pelvic diaphragm. The pubococcygeus has a convex shape due to the pressure of the surrounding ischiorectal fat tissue, which helps to press it against the rectum. (Redrawn from Nichols DH and Milley P: Clinical anatomy of the vulva, vagina, lower pelvis, and perineum. In Sciarra J, editor: Gynecology and obstetrics, New York, 1977, Harper & Row.)

replacing the prolapse within the pelvis, the examiner lets the tissue rest for 1 or 2 minutes, then asks the patient to strain and see what tissues appear first. If the cystocele and rectocele appear first, followed by the vaginal vault, the primary site of damage is probably in the supports of the lower portion of the vagina (i.e., the pelvic and urogenital diaphragms). If the vaginal vault appears first, followed by a cystocele and rectocele, the site of primary damage is probably in the upper suspensory system of the vagina and pelvis.

With an extreme degree of prolapse of the full length of the vagina, there is some stretching or avulsion of the paravaginal or lateral supporting tissues (Figure 6.7), including some of the fibers of Luschka, which attach the anterior vaginal sulcus to the arcus tendineus (Figures 6.8 to 6.10). This circumstance was first appreciated as a clinical problem by White in 1909.[8] The presence of this lateral or paravaginal detachment can be demonstrated by replacing the vaginal vault into the hollow of the sacrum, holding it there, and asking the patient to strain. This maneuver may demonstrate disappearance or descent of the lateral vaginal sulcus. The lateral sulcus displacement is then reduced by mechanical or digital support, and the patient is asked to strain again while the examiner notes whether or not the cystocele returns. If it does not return, one has identified a probable defect in the lateral or paravaginal supporting tissues. If the cystocele persists with straining, even though the anterior sulcus is supported on both sides, the defect is present in the midline supporting tissues of the vagina. The presence of significant lateral defect can be further evidenced with the Baden and Walker modification of this maneuver.[9] Asking the patient to stand, the gynecologist holds the vault in its proper place in the hollow of the sacrum. With the free hand, the examiner lightly palpates the anterior sulcus when the patient strains and once more when she voluntarily contracts her pubococcygei. Note is made of whether or not the vaginal sulcus rises in concert with the contraction. If it does rise, some residual anatomic connection of the bridge between the anterior sulcus and the arcus tendineus is implied, but if it

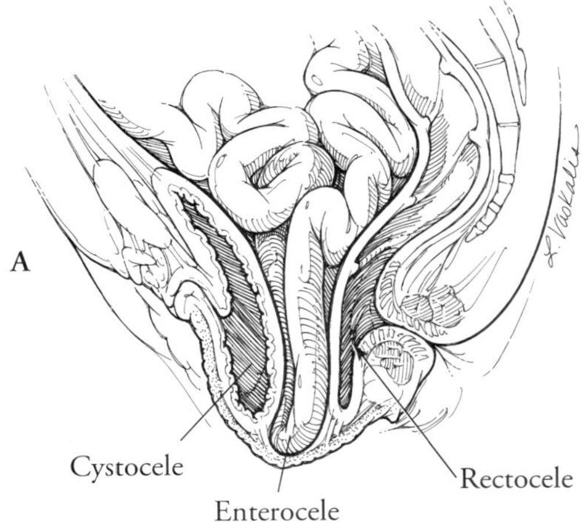

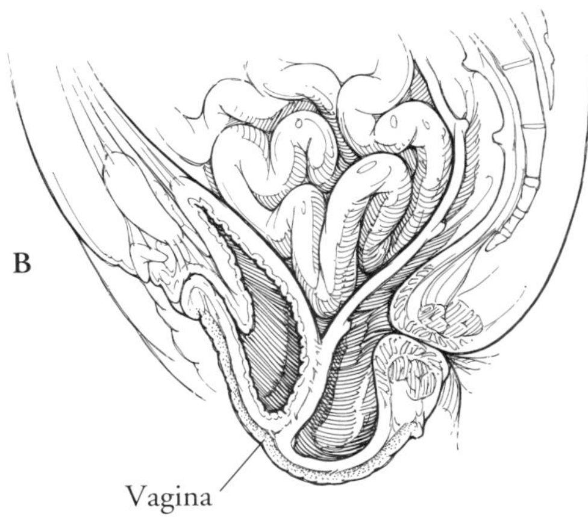

Figure **6.6** Massive eversion of the vagina with and without coincident enterocele. **A,** An enterocele is present in the majority of patients with massive eversion of the posthysterectomy vagina. **B,** Occasionally, however, the connective tissue capsule of the bladder is fused with that of the anterior rectum. Making the distinction is important during surgery because, in the absence of enterocele, further dissection in this area is unnecessary. If enterocele is present, identification, opening, excision, and closure of the neck of the enterocele removes it from the operative field. If it is present but undiagnosed and untreated, it will progress over a period of time, usually necessitating still another operative procedure.

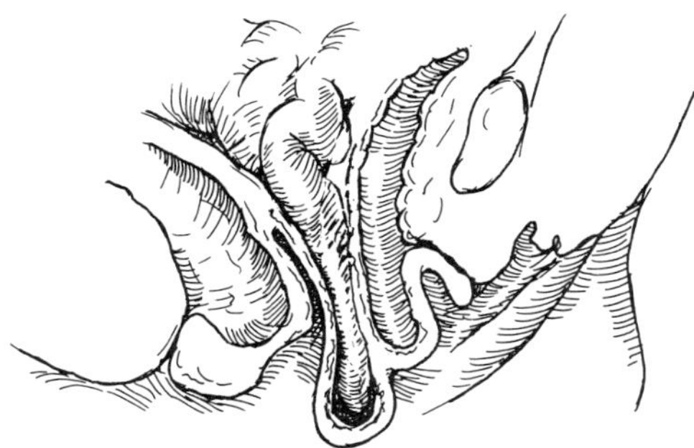

Figure **6.7** Posthysterectomy eversion of the vagina is shown. There is rectocele, enterocele, and cystocele. The vaginal prolapse has stretched the attachments of the anterior fornix to the arcus tendineus, as well as elongated the attachments of the anterior vaginal wall to the urogenital diaphragm, producing a combined lateral and midline defect in support. (Redrawn from Nichols DH: Obstet Gynecol 40:257, 1972.)

does not rise, it may be assumed that there is great likelihood of avulsion of the vaginal sulcus from the arcus tendineus at such a site.

Pertinent specialized laboratory studies are related to an identification of possible disturbance in neuromuscular physiology. These urodynamic assessments may include a urethrocystometrogram if urinary continence is a question[5] and electromyography of the striated muscles of the pelvic floor, pudendal nerve motor latency study, rectal manometry, and x-ray defecogram if rectal incontinence is present.

Disturbances in function of the voluntary muscles and inability to voluntarily contract the pubococcygei strongly suggest that contributory pudendal neuropathy is likely. If there is complete paralysis of the pelvic diaphragm and the external anal sphincter, rectal continence may be maintained solely through action of the involuntary internal anal sphincter, a sometimes fragile remaining source of continence, the integrity of which must be retained at all costs.

Choice of Operation

Surgical reconstruction should involve a primary transvaginal approach, or a transabdominal one, or a combination of the two, depending on the experience of the operator and the availability of skilled surgical assistance. For the experienced reconstructive surgeon, the transvaginal approach holds many attractions. It permits appropriate enterocele excision, an-

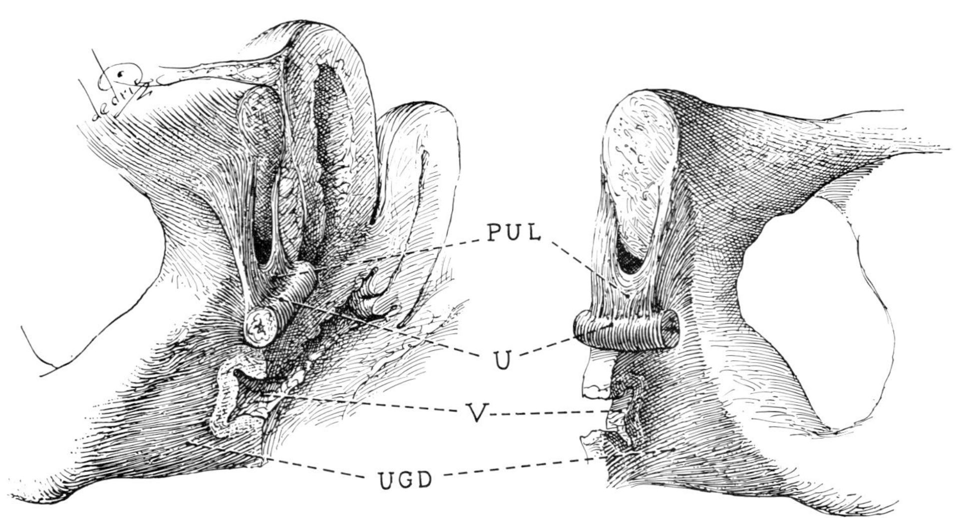

FIGURE 6.8 The relationship between the pubourethral ligament *(PUL)* and the urogenital diaphragm *(UGD)* is shown in the sagittal drawing. Note further the relationship between the urethra *(U)* and vagina *(V)* to the urogenital diaphragm and to the bladder, which has been sketched into the drawing at the left. (From Milley PS and Nichols DH: Anat Rec 170:281, 1971.)

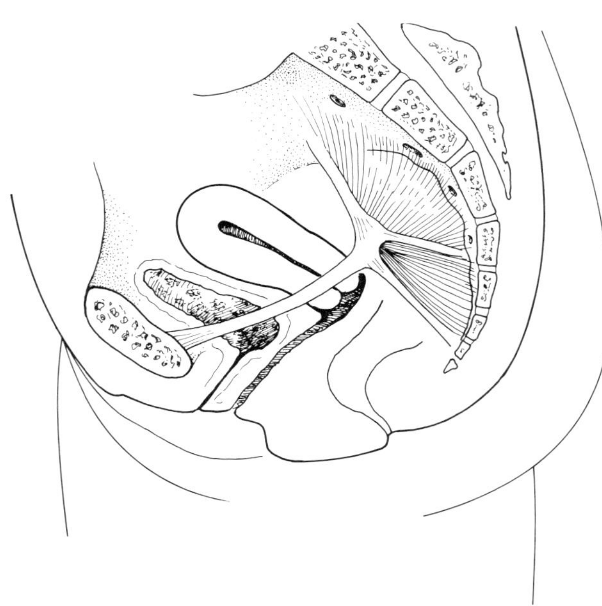

FIGURE 6.9 The relationship between the arcus tendineus (one on each side of the pelvis) and the normal vaginal axis is shown in this schematic drawing. The anterior sulcus is attached to the arcus tendineus by an intermediate bridge of connective tissue that varies in length between the proximal and distal portions of the vagina. (Redrawn from Nichols DH and Randall CL: Vaginal surgery, ed 4, Baltimore, 1996, Williams & Wilkins.)

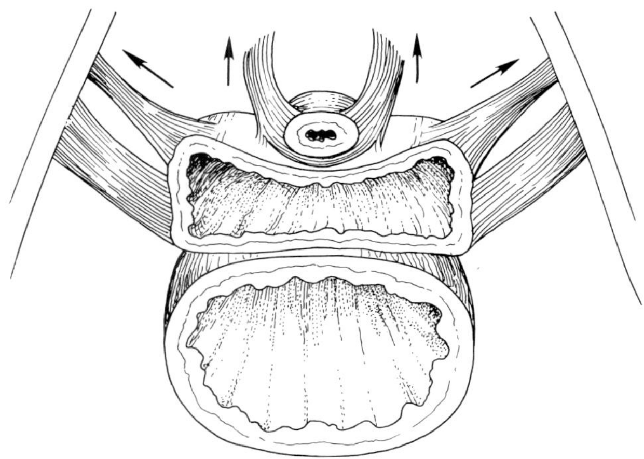

Figure 6.10 The urethra is both suspended by the urogenital diaphragm (as shown by the *central arrows*) and supported by the anterior vaginal wall, which is itself attached to the arcus tendineus on each side by a connective tissue bridge (as indicated by the *lateral arrows*). (Redrawn from Nichols DH and Randall CL: Vaginal surgery, ed 4, Baltimore, 1996, Williams & Wilkins.)

terior and posterior colporrhaphy, including restoration of midline and paravaginal defects, and perineorrhaphy, all through the same operative exposure. If a perineal descent syndrome has been noted, a retrorectal levatorplasty may be performed as well.

Vaginal hysterectomy and repair may be the treatment of choice in the patient in whom the uterus is still present. Strong but surgically useful uterosacral ligaments may be shortened and employed to suspend the vault. A McCall-type cul-de-plasty will restore length and proper axis to the upper portion of the vagina (see Chapter 9). For the patient with previous hysterectomy, the uterosacral ligaments of a prolapsed vagina will generally have undergone atrophy and will be neither surgically useful nor dependable.

In some instances a primary abdominal approach for the support of the prolapsed vaginal vault is preferred. Indications for the abdominal route include the presence of an adnexal mass that must be investigated, rerecurrent vaginal vault eversion in a patient with severe chronic respiratory disease, the rare vaginal vault eversion in a patient with a short vagina that will not reach the sacrospinous ligament, or the extreme anterior displacement of the vagina that may follow ventral suspension or less commonly the Burch procedure,[10] in which a wide and unprotected cul-de-sac of Douglas was not separately obliterated.

Ventral fixation with obliteration of the cul-de-sac is an effective treatment for the rare parous prolapse patient born with bladder exstrophy, provided that the patient has been sterilized by either hysterectomy or tubal ligation.

Techniques of Reconstruction

Vaginal Hysterectomy and Repair

The prolapse is carefully examined under anesthesia and a tenaculum placed on the posterior lip of the cervix to which traction is applied. Digital palpation carefully determines the site and width of the base of the cul-de-sac of Douglas and the length and strength of the uterosacral ligaments (Figures 6.11 and 6.15). In most instances, the latter will be strong, though elongated. If surgically shortened during the procedure, the uterosacral ligaments will be useful in supporting the vaginal vault postoperatively. The surgeon then proceeds with a Heaney-type vaginal hysterectomy. If there has been a previous ventral suspension of the uterus, the fundus must be surgically detached from the underside of the anterior abdominal wall. The ovaries are carefully examined. They may be removed if there is any pathologic condition present or, with her permission if the patient is

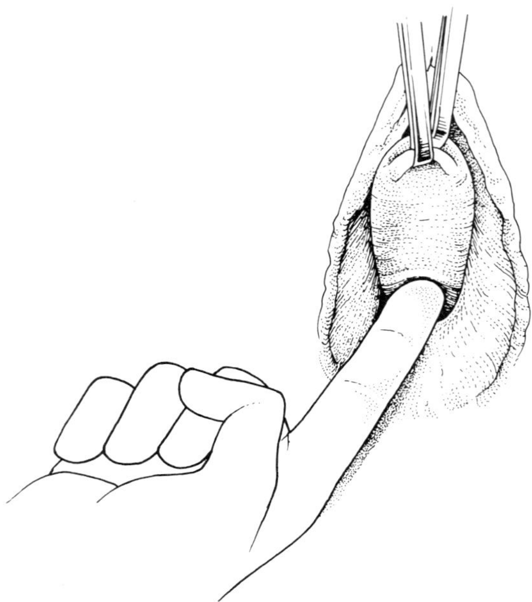

FIGURE 6.11 When traction is made to a tenaculum applied to the posterior lip of the cervix, one can palpate both the length and strength of the uterosacral ligaments, as well as the base of the cul-de-sac of Douglas. (Redrawn from Nichols DH and Randall CL: Vaginal surgery, ed 4, Baltimore, 1996, Williams & Wilkins.)

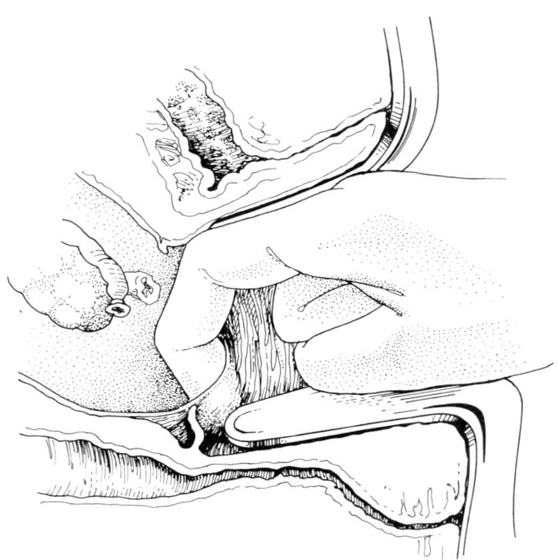

FIGURE 6.12 Redundant peritoneum of the cul-de-sac that should be excised can be demonstrated by hooking a finger into this pocket of peritoneum. It should be mobilized and excised back to its junction with the peritoneum overlying the anterior surface of the rectum, indicated by the yellow prerectal fat attached to the underside of the peritoneum. (Redrawn from Nichols DH and Randall CL: Vaginal surgery, ed 4, Baltimore, 1996, Williams & Wilkins.)

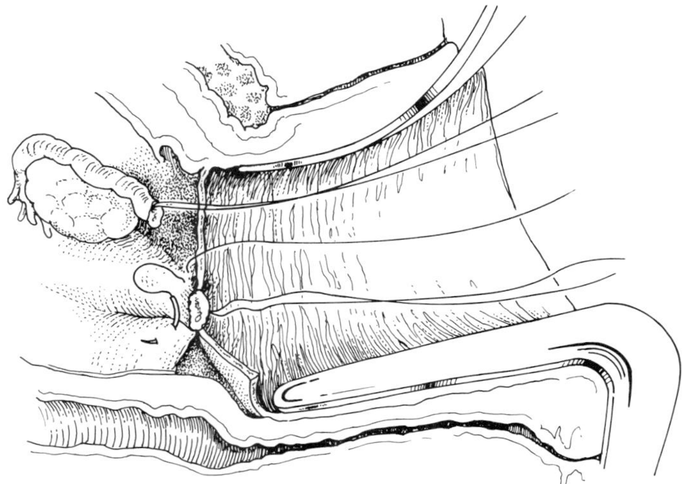

Figure 6.13 High peritonealization is begun by a suture through the peritoneal side of the left uterosacral ligament, which proceeds in a clockwise fashion through the peritoneum overlying the rectum, the right uterosacral ligament, peritoneal side of the right round ligament, anterior peritoneum, and left round ligament. The suture avoids damaging the blood vessels within the cardinal ligament and brings together both the peritoneum and the subperitoneal retinaculum. (Redrawn from Nichols DH and Randall CL: Vaginal surgery, ed 4, Baltimore, 1996, Williams & Wilkins.)

postmenopausal, in the absence of a pathologic condition.

Any enterocele sac is carefully identified and dissected from the surrounding tissue up to the point where the yellow prerectal fat is attached to its underside[11] (Figure 6.12). The excess peritoneum is excised. One or more McCall-type sutures are placed taking a bite through one side of the posterior vaginal vault, the cut edge of the peritoneum, and the peritoneal surface of the homolateral uterosacral ligament. The suture is anchored to the prerectal peritoneum in the midline, then made to penetrate the same structures on the opposite side in reverse order. A second or third McCall's stitch may be placed successively higher on the uterosacral ligaments as the path of the ureters courses more anterolaterally.

If the posterior vaginal vault is unusually wide, it should be narrowed by excision of a V-shaped wedge, the sides of which are approximated with full-thickness sutures. The peritoneal cavity may be closed by one or more purse-string sutures (Figure 6.13). The McCall stitches are tied, bringing the posterior vault of the vagina into firm contact with the underside of the uterosacral ligaments grasped by the McCall stitches. The vagina is thus elongated and restored to its natural position in the hollow of the sacrum. Next, appropriate full-length anterior colporrhaphy is usually accomplished with special efforts expended to preserve and accentuate the cystourethral angle, so that it is restored to a position within the pelvis approximating the junction of the lower third and upper two thirds of the back of the pubis. Finally, any rectocele and perineal defect are repaired. At the conclusion of the operation, the patient should have an effective restoration of a normal vaginal depth and axis. Because of the increased proximity of the ureters to the operative field in genital prolapse, it is reassuring to verify ureteral patency at the end of the procedure. The patient is given one ampule (5 ml) of IV indigo carmine, the bladder emptied of urine, and 250 ml of sterile saline instilled. Observation cystoscopy is performed while the patient is still under anesthesia. Usually in less than 5 minutes from the time of IV indigo carmine injection, the operator will note violet-stained urine spurting from each ureteral orifice. Should patency not be thus demonstrated after a wait of 10 or 15 minutes, it is appropriate to investigate the reasons for apparent absence of ureteral patency. An infusion pyelogram may be per-

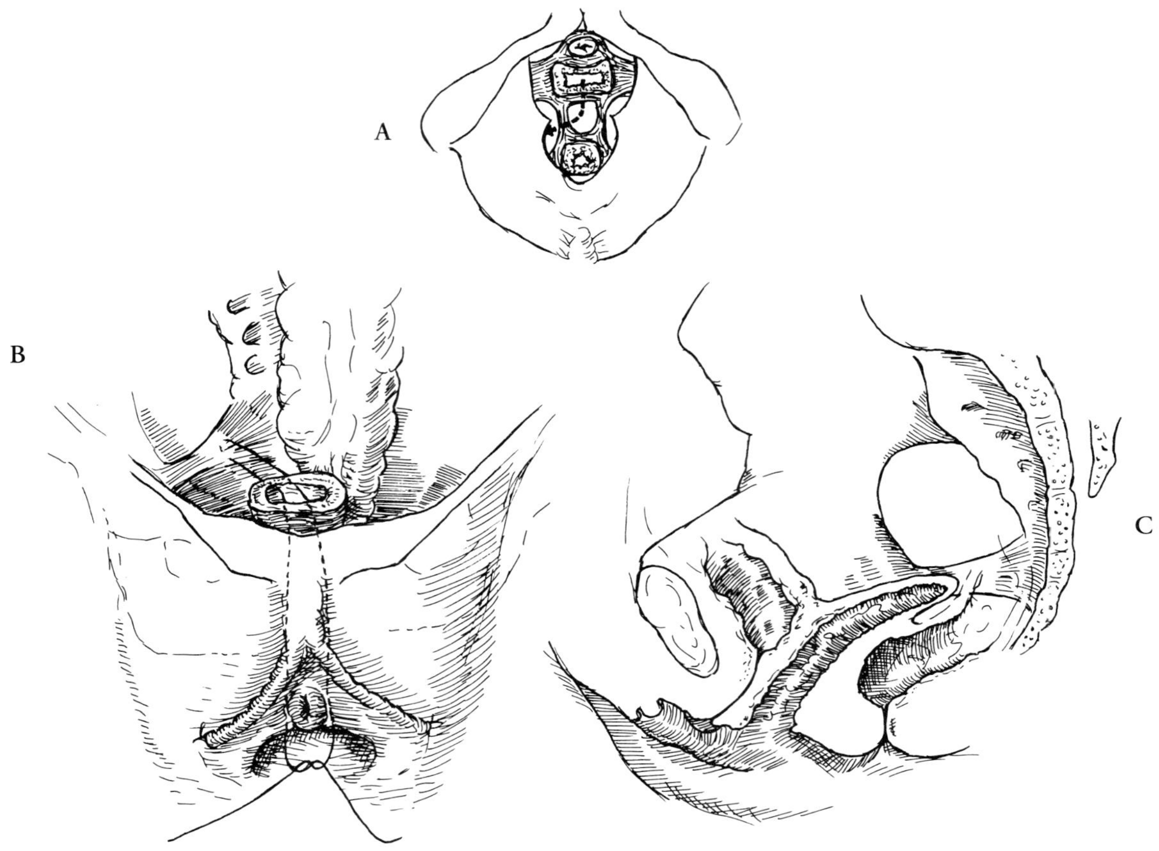

FIGURE 6.14 Technique of right sacrospinous colpopexy. A path of dissection occurs through the posterior vaginal wall into the rectovaginal space and then through a window in the descending rectal septum into the right pararectal space (**A**). The dissection always proceeds toward the ischial spine in the lateral wall of the pararectal space. The vagina is sewn to the right sacrospinous ligament–coccygeus muscle complex at a point one and one half fingerwidths medial to the right ischial spine, as shown in **B**. After the fixation stitches have been tied, the attachment of the vagina to the right sacrospinous ligament is shown in **C**, indicating, after appropriate colporrhaphy, a fairly normal vaginal depth and axis.

formed while the patient is still on the operating table, and any obstruction can be confirmed by resistance to the passage of a ureteral catheter. If a ureter has been ligated, deligation without delay with probable catheterization of the ureter by a ureteral stent should be an effective remedy.

Transvaginal Sacrospinous Colpopexy

For patients in whom the uterosacral-cardinal ligament complex is too attenuated to be of use in supporting the vagina, transvaginal sacrospinous colpopexy is useful[12-16] using the newer synthetic but nonabsorbable sutures (Figure 6.14). Coincident excision of any enterocele is easily done, and any necessary colporrhaphy may be performed through the same operative exposure.

Transvaginal sacrospinous colpopexy immediately following vaginal hysterectomy in patients with uterine prolapse without strong uterosacral-cardinal ligament support (Figures 6.15 and 6.16) is surprisingly easy. The opera-

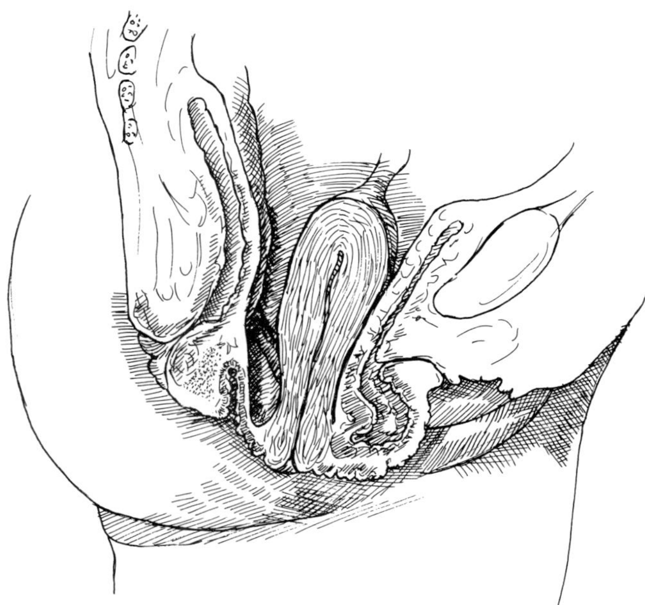

FIGURE 6.15 The more common uterovaginal or sliding prolapse is shown. There is enterocele but no significant rectocele, because there is no direct involvement of the anterior rectal wall in this prolapse. The uterosacral ligaments are long and strong, and the cervix is elongated. (Redrawn from Halban J and Tandler J: Änatomie und Atiologie der Genitalprolapse beim Weibe, Vienna, Austria, 1907, Braumuller.)

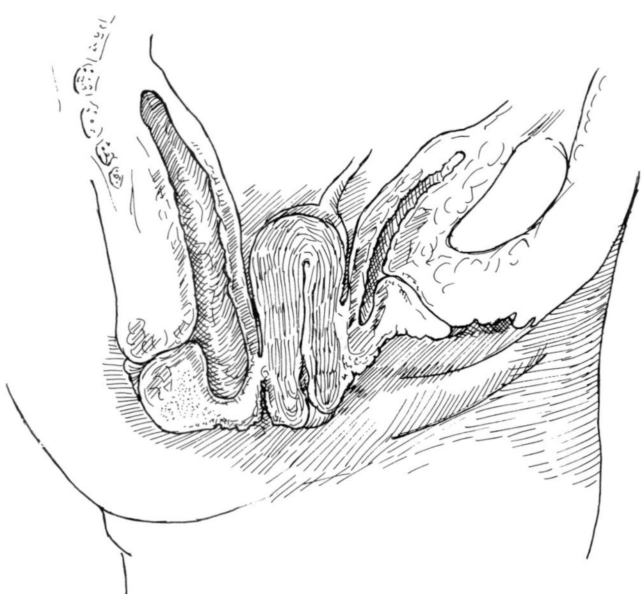

FIGURE 6.16 The less common general postmenopausal prolapse is shown in sagittal section. All endopelvic supporting tissues are atrophied and weakened. A rectocele and a descent of the cul-de-sac are shown but no enterocele. There is an obvious defect in the supports of the anterior rectal wall. The uterosacral ligaments are weak and hard to define by palpation. The cervix is not elongated. (Redrawn from Halban J and Tandler J: Änatomie und Atiologie der Genitalprolapse beim Weibe, Vienna, 1907, Braumuller.)

tion can be accomplished within an additional 15 minutes of operating time. The sequence of events in this instance is as follows:

1. Perform vaginal hysterectomy.
2. Excise any enterocele with high ligation of the sac and closure of the peritoneal cavity.
3. Perform anterior colporrhaphy.
4. Make an incision in the perineum and open the rectovaginal space.
5. Penetrate the right rectal pillar overlying

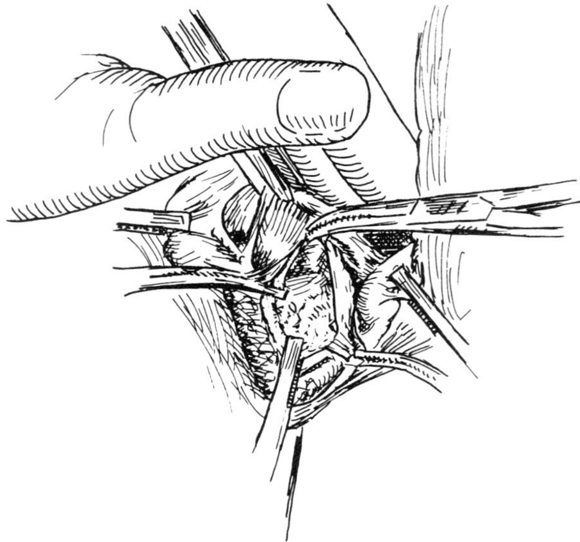

Figure 6.17 An enterocele has been identified, opened, and mobilized before resection.

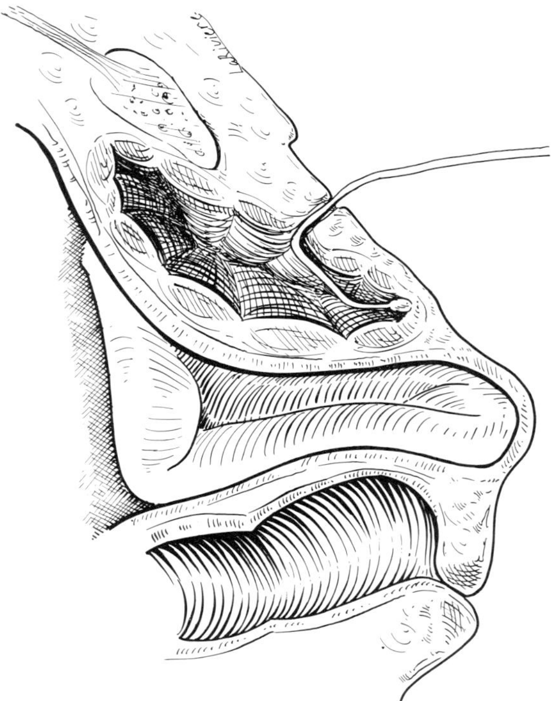

Figure 6.18 If the limits of a partly filled bladder cannot be determined precisely, palpating the tip of a bent uterine sound can identify at surgery the site where the bladder and the wall of an enterocele sac come together. (From Nichols DH, editor: Gynecologic and obstetric surgery, St Louis, 1993, Mosby.)

the right ischial spine to open the right pararectal space. (The ischial spine and the sacrospinous ligament–coccygeus muscle complex form a portion of the lateral wall of the pararectal space.)

6. Perform sacrospinous colpopexy.
7. Start posterior colporrhaphy.
8. Tie colpopexy stitches.
9. Complete posterior colporrhaphy and perineorrhaphy.

In the likely event that the uterus has been removed before this procedure and there is massive posthysterectomy eversion of the vaginal vault, the sequence and techniques are as follows:

1. Initial surgical incision is through the perineum and posterior vaginal wall with entry into the rectovaginal space.
2. Any enterocele is identified and opened (Figure 6.17), and the neck of the enterocele sac is carefully palpated for any usable uterosacral ligament strength. Usually this is found lacking. The neck of the sac is closed by a purse-string suture, the sac is excised, and the operator may proceed with sacrospinous colpopexy. At times, consequent to scarring from previous surgery, it is difficult to determine by physical examination whether an enterocele coexists between the bladder and the rectum. Palpating the tip of a bent uterine sound introduced through the urethra (Figure 6.18) will identify the lower limit of the bladder. This will make the dissection safer and protect against unexpected accidental cystotomy.
3. When the rectum has been carefully displaced by an appropriate retractor to the opposite side of the pelvis, the ischial spine is carefully palpated. To approach the sacrospinous ligament, the surgeon must make a window through the descending rectal septum over the ischial spine. This window can be established by blunt penetration with the operator's finger or by the closed tips of curved Mayo scissors or a sharp pointed hemostat (Figure 6.19).
4. Once established, the window is gen-

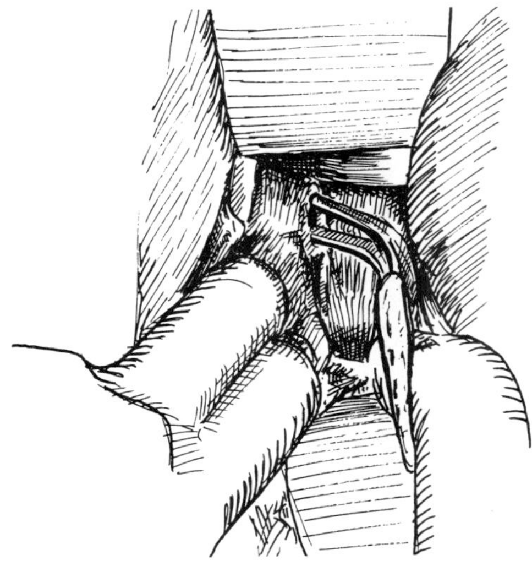

Figure 6.19 While the upper retractor displaces the cardinal ligament and ureter and the lower retractor holds the rectum to the patient's left, the right rectal pillar has been penetrated by the tips of a long pointed forcep, providing entry to the right pararectal space at a point overlying the right ischial spine.

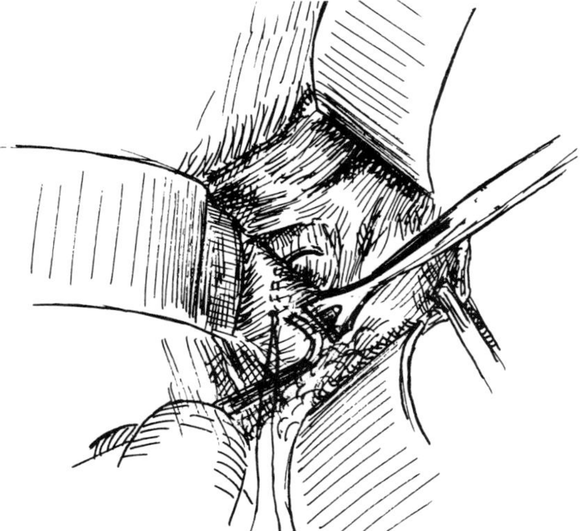

Figure 6.20 The opening through the right rectal pillar has been enlarged and the sacrospinous ligament–coccygeus muscle complex grasped with a long-handled Babcock's clamp. At a point about one and one half fingerwidths medial to the right ischial spine, the sacrospinous ligament and coccygeus muscle have been penetrated by the suture-bearing tip of a long-handled Deschamps' ligature carrier.

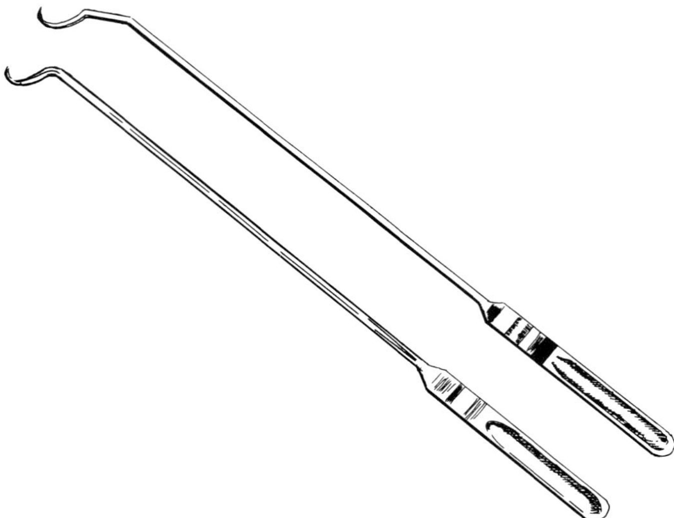

Figure 6.21 Long-handled Deschamps' ligature carriers for the right hand are shown. The angled modification (suggested by Rosenshein) at the top is useful when the sacrospinous ligament is unusually deep. The handle must be swung through a wide arc. (These instruments are available from BEI Medical Systems/Zinnanti Surgical Instruments, Chatsworth, CA 91311, and on special order from Codman and Shurtleff, Custom Device Department, New Bedford, MA 02745, or from William Merz, American V. Mueller Company, Chicago, IL 60648.)

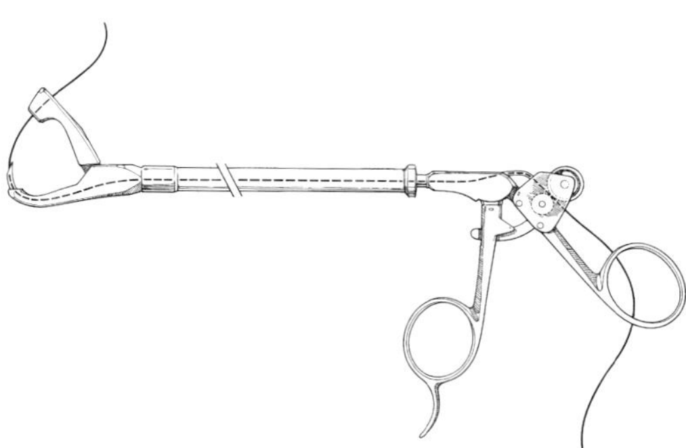

Figure 6.22 The Shutt punch is shown in phantom drawing. A single monofilament suture is threaded through a small opening near the handle of the instrument, and the suture is made to advance along the path of the *dashed line* by counterclockwise rotation of the friction wheel until the suture appears at the tip of the hollow needle as shown. The rotation of the friction wheel is reversed until the tip of the suture is just within the needle tip. (Available from Linvatec, Largo, FL, 34643.) (Redrawn from Nichols DH and Randall CL: Vaginal surgery, ed 4, Baltimore, 1996, Williams & Wilkins.)

tly enlarged with the fingers. This stretching of the window provides a clear view and easy palpation of the upper surface of the pelvic diaphragm, the ischial spine, and sacrospinous ligament–coccygeus muscle complex. One retractor is placed in the 12 o'clock position holding the cardinal ligament containing the ureter out of harm's way. Another retractor holds the patient's rectum to the side opposite the dissection, and a shorter retractor may compress the distal portion of the pelvic diaphragm along the lateral wall of the pelvis. Because the surgeon is working in a confined area, essentially in the hollow of the sacrum, supplemental illumination by a fiberoptic headlight is useful.

5. At a point one and one half to two fingerbreadths medial to the ischial spine, the sacrospinous ligament–coccygeus muscle complex is penetrated by the blunt tip of a long-handled Deschamps' ligature carrier (Figures 6.20 and 6.21), the Shutt punch[21] (Figures 6.22 and 6.23), or the Nichols-Veronikis ligature carrier

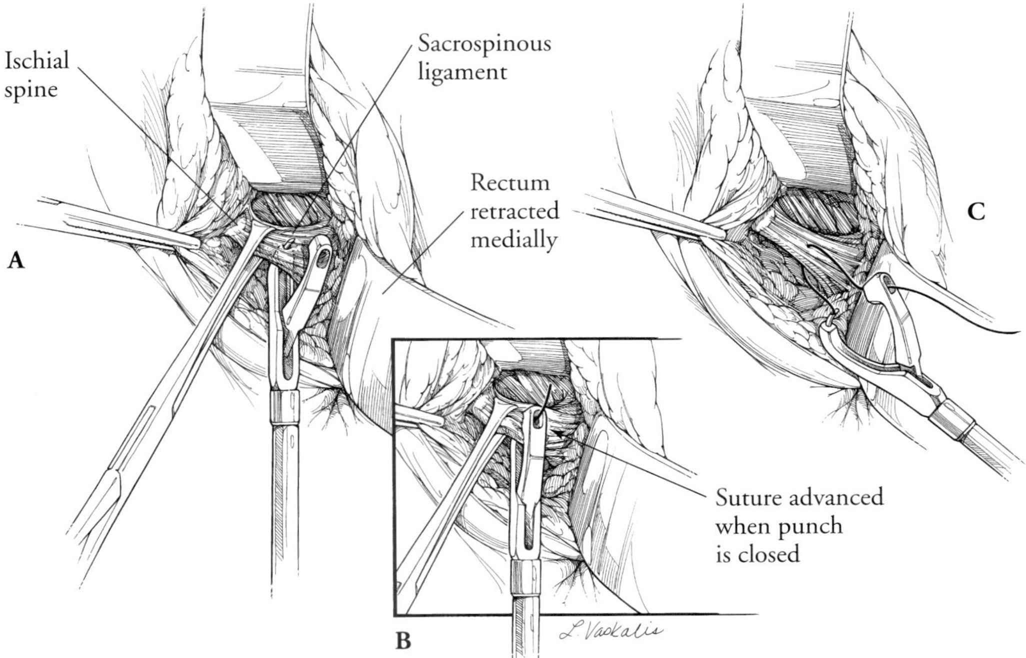

FIGURE 6.23 Penetration of the sacrospinous ligament using the Shutt punch. **A,** The right pararectal space has been entered and the ischial spine identified. The sacrospinous ligament–coccygeus muscle complex running posteromedially from the ischial spine to the sacrococcygeal area is exposed and grasped by a long-handled Allis' or Babcock's clamp as shown. The tip of the Shutt punch is pushed under and through the ligament-muscle complex, the cardinal ligament being held out of harm's way by an anterior retractor as shown, and the rectum held medially by a second retractor. **B,** The jaws of the punch are closed, and the friction wheel rotated to propel the suture through the hollow needle and the fenestration in the upper jaw of the punch. **C,** The free end is grasped with a hemostat, the punch opened and removed, and the suture disengaged from the ligature carrier. Additional stitches may be placed as necessary. The long-handled Allis or Babcock clamp is removed. (Redrawn from Nichols DH and Randall CL: Vaginal surgery, ed 4, Baltimore, 1996, Williams & Wilkins.)

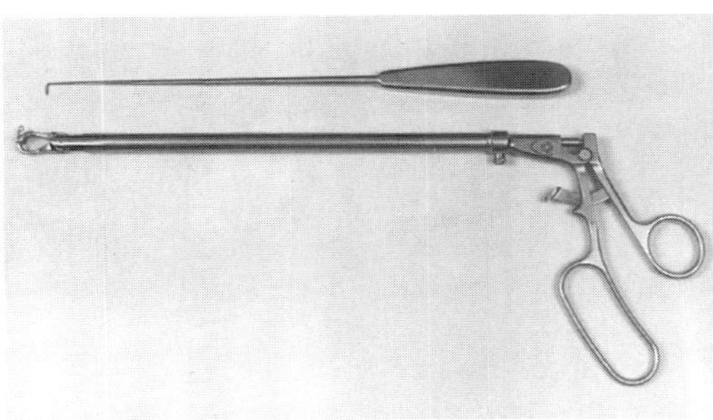

FIGURE 6.24 The Nichols-Veronikis ligature carrier is shown with the jaws in the closed position along with the suture-catching hook used to retrieve the suture loops. (Available from BEI Medical Systems/Zinnanti Surgical Instruments, Chatsworth, CA 91311.)

(Figures 6.24 to 6.26) holding full lengths of a synthetic nonabsorbable suture, such as size 0 polypropylene (Prolene, Surgilene) or polybutester (Novafil), and a heavy polyglycolic acid–type suture, such as polydiaxanone (PDS) or size 2 Dexon or Vicryl.

In the rare instance that visual exposure is difficult, penetration of the ligament can be done safely by palpation using the following maneuver: If the penetration is made through the right sacrospinous ligament–coccygeus muscle complex, the index and middle fingers of the surgeon's left hand are inserted through the

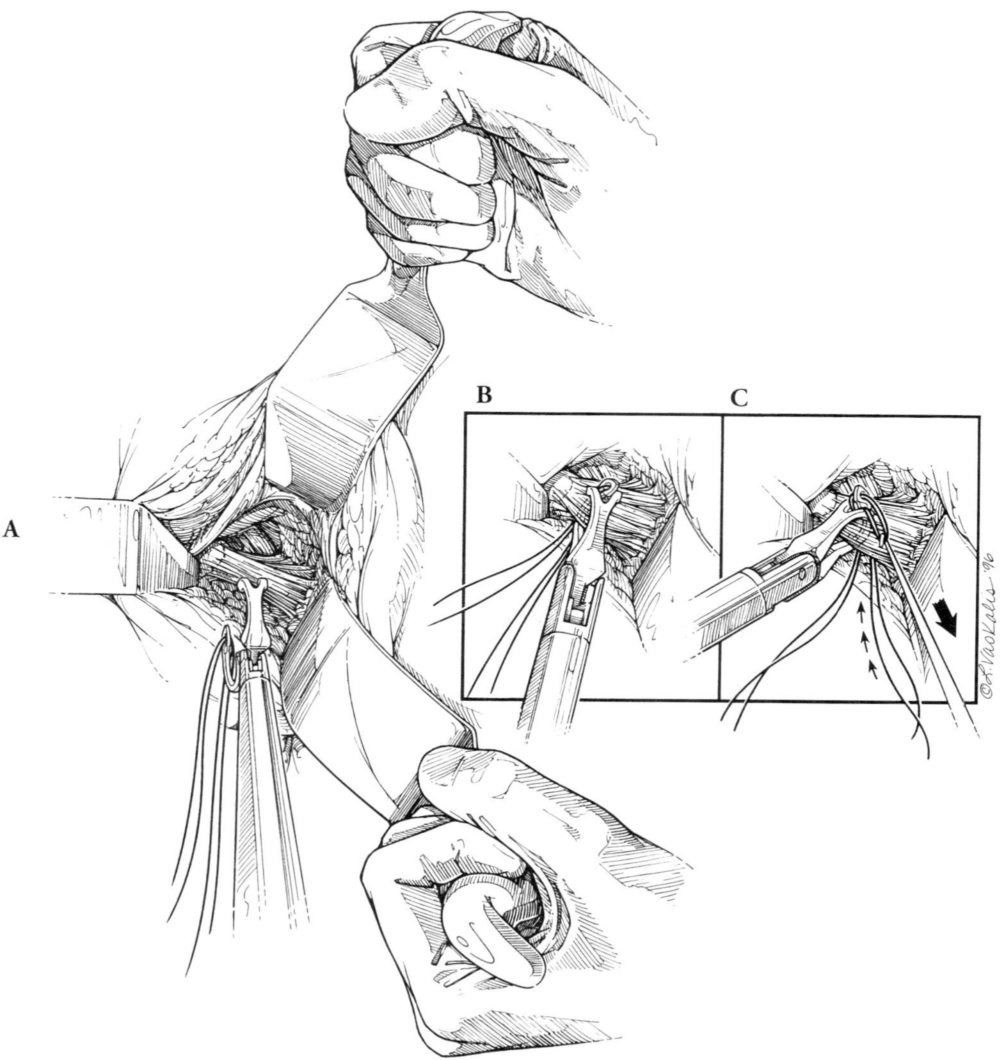

FIGURE 6.25 Placement of the Nichols-Veronikis ligature carrier under effective, direct illumination as furnished by a fiberoptic headlight. An opening has been made into the right pararectal space by creation of a window through the right rectal pillar, exposing the surface of the right coccygeus muscle containing the sacrospinous ligament. Suitable retraction is obtained in **A** and at a point well removed from the ischial spine the muscle-ligament complex may be grasped by a long Allis' or Babcock's clamp. At a point at least one and one half fingerbreadths medial to the spine the tip of the lower jaw of the opened ligature carrier is pushed gently beneath the lower margin of the complex, and the jaws of the carrier closed, advancing the needle tip holding *two* sutures through the ligament as shown in **B**. The suture loops are grasped by a fine-pointed suture hook. Traction to the hook, as shown in **C**, brings one end of the pair of sutures through the ligament. The ligature carrier is opened and removed.

window in the rectal pillar into the pararectal space. The tip of the middle index finger is made to touch the medial surface of the right ischial spine.

The long-handled Deschamps' ligature carrier, holding a proper suture, is grasped in the right hand, and the curved tip of the carrier is gently slid down the undersurface of the left index finger to the posteroinferior border of the sacrospinous ligament–coccygeal muscle complex at a spot one and one half to two fingerbreadths medial to the ischial spine, which is still being palpated by the

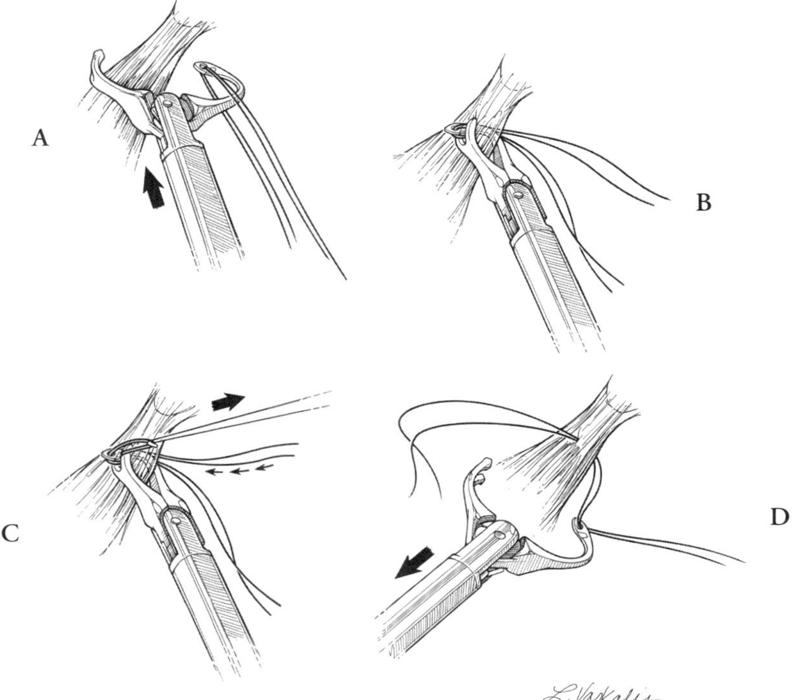

Figure 6.26 A similar procedure can be employed using the patient's left sacrospinous ligament–coccygeus muscle complex.

middle finger of the left hand (Figure 6.27). Pressure is made pushing the tip of the ligature carrier beneath the under edge of the muscle complex, and the tip is rotated in a clockwise direction; a significant resistance should be encountered, indicating that the carrier has been placed *through* the ligament, and neither superficial nor deep to it. At the same time, the handle of the ligature carrier is moved in an independent clockwise direction permitting vertical penetration of the ligament (Figure 6.28). A gentle tug to the ligature carrier or to the suture (Figure 6.29), which has been grasped by a hook, should actually move the patient a small degree on the table. Proper placement of the suture through the substance of the sacrospinous ligament is thus indicated. Direct palpation of the suture and of the ischial spine confirms the required distance between the two. If the suture seems too close to the ischial spine, traction is made on it, and a new suture is placed medial to the offending suture, which is then removed. An additional suture or two of a synthetic absorbable polydiaxanone (PDS) or polyglycolic acid-type (no. 1 or 2 Dexon or Vicryl) can be inserted through the muscle-ligament complex medial to the first suture, if extra support is desired.

6. Sacrospinous colpopexy may be performed on both sides if the vaginal vault is wide (Figure 6.30). Bilateral colpopexy may be of value using two synthetic sutures to each side to lessen the chance of recurrence of prolapse in a patient with coincident obstructive pulmonary disease (smoker, chronic bronchitis, asthma) or a lifestyle that requires heavy lifting or the postmenopausal patient with atrophic vaginal connective tissues often without the benefit of estrogen replacement therapy. Less-than-optimal pelvic connective tissue can be predicted, probably on an inherited basis, in a patient

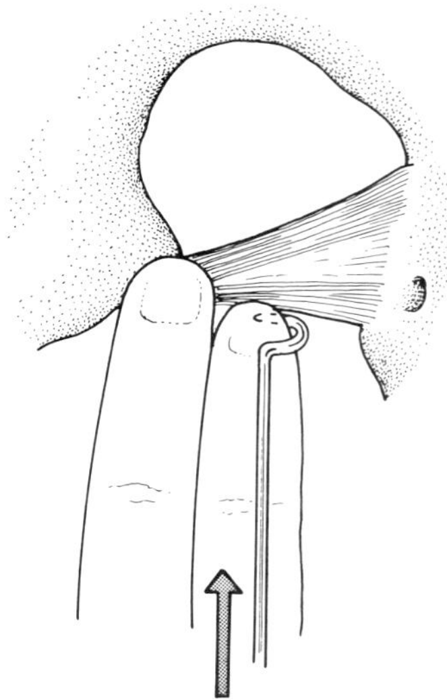

FIGURE 6.27 Through a window between the rectovaginal space and the right pararectal space, the middle finger of the operator's left hand has been placed against the medial edge of the left ischial spine, and the tip of the Deschamps ligature carrier slid beneath the left index finger, as shown, until it is in contact with the lower border of the sacrospinous ligament–coccygeus muscle complex. It is pushed in the direction of the *arrow* beneath this complex at this point. (Redrawn from Nichols DH and Randall CL: Vaginal surgery, ed 4, Baltimore, 1996, Williams & Wilkins.)

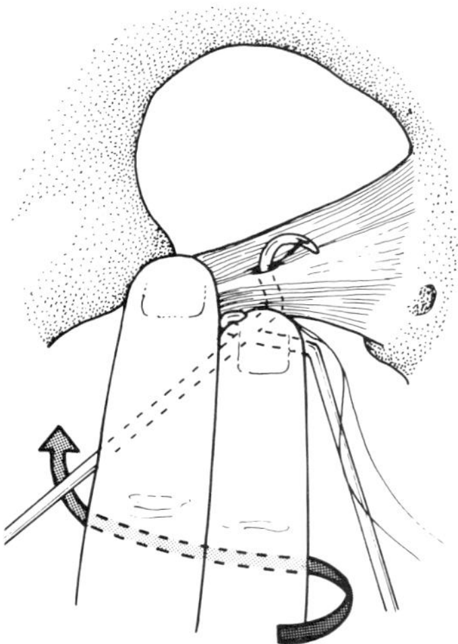

FIGURE 6.28 The tip of the ligature carrier is rotated so as to penetrate this complex from below upward *(arrow)* at the same time as the handle of the ligature carrier is rotated in a clockwise direction beneath the palm of the left hand. (Redrawn from Nichols DH and Randall CL: Vaginal surgery, ed 4, Baltimore, 1996, Williams & Wilkins.)

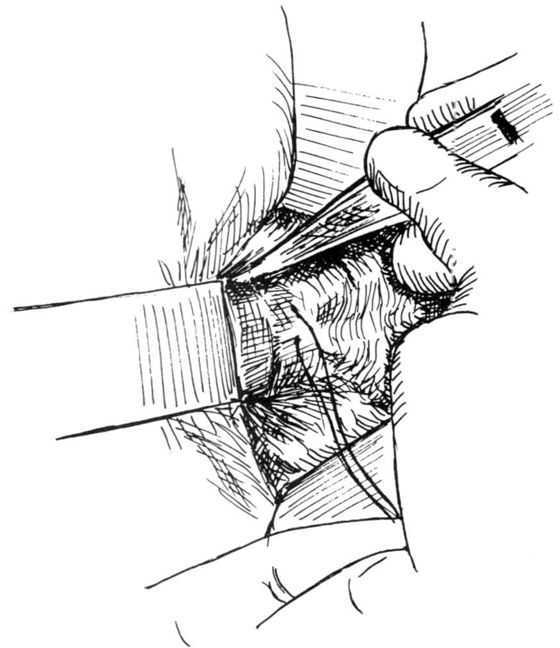

FIGURE 6.29 The ligature carrier and the Babcock clamp have been removed. The drawing shows the placement of the suture through the ligament-muscle complex. Traction to the suture will move the patient a slight amount on the table, indicating that the suture has been properly placed. The right ischial spine is at the tip of the forceps, indicating the position of the suture placement 2 to 3 cm medial to the ischial spine and safely removed from the location of the pudendal nerve and artery.

with multiple wide abdominal striae. Major genital prolapse and risk of recurrence are more common in such a patient.

Two synthetic sutures are used for each side of the colpopexy. A permanent monofilament (Novafil or Prolene) is placed through the full thickness of the fibromuscular wall of the vagina, but not through the squamous epithelial surface. A second long-lasting absorbable suture (PDS, Dexon, or Vicryl) through the full thickness of the often thin and atrophic vaginal vault creates a "bolster" of vaginal wall between the entry and exit points of the suture. This double suture provides a safety component in case one suture should be broken or the knot become untied, as well as providing a scar stronger by two sutures instead of one (see Figure 6.34).

With a unilateral colpopexy, a wide vault must be surgically narrowed (Figure 6.31). The vagina,

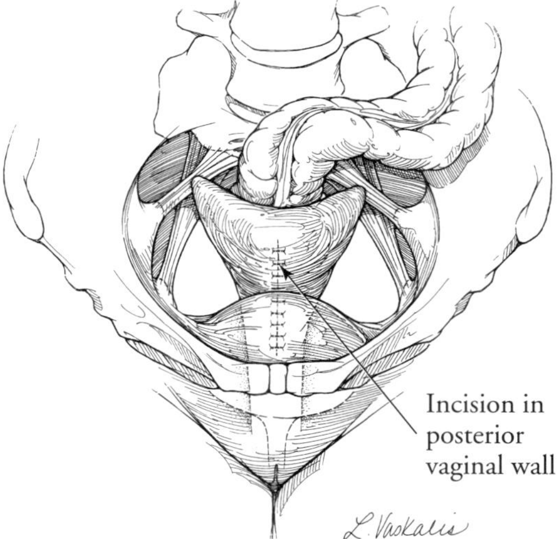

Figure 6.30 Bilateral sacrospinous colpopexy. The end result of bilateral sacrospinous colpopexy is shown in a phantom drawing. The vaginal vault is wide enough to reach between the ischial spines, as shown. Any enterocele has been excised previously, and any anterior colporrhaphy accomplished. The site of the posterior colporrhaphy closure is shown in the phantom suture line in the posterior vaginal wall. (Redrawn from Nichols DH and Randall CL: Vaginal surgery, ed 4, Baltimore, 1996, Williams & Wilkins.)

which is now an instrument of coitus and not for parturition, is thus converted to a cylinder of uniform diameter.

7. By a free needle, each suture is sewn to the undersurface of the midportion of the vaginal vault (Figures 6.32 to 6.34), but the colpopexy stitches are not tied until later in the operation.
8. Any necessary anterior colporrhaphy is accomplished. Full-length anterior colporrhaphy with special attention to the supports of the cystourethral junction is performed almost without exception. Such support usually includes plication of the pubourethral "ligament" portion of the urogenital diaphragm beneath the urethra using a permanent or a long-acting absorbable suture such as polydiaxanone-type (PDS or Maxon). Colporrhaphy by this method will effectively treat or prevent postoperative SUI or prevent postoperative incontinence that could result from the change in the vaginal axis that occurs with the sacral colpopexy. A coincident uncommon low-pressure urethra may require a vesicourethral sling procedure to effectively elevate intraurethral pressure under stress to a continent level.
9. The upper portion of the posterior colporrhaphy is begun at the vault of the vagina by a side-to-side, running spiral, subcuticular suture that in-

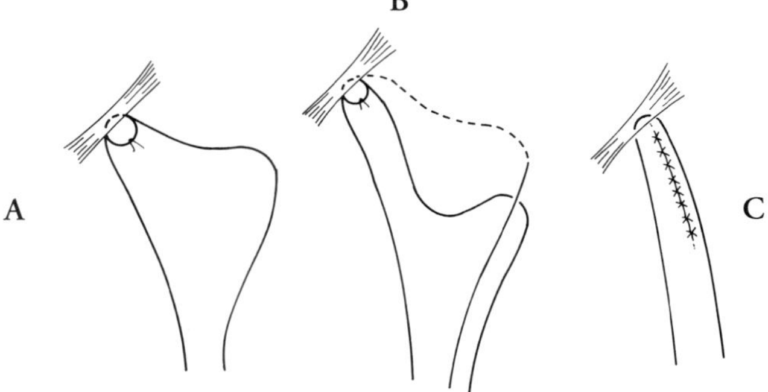

Figure 6.31 **A**, A wide vaginal vault illustrated at the left following sacrospinous colpopexy. The result of failure to narrow this wide vault is shown in **B**, in which there may be prolapse of the left side. The result of narrowing this wide vault by excision of a proper width tissue from the anterior and posterior vaginal wall is shown in **C**, which has converted the shape of the vagina to that of a cylinder of more or less uniform diameter. It is now an instrument of coitus and not parturition. (Redrawn from Nichols DH and Randall CL: Vaginal surgery, ed 4, Baltimore, 1996, Williams & Wilkins.)

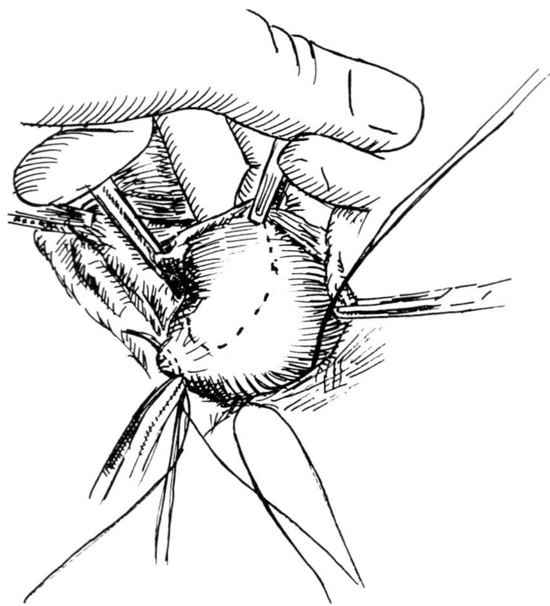

Figure 6.32 The free end of the colpopexy suture is sewn through the undersurface of the fibromuscular wall of the vagina at the site of the new vaginal apex.

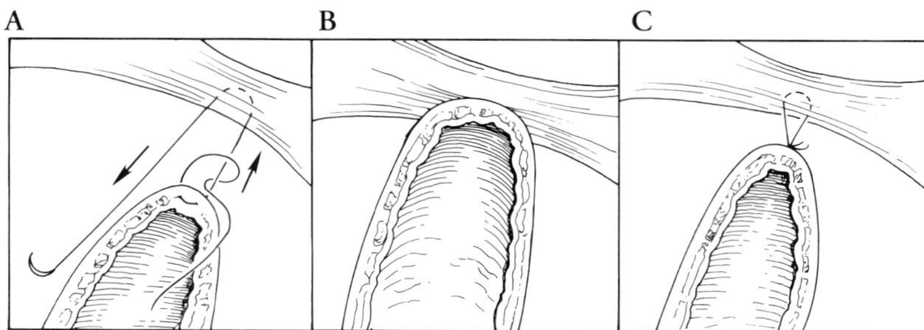

Figure 6.33 The "pulley" stitch is shown. One end of the suture through the sacrospinous ligament has been sewn to the undersurface of the cut edge of the vaginal vault and the stitch tied (**A**). Traction to the other end of the suture draws the vagina up and laterally to the surface of the ligament. When the ends have been tied together, the vagina is fixed to the surface of the sacrospinous ligament–coccygeus muscle complex at this point (**B**). A second or "safety" stitch for reinforcement of this attachment may be placed through the ligament. Failure to tie this stitch snugly will result in a suture bridge (**C**), which should be avoided, if possible, because the weak scar that results threatens the security of the attachment. (Redrawn from Nichols DH and Randall CL: Vaginal surgery, ed 4, Baltimore, 1996, Williams & Wilkins.)

corporates the full thickness of the posterior vaginal wall yet carefully avoids the anterior wall of the rectum to prevent obliteration of the rectovaginal space. This stitch continues to the midportion of the posterior vaginal wall.

10. At this point, the sacrospinous colpopexy stitches are tied, firmly attaching the vagina to the surface of the sacrospinous ligament–coccygeus muscle complex with no intervening bridge of suture material (Figure 6.33).
11. Posterior colporrhaphy is completed.
12. Any necessary perineorrhaphy is accomplished.
13. Rectal examination confirms integrity of the rectum, and vaginal packing may be inserted overnight, if desired.

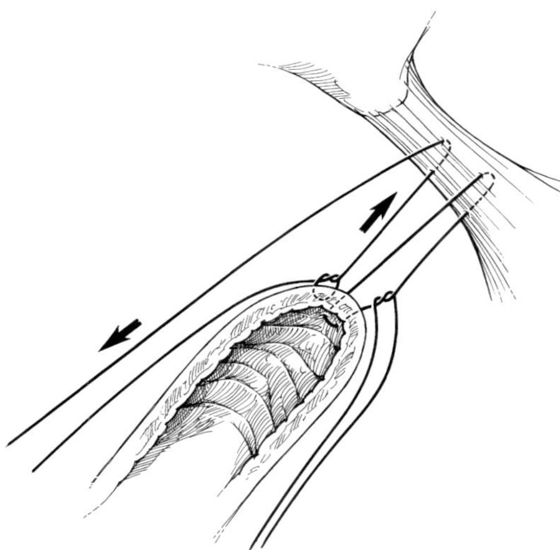

FIGURE 6.34 Tying the colpopexy sutures, knots buried. The nonabsorbable monofilament suture may be placed as a pulley stitch, as shown. The monofilament absorbable suture may be placed through the full thickness of the posterior wall with two penetrations about 1 cm apart for tying after the pulley stitch has been tied. The thin vaginal wall between the penetrations acts as a bolster. (Redrawn from Nichols DH and Randall CL: Vaginal surgery, ed 4, Baltimore, 1996, Williams & Wilkins.)

When the patient has a history of previous surgery in this area, the anatomic relationships are often distorted by fibrosis and adhesions. This distortion complicates the ease with which the surgeon can find the lateral wall of the pararectal space. Nevertheless, when one follows the previous steps, identification and entry into the pararectal space is anatomically and surgically precise. Alternatively, the space and structure of the patient's left side may be used.

The longer a massive eversion has been present, the greater the length as well as width of the vagina. Such a long vagina must be reduced in length and width to prevent recurrent cystocele in the patient having transvaginal sacrospinous colpopexy with colporrhaphy.

Transabdominal Repair

If the operator is more comfortable with transabdominal surgery, and especially if there is some pressing reason for a transabdominal approach such as the presence of a suspicious lesion of the adnexa, hysterectomy and colpopexy can be performed by the abdominal route. When there is a minor degree of vault prolapse, the McCall-type cul-de-plasty can be used transabdominally as well with great effectiveness, provided that the uterosacral ligaments are strong. Any pathologic widening of the vaginal vault should be corrected by excision of an appropriate wedge from either posterior or anterior vaginal wall, with reapproximation of the cut edges of each by a running suture. A deep cul-de-sac should be obliterated by either the sagittally placed sutures of Halban[1,17] or the circumferential sutures of Moschcowitz,[18] either of which will lessen the tendency toward future enterocele. Any remaining cystocele or rectocele should be repaired by appropriate colporrhaphy, whether the hysterectomy was transvaginal or transabdominal. With transabdominal hysterectomy and the McCall or New Orleans–type cul-de-plasty, the surgeon must be particularly mindful of the possibility of interference with the path of the ureter, because it is more vulnerable in the transabdominal approach when cul-de-plasty stitches have been placed more laterally. The position of the ureter should be verified before the passage and tying of each stitch. At the conclusion of the procedure, it is helpful to give the patient 5 ml of IV indigo carmine and perform an observation cystoscopy 5 or 6 minutes later to observe the efflux of dye from each of the ureteral orifices. Such verification of ureteral patency is easily accomplished if the abdominal procedure has been performed with the patient in Allen stirrups.

In a patient with massive posthysterectomy eversion of the vagina in whom a transabdominal approach is desired, it is possible to support the vault of the vagina by a ligament attaching it to the periosteum in the hollow of the sacrum through a retroperitoneal tunnel.[19,20] In this transabdominal sacral colpopexy, the surgeon may once again use fascia lata, but many will prefer to save the patient the attendant painful leg and use a synthetic plastic such as Mersilene mesh. The mesh should be attached by multiple nonabsorbable sutures both to the vaginal vault and to the presacral ligament (Figure 6.35). Simultaneous

Text continued on p. 86.

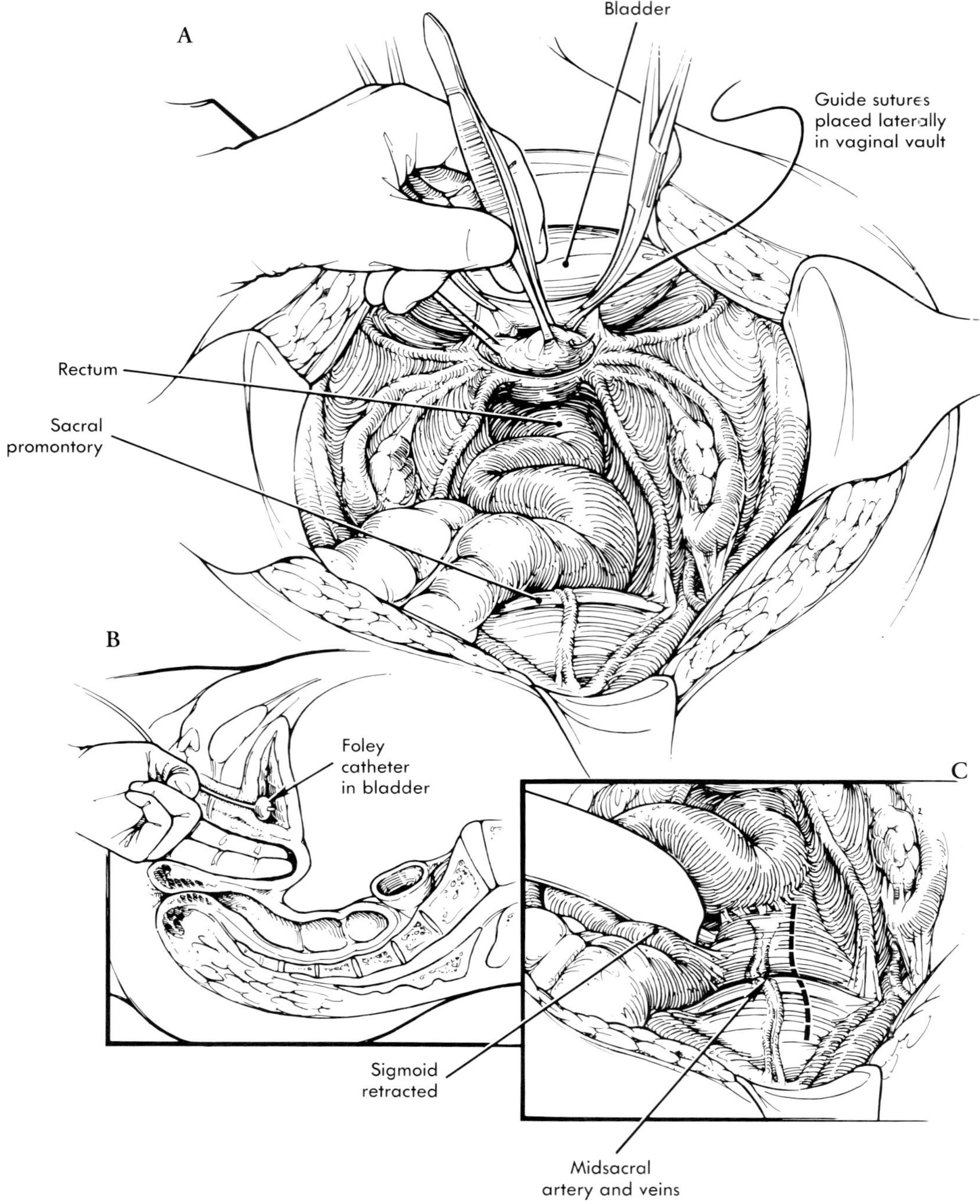

FIGURE 6.35 Transabdominal sacral colpopexy. **A**, The abdomen has been opened by a midline incision. The vaginal vault is manually elevated, as shown (**B**) and the peritoneum covering it is incised transversely (**A**). Bowel is packed out of the way, and the promontory of the sacrum is exposed. The peritoneum overlying the promontory is incised as shown by the *broken line* (**C**).

Continued.

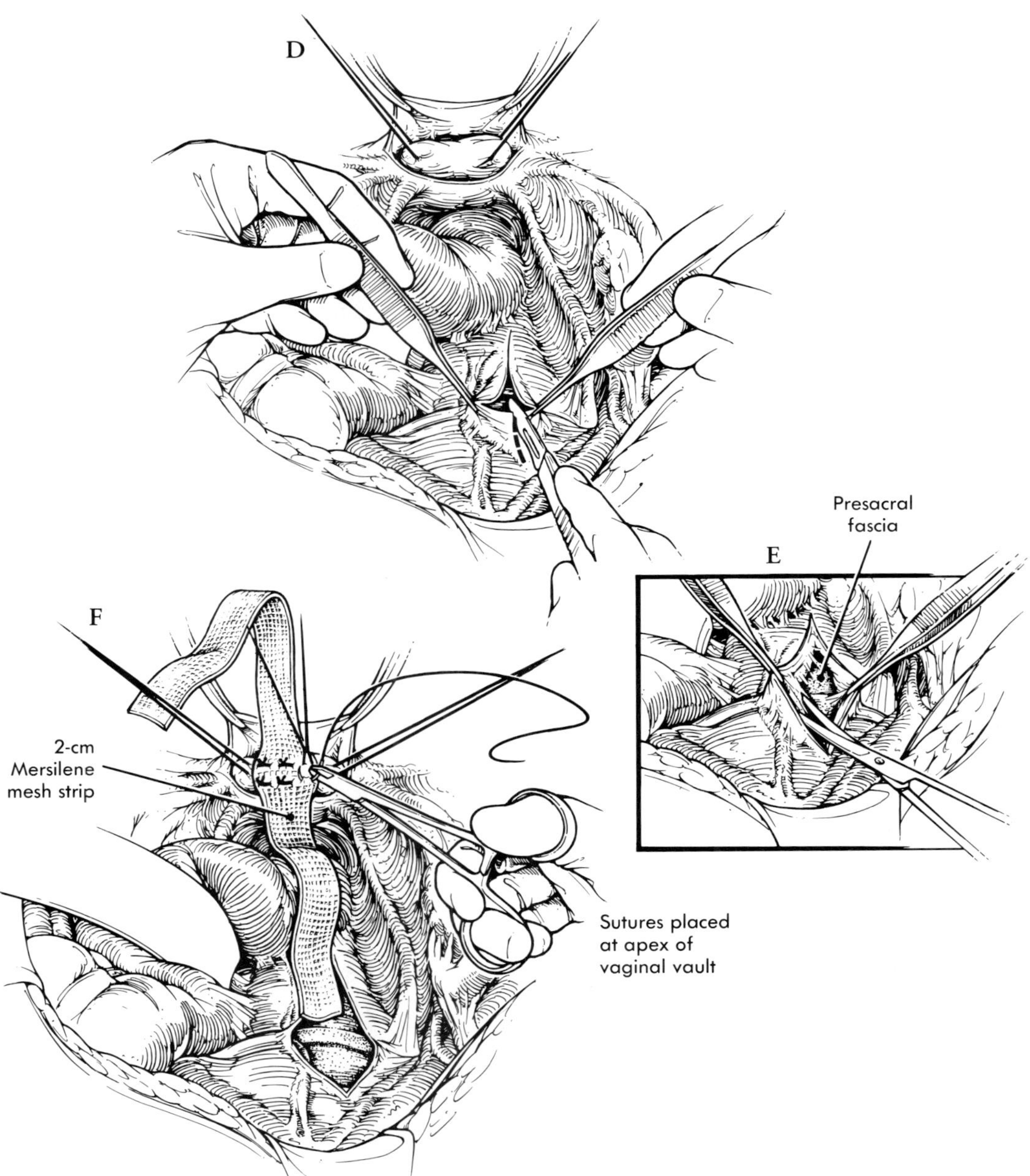

FIGURE 6.35, cont'd. The tissues are carefully separated (**D**), exposing the presacral fascia (**E**). The central belly of a precut band of polyester (Mersilene) or fascia lata is sewn to the vaginal vault (**F**).

Continued.

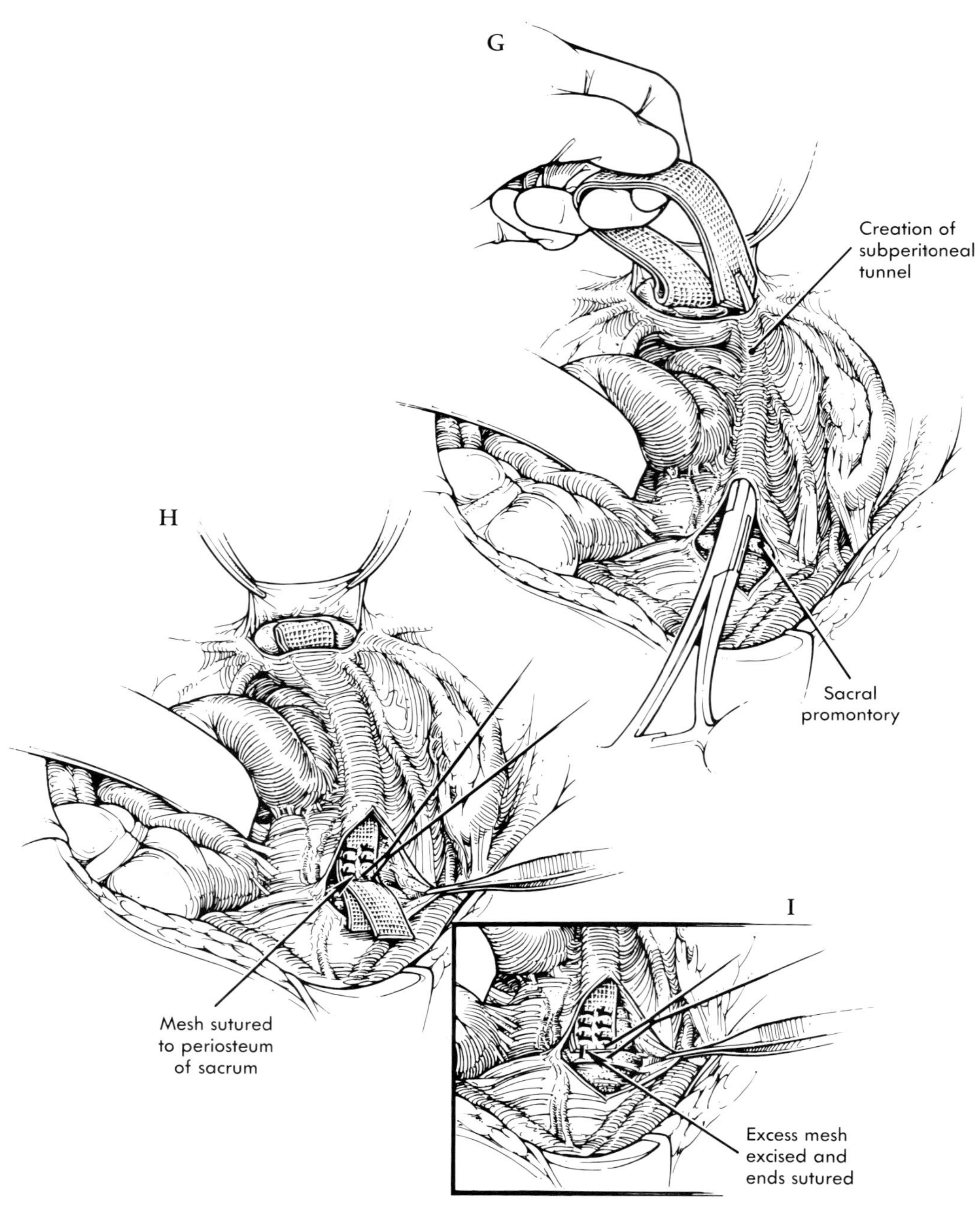

FIGURE 6.35, **cont'd.** A subperitoneal tunnel beneath the peritoneum has been established, and a long Kelly's forceps is introduced to grasp the free ends of the polyester or fascia (**G**), which is drawn through the tunnel and sewn to the presacral fascia and periosteum (**H**). The excess mesh is excised (**I**).

Continued.

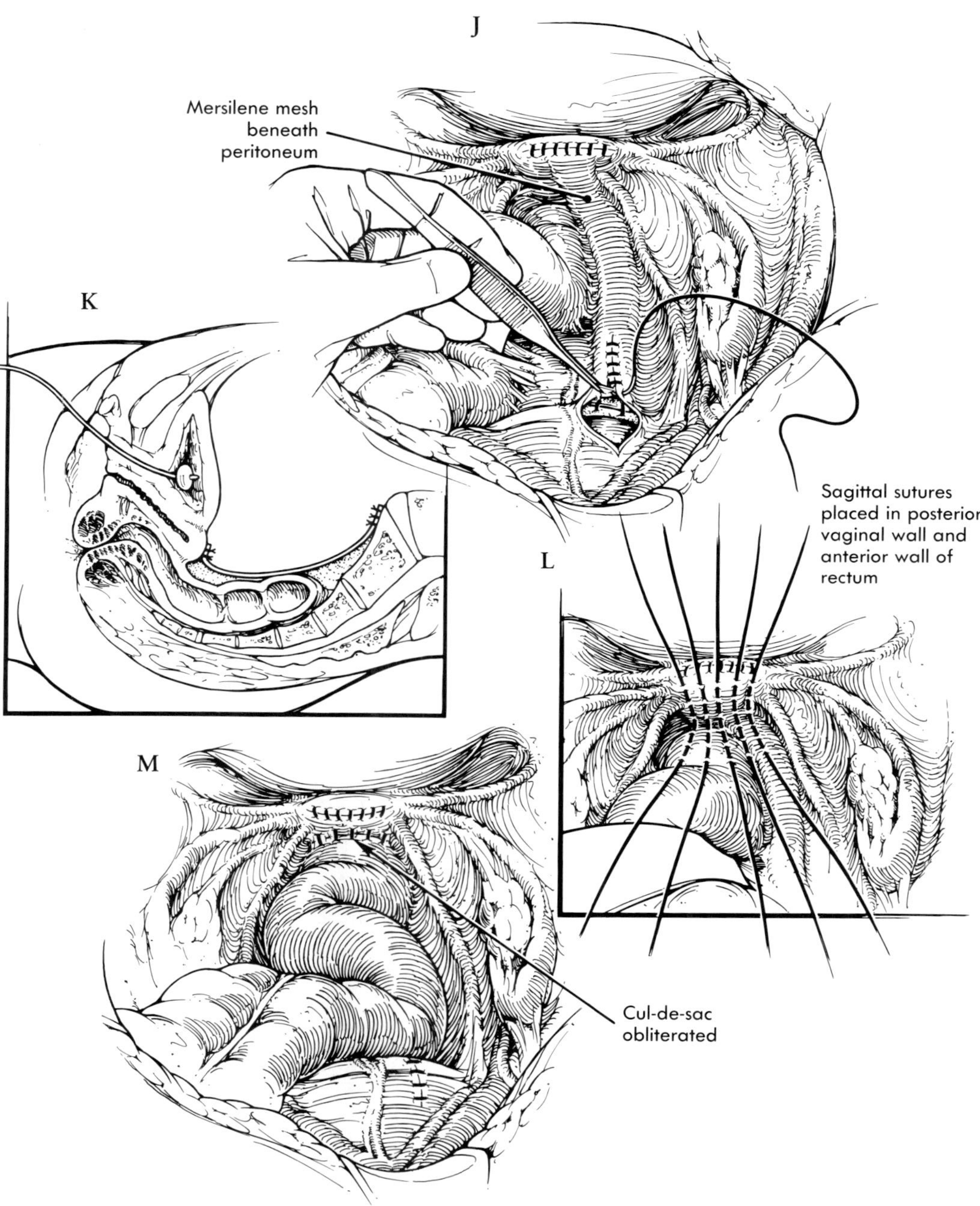

FIGURE 6.35, **cont'd.** The peritoneum is closed (J). Sagittal view (**K**) shows the end result of the sacral colpopexy. The surfaces of the cul-de-sac of Douglas are approximated by sagittally placed sutures (**L**), thus obliterating the cul-de-sac (**M**), and the abdomen is closed. (From Nichols DH, editor: Gynecologic and obstetric surgery, St Louis, 1993, Mosby.)

appropriate colporrhaphy may correct any significant cystocele and rectocele, and coincident enterocele can be excised along with the primary procedure.

Other Techniques

For the occasional patient, often one who is bedridden, is infirm, and can no longer wear an intravaginal pessary, conservation of vaginal function may no longer be a prerequisite. In such cases, there is a place for the Le Fort colpocleisis (Figure 6.36) if the uterus is present or colpectomy[1,19] (Figure 6.37) if the uterus has been removed. Rarely, the surgeon may elect vaginal hysterectomy with colpectomy as a means of providing permanent obliteration of the vaginal canal.

With Le Fort's colpocleisis (or partial colpectomy), a rectangle of tissue is removed from the upper anterior vaginal wall and the upper posterior vaginal wall. The posterior surface of the bladder is then sewn directly to the anterior surface of the rectum, leaving a permanent lateral drainage canal across the vault and along both sides of the centrally obliterated vagina.

The operation is relatively simple but has three principal disadvantages:

1. The coital use of the vagina and the patient's concept of her vagina as a part

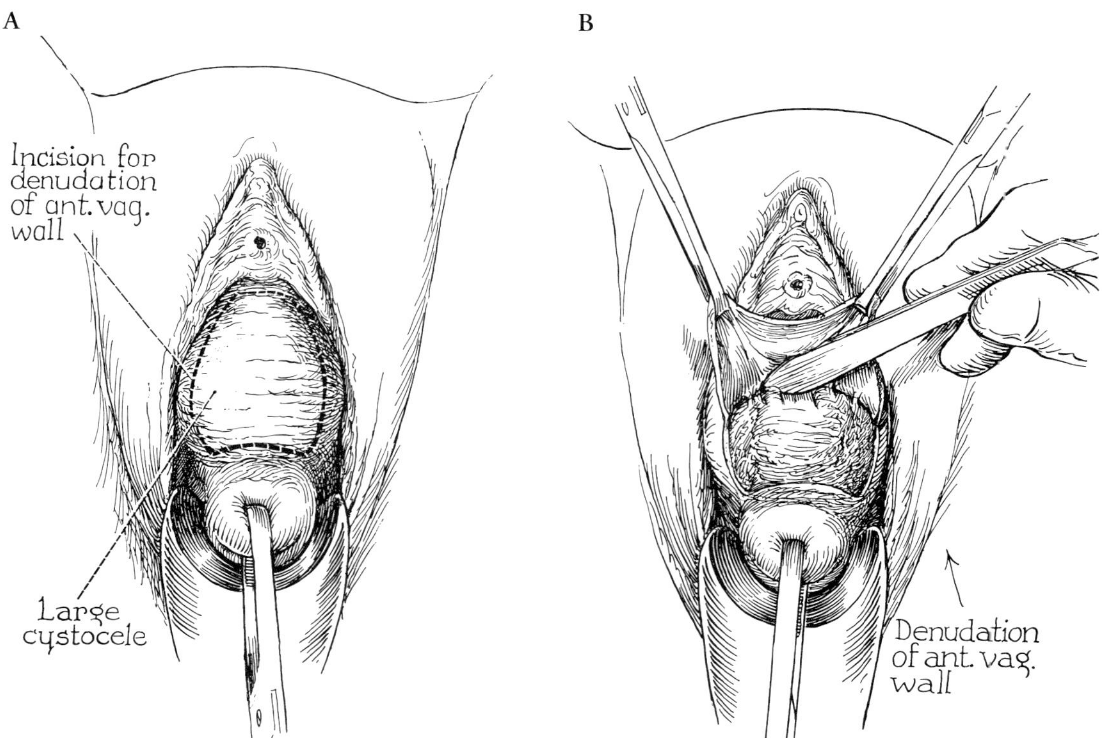

FIGURE 6.36 **A,** An area to be denuded is outlined from the external urinary meatus to the bladder reflection on the cervix. Along the outline, an incision is made that extends through the mucosa and superficial musculature of the vaginal wall. **B,** The area is now denuded of mucosa, leaving as much of the muscular wall as is possible while dissecting in this unnatural line of cleavage. Considerable general oozing may be encountered despite the fact that patients subjected to this procedure are postmenopausal.

Continued.

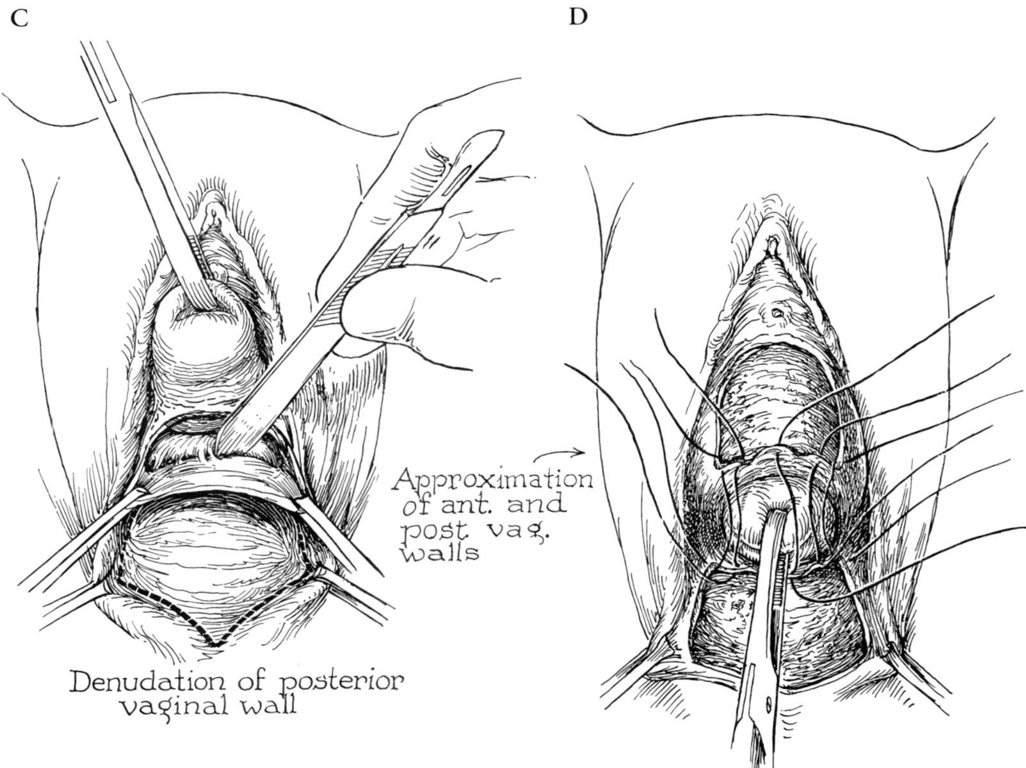

FIGURE 6.36, cont'd. **C,** A similar area is denuded posteriorly but also including a triangular area of the skin of the perineum. Bilateral strips of mucosa are left. **D,** Using interrupted sutures of 00 polyglycolic acid, the mucosa of the vault is approximated over the cervix. After the anterior wall has been united to the posterior, the lateral edges on each side are approximated.

Continued.

of her intrinsic femininity may be destroyed.

2. If there is an enterocele present, it will still be present postoperatively, because the operation is essentially extraperitoneal. The persistent enterocele may progress and ultimately continue downward to distend the perineum, with as many symptoms as were present with the original prolapse.
3. Occasionally a patient will develop postoperative SUI following a Le Fort's colpocleisis. This can be most difficult to treat, because the base of the bladder is fused to the anterior surface of the rectum, straightening out the cystourethral angle.

A disadvantage of colpectomy, on the other hand, is the sometimes generous blood loss associated with transection of the vaginal blood supply at its lateral margins. To combat this problem the surgeon may, following excision of the vagina, bring together the covering fascia of the levatores ani in the midline and thoroughly pack the remaining pelvic cavity with iodoform gauze. Starting on the fifth postoperative day, the gauze packing is gradually removed a little bit at a time over a period of several days. The residual cavity will quickly shrink, become covered with healthy granulation tissue, and finally be obliterated over a period of several weeks. The process is less complicated than seeking to

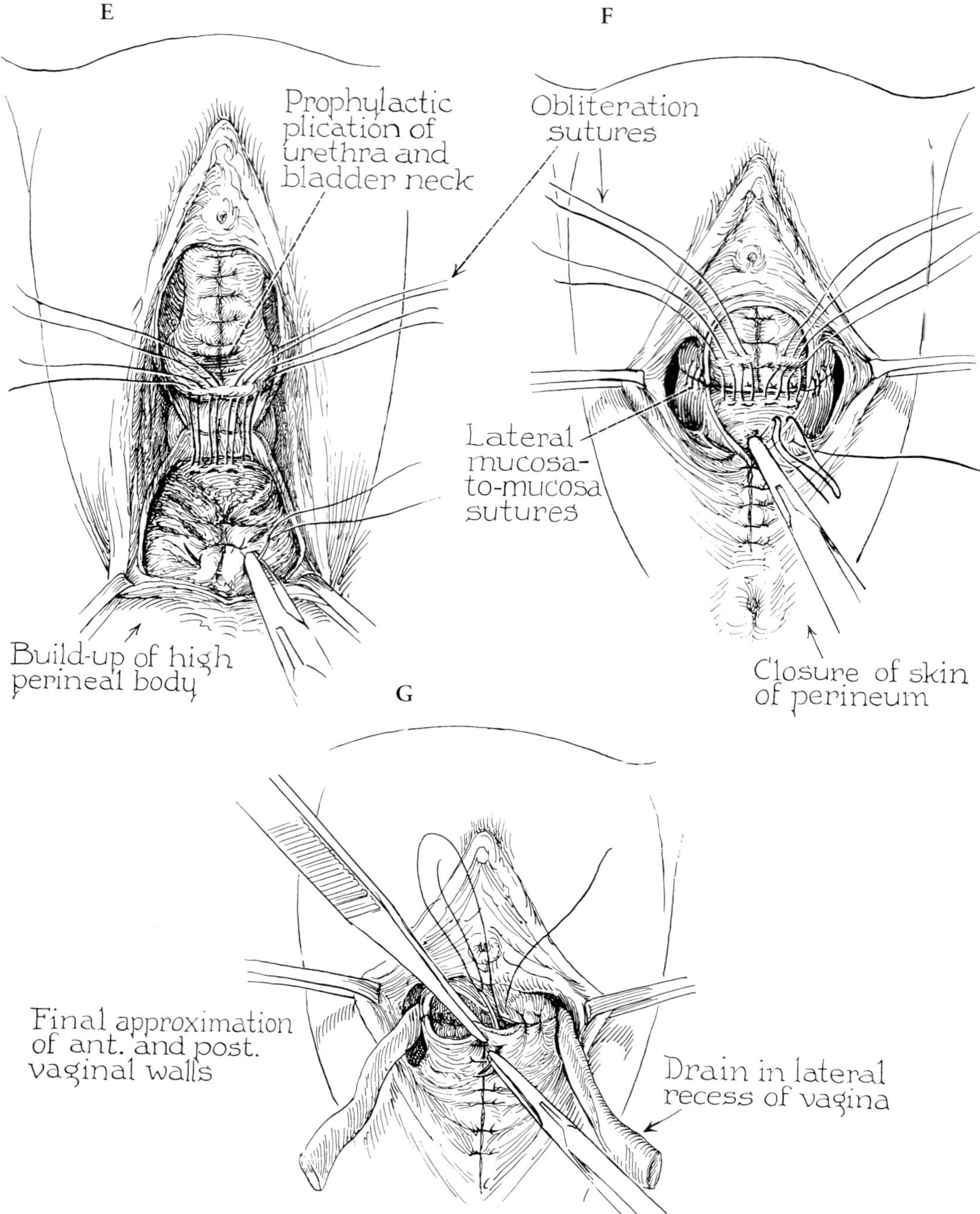

FIGURE 6.36, cont'd. E, The denuded vaginal wall is approximated anteroposteriorly by a series of mattress sutures in conjunction with the mucosal closure. When the area of the bladder neck is reached, this is plicated not only in the event of stress incontinence, but also for prophylactic purposes. F, The musculature of the perineal body is built up with interrupted sutures to aid in the obliteration of the genital aperture. Successive rows of mattress sutures continue the obliteration of the vaginal canal. The skin of the perineum is approximated in the midline by interrupted sutures. G, The remainder of the anteroposterior approximation is done, and drains are placed in both of the lateral tunnels of the vagina that result. (From Ball TL: Gynecologic surgery and urology, St Louis, 1963, Mosby.)

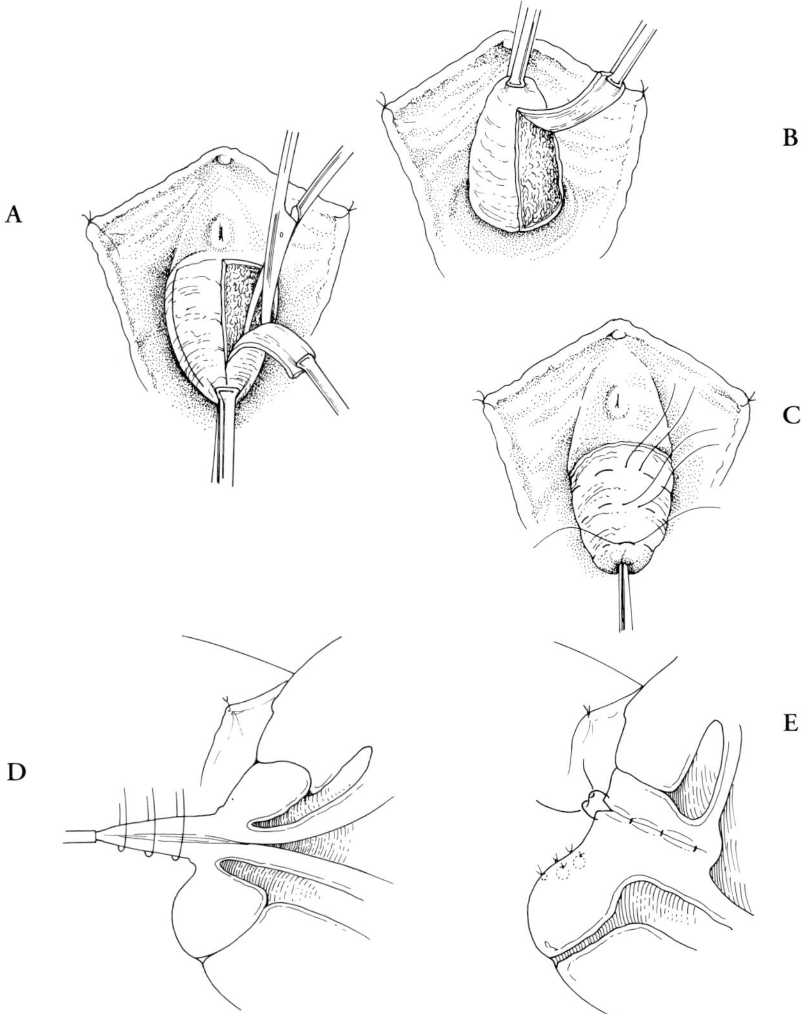

Figure 6.37 The technique of total colpectomy. After subcutaneous infiltration by 0.5% lidocaine in 1:200,000 epinephrine solution, the vagina is circumscribed by an incision at the hymen and marked into quadrants, each of which is separately removed by sharp dissection (**A** and **B**). A series of purse-string, synthetic absorbable sutures is placed (**C**) and tied, with progressive inversion of the soft tissue before tying each suture (**D**) so that the final result is as shown in **E.** An appropriate perineorrhaphy may complete the operation. (Redrawn from Nichols DH and Randall CL: Vaginal surgery, ed 4, Baltimore, 1996, Williams & Wilkins.)

obliterate the vaginal cavity by sewing it tightly shut in its entirety. This latter feat is rather difficult to achieve without leaving little pockets of dead space in which troublesome postoperative hematoma or seroma may form.

For the symptomatic prolapse patient awaiting future surgery or for the occasional patient at high operative risk, insertion of a proper-sized Gellhorn's pessary provides temporary pelvic support and relief of discomfort, presuming that the pelvic diaphragm is effectively able to contract and permit the pessary to be retained (Figure 6.38).

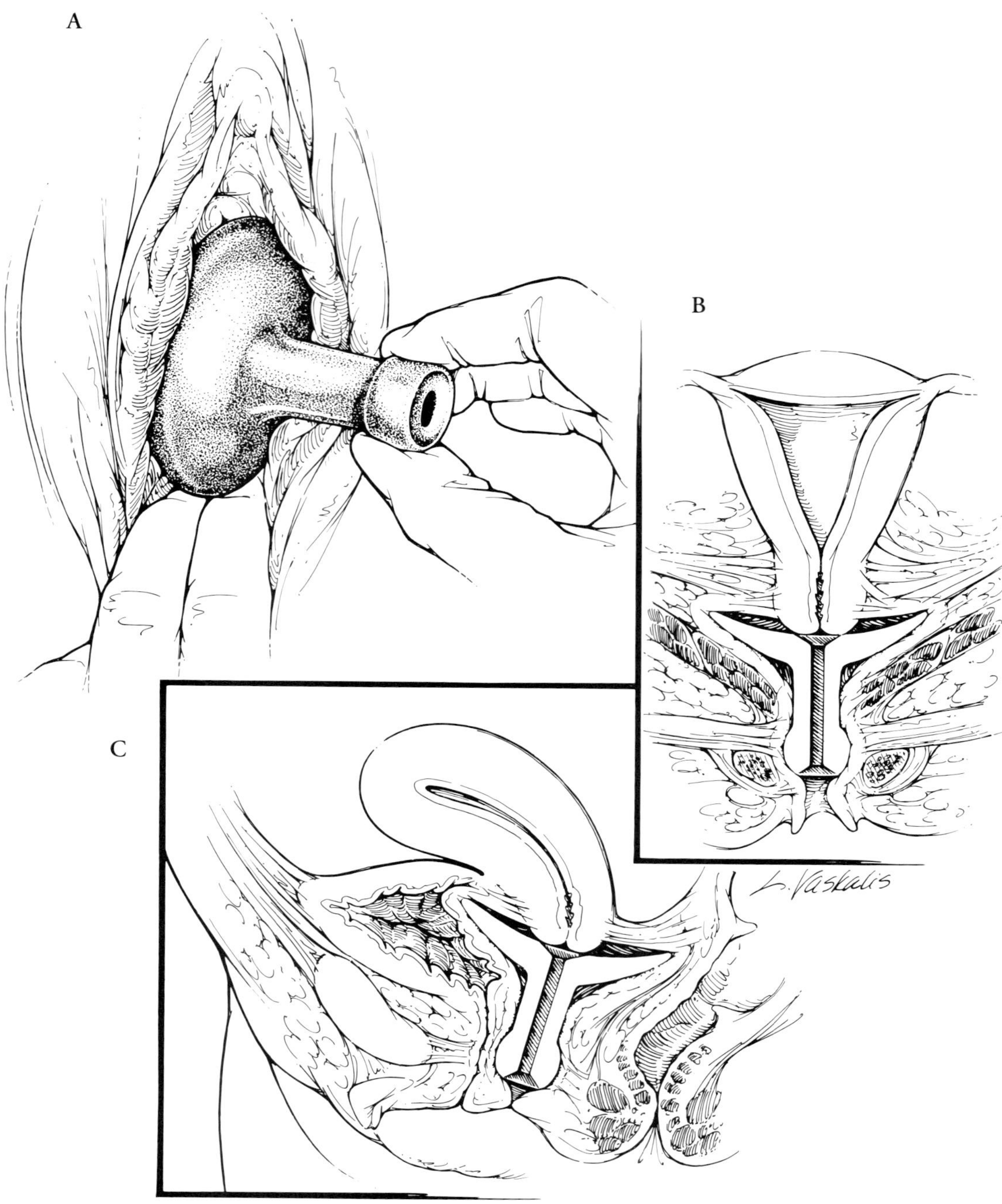

Figure 6.38 Insertion of a Gellhorn's pessary. **A,** The perineum is depressed, and the disk portion of the pessary is inserted using downward pressure against the perineum. **B,** It should rest comfortably, being retained above an effective pelvic diaphragm. **C,** Notice in sagittal section that the properly fitted pessary elevates the vaginal vault and uterus to a position once again within the pelvis and, at the same time, relieves some of the distension of the cystocele and rectocele. (From Nichols DH, editor: Gynecologic and obstetric surgery, St Louis, 1993, Mosby.)

REFERENCES

1. Nichols DH and Randall CL: Vaginal surgery, ed 4, Baltimore, 1996, Williams & Wilkins.
2. Given FT Jr: Is posthysterectomy vaginal vault prolapse preventable? J Gynecol Surg 8:201, 1992.
3. Given FT Jr, Muhlendorf IK, and Browning GM: Vaginal length and sexual function after colpopexy for complete uterovaginal eversion, Am J Obstet Gynecol 169:284, 1993.
4. Wall LL and Hewitt JK: Urodynamic characteristics of women with complete posthysterectomy vaginal vault prolapse, Urology 44:336, 1994.
5. Rosenzweig BA and others: Prevalence of abnormal urodynamic test results in continent women with severe genitourinary prolapse, Obstet Gynecol 79:539, 1992.
6. Nichols DH, Milley PS, and Randall CL: Significance of restoration of normal vaginal depth and axis, Obstet Gynecol 36:241, 1970.
7. Bonney V: The sustentacular of the female genital canal, the displacements that result from the yielding of its several components, and then appropriate treatment, J Obstet Gynaecol Br Emp 45:328, 1914.
8. White GR: An anatomical operation for the cure of cystocele, JAMA 53:1707, 1909.
9. Baden WF and Walker TA: Physical diagnosis in the evaluation of vaginal relaxation, Clin Obstet Gynecol 15:1060, 1972.
10. Burch JC: Urethrovaginal fixation to Cooper's ligament for stress incontinence, Am J Obstet Gynecol 81:2, 1961.
11. Symmonds R and others: Posthysterectomy enterocele and vaginal vault prolapse, Am J Obstet Gynecol 140:852, 1981.
12. Carey MP and Slack MC: Transvaginal sacrospinous colpopexy for vault and marked uterovaginal prolapse, Br J Obstet Gynaecol 101:536, 1994.
13. Nichols DH: Sacrospinous fixation for massive eversion of the vagina, Am J Obstet Gynecol 142:901, 1982.
14. Richter K and Albrich W: Long-term results following fixation of the vagina on the sacrospinal ligament by the vaginal route (vaginaefixatio sacrospinalis vaginalis), Am J Obstet Gynecol 141:811, 1981.
15. Richter K: Massive eversion of the vagina: pathogenesis, diagnosis, and therapy of the "true" prolapse of the vaginal stump, Clin Obstet Gynecol 25:897, 1982.
16. Sederl J: Zur Operation des Prolapses der blind endigenden Scheide, Geburtshilfe Frauenheilkd 18:824, 1958.
17. Halban J: Gynäkologische Operationslehre, Vienna, 1932, Urban & Schwarzenberg.
18. Moschcowitz AV: The pathogenesis, anatomy, and care of prolapse of the rectum, Surg Gynecol Obstet 15:18, 1912.
19. Nichols DH, (editor): Gynecologic and obstetric surgery, St Louis, 1993, Mosby.
20. Parsons L and Ulfelder H: An atlas of pelvic operations, ed 2, Philadelphia, 1968, WB Saunders Co.
21. Sharp TR: Sacrospinous suspension made easy, Obstet Gynecol 82:873, 1993.

7

Recurrent Cystocele

GEORGE B. MCCLURE
DAVID H. NICHOLS

When bulging of the anterior vaginal wall consistent with recurrent cystocele occurs after previous surgery to repair the same, the pelvic surgeon's challenge is to make a thorough assessment of the defect, to determine factors that might have predisposed toward the recurrence, and to develop a treatment plan that will give the greatest likelihood of a permanent and effective repair. The patient experiencing recurrent cystocele may have an ill-defined feeling of fullness in her vagina. These feelings may worsen over the course of the day, due to the effects of gravity, and are usually relieved by lying down. In many cases, however, recurrent cystocele may be asymptomatic and may be appreciated only during routine annual examination. In either instance when it has been demonstrated, the recurrent cystocele should be followed by periodic examination, and the care provider should develop a plan for evaluation of the rate of progression and its possible future treatment.

PERSISTENCE VERSUS RECURRENCE

Upon noting a "recurrent" cystocele, the surgeon should determine whether this is truly a recurrent cystocele or in fact a persistent one. The time when the cystocele was first noted postoperatively is significant in determining this. If the cystocele is noted at the first postoperative examination, it is probably the consequence of inadequate initial anterior colporrhaphy. In evaluating the problem, the surgeon should consider whether the recurrence is due to an incorrectly chosen initial procedure, whether the surgery was inexpertly performed, and whether the choice of a short-acting catgut suture contributed to poor scar formation as opposed to the use of a long-lasting synthetic or even permanent suture material that might be associated with a stronger scar. The cystocele seen for the first time 2 years or more after the original surgery is more likely to be a recurrent one. The surgeon should ask over how long a period of postoperative time it developed and whether it is continuing to progress. The examiner should determine if it is accompanied by any other signs of pelvic herniation or weakness. Does it appear to be a consequence of the continuation of the normal aging process or of a lifestyle persistently characterized by increased intraabdominal pressure (e.g., chronic constipation, heavy lifting, chronic respiratory disease, or smoking)? Do these findings represent an extension of a herniation process beyond that which was present at the time of the initial surgery? Additionally, might the recurrent cystocele represent the consequence of failure to repair coexistent accessory damage such as previously unrecognized partial eversion of the vaginal vault, a large rectocele, or a paravaginal or perineal defect that may have been present at the time of the initial surgery? To make such determinations, the surgeon should obtain a copy of the surgical dictation from each of the previous operative experiences to correlate them with the present findings on examination.

EVALUATION

History

A thorough history should be taken from an individual experiencing the recurrence of a cystocele. Pertinent questions might include some or all of the following:

General
Is the patient postmenopausal?
If so, is she receiving the necessary estrogen supplementation?
Is estrogen supplementation being given vaginally, systemically, or both?
Is the estrogen dose appropriate?
How long has the patient been receiving estrogen replacement therapy?
Bladder
Does the bladder empty completely?
Is there evidence of stress incontinence?
Is this of new onset?
Does the patient report frequency and/or urgency?
Is there a history of recurrent UTI?
If so, is there a trigger for these?
Does the patient have nocturia?
If so, how many episodes per night?
Bowel
Does the patient suffer from constipation?
Does the patient strain at stool?
Are movements incomplete?
Do they require manual expression?
Is there any anal incontinence of either stool or gas?
Vaginal
Is the patient sexually active?
If so, does she report dyspareunia or vaginal dryness?
Respiratory
Does the patient suffer from any respiratory illness that would lead to chronic coughing?
Does she engage in any activity that would lead to persistent increases in intraabdominal pressure?

Physical Examination

A careful and thorough physical evaluation should be performed and the findings correlated with the patient's symptoms. The surgeon should identify all sites of weakness, including cystocele, hypermobility of the vesicourethral junction, paravaginal defect, vaginal detachment, uterine prolapse, prolapse of the vaginal vault, enterocele, rectocele, and perineal defect. The axis and the depth of the vagina should be determined with the patient at rest, then straining by a Valsalva maneuver. Using a single examining finger, the surgeon should note the strength, the symmetry, and the effectiveness of the pubococcygei, first with the patient at rest and then with the patient straining by a Valsalva maneuver. Palpation of the pelvic diaphragm around the vaginal hiatus while the patient is contracting or "holding" will frequently identify a defect in the integrity of the pelvic diaphragm, often a result of avulsion during childbirth many years ago. During a repetition of these maneuvers (i.e., with the patient relaxing, then squeezing, then holding), the surgeon palpates the anterior vaginal sulci[1] to identify any lateral detachment of the vaginal periurethral tissues from the bridge of connective tissue that attaches the vagina to the arcus tendineus. The surgeon should take note whether there is damage on one or both sides. The assessment may be aided by using ovum forceps or another instrument to hold the vaginal sulci bilaterally against the acrus tendineus to assess the degree to which the cystocele is corrected by this maneuver. The patient's recurrent cystocele thus may be due to a midline defect, a paravaginal defect, or a combination of the two with or without coincident vault prolapse.

Pelvic examination is then repeated with the patient in a standing position. All of the previous observations are confirmed or modified. The standing position is, of course, the one in which the effects of gravity are added to the patient's demonstrated weaknesses. The most important single consideration is whether or not the vault of the vagina descends either to mimic cystocele or, by bringing with it portions of the anterior vaginal wall, to cause a displacement-type cystocele. The only restorative treatment for a vault prolapse is effective colpopexy,[2] usually using the transvaginal route, but occasionally through a transabdominal approach.

The surgeon should estimate in centimeters the extent to which the bladder sags beneath the inferior margin of the pubis when the standing patient strains.

With the patient in the standing position, the rectum is examined for weakness of the posterior vaginal wall and coincident rectal prolapse. The surgeon places one finger in the patient's rectum and the thumb in the vagina and has the patient strain. This examination can determine not only the presence of a previously unsuspected and undetected vault prolapse, but by spreading the fingertip and

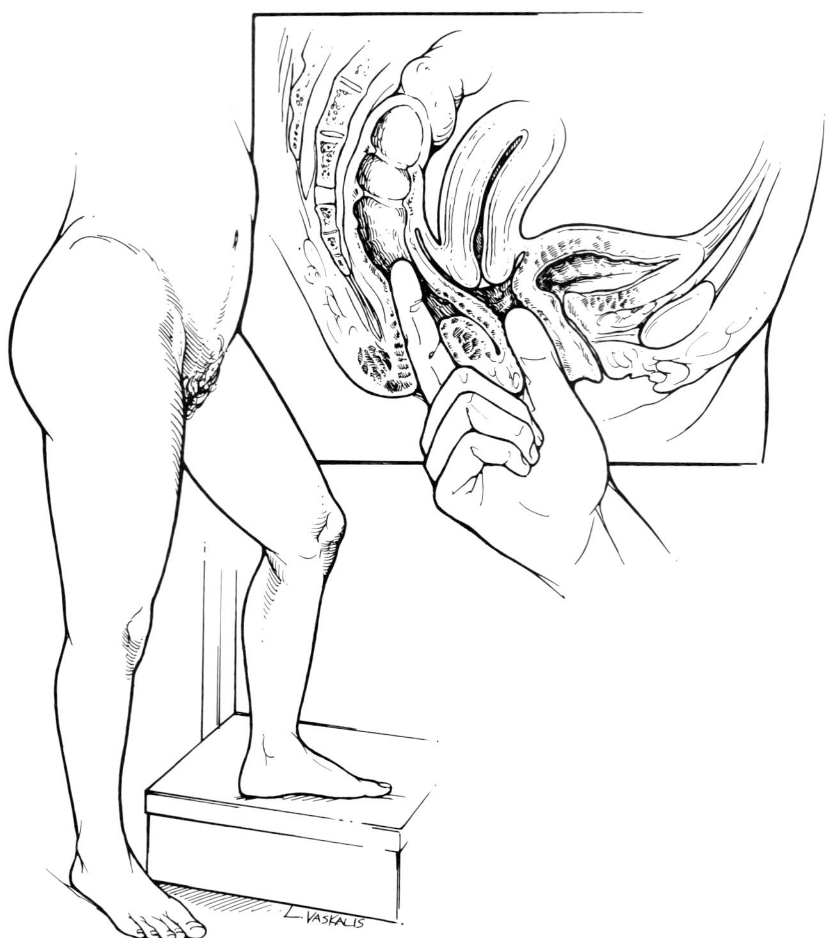

Figure 7.1 Examination of the patient in the standing position permits the thumb in the vagina to note and replace any descent of the vaginal vault, while the index finger introduced into the rectum permits evaluation of any possible rectocele. When the patient strains, any enterocele present is evidenced by palpation of a bowel-filled sac prolapse dissecting the rectovaginal septum. (From Nichols DH: Gynecologic and obsteric surgery, St Louis, 1993, Mosby.)

thumb and asking the patient to strain, the physician can also palpate an enterocele between the thumb and index finger (Figure 7.1).

Urodynamic Evaluation

Urinary incontinence after anterior colporrhaphy in patients previously continent may unmask a previously undiagnosed urethral sphincter weakness. This is particularly evident among older women, in whom it is not uncommonly related to a low urethral closure pressure.[3] Lacking sophisticated testing equipment, this possibility can be predicted by packing the vagina during preoperative evaluation, which will temporarily relieve the urethral kinking produced by the cystocele, and asking the patient to perform a series of Valsalva maneuvers and observe whether or not there is coincident leakage of urine.[4] This possibility can be further suspected if it possible to draw the partly inflated (0.5 ml) bulb of no. 8 pediatric Foley catheter through the urethra with ease.[2] The likelihood of a clinically significant low urethral closure pressure is so great that such as patient should undergo urodynamic testing to include assessment of the urethral pressure profile.

When symptoms warrant and surgical intervention for the recurrent cystocele is contemplated, preoperative complex urodynamic evaluation in the laboratory is warranted. This recommendation is made even if the history does not reveal symptoms of urinary incontinence. The rationale for such a recommendation is twofold. First, urodynamic assessment of the incontinence mechanism(s) in effect preoperatively may help the reconstructive surgeon predict which patients might become incontinent after reconstruction. With this information the surgical plan could be augmented to offer some prevention against this occurrence. Secondly, the urodynamic assessment in the previously operated patient may provide the surgeon with some insight into the reason for the initial failure, particularly if incontinence was an indication for the primary procedure. Again, with this knowledge, the surgeon could offer a prudent and rational operative plan to the patient and describe the likelihood of its success.

Components of a complex urodynamic evaluation that might affect a reoperative surgical plan are described in the following discussion.

Cystometry. Cystometry can be best described as an assessment of the pressure within the bladder during a period of filling and storage. The filling medium may be fluid or gas, preferably the former as liquid is noncompressible. There are a variety of methods from which to choose, ranging from "simple" office techniques (Figure 7.2) to multichanneled, subtractive, computer-enhanced techniques. The surgeon preparing for repair of a recurrent cystocele should use cystometry to look for the presence of uninhibited detrusor muscle contractions, a condition also known as detrusor instability. Cystocele repair would not be expected to improve urinary incontinence determined preoperatively to be due to detrusor instability. Conversely, when recurrent cystocele and urinary incontinence coexist in the absence of detrusor instability, appropriate colporrhaphy should help rectify the situation.

Urethral Pressure Profile. The urethral pressure profile is performed using multichannel subtractive urodynamic techniques. A dual microtransducer catheter allows for the simultaneous measurement of bladder (P_{ves}) and urethral (P_{ure}) pressure. The difference between these two $P_{ure} - P_{ves}$ is known as the urethral closure pressure. By withdrawing the

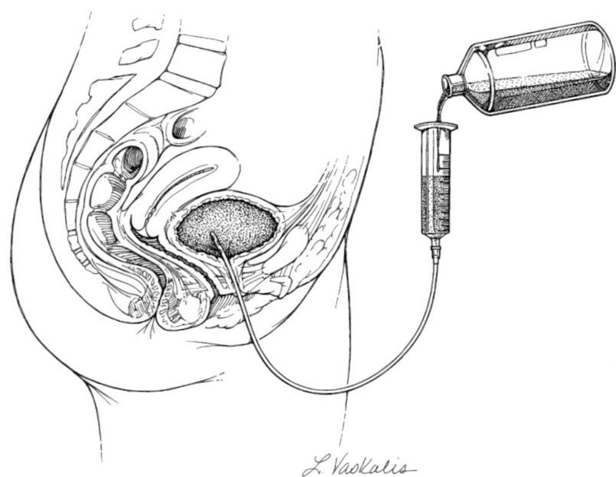

Figure 7.2 Simple "eyeball" cystometry can be done in the office setting. Increments of sterile saline are instilled through an open-ended Asepto syringe barrel as shown, the observer watching the fluid level. A rise in the fluid level would signal a provoked detrusor contraction, suggesting the possibility of detrusor instability as a cause of the incontinence.

catheter through the full length of the urethra and recording all pressures, the surgeon obtains the urethral pressure profile and can calculate the maximum urethral closure pressure (MUCP) and the functional urethral length (FUL). Studies by McGuire have shown that an MUCP of less than 20 cm H_2O is indicative of a low urethral closure pressure.[5] Patients with such a finding have a significant risk for postoperative urinary incontinence if the low-pressure urethra is not addressed surgically with an appropriate procedure (such as a vesicourethral sling) at the time of recurrent cystocele repair. Additionally, the relative amount of abdominal pressure exerted on the bladder and the urethra can be measured by simultaneously recording the pressure in each structure during coughing. *Change* in urethral pressure divided by the *change* in bladder pressure, expressed as a percentage, is known as the pressure transmission ratio (PTR). In normal continent women any increase in the abdominal pressure should be equally distributed to the bladder and the urethra, and thus the PTR should approach 100%. Pressure transmission ratios of less than 90% have been shown to be a sensitive indication of genuine stress incontinence.[6] Furthermore, the higher the postoperative PTR, the more likely it is for the surgery to be successful when an anticontinence procedure has been performed.

Voiding Mechanism. Prior to performing any procedure where the intent is to partially obstruct the urethra for the maintenance of continence, it is helpful to determine the mechanism(s) by which the patient voids. This can be determined by measuring the pressure while the patient voids, with microtip pressure transducers in the bladder and in the vagina (the latter an indication of abdominal pressure). By comparing the measured detrusor pressure with the abdominal pressure, the surgeon can readily determine whether the patient voids by detrusor contraction, Valsalva maneuver, or a combination of these. This information should be useful to predict which patient may require prolonged bladder drainage[7] postoperatively. Additionally, patients who void using a significant Valsalva mechanism and are to undergo a suburethral sling procedure as part of the recurrent cystocele repair must be made aware that continued bearing down at urination postoperatively will result in closure of the urethra and urinary retention. This should be avoided by giving preoperative instructions in alternate voiding mechanisms involving relaxation rather than bearing down.

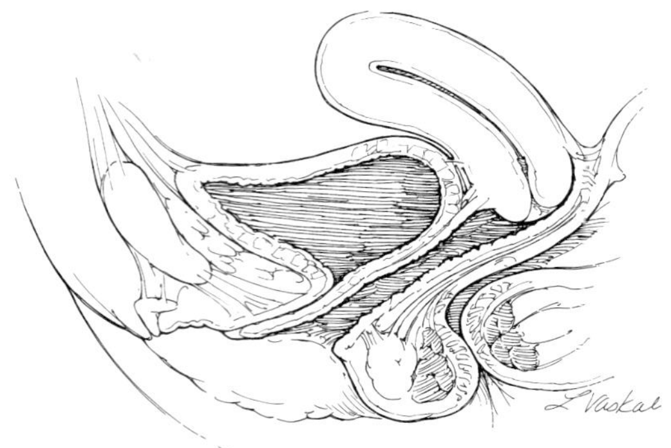

FIGURE 7.3 Rotational descent of the bladder neck.

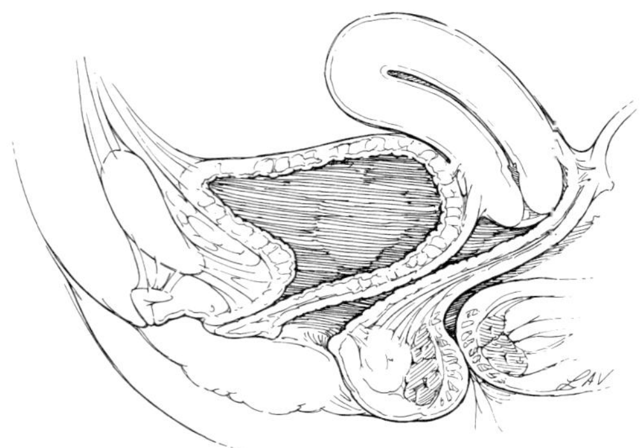

FIGURE 7.4 Funneling of the urethra and rotational descent of the vesicourethral junction.

TYPES OF RECURRENT CYSTOCELE

There may be a somewhat diverse origin or combination of factors leading to cystocele. The distention cystocele is fundamentally a hernial weakness of the vagina that permits the bladder to overdistend and follow the altered vaginal contour. This type of recurrence may be due to one or a combination of types of defects in the anterior vaginal wall.

Anterior cystocele,[8] occurring anterior to Mercier's bar (the interureteric ridge), is fundamentally a rotational descent of the bladder neck and when present at rest represents a significant alteration in the supports of the vesicourethral junction (Figure 7.3). It may occur with or without urethral funneling (Figure 7.4). When the latter is present, the incidence of coincident SUI is increased.

Posterior cystocele,[8] on the other hand, represents herniation of the bladder into the vagina behind the interureteric ridge (Figure 7.5). It may be the consequence of overdistention at childbirth with compromise of the normal elasticity of the vagina. Diminution in rugal folds of the vagina and pathologic thinness of the central portion of the vaginal wall are often features. The defect may represent literally a hernial weak spot, or "blowout," in the vaginal wall itself. The floor of the bladder follows the weakness of the anterior vaginal wall, a secondary damage. Posterior cystocele and urethral detachment may coexist (Figure 7.6).

Compromise of the connective tissue bridge between the vagina and the arcus tendineus (Figure 7.7), either by stretching or avulsion, is not rare and can be determined by noting the disappearance of the anterior sulcus of the vagina on one or both sides and by the failure of the tissue in this area to elevate when the patient voluntarily contracts her pubococcygeal muscles. The paravaginal defect may

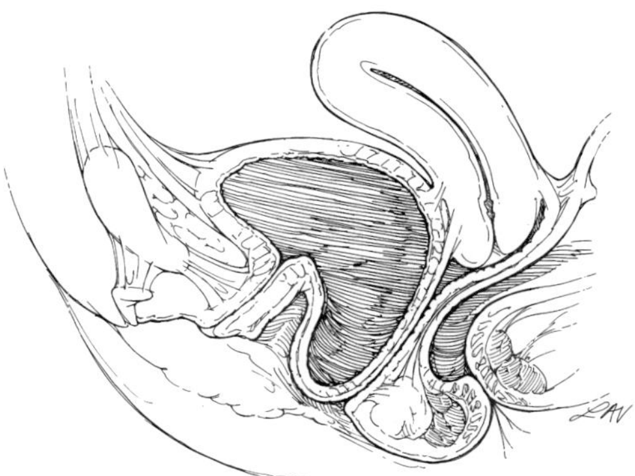

FIGURE 7.5 Posterior distention-type cystocele.

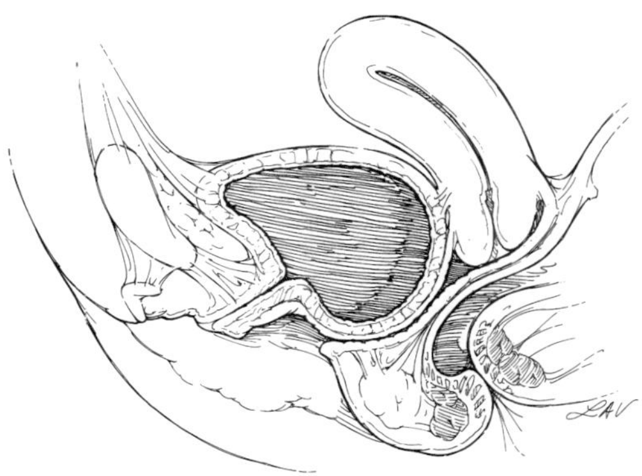

FIGURE 7.6 Urethral detachment may coexist with cystocele.

occur at any level in the vagina or at all levels (Figure 7.8).

Its presence can be demonstrated by elevating the anterior vaginal wall with the tips of a modified sponge or dressing forceps held adjacent to the arcus tendineus. The patient is asked to strain, and the surgeon observes whether or not the cystocele persists. If the cystocele is eliminated by this maneuver, the defect is located primarily in the paravaginal tissues.[1] If the cystocele persists during this maneuver, the defect must be located in the central portion of the vaginal wall. These defects in the lateral or paravaginal supports of the vagina may have been present and unrecognized at the time of the original anterior colporrhaphy. The primary surgeon may have performed a midline colporrhaphy without recognizing that damage had been done to the connective tissue attachment between the anterior vaginal sulcus and arcus tendineus.

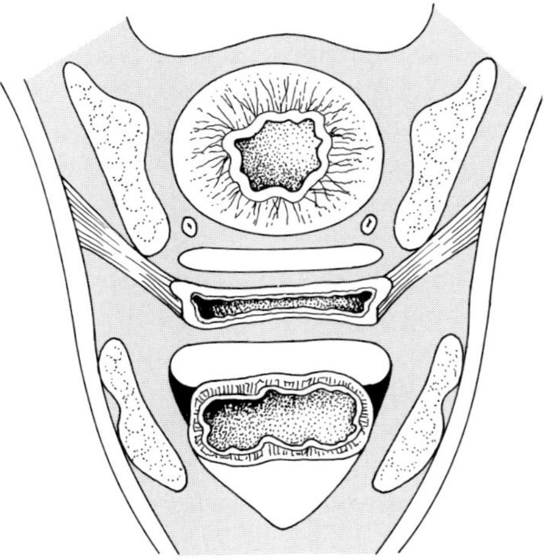

FIGURE 7.7 Connective tissue septa and spaces of the pelvis. Notice particularly the vesicovaginal space between the bladder and the rectum. There is an attachment of the vaginal sulci to the arcus tendineus and the sidewall of the pelvis. (Redrawn from Nichols DH and Randall CL: Vaginal surgery, ed 4, Baltimore, 1996, Williams & Wilkins.)

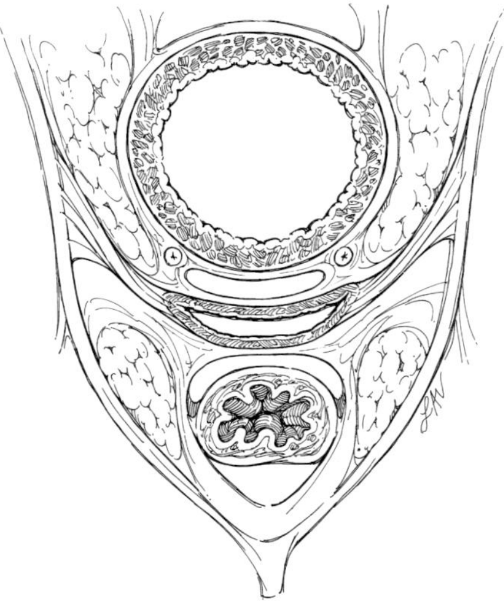

FIGURE 7.8 The paravaginal defect evidenced by the marked elongation of the attachment of the vaginal sulci to the arcus tendineus.

Paravaginal reattachment during the original surgery would probably have prevented this recurrence. Likewise, failure to do so has contributed to the recurrence.

One particular type of recurrent distension cystocele deserves to be noted and that is one seen following a previous colpopexy, either a sacrospinous colpopexy or a sacral colpopexy. This type of recurrent cystocele is seen more frequently following the transvaginal operation, most likely due to the fact that the distance from the introitus to the site of the new vaginal vault is shorter than with the transabdominal procedure. If the surgeon does not take special measures to shorten as well as to narrow a long anterior vaginal wall and cystocele, residual tissue in the long axis of the vagina will probably lead to recurrence of cystocele. The transabdominal sacral colpopexy provides for a longer vaginal length, thus less shortening would be required during the cystocele repair. To lessen the incidence of this usually asymptomatic but aesthetically displeasing postcolpopexy recurrent cystocele, one should take steps not only to correct the excessive width but to shorten a pathologically long vagina and the bladder beneath it at the same time (Figure 7.9).[9]

Displacement Cystocele

A displacement cystocele occurs if there is failure of the support mechanisms of the vaginal wall and vault after hysterectomy, or of the uterus if it is in situ, and the vagina vault eversion or uterine descent brings or displaces the underlying bladder with it. This condition is best diagnosed when the patient is examined standing. It is often associated with a previously unsuspected partial eversion of the vaginal vault. This undiagnosed and unsuspected vault eversion is by no means uncommon. Moreover, its occurrence is so frequent it should be again sought in the operating room during examination under anesthesia by applying traction to the vault with one or more Allis' clamps applied to the site at which the uterine cervix had been attached. When traction pulls the vault down in the midportion of the vagina, a partial eversion of the vault is assuredly present. By careful observation the surgeon should notice whether or not the cystocele disappears when the vault has been momentarily restored to its usual position. The cystocele is thus recognized to be due to displacement. Displacement cystocele may be seen in up to two thirds of patients with eversion of the vaginal vault.[10]

Combination

Recurrent cystocele is frequently the consequence of a number of these weaknesses, which

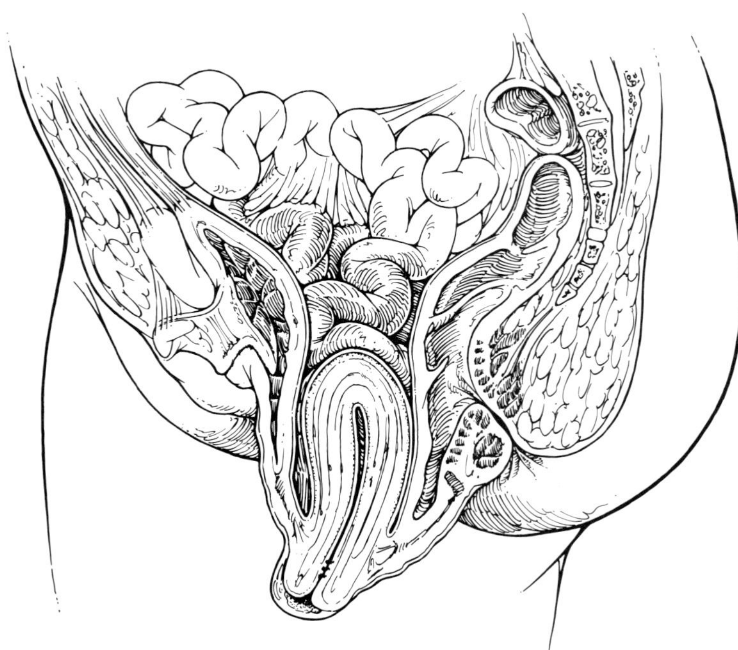

FIGURE 7.9 A pathologically long vagina requires both shortening and narrowing. (From Nichols DH: Gynecologic and obstetric surgery, St Louis, 1993, Mosby.)

may appear in an almost limitless variety of combinations. The most successful surgeon recognizes and seeks to correct each of the contributing factors and anatomic weaknesses.

Look-alikes

Care should be taken to ensure that a cystocele is not diagnosed incorrectly when in fact none exists. "Apparent cystocele" is an entity in which a pathologic exposure of the anterior vaginal wall due to an unrepaired but marked perineal defect appears to be a cystocele. Examination reveals that the tissues do not extend caudal to the inferior margin of the pubis. Thus apparent cystocele is a visual misconception representing the consequence of overexposure of the anterior vaginal wall.

Anterior enterocele (see Figure 9.15) is another defect occasionally seen masquerading as a cystocele.[2] It may be accompanied by a feeling of pelvic pressure and fullness when the patient is on her feet and straining. It is often the consequence of incomplete diagnosis and repair of an enterocele found at the initial surgery or of a failure to have resected excess anterior peritoneum at the time of reperitonealization following hysterectomy. In the latter circumstance, the surgeon may have encountered some difficulty in identifying the anterior vesicouterine peritoneal fold at the time of hysterectomy and dissected the anterior peritoneum from the lower uterine segment and body of the uterus well above the vesicouterine peritoneal fold before entering the peritoneal cavity. There is nothing wrong with this approach to the anterior colpotomy, as long as the surgeon recognizes the presence of this excess peritoneum and excises it carefully at the time of peritonealization.

Anterior enterocele is often unsuspected preoperatively but may be recognized at the time of the planned anterior colporrhaphy for "recurrent cystocele." The surgeon finds a sac of peritoneum at the site where the bladder is presumed to be. When its exact nature has been proved beyond a shadow of a doubt, as by delineating the bladder margin transurethrally with a uterine sound bent into a U shape, the sac is opened and the true nature of the herniation determined. The treatment is mobilization of the sac, high ligation of its neck, and resection of the excess peritoneum.

The most common cystocele "look-alike" is eversion of the vaginal vault. The consideration is whether the vault of the vagina descends to mimic a recurrent cystocele or actually brings the bladder along as a displacement cystocele as discussed earlier.

SURGICAL ANATOMY

The vagina is a fibromuscular tube lined by stratified squamous epithelium with rugal folds, permitting some accordion-like distensibility without laceration. A thin but dense layer of elastic fibers is found immediately beneath the epithelium. The fibromuscular layer is a meshwork of smooth muscle fibers oriented predominantly in a longitudinal direction in the innermost layer but arranged circularly toward the periphery. The fibrous connective tissue capsule external to this muscular coat is rich in elastic fibers and large venous plexus. The vagina is attached to the lateral pelvic walls by condensations of connective tissue and smooth muscle intimately adherent to the adventitia of the vaginal blood vessels. The rectovaginal septum (the fascia of Denonvilliers) is fused to the undersurface of the posterior vaginal wall and can be identified as the anterior lining of the rectovaginal space.[2]

Since the cervix is incorporated in the anterior vaginal wall, the length of the anterior wall plus cervix approximates the length of the posterior wall. The connective tissue adventitia of the vagina is continuous with that of the cervix. The connective tissue lateral to the lower third of the vagina is attached to the pubococcygeal muscle by the fibers of Luschka. At the vesicourethral junction, it is fused with the fibers of the urogenital diaphragm.

Its blood vessels enter the vagina from each side. Their surrounding connective tissue condensations and perivascular sheaths are arranged laterally in tissue that also includes some smooth muscle. The anterior portion of this connective tissue bridge is attached to the arcus tendineus, which is the site of origin of the lateral portion of the levator ani from the surface of the obturator internus.

There is an avascular plane or potential

space between the connective tissue capsule of the anterior vagina and the adventitia of the bladder. This vesicovaginal space has strong functional significance in that it permits the bladder and vagina to distend and function independently of each other. The space ends caudally at the vesicourethral junction, since the urethra acts mainly as a conduit of urine and requires only limited distensibility.

The upper limit of the vesicovaginal space is the fusion between the connective tissue capsule of the vagina and that of the bladder near the cervix. This area of fusion has been called the *supravaginal septum.*[11]

The urethra is secured laterally by fibers of the urogenital diaphragm. A condensation of fibers in the urogenital diaphragm forms the so-called pubourethrovaginal ligaments. These attach primarily to the lateral sides of the urethra, but the condensations run to the back portion of the pubis (see Figure 6.10) as well and have two components: (1) an anterior ligament, the homologue of the suspensory ligament of the penis, and (2) a posterior ligament that runs to the vesicourethral junction. The posterior pubourethral (or pubourethrovaginal) ligaments aid significantly in the midline support of the proximal urethra.[12,13] Because they contain smooth muscle fibers, the ligaments are capable of relaxation during the normal voiding process and thus permit a physiologic descent of the vesicourethral junction.[14] They are susceptible to damage from obstetric trauma and, when pathologically elongated, permit a rotational descent of the bladder neck even in the resting phase. This anatomic situation is conducive to a decreased urethral tone and in some patients is etiologically significant in the production of SUI, because the urethrovesical junction has been displaced from its retropubic position at which it was responsive to increases in intraabdominal pressure coincident with laughing, sneezing, coughing, or changing position.

In addition, the urethra receives considerable support from the underlying anterior vaginal wall. The anterior sulcus of each side of the anterior vaginal wall is normally attached to the arcus tendineus on each side by an intermediate bridge of connective tissue, which can similarly be damaged by a number of factors. Obstetric trauma is the principal culprit, but chronic increases in intraabdominal pressure may also play a role. Thus, the urethra is both suspended and supported: suspended by the pubourethral portion of the urogenital diaphragm and supported by the anterior vaginal wall.[2]

The pubococcygeal muscle plays a considerable role in the normal voiding mechanism, as was described by Muellner, who emphasized the importance of voluntary skeletal muscle in the mechanism of continence[15]:

> Before urination begins, the diaphragm and the muscles of the abdominal wall contract. The intra-abdominal pressure rises, and the pubococcygei relax. As the pubococcygei relax, the neck of the bladder moves downward. This downward movement activates or initiates the contraction of the detrusor. At the same time, the contraction of the longitudinal fibers of the urethra, which are continuous with those of the detrusor, shortens the urethra and thereby widens and opens the internal urethral orifice. Urine is then expelled from the bladder. At the conclusion of voiding, a contraction of the pubococcygei raises the neck of the bladder, the detrusor and urethral musculature relax, the urethra lengthens, the internal urethral orifice narrows and closes, and urination stops.

Gosling has described the relationship between the levator ani muscles and the urethral wall and urethral junction[14]:

> The medial parts of the levator ani muscles (sphincter vaginae) are related to (but structurally separate from) the urethral wall. These periurethral fibers consist of an abundance of large-diameter fast- and slow-twitch fibers, together with muscle spindles. Therefore, unlike the rhabdosphincter, periurethral muscle possesses morphologic features that are similar to other "typical" voluntary muscles.
>
> The levator ani plays an important part in urinary continence by providing an additional occlusive force on the urethral wall, particularly during events that are associated with an increase in intra-abdominal pressure, such as coughing and sneezing. This urethral occlusive force in the female is maximal at the level immediately distal to the maximum urethral pressure generated by the external urethral sphincter. Thus, in addition to providing support for the pelvic viscera, the periurethral parts of the levator ani also play an important active

> role in the urethral mechanisms that maintain continence of urine.
>
> For micturition to occur, the pressure differential between the bladder and urethra muscle overcomes the elastic resistance of the bladder neck. Immediately before the onset of micturition, the tonus of the rhabdosphincter is reduced by central inhibition of its motor neurons located in the second, third, and fourth sacrospinal segments. Such inhibition is mediated by descending spinal pathways originating in higher centers of the central nervous system. Concomitantly, other descending pathways activate (either directly or via sacral interneurons) the preganglionic parasympathetic motor outflow to the urinary bladder. This central integration of the nervous control of the bladder and urethra is essential for normal micturition. . . . Periurethral fibers are innervated by the pudendal nerve and consist of an admixture of large-diameter fast- and slow-twitch fibers.

More recently, DeLancey has confirmed, through microscopic cadaveric observation, the work of other anatomists and surgeons. He has described and characterized histologically the type of tissue and method of support present throughout the pelvic floor. While the various support mechanisms are continuous in nature from the lower vagina up the uterosacral/cardinal complex, he has delineated various levels of support to highlight the differences present at each and to facilitate understanding. Clearly, when the mechanism of support is understood the appropriate surgical correction of the defect can be effected. *Level I* represents suspensory mechanisms present in the cephalic 2 to 3 cm of the vagina. *Level II* represents attachments of the vagina to the pelvic sidewall via the arcus tendineus fasciae pelvis. It is this level that provides support for the bladder and vesical neck. *Level III* represents the lower 2 to 3 cm of the vagina and is characterized by fusion with the surrounding structures to include the perineal body posteriorly and the urogenital diaphragm anteriorly.[10]

It seems therefore that the recurrent cystocele may be due to defects at Level II, leading to the previously described distention type of cystocele, or a failure at Level I, leading to vault eversion and a displacement type of cystocele, or a combination of the two. It is incumbent upon the reconstructive surgeon to identify all the defects present and correct each with an appropriate repair.

Conservative Management

Prevention

Prevention of recurrent cystocele should be achieved when at all possible. Once a primary reconstruction has been completed, the patient must be aware that necessary changes in her lifestyle must be accomplished. These include the avoidance of heavy lifting, greater than 25 lb as a general rule. These women often have been accustomed to compulsively "doing what needed to be done." Postoperatively the patient must learn to ask for assistance and avoid any prolonged or excessive increases in intraabdominal pressure, including chronic constipation. If she must lift, it should be done by bending her knees while keeping her back straight. Additionally, keeping the shoulders back and the spine straight will permit the pelvis to rotate to a more effective axis.

The use of a timely and adequate episiotomy that is properly repaired in the obstetric patient with reduced tissue elasticity (e.g., the presence of multiple wide striae of the anterior abdomen or the primigravida who is older than 25 years of age) may prevent damage to the support mechanisms of the pelvis. Furthermore, it should be remembered that pregnancy, labor, and delivery all traumatize the supports of the anterior vaginal wall, especially in the patient with a wide pubic arch. Therefore colporrhaphy should be reserved generally for the patient who has completed her childbearing. Repeated surgery after subsequent obstetric damage to these tissues is never as effective as a properly executed primary procedure. Reoperation in the former case necessitates dealing with alterations caused by postsurgical scar tissue. In the latter case, scarring is either nonexistent or at least less extensive.

When a postmenopausal patient demonstrates atrophy of the vaginal skin, the surgeon may assume that the subepithelial tissues also are hypoestrogenic with a reduction in subepithelial elastic tissue as well as in blood supply. These atrophic changes can be slowed, arrested, and at times reversed by long-term adequate estrogen supplementation or replacement.

Nonsurgical Intervention

The pubococcygeal muscle plans a considerable role in the normal voiding mechanism, as was described by Muellner[15] who emphasized the importance of voluntary skeletal muscle in the mechanism of continence. Kegel[16] described the positive effects of perineal muscle resistive exercises on restoring muscle tone and mass to the striated voluntary muscle of the urogenital diaphragm. He suggested that if the descent of the cystocele is less than 4 cm below the inferior margin of the pubic symphysis (of the standing patient), much can be expected from a long course of perineal resistive exercises, and if the symptoms are relieved, surgery may be unnecessary. If the descent of the bladder is greater than 4 cm, then surgery is suggested as the treatment of choice for the symptomatic patient. An appropriate exercise regimen consists of 15 strong, 3-second isometric pubococcygeal squeezes in a row, performed 6 times daily. After 2 or 3 months, there will be a considerable improvement in pubococcygeal strength, which should many times help in the support of the vagina and indirectly in the support of the bladder and urethra.

Recently, visual and/or auditory feedback has been provided to the patient who is performing perineal resistive exercises in an effort to increase the effectiveness of this treatment. This form of biofeedback has proven to be efficacious particularly in those patients who continue to perform the exercises after the interventional period.[17-19]

Specifically designed weighted vaginal cones may be used to assist pelvic muscle training. The lighter weighted cone is placed in the vagina, and the patient then contracts the pelvic muscles in order to retain it. When the patient is able to retain the cone for 15 minutes on two occasions, she can graduate to the next heavier cone.[20]

Another method for increasing the strength of perineal muscles that has become available in the United States is functional electric stimulation. It is believed that this nonsurgical therapy provides stimulation to *both* smooth and skeletal muscle in contrast to Kegel's perineal resistive exercises, which affect only voluntary striated muscle.[21] Its effectiveness in improving muscle strength has recently been demonstrated by Sand and others.[22]

For the symptomatic patient who refuses surgery, an intravaginal pessary, such as the Gellhorn, the ring, the Gehrung or the rubber doughnut, can be used. The pessary must, however, be taken out, the vagina inspected for irritation or ulceration, and the pessary replaced at intervals for the balance of the patient's life. Compared with surgery, it is a poor second choice.

Surgical Management

Choice of Procedures

An important goal of surgery is the reestablishment of normal anatomic relationships between the vagina, bladder, urethra, and their supporting structures, including the urogenital diaphragm and pelvic diaphragm, cardinal ligaments, other genital organs, and bony pelvis. Careful and thorough preoperative physical evaluation should be performed and the findings correlated with the patient's symptoms. The surgeon should identify all sites of weakness, including urethral detachment, vaginal detachment, uterine prolapse, prolapse of the vaginal vault, enterocele, rectocele, and perineal defect.

The choice of the procedure or combination of procedures to be performed for an individual patient depends on the types and extent of the various defects that are present. There is no such thing as a "standard" patient or a "standard procedure." Each case must be individualized. Some general guidelines are in order, however.

For the patient with a uterus who has a partial or complete prolapse of the vaginal vault accompanying her recurrent cystocele, effective treatment must reestablish the support of the vault. If the cardinal-uterosacral ligament complex is strong, the simplest way to correct the prolapse is via vaginal hysterectomy with shortening of the cardinal-uterosacral ligament complex, which are then reattached to the vaginal vault. A McCall or New Orleans type of cul-de-plasty, if the ligaments are strong but elongated, will reinforce the reconstruction and act to prevent subsequent enterocele formation.[2] Appropriate colporrhaphy is then carried out.

For the patient in whom retention of the uterine corpus is requested or desired for future reproduction, a Manchester-Fothergill procedure may be considered if the prolapsed vault is of the uterovaginal type with demonstrable cervical elongation.[2] In such a technique the uterosacral and cardinal ligaments are mobilized, the cervix is amputated, and the shortened ligaments are crossed in front of the remaining cervical stump to aid in its support. Appropriate anterior and posterior colporrhaphy follows. This procedure is not as popular in America as it once was, possibly because of the high contemporary use of postmenopausal hormone replacement and subsequent bleeding. If the premenopausal patient understands and accepts the hazards of cervical amputation with its increased risk of premature labor, infertility, dysmenorrhea, and possible difficulty of assessing future uterine bleeding because of cervical stenosis, the procedure may be considered for her.

When it is evident that the cardinal-uterosacral complex is weak and cannot be relied on with confidence to support the vaginal vault, an alternative method of colpopexy should be considered. For the experienced vaginal surgeon, the procedure of choice is usually a transvaginal sacrospinous colpopexy, in which the vaginal vault is attached to sacrospinous ligament at a point one or more fingerbreadths medial to the ischial spine. If the vaginal vault is widened, the procedure may be accomplished bilaterally. A satisfactory result is achieved, however, when it is performed unilaterally provided that the vaginal cylinder narrowed to an appropriate width during the coincident colporrhaphy.

In cases of pure displacement cystocele, reconstructive surgery to support the vaginal vault may be all that is required to reduce the cystocele. The surgeon who chooses not to perform a coincident colporrhaphy must be confident that straightening of the anterior vaginal wall from a colpopexy will not result in SUI.[23]

In spite of the preoperative assessment in the examining room, the extent of colporrhaphy required to correct the recurrent cystocele must be reconfirmed during the examination under anesthesia immediately preceding surgery. The effect of vaginal vault suspension on the anterior vaginal wall becomes apparent when a tenaculum, such as a long Allis' clamp, is attached to the vaginal vault at the site that will become the new apex, and the vault is replaced into the hollow of the sacrum adjacent to the ischial spine. If the patient is awake under spinal anesthesia, she can be asked to strain or cough. The extent to which residual cystocele is apparent after replacement of the vault is the extent to which the displacement cystocele will require concident colporrhaphy to effect an adequate repair. When performed along with sacrospinous colpopexy, the anterior colporrhaphy is usually completed first; hence the need for skillful clinical judgment so that the postoperative vagina will be neither too large nor too small. The former case would encourage rerecurrent prolapse, the latter, dyspareunia.

If the surgeon is uncomfortable with the transvaginal colpopexy, the transabdominal route by transabdominal sacral colpopexy alternatively may be chosen. The apex of the vagina is attached to the periosteum of the sacrum just caudal to the sacral promontory via an intervening bridge of fascia lata or synthetic mesh such as uncoated polyester (Mersilene).[2] Although sacral colpopexy will to some degree eliminate a displacement cystocele and rectocele, it will not effectively treat the more common coincident distention type of cystocele and rectocele. These must be treated separately by colporrhaphy. Even though it will necessitate a two-stage procedure, most operators will prefer to perform the colporrhaphy vaginally since only the transvaginal route will allow the concomitant repair of an accompanying low rectocele and perineal defect.

Alternatively, an occasional high cystocele and rectocele can be repaired from above (transabdominally) by excision of a wedge of tissue from the anterior and posterior walls of the vagina, respectively. Since the sacral colpopexy has a tendency to straighten the urethrovesical junction, a prophylactic urethropexy, such as the vesicourethral sling, the Marshall-Marchetti-Krantz operation, or Burch procedure, may be performed to support a hypermobile vesicourethral junction before the abdomen is closed. We do not recommend Pereyra-type needle suspension because of the high incidence of subsequent recurrence. If a paravaginal defect has been demonstrated, a transabdominal paravaginal repair attaching the anterior vaginal sulci to the arcus tendineus can be carried out.[24]

Surgical Procedures

Transvaginal Colporrhaphy

It is important for the surgeon to estimate the extent to which there is an excess of anterior vaginal wall, both in width and in length, so that excision of an appropriate amount can be effectively gauged before any vaginal wall has been excised. The surgeon should similarly establish whether the damage for which reoperative surgery is being performed involves primarily the midline suspensory tissues (a hernial weakness in the central part of the anterior vaginal wall) or a paravaginal defect or both. Although a paravaginal defect is suspected from the initial pelvic examination, it can be confirmed in the operating room as well by pressing each anterior vaginal sulcus against the tissues of the arcus tendineus on each side and observing what happens to the anterior vaginal wall. In the event of demonstrated paravaginal or lateral vaginal contributory weakness, coincident paravaginal colpopexy can be incorporated in the operative procedure.

Midline Defects. For adequate mobilization of the affected tissues, the operator should proceed directly into the vesicovaginal space so that the full thickness of the anterior vaginal wall can be identified, mobilized, resected, and repaired. Sometimes this space will have been compromised by scarring from the previous surgery, so the operator must proceed with caution to avoid an uinintentional cystotomy. The bladder is emptied of urine. An indwelling no. 16 silicone-coated Foley catheter is inserted for identification of the vesicourethral junction and urethra during the course of surgery. The midpoint of the anterior vaginal wall underlying the cystocele is grasped between two transversely placed Allis' clamps about 1.5 cm apart. The anterior vaginal wall between the clamps is massaged to displace the vagina from the underlying bladder. A vertical incision through the anterior wall is made between the Allis' clamps directly into the vesicovaginal space (Figure 7.10, *A*). The position of the Allis' clamps is rotated so that they now

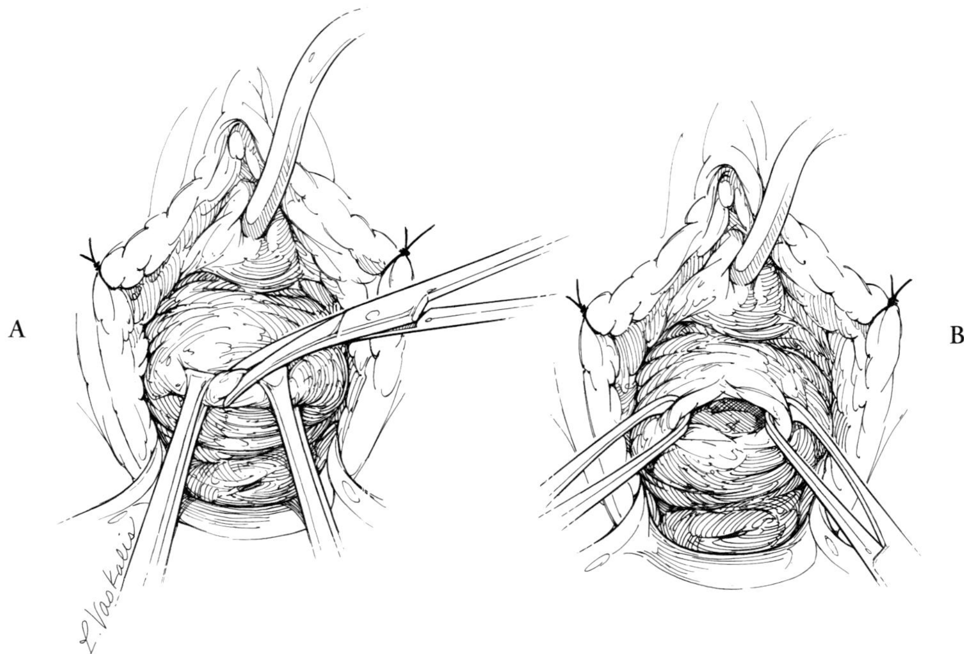

Figure 7.10 The anterior vaginal wall is grasped between two Allis' clamps, and a vertical incision is made directly into the vesicovaginal space (**A**). The position of the Allis' clamps is changed to encompass the full thickness of the anterior vaginal wall (**B**).

grasp the full thickness of the cut edge anterior vaginal wall (Figure 7.10, *B*), which is incised for the full length of the vesicovaginal space beneath the cystocele.[2] The surgeon next establishes a plane of cleavage between the anterior vaginal wall and urethra and separates the vaginal wall from the undersurface of the urethra for most of its length, to within 1 or 1.5 cm of the external urethral meatus. Appropriate Allis' clamps are placed along the edges of the vaginal wall for traction and exposure. The vagina is freed from the undersurface of the urethra through the site of the urogenital diaphragm, being careful to avoid skeletonizing the urethra lest the surgeon compromise its blood and nerve supply. A gentle tug on the Foley catheter will identify the vesicourethral junction. Any urethral finding that has been demonstrated (Figure 7.11) is corrected by one or more Kelly-type[25] urethral wall plication stitches (Figure 7.12) using a long-acting synthetic suture material of the polyglycolic acid or polydioxanone type. If there is hypermobility of the urethra with coincident rotational descent of the bladder neck, this should be repaired by pubourethrovaginal ligament plication[12] (Figure 7.13) using a long-lasting or a nonabsorbable synthetic suture, which, when tied, should displace the vesicourethral junction cranially until it is once again retropubic in its normal position at about the junction of the lower third with the upper two thirds of the back of the pubis. If one suture is insufficient to achieve this goal, a second should be placed lateral to the first. The suture is tied, and a bite taken to the undersurface of the vaginal wall, reestablishing fusion of the urogenital diaphragm and the vagina.

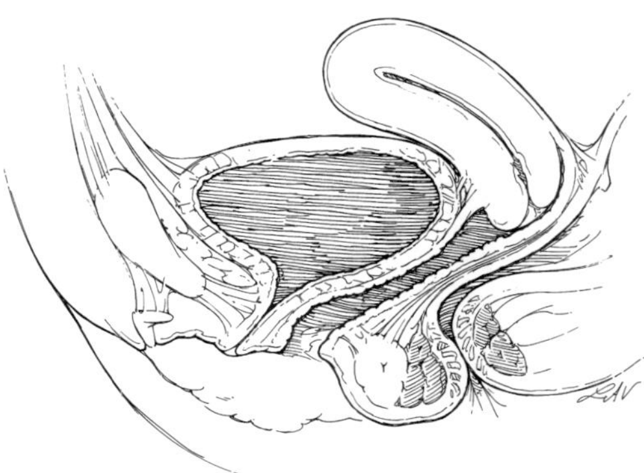

Figure 7.11 Funneling of the urethra without rotational descent of the bladder neck.

The vesicovaginal space is dissected the full limit of its lateral extent to separate fully the unsplit anterior vaginal wall from the underlying bladder. The width and length of the connective tissue capsule of the bladder are reduced by one or more layers of running locked permanent sutures or polyglycolic acid or polydioxanone, the stitch at the top of the vagina incorporating some of the tissue at the site of each uterosacral ligament. Occasionally this bladder plication is accomplished using a "tobacco pouch" purse-string suture. The neck of such a purse-string suture must always be reinforced by an additional layer of mattress sutures in case strength is lost at the time of absorption of the suture material of the purse string. Any additional trapezoid-type mattress stitches are placed to further reduce the size of a large cystocele.

When it is evident that the cystocele should be reduced in length as well as width, the reconstructive surgeon should place a purse-string suture using a permanent or long-lasting polyglycolic type of suture. The closed bladder neck of the inverted sac of the bladder is reinforced with overlying interrupted sutures, generously plicating the tissue front to back (Figure 7.14). When the defect is of

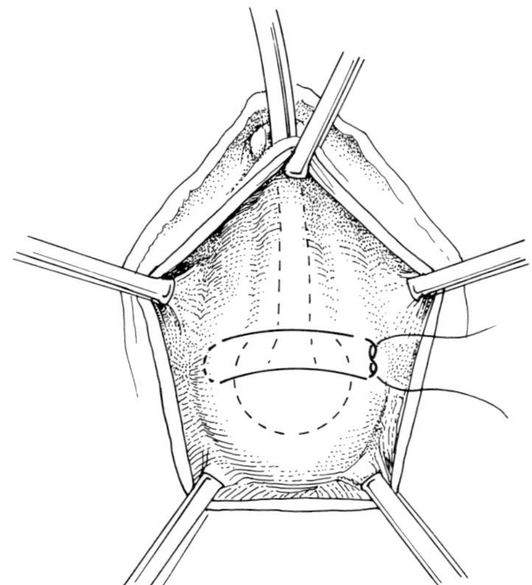

Figure 7.12 The original Kelly stitch. It had been introduced to plicate a presumed internal urethral sphincter. One or more may be placed at the vesical neck. Note the inflated bulb on the Foley catheter *(dashed line)*. (Redrawn from Nichols DH and Randall CL: Vaginal surgery, ed 4, Baltimore, 1996, Williams & Wilkins.)

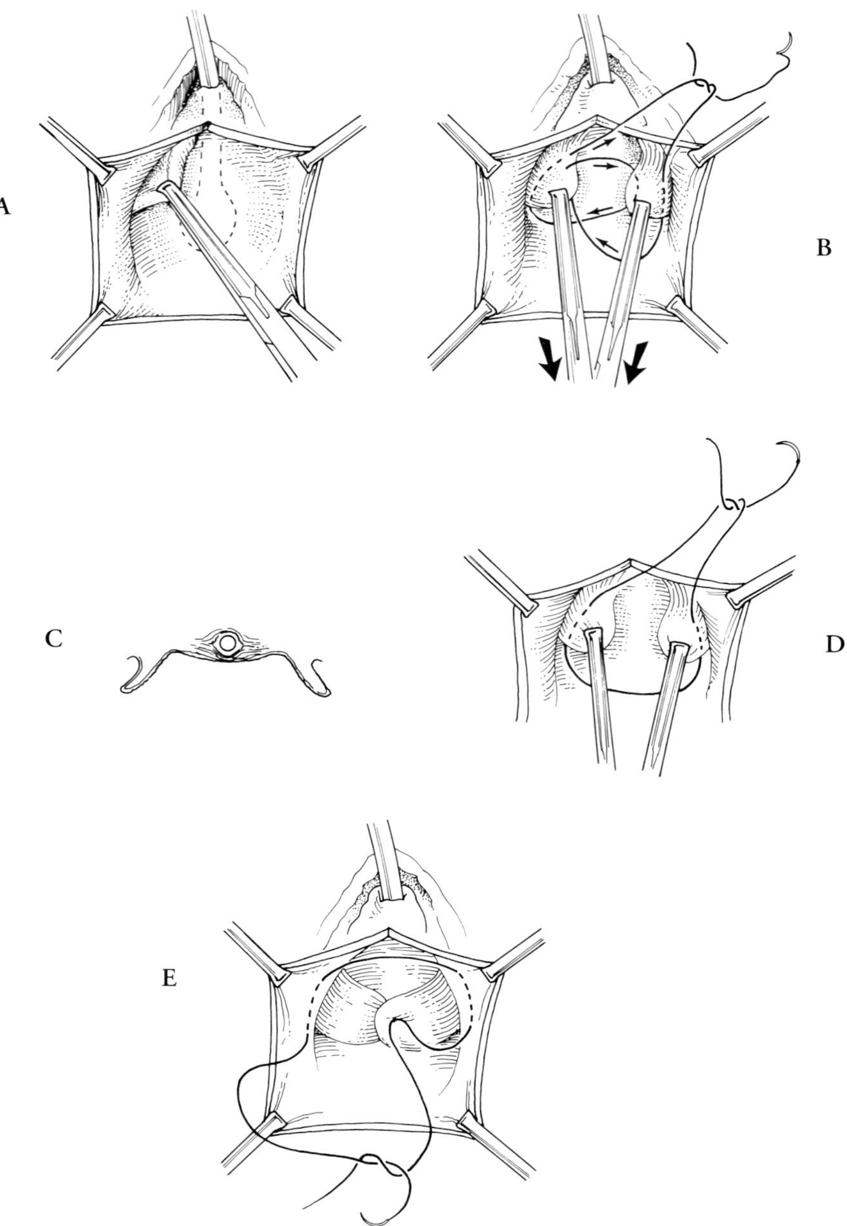

FIGURE 7.13 Pubourethral "ligament" plication. The anterior vaginal wall has been incised in the midline into the vesicovaginal space and the dissection carried anteriorly beneath the urethra (**A** and **B**). Notice that the proper depth of the urethral dissection does not skeletonize the urethra (**C**) so as not to overly disturb its blood and nerve supply. In **A** the paraurethral tissue of the urogenital diaphragm has been grasped in a Kocher's hemostat closed only one notch of its ratchet. Traction to the forceps in the line indicated by the *arrows* (**B**) will actually move the patient to a small degree on the table. A polydioxanone suture is placed through each side of the ligament (**B**) in a far-near-near configuration. An alternative method (**D**) may be used when synthetic nonabsorbable sutures are applied. After the ligaments have been plicated, the same suture takes a bite of the vaginal wall (**E**), reestablishing the fusion between the vagina and the urogenital diaphragm. (Redrawn from Nichols DH and Randall CL: Vaginal surgery, ed 4, Baltimore, 1996, Williams & Wilkins.)

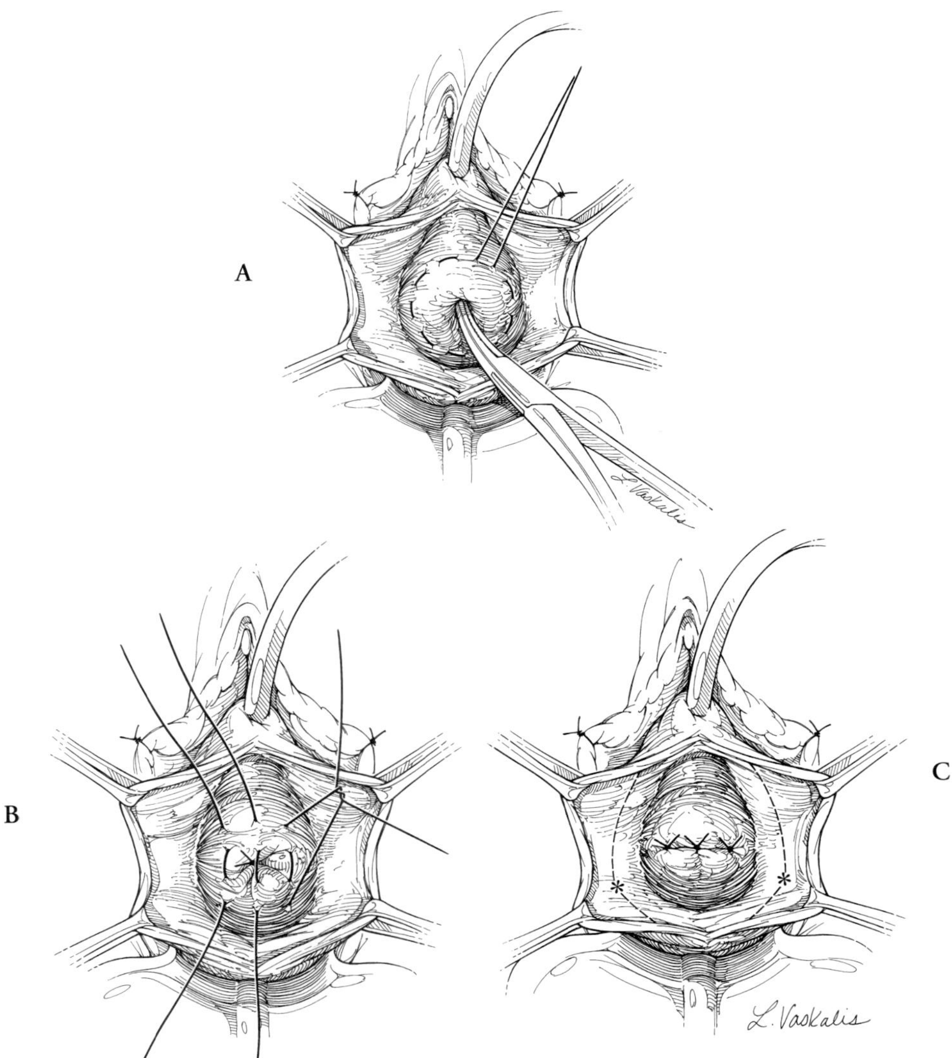

FIGURE 7.14 A, Halban purse-string suture placed wide and the cystocele inverted. Reinforcing transverse plication sutures are placed (**B**). The sutures are tied (**C**) and the full thickness vagina trimmed as indicated by the *dashed line*. The *asterisks* indicate the new vaginal vault, shortening the vagina when they are brought together.

Continued.

increased length alone, but not width, as in the previously operated patient, one or more layers of transversely placed suture will achieve a similar result. The excessive anterior vaginal wall is trimmed appropriately in both length and width (Figure 7.15).[9]

It is important for the operator to correct most of the secondary damage to the wall of the bladder by this colporrhaphy but to guard carefully against overcorrection lest the posterior urethrovesical angle be straightened out pathologically and the patient given an anatomic predisposition for postoperative SUI (Figure 7.16).[23] As discussed earlier, preoperative determination of the urethral pressure profile, specifically, the MUCP, should help in the avoidance of this complication. If the MUCP is found to be less than 20 cm H_2O, it should be addressed with a separate procedure at the time of reoperation (e.g., coincident vesicourethral sling operation if there is hypermobility of the vesicourethral junction). If sacrospinous colpopexy is to be performed, the extent of excess anterior vaginal wall to be excised should be very carefully estimated by holding the vaginal vault adjacent to the ischial

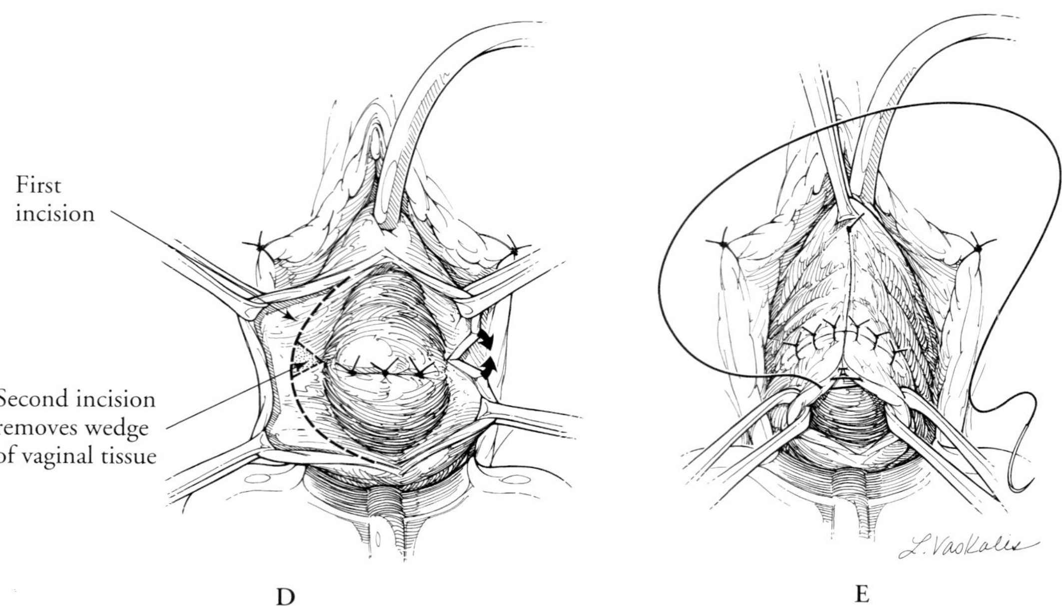

FIGURE 7.14, cont'd. Alternatively, when the vagina has been narrowed by excision along the path of the *dashed line*, a wedge on each side of the remaining vagina may be excised as shown (**D**) and the edges reapproximated by interrupted sutures. The midline incision is closed by a running subcuticular suture (**E**).

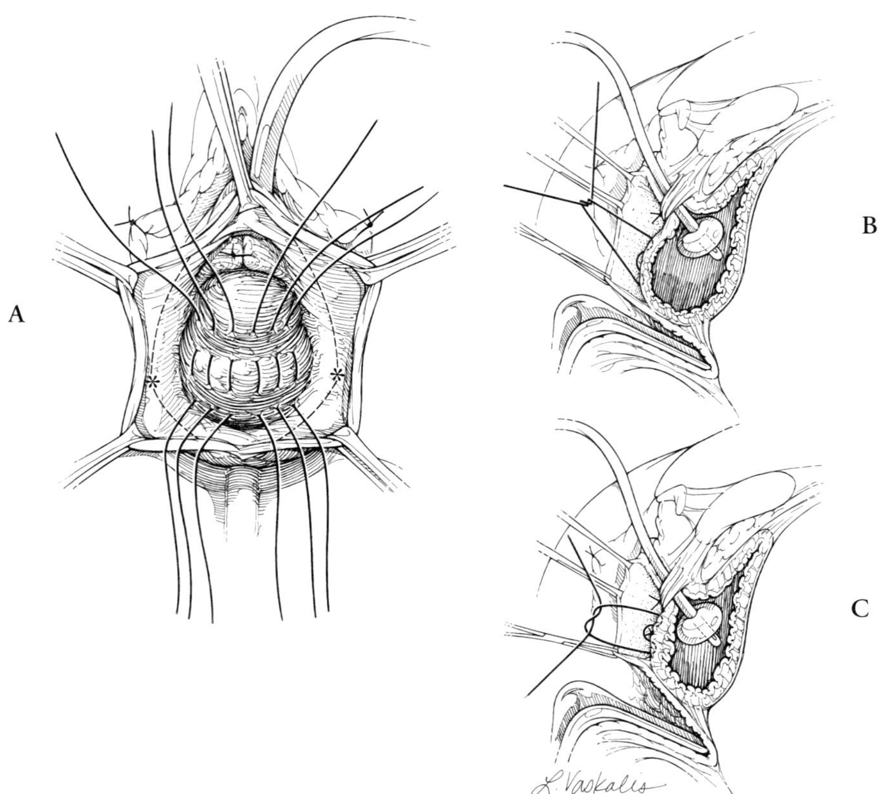

FIGURE 7.15 Transverse plication sutures placed over the previously placed purse-string suture to shorten a pathologically long vagina. Transverse plication sutures can be placed in the bladder muscularis (**A**) to shorten a pathologically long vagina. The vagina is trimmed along the path of the *dashed lines*, and the tissue indentified by the *asterisks* is brought to the new vault, shortening the vagina. These stitches in the bladder muscularis are shown in sagittal section (**B**). An additional layer may be inserted if necessary (**C**).

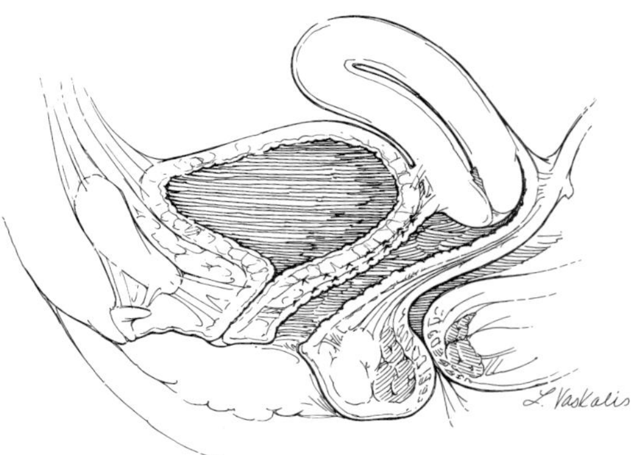

FIGURE 7.16 Overcorrection of the cystocele has straightened the posterior vesicourethral angle. (Redrawn from Nichols DH and Randall CL: Vaginal surgery, ed 4, Baltimore, 1996, Williams & Wilkins.)

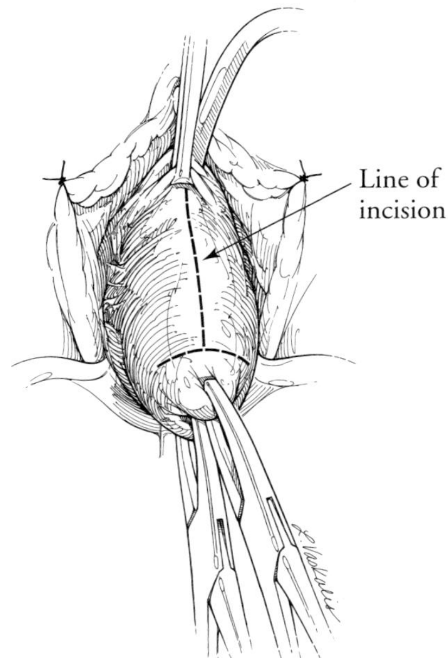

FIGURE 7.17 Vaginal paravaginal repair. The cervix or vaginal vault is grasped, traction applied, and an incision made along the pathway indicated by the *dashed line*.

spine, and the full thickness of the excess vagina can be excised. The anterior vaginal walls are then reapproximated in the midline by a spiraling subcutaneous subcuticular suture of size 00 polyglycolic acid or polydioxanone suture. The suture starts at either end of the dissection and brings the sides of vagina together for the full length of the incision. Each pass of the suture incorporates the full thickness of the vaginal wall with the exception of penetration of the superficial layer of the epithelium; that is, the suture material remains subcuticular and does not actually perforate the "mucosa." Since the vaginal wall has not been split, its blood supply has not been disturbed, and the integrity of the subepithelial coat of the vagina adds its full strength to the repair.

Paravaginal Defects. If the recurrent cystocele demonstrates a coincident paravaginal defect, before any vaginal wall is resected and the midline bladder defect repaired, the dissection of the anterior vaginal wall from the bladder is continued laterally beyond the lateral margins of the vesicovaginal space to expose the fascia covering the obturator internus and the arcus tendineus (Figures 7.17 and 7.18). Interrupted stitches (usually synthetic permanent suture) are placed in series in the tissues of each arcus tendineus or at this site on the obturator fascia. The sutures, which are held long, are then individually sewn to the subepithelial fibromuscular wall of the vagina at the site of the vaginal sulci (Figure 7.19). After the sutures on one side have been individually tied, a similar fixation is usually necessary on the opposite side. Only after paravaginal repair is complete is any midline bladder defect repaired and any excess anterior vaginal wall trimmed. The surgeon then closes the midline incision with the spiraling continuous subcuticular suture.

In the uncommon instance when the patient has no demonstrable midline defect, the paravaginal repair may be approached through parallel incisions in the anterior vaginal wall, as originally suggested by White[26] and popularized more recently by Shull and Baden.[27] Preliminary infiltration of the area with saline or a liquid tourniquet such as 1:200,000 epinephrine in 0.5% lidocaine solution will diminish the blood loss during the dissection. Absorbable stitches in the arcus tendineus are placed,[28] then brought through the cut edges of the vagina. When all have been placed, they are tied one by one. This is completed first on one side and then on the other. Recently Grody and others[29] have reported using a paravaginal cystopexy and paraurethral fascial sling urethropexy to restore the normal anatomic positioning of the anterior vaginal wall. The initial approach is similar to that de-

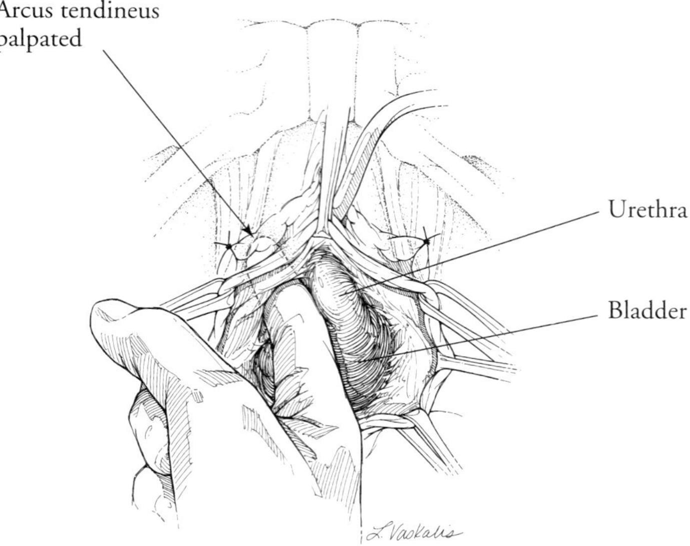

Figure 7.18 The dissection of the anterior vaginal wall is continued laterally beyond the lateral margins of the vesicovaginal space. The index finger palpates the site of the arcus tendineus.

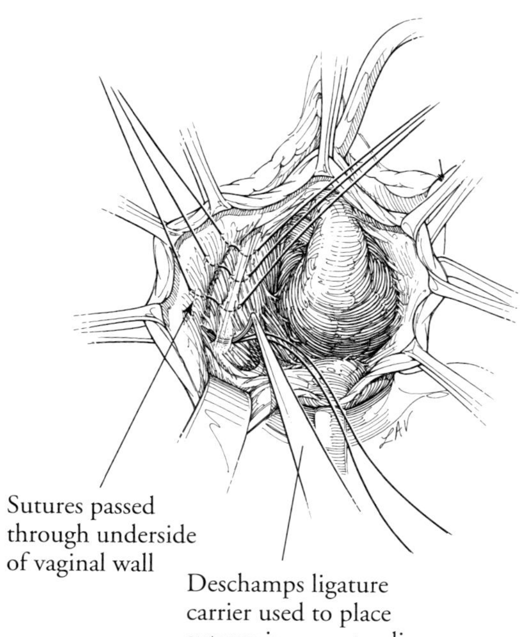

Figure 7.19 The paravaginal repair. Interrupted stitches are placed in series in the tissue of each arcus tendineus, then each is affixed to the subepithelial fibromuscular wall of the vagina at the site of the undersurface of the vaginal sulci.

scribed previously in this chapter. Once the paraurethral tissues have been plicated under the urethra, the paravesical connective tissue is sutured to the fascia of the internal obturator muscle at the level of the arcus tendineus fasciae pelvis. An anterior bladder wall plication completes the procedure. The initial results appear promising.

Unusually Thin Vagina. We occasionally encounter a patient who has previously undergone numerous transvaginal reconstructive procedures and now has marked atrophy and thinning of the anterior portion of the vagina that has not responded sufficiently enough to estrogen and supplementation to have restored adequate thickness to the vaginal wall. The patient, who is usually postmenopausal, may be sexually active, making the surgeon most reluctant to resect any more vaginal tissue. Too much may already have been removed by previous colporrhaphy to permit bilateral paravaginal fixation. One alternative repair for such a large thin-walled cystocele is using a subepithelial prosthetic mesh such as Mersilene to create an additional tissue layer.[2] When cut to size, the Mersilene mesh is fixed in place by interrupted nonabsorbable sutures. It may be insulated from the overlying vaginal wall by either a vaginal lapping operation (Figure 7.20) or by the use of a broad-based bulbocavernosus fat pad transplant.[2] Alternatively, and in the event that all excess vaginal mucosa that has been previously excised during colporrhaphy has been saved, a patch can be cut from the full thickness of the freshly excised vaginal mucosa, cut to fill the defect, and sutured into placed as described

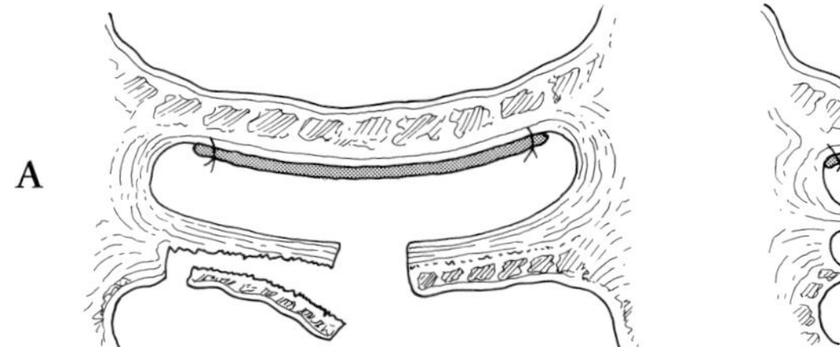

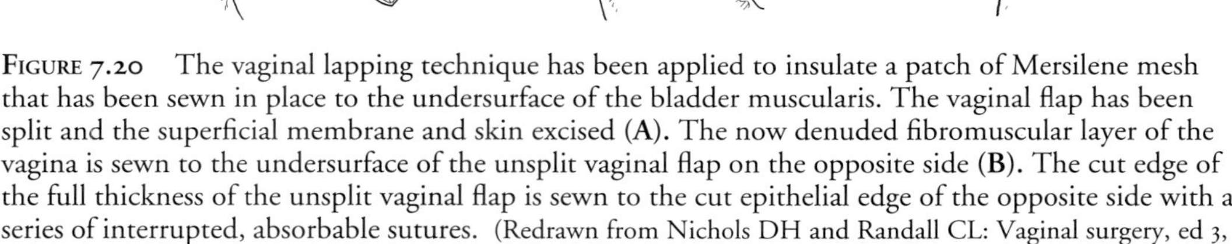

Figure 7.20 The vaginal lapping technique has been applied to insulate a patch of Mersilene mesh that has been sewn in place to the undersurface of the bladder muscularis. The vaginal flap has been split and the superficial membrane and skin excised (**A**). The now denuded fibromuscular layer of the vagina is sewn to the undersurface of the unsplit vaginal flap on the opposite side (**B**). The cut edge of the full thickness of the unsplit vaginal flap is sewn to the cut epithelial edge of the opposite side with a series of interrupted, absorbable sutures. (Redrawn from Nichols DH and Randall CL: Vaginal surgery, ed 3, Baltimore, 1989, Williams & Wilkins.)

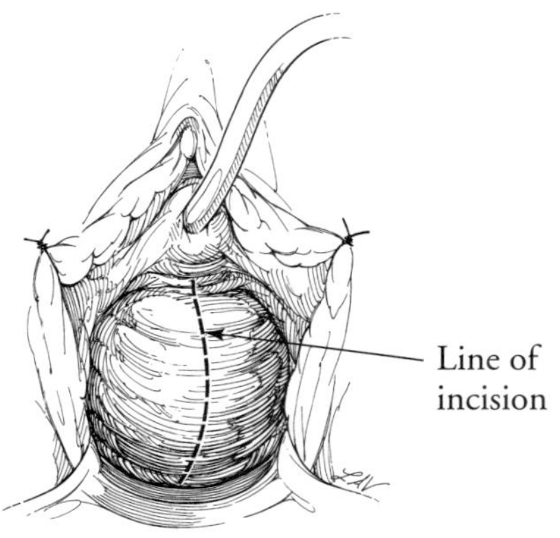

Figure 7.21 A vaginal patch. An incision is made in the midline along the path indicated by the *dashed line.*

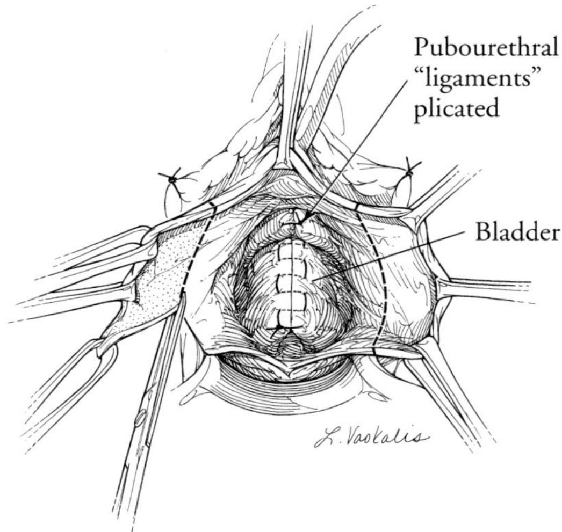

Figure 7.22 The pubourethrovaginal portion of the urogenital diaphragm has been plicated as shown. The cystocele has been reduced by a running mattress suture, and the excess but thin vaginal wall excised along the pathway of the dashed lines. The larger flap *(stippled)* will be saved for creation of the patch.

previously[2,30](Figures 7.21 and 7.22). To further thicken the anterior vaginal wall the patch, sewn to the bladder capsule at the lateral limits of the vesicovaginal space, is insulated by approximating the resected edges of the anterior vaginal wall over it, without tension (Figure 7.23). The anterior vaginal wall should be closed without tension with a running subcuticular suture or by interrupted sutures. If there is any question as to the presence of tension in this suture line, bilateral vaginal relaxing incision should be made at the 3 or 9 o'clock position as described in Chapter 22. These will effectively take the tension from the anterior suture line.

Another interesting alternative procedure in such a patient, should she still retain a well-supported uterus, would be the Ocejo[31] modification of the Watkins-Wertheim bladder transposition operation. In this procedure, the fundus of the uterus, from which all endometrium has been excised, is interposed between the bladder and the anterior vaginal wall. The excision of the endometrium removes the site and source of future uterine bleeding and its attendant problems.

Posterior Colporrhaphy

The length of the urethra is approximately the same as the length of the perineal body. If, therefore, the patient who is undergoing anterior colporrhaphy for a recurrent cystocele has

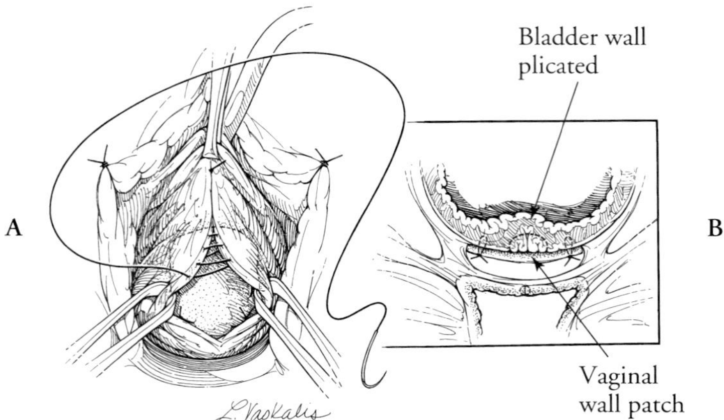

FIGURE 7.23 A tailored patch is sewn in place, and the anterior vaginal wall is approximated over it, without tension (**A**). The final result is seen in coronal section (**B**).

a coincident defect of the perineum or posterior vaginal wall, the coincident rectocele or perineal defect should be repaired, because such a repair will aid considerably in the postoperative long-term support of the anterior vaginal wall.

POSTOPERATIVE CARE

Hospitalization

Patients undergoing repeat anterior colporrhaphy should have the bladder drained by catheter for at least 60 hours postoperatively. A no. 16 transurethral silicone-coated Foley is recommended because the urethral mucosa has less affinity for silicone than rubber. The silicone-coated catheter therefore will cause less mucosal edema. The transurethral route is preferred over the suprapubic one for patient comfort, and the time the bladder is to be drained is short. Those patients who do not resume normal voiding begin a course of intermittent self-catheterization using the female no. 14 Mentor soft plastic catheter. This technique is taught preoperatively to all patients who are willing to learn it. Alternatively, in the patient unwilling or unable to perform self-catheterization, a transurethral Silastic-coated Foley catheter may be reinserted for 2 weeks and clamped and opened as necessary. It is removed at home.

As few of the procedures for repair of a recurrent cystocele involve significant manipulation of the bowel and most are usually completed under spinal anesthesia, the patient may be given "diet as tolerated" immediately after recovery from anesthesia. Any vaginal packs are removed as soon as the risks of emesis or significant retching have abated. Patients are encouraged to ambulate the morning after surgery.

Discharge

Patients undergoing procedures are given 500 mg of ascorbic acid daily for a 3- to 6-month minimum to inhibit formation of collagenase, which may impede wound healing. Suitable estrogen replacement (in every postmenopausal patient), both systemically and intravaginally, should be used unless contraindicated. A long-term course of Kegel perineal resistive exercises[16] should be continued at least 3 months postoperatively. Additionally, the patient should be counseled that convalescence is a slow process. Physical activities should be rather conservative for the first month after surgery. She should be cautioned against heavy lifting, lifting no more than 5 to 10 lb during the first 6 weeks and no more than 25 lb thereafter. She should also avoid chronic constipation because chronic bearing down in connection with defecation can compromise a nice repair.

REFERENCES

1. Baden WF and Walker TA: Evaluation of the stress incontinent patient. In Cantor EG, editor: Female urinary stress incontinence,

Springfield, Ill, 1979, Charles C Thomas, Publisher.

2. Nichols DH and Randall CL: Vaginal surgery, ed 4, Baltimore, 1996, Williams & Wilkins.
3. Horbach NS and Ostergard DR: Predicting intrinsic sphincter dysfunction in women with stress urinary incontinence, Obstet Gynecol 84:188, 1994.
4. Ghoniem GM, Walters F, and Lewis V: The value of the vaginal pack test in large cystoceles, J Urol 152:931, 1994.
5. McGuire EJ: Urodynamics findings in patients after failure of stress incontinence operations, Prog Clin Biol Res 78:381, 1981.
6. Bump RC, Fantl JA, and Hurt WG: Dynamic urethral pressure profilometry pressure transmission ratio determinations after continence surgery: understanding the mechanism of success, failure and complications, Obstet Gynecol 72:870, 1988.
7. Bhatia NN and Bergman A: Urodynamic predictability of voiding following incontinence surgery, Obstet Gynecol 631:85, 1984.
8. Ball TA: Anterior and posterior cystocele, Clin Obstet Gynecol 9:1062, 1966.
9. Nichols DH: Anterior coloporrhaphy technique to shorten a pathologically long vaginal wall, Int Surg 64(5):69, 1979.
10. DeLancey JOL: Anatomic aspects of vaginal eversion after hysterectomy, Am J Obstet Gynecol 166:1717, 1992.
11. Von Peham H and Amreich J: Operative gynecology, Philadelphia, 1934, JB Lippincott Co (Translated by LK Ferguson).
12. Nichols DH and Milley PS: Identification of pubourethral ligaments and their role in transvaginal surgical correction of stress incontinence, Am J Obstet Gynecol 115:123, 1973.
13. Zacharin RF: The suspensory mechanism of the female urethra, J Anat 97:423, 1963.
14. Gosling JA: The structure of the female lower urinary tract and the pelvic floor, Urol Clin North Am 12:207, 1985.
15. Muellner SR: The anatomies of the female urethra, Obstet Gynecol 14:429, 1959.
16. Kegel AH: Physiologic therapy for urinary stress incontinence, JAMA 146:915, 1951.
17. Burgio KL, Robinson JC, and Engel BT: The role of biofeedback in Kegel exercise training for stress urinary incontinence, Am J Obstet Gynecol 154(1):58, 1986.
18. Dougherty MC and others: Graded pelvic muscle exercises: effect on stress urinary incontinence, J Reprod Med 38(9):684, 1993.
19. Ferguson KL and others: Stress urinary incontinence: effect of pelvic muscle exercise, Obstet Gynecol 75(4):671, 1990.
20. Peattie AP, Plevnik S, and Stanton SL: Vaginal cones: a conservative method for treating genuine stress incontinence, Br J Obstet Gyneacol 95:1049, 1988.
21. Huffman JW, Osborne SL, and Sokol JK: Electrical stimulation in the treatment of intractable stress incontinence, Arch Phys Med 33:674, 1952.
22. Sand PK and others: Pelvic floor electrical stimulation in the treatment of genuine stress incontinence: a multicenter, placebo controlled trial, Am J Obstet Gynecol 173(1):72, 1995.
23. Symmonds RE and Jordan LT: Iatrogenic stress incontinence of urine, Am J Obstet Gynecol 82:1231, 1961.
24. Richardson AC, Lyons JB, and Williams NL: A new look at pelvic relaxation, Am J Obstet Gynecol 126:568, 1976.
25. Kelly HA: Incontinence of urine in women, Urol Cutan Rev 1:291, 1913.
26. White GR: Cystocele: a radical cure by suturing lateral sulci of the vagina to the white line of pelvic fascia, JAMA 53:1707, 1909.
27. Shull BL and Baden WF: A six-year experience with paravaginal defect repair for stress urinary incontinence, Am J Obstet Gynecol 160(6):1432, 1989.
28. Figurnov KM: Surgical treatment of urinary incontinence in women, Akush Ginekol (Mosk) 6:7, 1949.
29. Grody MHT and others: Paraurethral fascial sling urethropexy and vaginal paravaginal defects cystopexy in the correction of urethrovesical prolapse, Int Urogynecol J 6:80, 1995.
30. Zacharin RF: Free full-thickness vaginal epithelium graft in correction of recurrent genital prolapse, Aust NZ J Obstet Gynaecol 32(2):146, 1992.
31. Gallo D: Ocejo modification of interposition operation. In Urologica ginecologica, Guadalajara, Mexico, 1969, Gallo.

8

Recurrent Rectocele

David H. Nichols

Recurrent rectocele is a frustration for both the patient and her surgeon. Although it may be an extension of the naturally progressive aging process, it usually indicates an initial misdiagnosis as to the extent of the patient's weakness, failure to have correlated the anatomic damages with the patient's symptoms, or performance of an inadequate repair. The surgeon must decide whether only the patient's symptoms are recurring or whether an actual rectocele and/or perineal defect has recurred.

Posterior vaginal repair is among the most poorly understood and poorly performed of the common gynecologic surgical procedures. Although rectocele is fairly common among multiparous women, there is considerable confusion and divergence of opinion concerning not only the related symptoms and indications for repair but also the anatomic goals sought by the repair and therefore the specific techniques used to achieve them. Perineal defect generally is identified by a gaping perineum and may occur with or without coincident rectocele (Figure 8.1). Rectocele may be found in the lower third, middle third, or upper third of the vagina or all three, and it may or may not coexist with enterocele. When it is symptomatic, all elements of weakness should be repaired as part of the initial operation, or those sections left unrepaired will generally progress, requiring future surgical attention. Rectocele is fundamentally a defect of the vagina and its supports. The dilated rectum follows the vaginal defect rather passively, although the secondary damage to the wall of the rectum may become extreme over a long period of time, pathologically increasing the size of the rectal reservoir and requiring repair. Since the vagina is the primary site of damage, it is to the vagina that primary attention should be given and reconstruction directed when the patient is symptomatic.

Symptoms

Surprisingly, constipation is not necessarily a symptom of rectocele, though it may coexist. There are many women with constipation without rectocele, many more with rectocele who are not constipated, and some women with constipation who have rectocele. Posterior colporrhaphy per se will not necessarily relieve constipation, which may be essentially a functional disorder.[1-3]

The primary symptoms of rectocele include an inability to completely empty the bowel with defecation, often requiring manual vaginal or perineal expression to complete the process. Evacuation is often followed by postevacuation rectal discomfort probably related to venous engorgement consequent to straining. Such a tendency toward passive congestion may interfere with perineal circulation, and coincident hemorrhoids are frequent. Constipation per se is more likely the result of deranged bowel habits in which the patient has difficulty "unlocking" the anorectal valve and relaxing the internal anal sphincter.

It is important to review briefly the mechanism of rectal continence. The levator ani, or muscular portion of the pelvic diaphragm, is unique among human striated muscle in that it maintains sensory receptors that are stimulated by coincident rectal fullness. Stimulation of these sensors may reflexly influence the tone of the voluntary muscles of the pelvis but may also convey to the patient's sensorium a message of fullness. Although the levator ani is a voluntary muscle and can be contracted at will by the patient, it maintains a voluntary tone that is reflexly greater with increased rectal distention.

Both the levator ani and the external anal sphincter are innervated by the pudendal nerve and, most of the time, act in synergy. This

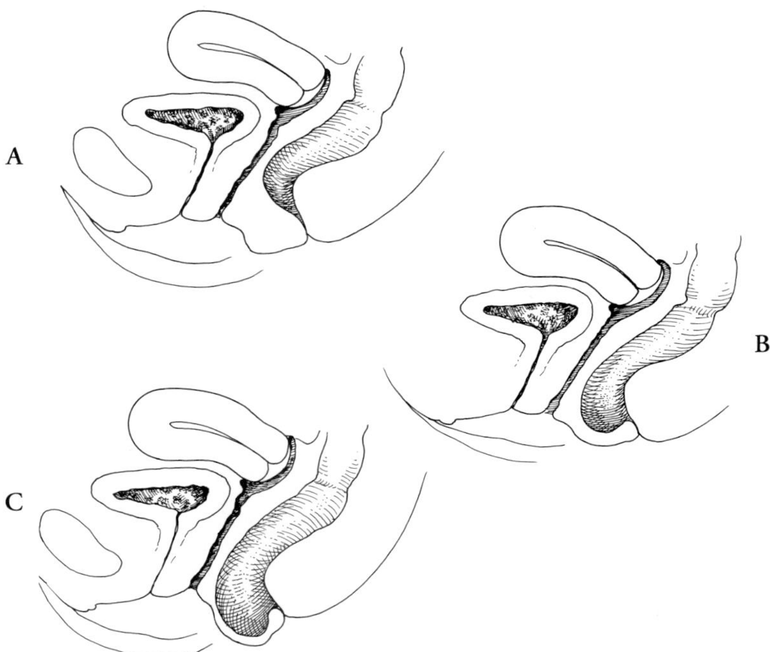

Figure 8.1 **A,** A normal relationship between the vagina, perineum, and rectum. **B,** A major perineal defect. There is no rectocele but restoration of the perineal body is indicated. **C,** A major perineal defect with rectocele. In this circumstance, perineorrhaphy should be accompanied by an appropriate posterior colporrhaphy. (Redrawn from Nichols DH and Randall CL: Vaginal surgery, ed 4, Baltimore, 1996, Williams & Wilkins.)

reflex tone is involuntary and constant, and for this reason we do not soil ourselves during the night, even though peristalsis constantly propels our intestinal content toward its ultimate site of expulsion. As it continues downward, the muscular wall of the large bowel becomes the internal anal sphincter, composed of smooth involuntary muscle. The internal sphincter is the backup system of continence to that offered by the external anal sphincter.

At certain times, usually in the morning, and following initiation of the gastrocolic reflex, a sensation of rectal fullness is conveyed to the sensory nervous system, and the patient may experience a desire to evacuate. If this desire is heeded, the patient in the course of evacuation relaxes the external anal sphincter and levator ani, straightening out the anorectal angle, and permitting direct access of intestinal content to the distal portion of the intestinal system. With intraabdominal pressure increased by a gentle voluntary Valsalva maneuver, this bolus is propelled, the internal anal sphincter relaxes, and defecation occurs.

Anal stricture, as is sometimes seen in posthemorrhoidectomy patients, might be estimated as that in which the anal diameter is less than a fingerbreadth. Overcoming it can require considerable straining and may be a chronic contributing factor for recurrent rectocele to which the stricture has provided an outlet obstruction. It is relieved by a proctotomy, usually at the 6 o'clock position, that includes a portion of the internal surface of the external anal sphincter, which enlarges the anal canal to at least two fingerbreadths.

Muscular dysfunction whereby the pubococcygei paradoxically contract instead of relaxing when a patient strains to achieve a bowel movement requires excessive intraabdominal pressure to overcome this resistance. This not only favors recurrence of rectocele but also risks a future pudendal neuropathy, which may be an etiologic factor in development of a perineal descent syndrome. The spastic dysfunction can generally be relieved by a course of biofeedback retraining exercises. It is possible that a patient's inability to contract her pubococcygei and external anal sphincter muscles may correlate with an established pudendal neuropathy, which might be demonstrated by a delayed pudendal nerve motor latency transmission test.

If any step of this process is deliberately or accidentally circumvented, the normal reflex pattern is disturbed, the internal anal sphincter will not unlock, and the tone of the levator ani and external sphincter system increases to avoid incontinence. When for the sake of personal convenience the patient persists in voluntary habitual inhibition of this reflex over a long period of time, the sensory mechanism is suppressed, and it may be difficult to reinitiate the reflexes leading toward evacuation. When these problems have been present for some time, the patient may develop a habit of overcoming them by excessive straining at stool. Voluntary massive increase in intraabdominal pressure by contraction of the anterior abdominal muscles to force content out of the bowel can result in damage to the resisting pelvic diaphragm and levator ani.

Once the normal evacuation system has been suppressed by voluntary interference with this normal reflex activity, it is difficult to reestablish a useful bowel pattern but is worth the trouble if the patient is to be cured of an annoying constipation. In hope that it will act as an intestinal stimulant, additional bulk in the stool may be provided by increased dietary fiber or various preparations. Peristalsis may be stimulated by the use of a laxative or cathartic. It is important that the patient maintain an adequate dietary liquid intake. Because thirst decreases with age, the older woman usually will consume less liquid in her diet than she did in her earlier and thirstier years. This relative dehydration promotes fecal hardness as the colon seeks to extract every possible bit of water from its content.

Since a long history of evacuation straining is associated with increases in intracolonic pressure, patients with this problem may also suffer from diverticulosis, which increases in frequency with age as well. Inducing adequate bulk by an increase in dietary fiber, such as bran, may coincidentally improve intestinal dysfunction associated with diverticulosis.

Another symptom of rectocele may be the partial retention of stool. The problem is mechanical, related not to constipation but to the trapping of stool in a pocket, which functions as a rather massive diverticulum of the anterior rectal wall. The harder the patient strains, the more intensely stool is packed into this pocket, preventing easy expulsion and producing congestion and discomfort.

Perineal Descent Syndrome

In the evaluation of the patient, it is important to note any tendency toward dropping of the perineum, which is called the perineal descent syndrome, because this may have great importance to the patient's future comfort.[4,5]

Perineal Defect

Rectocele and perineal defect are anatomically separate, but they may coexist. For an appropriate reconstruction, symptoms referable to each should be evaluated in concert with the specific anatomic pathologic condition demonstrated. Perineal defect may produce a wide and gaping perineum, which may at times subtract from coital satisfaction. The latter can be restored by perieorrhaphy, but the surgeon must be careful not to overtighten the outlet, because it may induce an anatomic coital obstruction. Perineorrhaphy, however, will not correct any marital discontent that is the result of interpersonal dissatisfaction or conflict, despite a patient's preoperative insistence to the contrary.

Normal Anatomy of Posterior Vaginal Wall and Its Supports

The S-shaped curve of the vagina terminates just anterior to the hollow of the sacrum (Figure 8.2). The vagina is separated from the rectum by the avascular rectovaginal space, more a potential space than an actual cavity. Because it permits the rectum and vagina to function independently of one another, the rectovaginal space should be preserved following surgery. The thin membranelike connective tissue, the fascia of Denonvilliers, is fused to the underside of the posterior vaginal wall.[6-9] It extends from the bottom of the cul-de-sac of Douglas to an attachment at the upper margin of the perineal body (Figure 8.3). When this attachment has been avulsed from the perineal body, the latter is destabilized anteriorly. Such a weakness is one cause of low rectocele and should be remedied by surgical reattachment during posterior repair.

The fascia of Denonvilliers has sufficient strength that it may be used effectively during posterior colporrhaphy to strengthen the posterior vaginal wall. It represents a peritoneal fusion layer of the obliterated extension of the cul-de-sac to the perineal body during fetal life. Failure of fusion of these two layers of peritoneum gives rise in adult life to a congenitally deep cul-de-sac of Douglas, and when filled with bowel or omentum, it constitutes congenital enterocele. Failure of fusion weakens this fascia of Denonvilliers and therefore its overlying posterior vaginal wall, a deficiency conducive to high rectocele. This weakness accounts in part for the frequent coexistence of high rectocele with the congenital type of enterocele (Figure 8.4). So frequent is this association that when one is found, the other should be sought and usually repaired at the same time before it progresses sufficiently to require subsequent surgery.

The more or less horizontal axis of the upper portion of the vagina is a consequence of its resting on a usually empty rectum, which, in turn, lies more or less passively on the levator plate, formed by the fusion of the right and left pubococcygeus posterior to the rectum.[10]

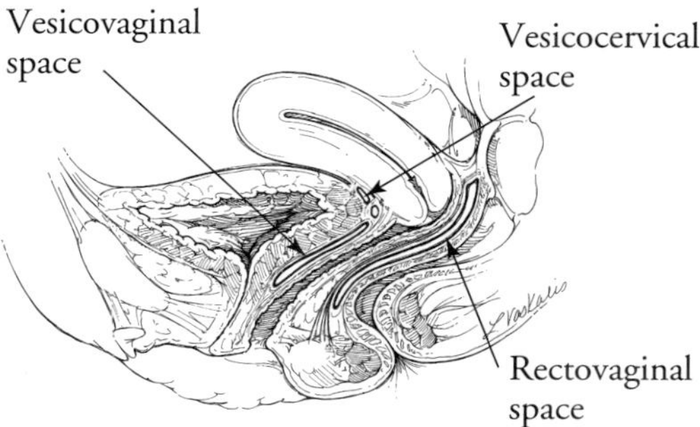

Figure 8.2 Sagittal section of the pelvis. Sagittal section of the normal adult pelvis shows a normal vaginal axis. The fascia of Denonvilliers (the rectovaginal septum) is fused to the undersurface of the posterior vaginal wall and forms the anterior wall of the rectovaginal space. The diagrammatic illustration of continuity between the rectovaginal septum (fascia of Denonvilliers) and the perineal body is shown. Note the rectovaginal, vesicovaginal, and vesicocervical spaces, which permit the organs to function somewhat independently of one another.

A

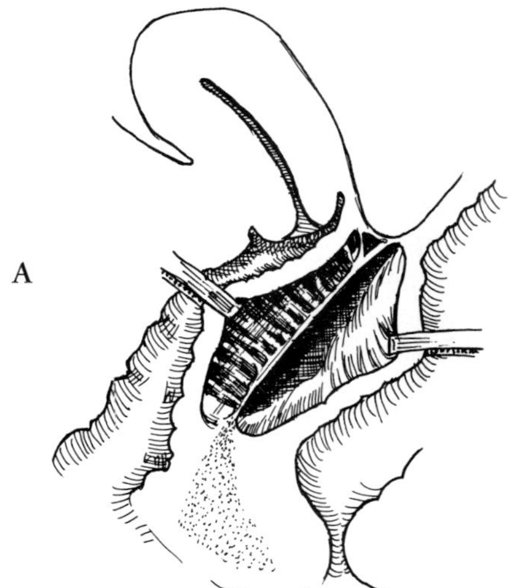

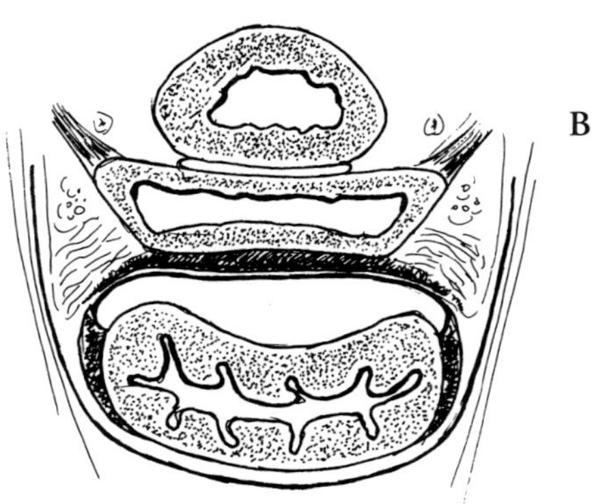

B

Figure 8.3 **A**, Rectovaginal septum, which is partly dissected from the undersurface of the vagina. It extends from the pouch of Douglas to the perineal body and forms the anterior surface of the rectovaginal space. Note the attachment of the perineal body to the fascia of Denonvilliers (**B**) as well as its adherence to the posterior vaginal wall along with its posterolateral curve. (Redrawn from Nichols DH and Milley PS: Am J Obstet Gynecol 108:17, 1970.)

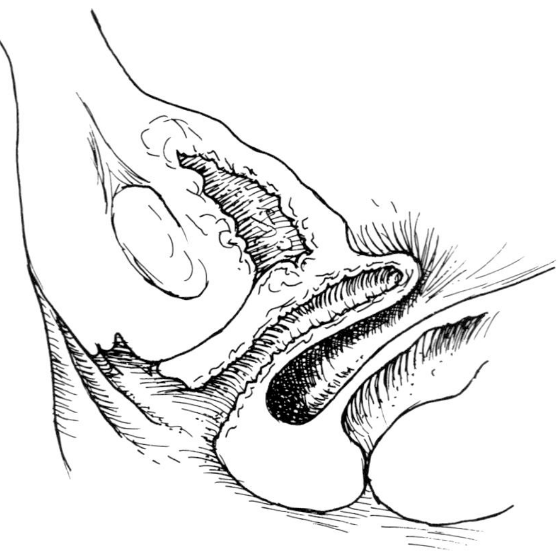

FIGURE 8.4 Posterior enterocele without eversion of the vagina in a posthysterectomy patient. (Redrawn from Nichols DH: Obstet Gynecol 40:257, 1972.)

Relatively few muscular fibers of the pubococcygeal converge anterior to the rectum. The lateral walls of the midportion of the vagina are attached to the medial borders of the pubococcygei by a connective tissue framework described as the fibers of Luschka. Therefore techniques of posterior repair that emphasize primarily a bringing together of the levatores ani between the vagina and rectum are essentially unanatomic and can create physically constricting ridges when sutures placed directly in the muscle bellies are later replaced by areas of painful fibrosis. It is these tender ridges that account for most of the postsurgical dyspareunia or apareunia reported by Jeffcoate.[11] So frequently was this seen in his practice (50% incidence of postoperative dysparunia, 25% incidence of apareunia) that he advised against posterior repair unless significant damage was confirmed by preoperative examination of the unanesthetized patient. Because anesthesia effectively paralyzes the skeletal muscles of the pelvis, an examination under anesthesia provides a false idea of anatomic weakness. Because of this temporary paralysis, the voluntary muscles cannot contract, "fight back," or resist effectively the forces of examination, and it appears as though every anesthetized woman has a rectocele.

In the days before intraperitoneal surgery and hysterectomy became relatively safe means of treating genital prolapse, an alternate treatment was the use of an intravaginal pessary, retained in the upper vagina cranial to the lateral pressures exerted by the levatores ani. With time, pressure against the pelvic diaphragm by the pessary caused the introitus to widen progressively. The patient could then no longer retain a pessary and was more uncomfortable than ever. Around the turn of the century, the introduction of prerectal levator plication as a feature of perineorrhaphy enabled such a patient once again to retain a pessary since the operation narrowed the levator or genital hiatus. Pessary use was gradually supplanted by vaginal hysterectomy and appropriate repair when these procedures became safer, more effective, and more popular for treatment of genital prolapse. Although pessary use has faded into the background, the procedures it helped engender have permitted the evolution of an erroneous concept suggesting that a firm perineum will function as a "cork in the neck of a bottle" and that perineorrhaphy would retard or prevent uterine prolapse. To the contrary, Kelly had previously observed that uterine prolapse was uncommon among the many women who had long before suffered unrepaired complete perineal tear.[12]

Rectocele and perineal defects most commonly develop from rapid overdistention of the vaginal wall during labor, although there

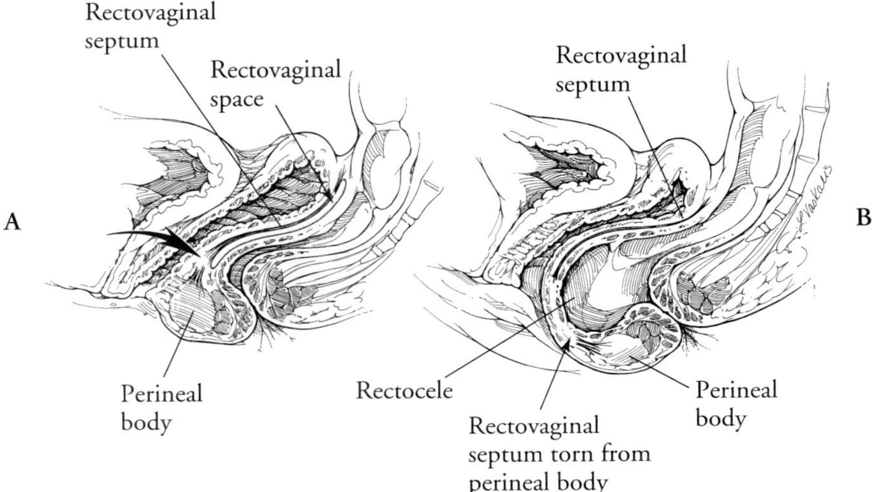

FIGURE 8.5 The potential effect of rupture of the rectovaginal septum. **A,** During childbirth and before hysterectomy, the rectovaginal septum has been torn from its attachment to the perineal body *(arrow).* **B,** This defect has permitted the development of a large low rectocele between the torn ends, which are now further apart. (Redrawn from Nichols DH and Randall CL: Vaginal surgery, ed 4, Baltimore, 1996, Williams & Wilkins.)

may be congenital perineal defects related to underdevelopment of the perineal body. There often may be traumatic detachment of the fascia of Denonvilliers (the rectovaginal septum) from the perineal body (Figure 8.5). The anterior rectal wall may herniate through this area of disruption, producing low rectocele that progressively enlarges. Such obstetric damage is more common in those patients in whom the elastic tissue component is reduced. It is more frequent in the primipara who is more than 25 years old and may be predicted as more frequent among persons with an abundance of wide abdominal striae, which imply a low elastic index.[13] The risk of subsequent rectocele and perineal defect may be lessened for such a patient by early and adequate episiotomy during labor and delivery, followed by a careful and meticulous repair bringing back together those tissues that have been cut. Weakness of the supports of the posterior vaginal wall may also develop coincident with massive eversion of the vagina attended by a shearing or avulsing of the fibers attaching the vagina to the pelvic diaphragm. This displacement of the vagina, another cause of rectocele, creates a large area of weakness into which the anterior rectal wall may expand, sometimes massively (Figure 8.6).

Preliminary pelvic examination of the unanesthetized patient should attempt to correlate the findings with the patient's symptoms. Examination of the patient when she is standing and straining (Figure 8.7) may disclose a coincident and often unsuspected prolapse of the vaginal vault. When found, remedy of this defect should be included as well in the plan for surgical reconstruction.

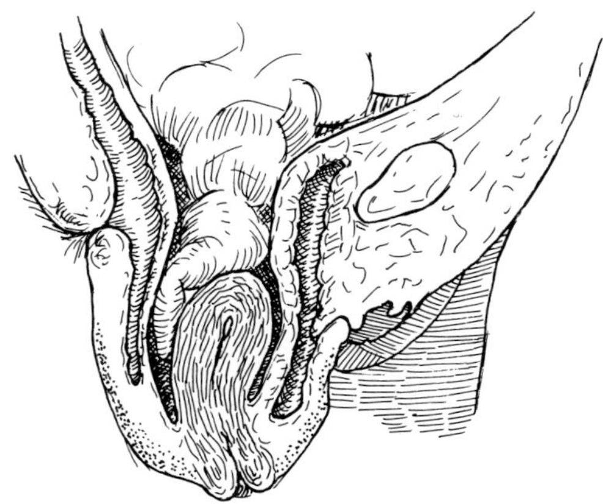

FIGURE 8.6 Procidentia may evolve as a result of unrestrained progression of any of the types of prolapse. (Redrawn from Nichols DH: Postgrad Med 46:183, 1969.)

Because the length of the perineal body approximates that of the female urethra, re-

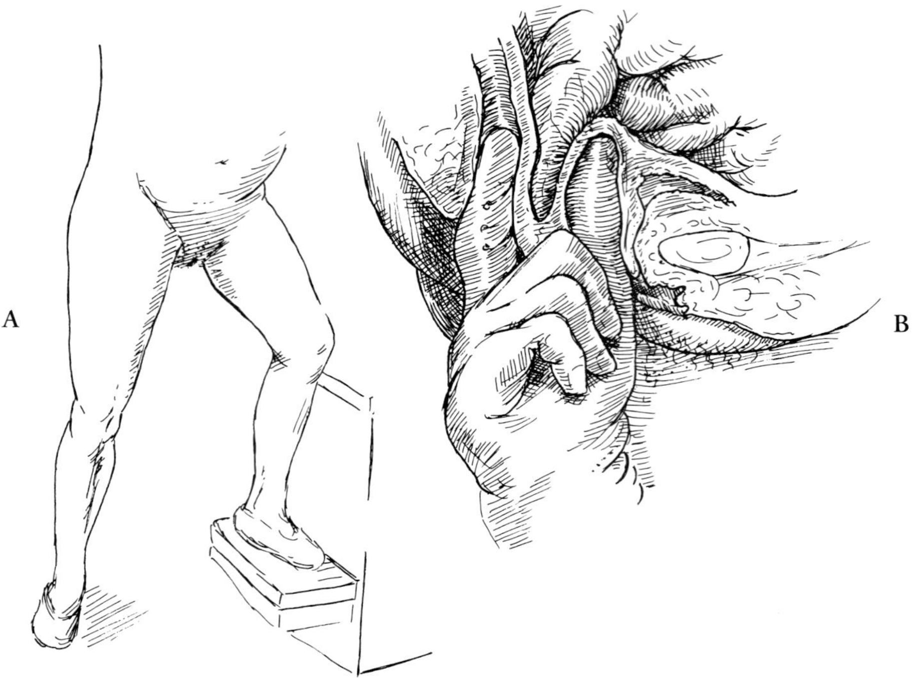

FIGURE 8.7 Examination of the patient in a standing position (**A**) permits the thumb in the vagina (**B**) to note and replace any descent of the vaginal vault while the index finger introduced into the rectum permits evaluation of any possible rectocele. When the patient strains, any enterocele present is evidenced by palpation of a bowel-filled sac dissecting the rectovaginal septum. (Redrawn from Nichols DH: Repair of enterocele and prolapse of the vaginal vault. In Barber H, editor: Goldsmith's practice of surgery, Woodbury, CT, 1981, Ciné Med.)

construction of a damaged perineum will improve urethral support and future function. Curiously, it will also lengthen the vagina.

TECHNIQUE OF REPAIR

The goals of reconstructive surgery are (1) relief of symptoms, (2) restoration of normal anatomic relationships, and (3) restoration of function. Surgical repair of the posterior vaginal wall should endeavor to recreate or duplicate a normal anatomic relationship in which there are an intact and effective perineal body, attachment of the upper margin of the perineal body to the fascia of Denonvilliers, and elimination of the weak spot in the midportion of an overdistended and thus enlarged vagina, but with preservation of the rectovaginal space that will permit continued independent function of the vagina and rectum. Secondary ballooning of the anterior rectal wall can be corrected by plication. If there is eversion of the vaginal vault, this should be corrected by coincident colpopexy, performed either transvaginally as in sacrospinous colpopexy or transabdominally as in sacral colpopexy. Any coincident enterocele should be surgically eliminated.

Long-acting but absorbable sutures of the polyglycolic acid type have replaced those of catgut in our practice, because they provide a longer period of support during wound healing, less edema and discomfort interfering with restoration of function, and elimination of batch-to-batch variability in suture strength. If postmenopausal, the patient is started preoperatively on a course of estrogen replacement using an intravaginal estrogen cream, which is continued for several months postoperatively. It will restore and improve vaginal elasticity and, by increasing the vaginal blood supply and thickening the vaginal wall, promote better wound healing.

Dissection and repair of rectocele should begin above the highest point of weakness. The undersurface of the perineal body is un-

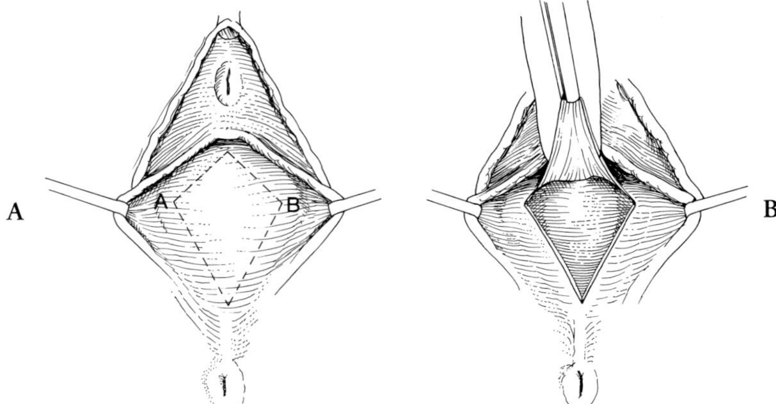

FIGURE 8.8 A, An initial V-shaped incision between points *A* and *B* is indicated by the *dashed line.* A flap will be mobilized by sharp dissection (**B**) and the incisions carried under and up the posterior vaginal wall to a point cranial to the rectocele. At the conclusion of the repair, the tissue identified by *A* will meet *B,* and the circumference of the introitus will be narrowed by the preselected distance *AB.* (Redrawn from Nichols DH and Randall CL: Vaginal surgery, ed 4, Baltimore, 1996, Williams & Wilkins.)

covered from beneath a V-shaped skin incision (Figure 8.8), the width of which is determined by the width of the introitus desired at the conclusion of the operation. Care should be taken to leave the introitus somewhat loose for the aging patient so that postoperative coital obstruction does not become a problem.

With the patient for whom perineorrhaphy is not necessary, a midline episiotomy will provide access to the lower portion of the vagina. The dissection is carried beneath the posterior vaginal wall, separating it from the vaginal surface of the perineal body, until the rectovaginal space is identified and opened. An appropriately wide strip of the full thickness of the posterior vaginal wall is removed to a point cranial to the rectocele (Figure 8.9). If high rectocele is present, the removal of this strip extends the full length of the vagina to the vault. Failure to correct rectocele for its full depth leaves a residual weakness in the midvagina that superficially resembles enterocele, but careful examination discloses the residual rectocele, which is often still symptomatic. Careful examination of the undersurface of the vagina at surgery will identify the fascia of Denonvilliers attached to it. The fascia can be identified by its blue-white color and by touch. It has a smooth peritoneum-like feel. If further dissection reveals the double fold of peritoneum so characteristic of an enterocele, the sac should be opened, the neck closed by high ligation, a second ligation placed 1 cm distal to the first (Figure 8.10), and the excess peritoneum excised.[3] This double ligation of the neck of the sac will not only take the tension from the initial closing stitch of the peritoneum but will also increase the thickness of the scar in this area, making it more resistant to recurrence of the enterocele. Closure of the neck of the enterocele sac not only brings together the thin me-

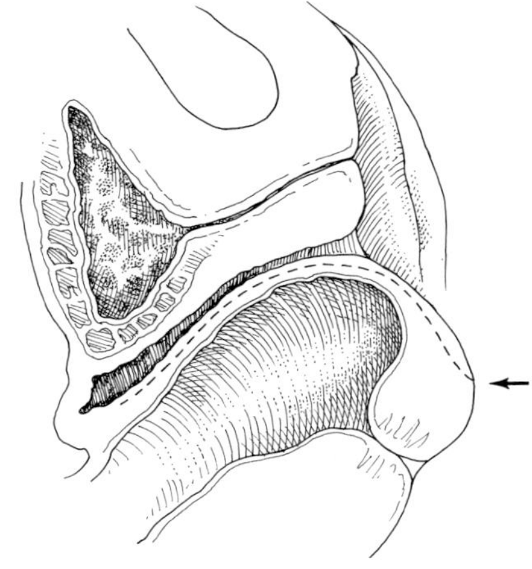

FIGURE 8.9 Sagittal section showing the initial line of dissection exposing the full perineum in the rectocele. Above the perineum, the dissection enters the rectovaginal space and continues to a point proximal and above the rectocele. The incision begins at the spot indicated by the *arrow,* and its course follows the *dashed line.* (Redrawn from Nichols DH and Randall CL: Vaginal surgery, ed 4, Baltimore, 1996, Williams & Wilkins.)

sothelial epithelium of the peritoneal cavity but also incorporates the rather strong subperitoneal retinaculum of connective tissue to increase the strength of the peritoneal flood. If strong uterosacral ligaments can be identified at the vault of the vagina, they should be sewn together in the midline.

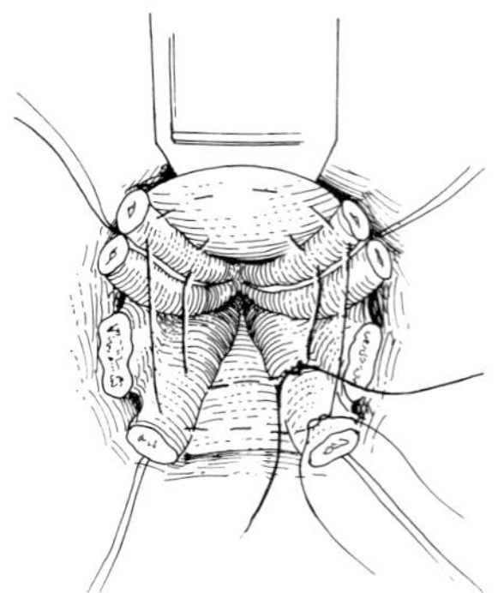

FIGURE 8.10 The enterocele sac has been resected, and the peritoneal cavity has been closed by a purse-string suture that incorporates the uterosacral and round ligaments. A second purse-string stitch, placed 1 cm distal to the first, reinforces the closure. (Redrawn from Nichols DH and Randall CL: Vaginal surgery, ed 4, Baltimore, 1996, Williams & Wilkins.)

Any ballooning of the anterior rectal wall and its fascia may be reduced by a layer or two of running locked suture continued to the perineum (Figure 8.11).

The cut edges of the vagina are brought together by a running subcuticular suture that goes well back into the fascia of Denonvilliers,[1,6] thickening the posterior vaginal wall (Figure 8.12). When the subcuticular vaginal wall suture has reached the site of the cranial edge of the perineal body, a separate figure-of-eight stitch should be taken in this cranial edge, reestablishing the attachment that is normally present between perineal body and fascia of Denonvilliers. At the conclusion of the posterior colporrhaphy and before the perineorrhaphy, the operator should be able to insert a finger into the rectovaginal space, demonstrating the freedom of the posterior vaginal wall from the rectum (Figure 8.13).

Some operators prefer to split the rectovaginal septum (including the fascia of Denonvilliers and a few fibers of the fibromuscular wall of the vagina to which the fascia is attached) from the vaginal wall and close this as a separate layer (Figure 8.14). The residual vaginal membrane is then trimmed appropriately and closed by subcuticular suture. This

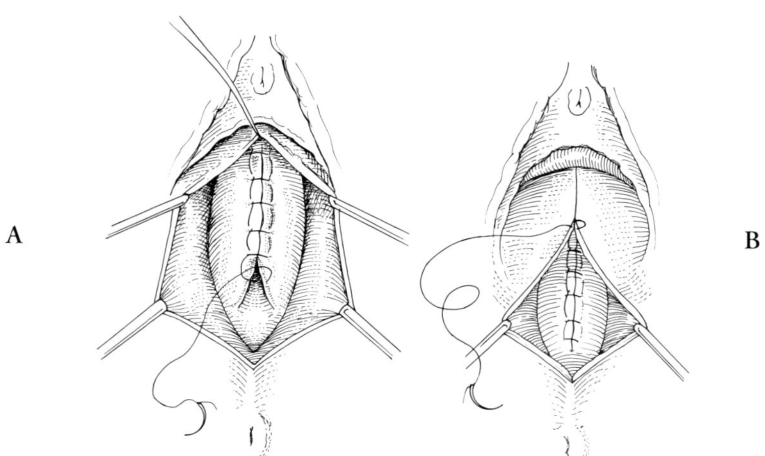

FIGURE 8.11 Any ballooning of the anterior rectal wall may be corrected by one or more layers of running, locked, fine absorbable suture commencing proximal to the defect and continuing distally for its full length. Reconstitution may be carried posterior to the site of the new perineal body, not yet restored (**A**). Side-to-side closure of the full thickness of the posterior vaginal wall is accomplished by running, subcuticular sutures (**B**). The cranial margin of the perineal body is reattached to the underside of the vagina at the bottom of the rectovaginal space. The perineal body is reconstructed by a series of interrupted stitches. (Redrawn from Nichols DH and Randall CL: Vaginal surgery. ed 4, Baltimore, 1996, Williams & Wilkins.)

method, particularly in the older patient, not only risks disturbing the vaginal blood supply with some increased postoperative fibrosis and longer wound healing but also renders less precise the amount of vaginal wall that should be removed. The amount of vagina to be excised with posterior colporrhaphy should be such that at the conclusion of the operation the vagina will admit three fingers, unless preoperative inquiry reveals that the patient's coital partner differs from this size.

During posterior colporrhaphy and recon-

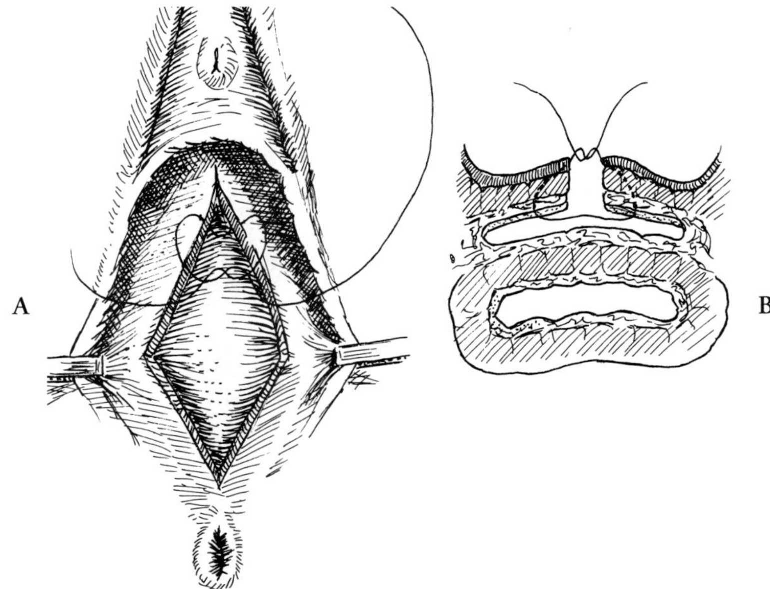

Figure 8.12 A full-thickness wedge of posterior vaginal wall has been excised, and the tissues, including a fused rectovaginal septum (the fascia of Denonvilliers), are closed from side to side (**A**) using a running, subcuticular suture (**B**).

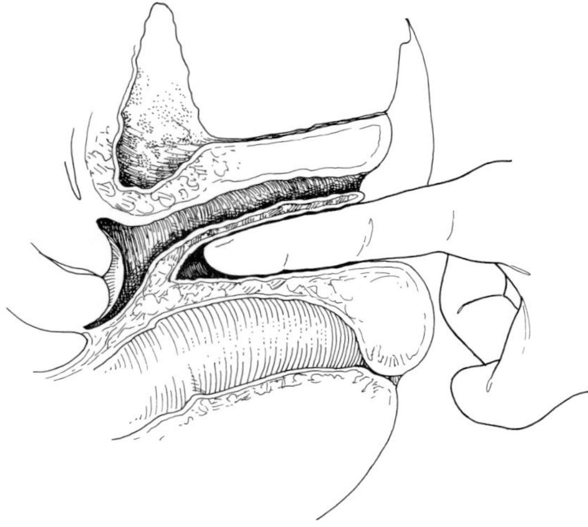

Figure 8.13 At the completion of the posterior colporrhaphy and before starting the perineorrhaphy, the operator should be able to insert an index finger between the posterior vaginal wall, to which the rectovaginal septum (fascia of Denonvilliers) is attached, and the anterior surface of the rectum, demonstrating the desired freedom of this space. (Redrawn from Nichols DH and Randall CL: Vaginal surgery, ed 4, Baltimore, 1996, Williams & Wilkins.)

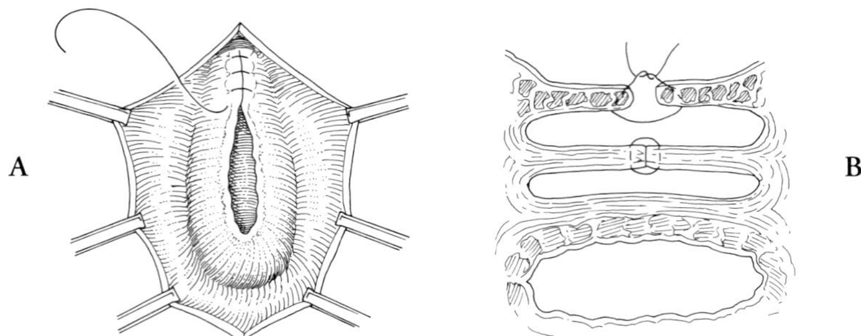

FIGURE 8.14 Bullard modification, in which the rectovaginal septum has been dissected from the posterior vaginal wall and closed as a separate layer between the rectum and the vaginal membrane (**A**). The excess vaginal skin is trimmed and the sides brought together by subcuticular suture (**B**). (Redrawn from Nichols DH and Randall CL: Vaginal surgery, ed 4, Baltimore, 1996, Williams & Wilkins.)

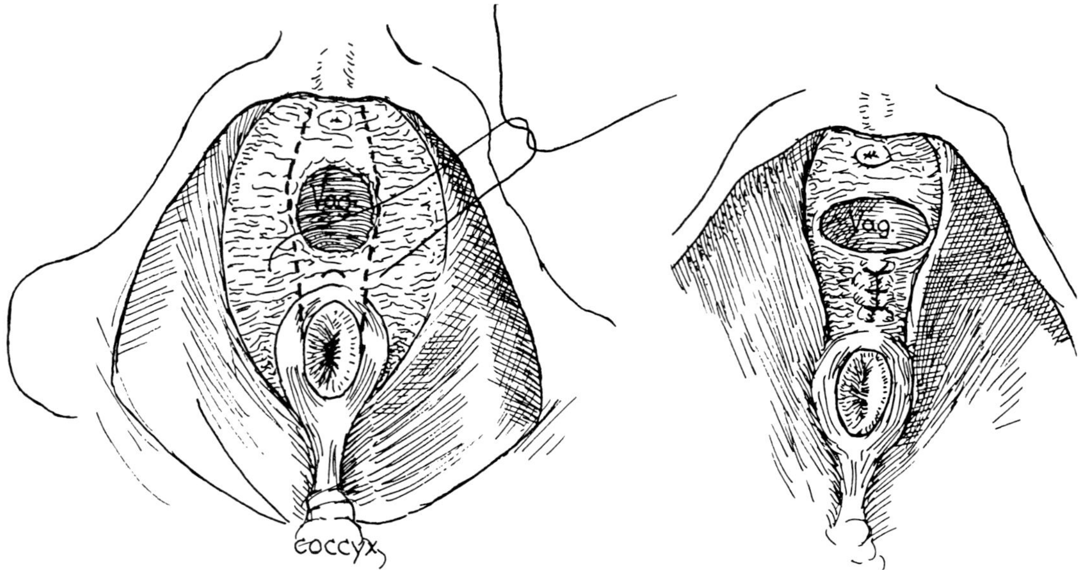

FIGURE 8.15 Perineorrhaphy may be accomplished without placement of stitches directly into the bellies of the pubococcygeal muscles, as shown with the wide genital hiatus in the drawing to the left. When the interrupted stitches in the perineal body have been tied, the lateral attachments of this tissue to the fascia of the pubococcygeal muscles bring the latter closer together, narrowing the genital hiatus, to a new position as noted by the *dashed line.* The end result is illustrated at the right. The genital hiatus has been effectively narrowed. No stitches have been placed directly into the pubococcygei. (Modified from Nichols DH and Randall CL: Vaginal surgery, ed 4, Baltimore, 1996, Williams & Wilkins.)

struction, the operator at all times should check frequently for the presence of palpable subepithelial ridges, which, if found, should be immediately relieved by cutting the offending suture. Such ridges will invariably remain postoperatively, often becoming symptomatic and tender and forming a coital obstruction. Because of their fibrosis, they can be very difficult to stretch.

The perineal body is reconstructed by a series of horizontal interrupted mattress stitches placed in the soft tissues medial to the pubococcygei and including the smooth muscle of the perineum (Figure 8.15). Although these stitches are not placed in the bellies of the levator muscles themselves, the tissues into which they have been put are attached to the medial borders of the pelvic

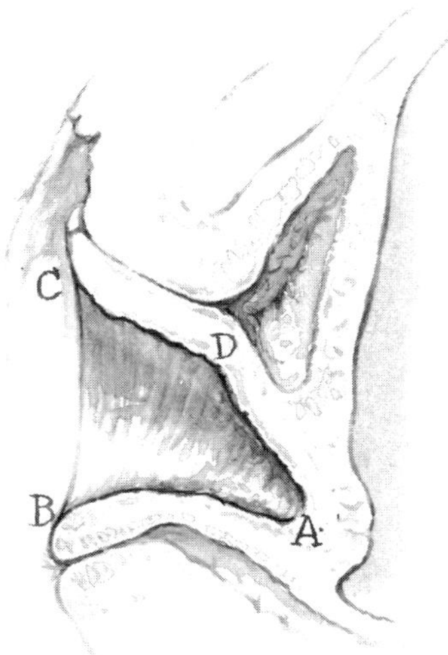

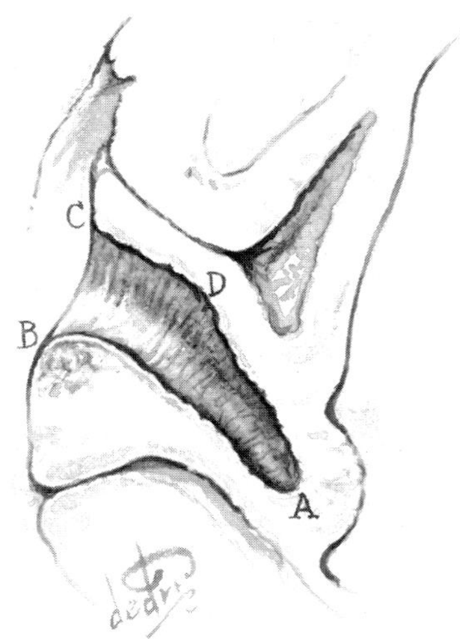

FIGURE 8.16 The effect of perineorrhaphy after lengthening the posterior wall is demonstrated. Sagittal drawing of the pelvis of a patient with a defective perineum is shown on the left. The anterior vaginal wall, *ADC,* is longer than the posterior wall, *AB.* The lengthening of the posterior vagina, *AB,* after perineorrhaphy is shown in the drawing to the right. The length of the anterior vaginal wall, *ADC,* is unchanged. (Modified from Nichols DH and Randall CL: Vaginal surgery, ed 4, Baltimore, 1996, Williams & Wilkins.)

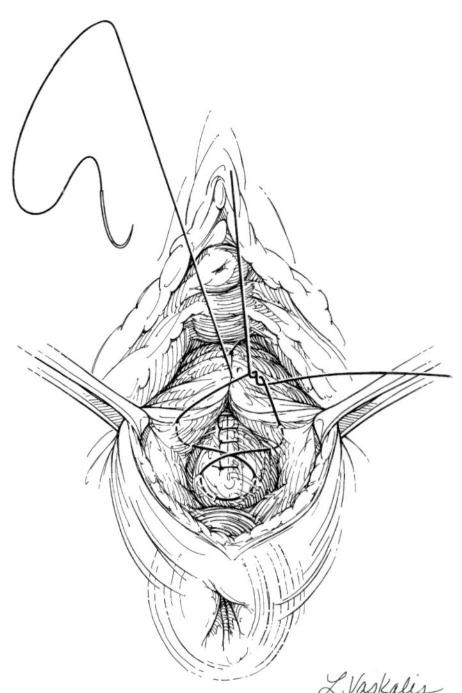

FIGURE 8.17 Reattachment of the fascia of Denonvilliers (rectovaginal septum) to the perineal body. Anterior rectal plication has reduced the size of the rectal reservoir for the full limit of the rectocele. A figure-of-eight stitch reattaches the fascia of Denonvilliers to the perineal body.

diaphragm. When these stitches are tied, they will effectively narrow the levator hiatus without the risk of levator spasm, fibrosis, and tenderness.

Reconstruction of a defective perineum by perineorrhaphy will actually lengthen the posterior vaginal wall (Figure 8.16). The fascia of Denonvilliers should be reattached to the perineal body by a figure-of-eight stitch (Figure 8.17). If the introitus has been narrowed by previous surgery, a troublesome stricture can be prevented by reconstitution of the perineal body by parallel "11" sutures (Figure 8.18). When the surgeon wishes to reduce both the width and length of the perineal body, a U-shaped suture may be used (Figure 8.19).

The perineal body of a long perineum can be reattached to the connective tissue capsule of the external anal sphincter by a separate figure-of-eight suture placed more posteriorly[14] (Figure 8.20). All of these stitches are useful in the correction of early perineal descent, identified when the anus is found to be the lowermost point on the perineum.

In an occasional patient, there is a perineal defect for which no soft tissues can be found to be brought together. In such a patient, "levator muscle stitches" can be placed, although the operator should check after each stitch for

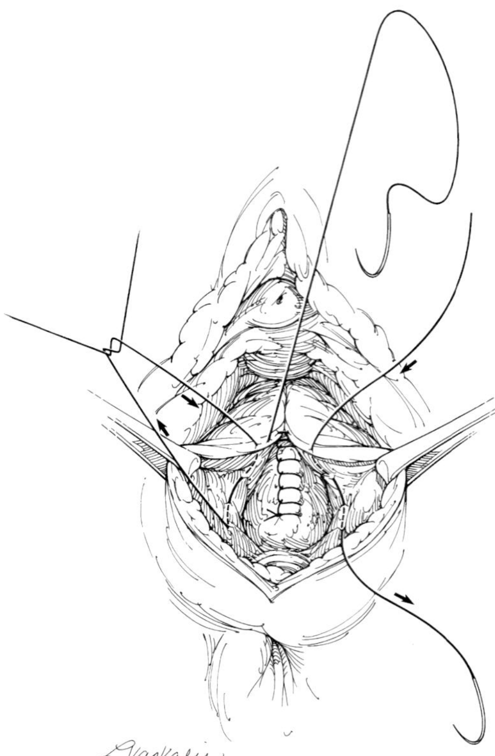

FIGURE 8.18 The "11" sutures. When the introitus has been previously narrowed, and occasionally in the presence of a perineal descent syndrome, the fascia of Denonvilliers may be reattached to the perineal body by two longitudinal interrupted sutures as shown. After both have been placed, they are tied. This will help restore the perineum without narrowing the introitus.

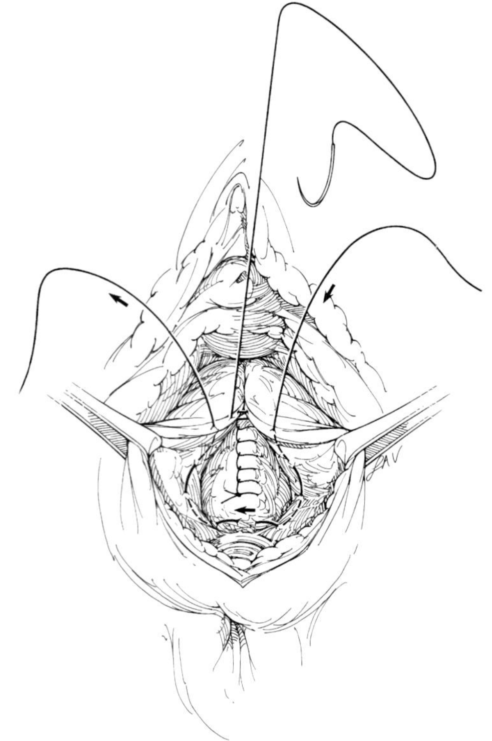

FIGURE 8.19 Reconstruction of the long and wide perineum. The full length of the increased rectal reservoir has been reduced by a running locked stitch that ends behind the site at which a new perineal body will be constructed. The underside of the fascia of Denonvilliers (rectovaginal septum) can be reattached to the widened site of the perineal body by a U-shaped suture configuration placed into it as shown. When this stitch has been tied, the perineum will have been reduced in width as well as in length.

ridge production (Figure 8.21). If a ridge is found, the stitch is removed and replaced by one located closer to the rectum. Levator stitches should never be tied tightly, because they may destroy the muscle in which they have been placed and convert it to a tender band of fibrous tissue, which may require future secondary perineotomy for relief.

The perineal skin is reapproximated in the midline by a running subcuticular suture. When monofilament absorbable suture has been used with colporrhaphy, it is desirable to bury the cut ends of the suture, removing the sharp points as a source of discomfort to the patient. The technique is simple and is illustrated in Figure 8.22. Finally, the caliber of the vagina is assessed carefully with consideration of future coital satisfaction. If it is unexpectedly constricted, appropriate full-thickness lateral vaginal wall relaxing incisions are made at the 3 or 9 o'clock position (or both). With relaxing incisions, a vaginal packing or postoperative vaginal obturator must be inserted to prevent postoperative constriction. The obturator is removed frequently for cleaning but is kept in place until a firm bed of granulation tissue has been formed and reepithelialization is underway.

Rectal examination is performed to confirm the integrity of the rectum. If a transgressing stitch is found, it is cut on the rectal side and allowed to retract. Cutting such a stitch lessens postoperative pain and the risk of rectovaginal fistula.

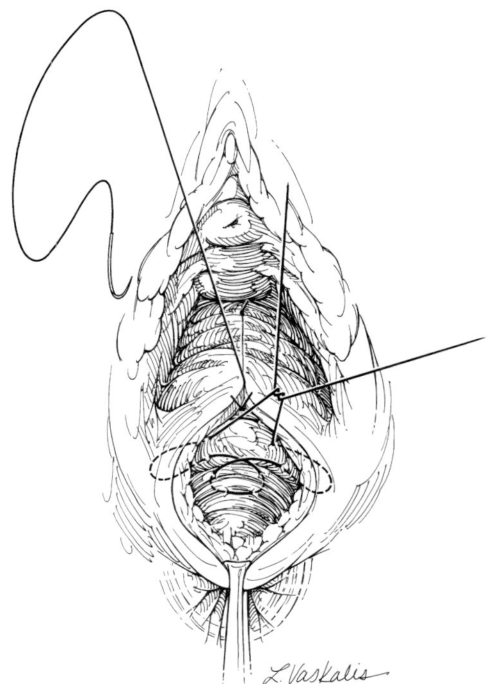

FIGURE 8.20 Correction of detachment of the anus from the perineal body. Detachment of the anal sphincter from the perineal body may be corrected by a buried figure-of-eight suture placed as shown. This will stabilize both the anus and the perineal body. (Redrawn from Nichols DH and Randall CL: Vaginal surgery, ed 4, Baltimore, 1996, Williams & Wilkins.)

Damage to the supports and attachments of the vagina and the stretching of its wall beyond the limits of elasticity permits the anterior rectal wall to herniate into the vagina, a condition termed *rectocele.* Secondary rectal herniation has increased the size of the rectal reservoir in some patients and is reflected by stretch damage to the strongest layer of the rectum, the submucosa,[15-17] causing it to become pathologically thin at the site of damage in the anterior rectal wall. When this is associated with inability to completely empty the bowel at the time of a movement, often requiring external manual pressure to the vagina or perineum, the condition can generally be remedied by an appropriate surgical repair consisting of posterior colporrhaphy and perineorrhaphy. In most instances the repair of coincident ballooning of the anterior rectal wall can be treated by reduction in rectal luminal size by suture imbrication of the anterior rectal wall using a running locked stitch placed directly into the perirectal fascial capsule and the rectal muscularis, restoring the rectal reservoir to near its former size and relieving the symptom of incomplete bowel movements. Such imbricating stitches are generally not placed in the rectal submucosal layer of tissue because of its proximity to the rectal mucosa. Occasionally, the resultant scar in the muscularis is insufficient to maintain reduction in the pathologic sizes of the reservoir after suture absorption, and the patient's symptoms of incomplete evacuation return even though the vagina and perineum have been restored to a normal anatomic relationship. This could be remedied by an endorectal reduction in size of the rectal reservoir[18-20] by longitudinal plication of the strong submucosal layer beyond its area of pathologic thinning. The majority of rectoceles are seen in the anterior rectal wall. Occasionally one may be found in the posterior rectal wall, and rarely one may be combined between anterior, posterior, and even lateral rectal walls (Figure 8.23). The techniques of endorectal repair are relatively simple and uncomplicated and can be applied to one or more quadrants simultaneously without disturbing the integrity of the posterior vaginal wall (Figures 8.24 and 8.25).

POSTOPERATIVE CARE

The patient follows a regular diet but uses stool softeners and gentle laxatives so as to avoid straining against the fresh repair while having a bowel movement. Ascorbic acid is given for 1 month or longer to promote wound healing, and postoperative estrogen supplementation is given if the patient is postmenopausal. Coitus may be resumed after 4 to 6 weeks of healing. On the first or second postoperative day the patient starts isometric perineal resistive exercises (15 strong voluntary pubococcygeal contractions, each of 3 seconds' duration, 6 times daily) to be continued for at least 3 months. This will aid both in reestablishing perineal circulation and in restoring physiologic bowel function and habits.

Text continued on p. 131.

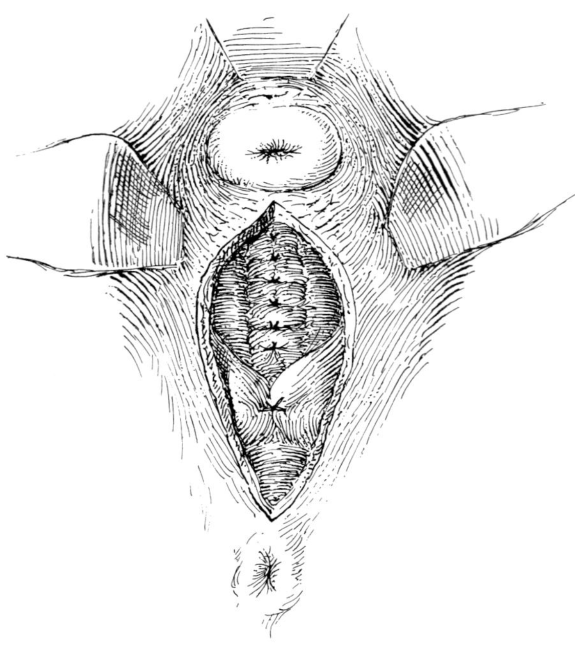

FIGURE 8.21 Optimal approximation of pubococcygeal fascia. In occasional instances of extreme perineal defect, it may be desirable to bring the fascia of each pubococcygeus together in the midline in front of the rectum; palpable ridges of tissue must be carefully avoided. (Redrawn from Nichols DH and Randall CL: Vaginal surgery, ed 4, Baltimore, 1996, Williams & Wilkins.)

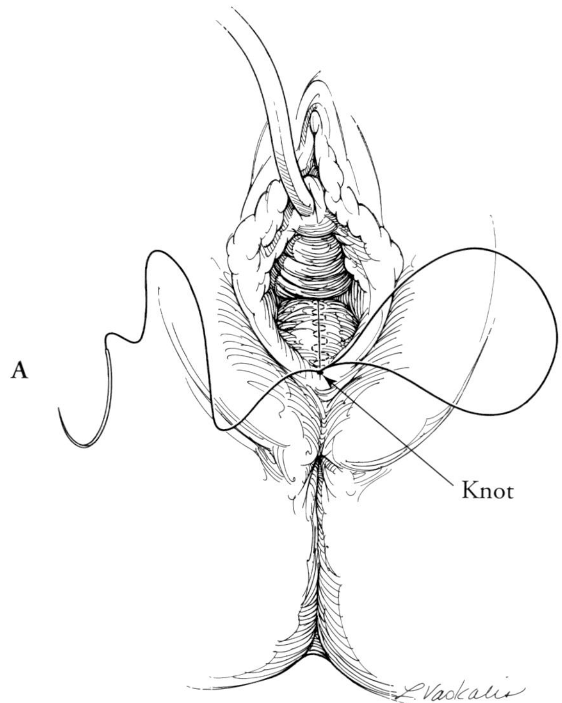

FIGURE 8.22 Method of burying the sharp ends of a monofilament suture. At the conclusion of a running subcuticular suture a knot is placed (**A**).

Continued.

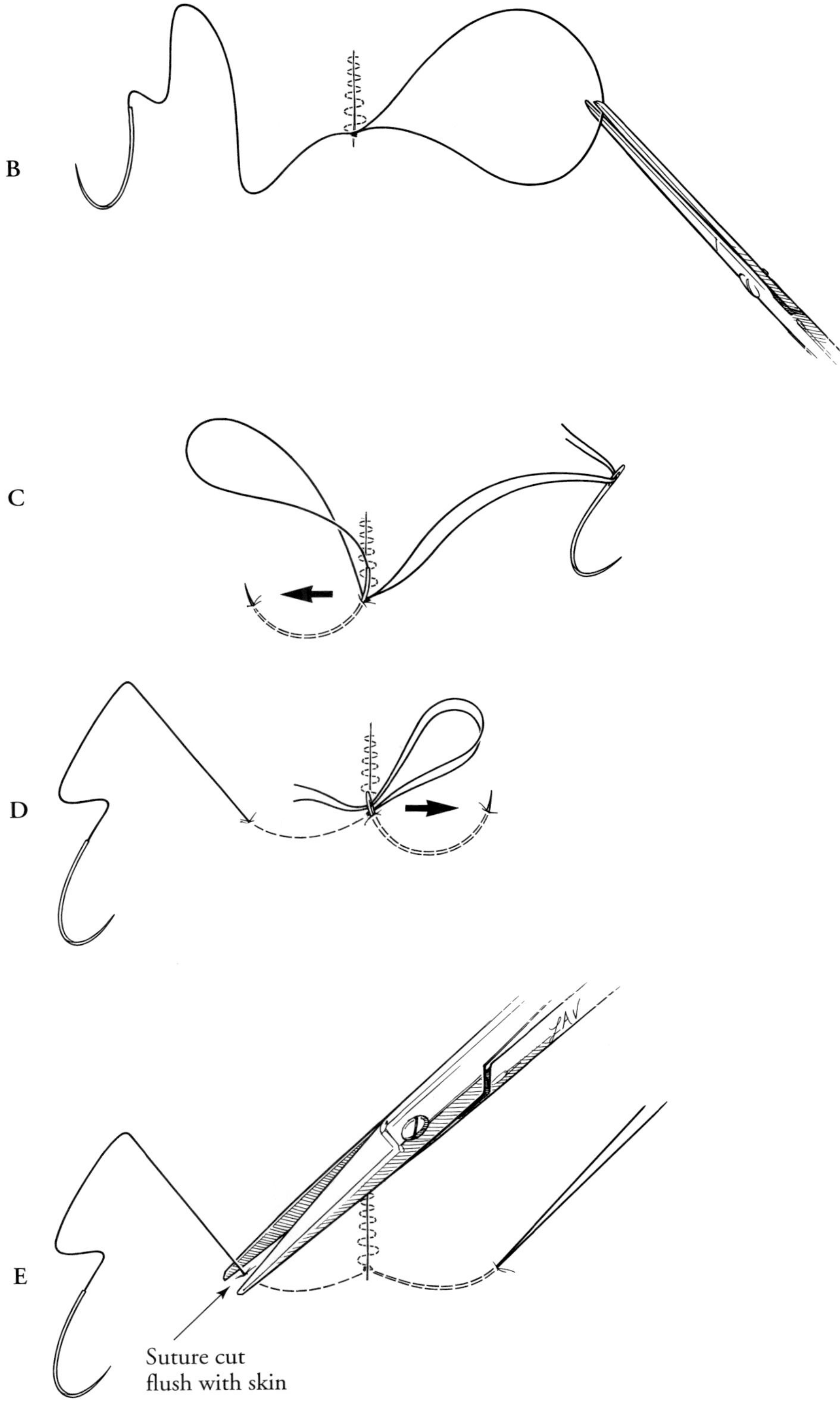

FIGURE 8.22, cont'd. The loop is cut (**B**) and threaded onto a free needle (**C**) while the opposite end of the suture with the swedged needle is passed laterally as shown. The free needle is passed (**D**) and traction made to the sutures on each side, at which time they are cut flush with the skin (**E**).

Continued.

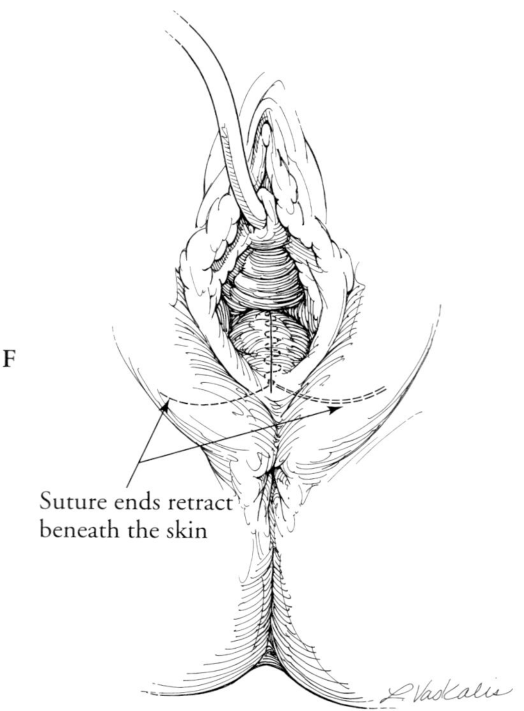

FIGURE 8.22, cont'd. The pointed ends of the suture retract beneath the skin's surface (F).

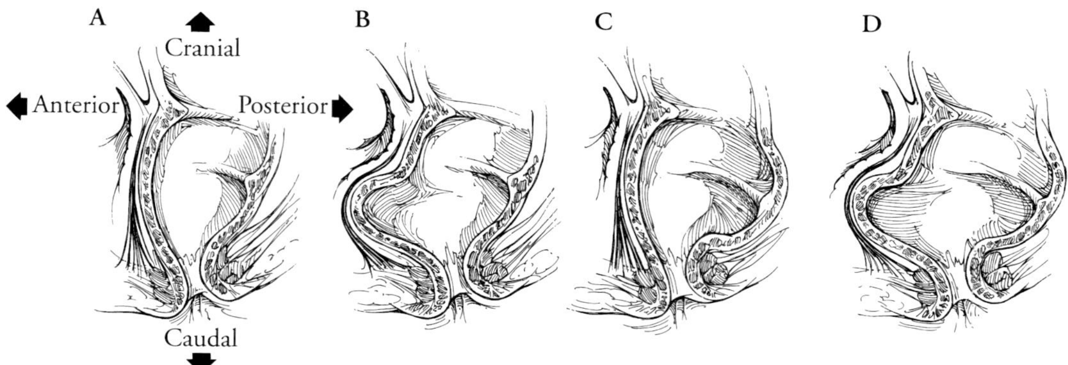

FIGURE 8.23 Sagittal views of types of rectocele. **A,** The normal rectum (the vagina is to the left). **B,** Anterior rectocele displacing the vagina. **C,** The rare posterior rectocele. **D,** Combined anterior and posterior rectocele. (Redrawn from Nichols DH and Randall CL: Vaginal surgery, ed 4, Baltimore, 1996, Williams & Wilkins.)

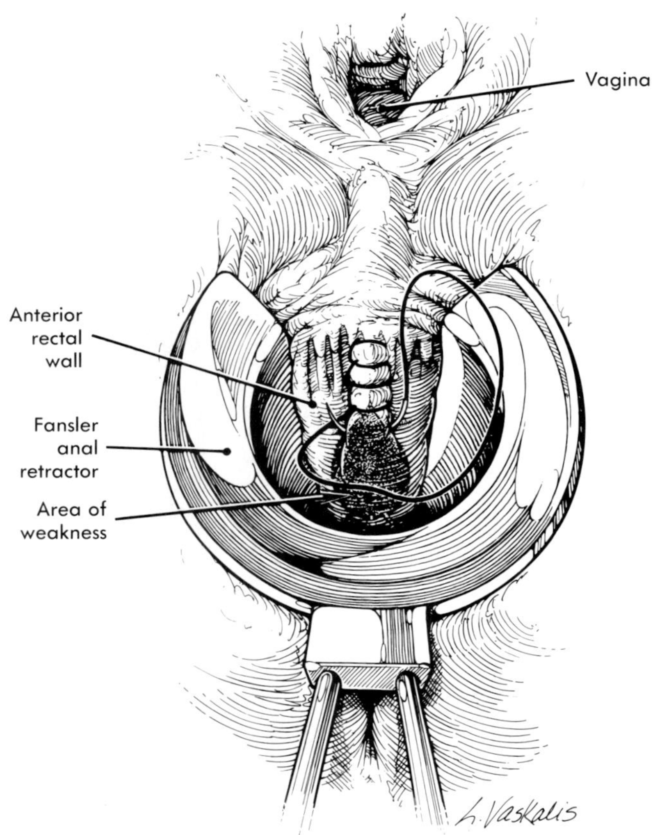

FIGURE 8.24 Endorectal repair of rectocele. A Fansler's rectal retractor has been inserted into the rectum, and the redundant mucosa and submucosa of the weakened anterior rectal wall have been identified. Starting just proximal to the mucocutaneous junction, a running locked obliterative suture has been started. The suture is placed through both mucosal and submucosal layers and includes the rectal muscularis. With each stitch the suture is tightly drawn. No portion of the intact vaginal wall is included in the suture. When the rectal tissue of the rectocele has been obliterated to a point cranial to the low or midvaginal rectocele, the direction of the suture is reversed and a second obliterative layer is placed, reinforcing the initial layer. (From Nichols DH: Gynecologic and obstetric surgery, St Louis, 1993, Mosby.)

SUMMARY

When a patient with rectocele and perineal defect receives only a perineorrhaphy as her surgical treatment, the unrepaired rectocele persists as such, and if she was previously symptomatic, the rectal symptoms of incomplete bowel movement and postevacuation pressure and aching remain. The physical appearance within the vagina masquerades as enterocele, but the true nature of the persistent rectocele is evident by rectovaginal examination, particularly in the standing patient who is bearing down. Failure to carry a rectocele repair high enough to a point beyond the upper limit of the defect produces this clinical and anatomic picture. It is corrected by transvaginal reoperation with more extensive rectocele repair, which is dissected and then repaired starting at the highest point of the rectocele.

Recurrent rectocele should be approached thoughtfully and evaluated with great care to ensure correlation between symptoms and findings. Physical examination should determine all areas of weakness so that their repair may be incorporated in the final surgical plan. A search for unexpected prolapse of the vaginal vault should be made by examination of the patient in a standing position. If found, it should be corrected. Any coincident enterocele should be identified and surgically repaired.

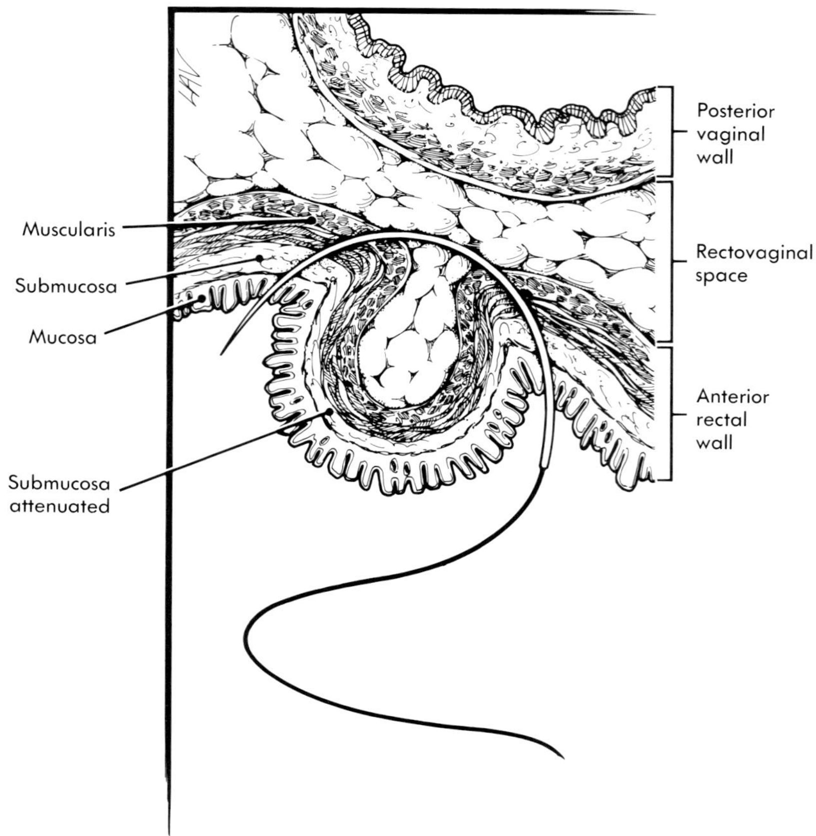

FIGURE 8.25 Section showing endorectal suture placement. The needle and suture are placed through the full thickness of the rectal wall, including the mucosa, submucosa, and muscularis. The unopened and unsewn vaginal wall is shown. (From Nichols DH: Gynecologic and obstetric surgery, St Louis, 1993, Mosby.)

REFERENCES

1. Nichols DH: Rectocele and perineal defect. In Nichols, DH, editor: Gynecologic and obstetric surgery, St. Louis, 1993, Mosby.
2. Nichols DH: Posterior colporrhaphy and perineorrhaphy: separate and distinct operations, Am J Obstet Gynecol 164:714, 1991.
3. Nichols DH and Randall CL: Vaginal surgery, ed 4, Baltimore, 1996, Williams & Wilkins.
4. Henry MM and Swash M: Coloproctology and the pelvic floor, ed 2, London, 1992, Butterworth.
5. Nichols DH: Retrorectal levatorplasty with colporrhaphy, Clin Obstet Gynecol 25:939, 1982.
6. Harrison JE and McDonagh JE: Hernia of Douglas' pouch and high rectocele, Am J Obstet Gynecol 60:83, 1950.
7. Milley PS and Nichols DH: A correlative investigation of the human rectovaginal septum, Anat Rec 163:443, 1969.
8. Tobin CE and Benjamin JA: Anatomical and surgical restudy of Denonvilliers' fascia, Surg Gynecol Obstet 80:373, 1945.
9. Uhlenhuth E and Nolley GW: Vaginal fascia, a myth? Obstet Gynecol 10:349, 1957.
10. Berglas B and Rubin IC: Study of the supportive structures of the uterus by levator myography, Surg Gynecol Obstet 97:677, 1953.
11. Jeffcoate TNA: Posterior colporrhaphy, Am J Obstet Gynecol 77:490, 1959.

12. Kelly HA: Operative gynecology, vol I, New York, 1898, Butterworth.

13. Magdi I: Obstetric injuries of the perineum, J Obstet Gynaecol Br Emp 49:687, 1942.

14. Kennedy JW and Campbell AD: Vaginal hysterectomy, Philadelphia, 1942, FA Davis Co.

15. Halsted WS: Circular suture of the intestine; an experimental study, Am J Med Sci 94:436, 1887.

16. Jansen A and others: The importance of the apposition of the submucosal intestinal layers for primary wound healing of intestinal anastomosis, Surg Gynecol Obstet 152:51, 1981.

17. Lord MG, Valies P, and Broughton AC: A morphologic study of submucosa of the large intestine, Surg Gynecol Obstet 145:155, 1977.

18. Block IR: Transrectal repair of rectocele using obliterative suture, Dis Colon Rectum 29:707, 1986.

19. Khubchandani IT and others: Endorectal repair of rectocele, Dis Colon Rectum 26:792, 1983.

20. Sehapayak S: Transrectal repair of rectocele: an extended armamentarium of colorectal surgeons, Dis Colon Rectum 28:422, 1985.

9

Recurrent Enterocele

David H. Nichols

When a primary repair has unsuccessfully correlated the cause of an enterocele with a technique of repair specifically designed to correct the cause, recurrence of the enterocele is not only possible, but likely, bringing with it a recurrence of both symptoms and physical findings. This necessitates re-repair but using a choice of more effective technique. The surgeon must decide whether the enterocele is truly recurrent or is only persistent.

For successful re-repair, it is desirable to determine the correct cause. This usually may be correlated with the findings on physical examination. These observations correlate, in turn, with the optimal specific surgical treatment.

Etiology

There are four principal causes of enterocele: (1) congenital, (2) pulsion, (3) traction, and (4) iatrogenic from a change in the vaginal axis.

Congenital Enterocele

Congenital enterocele is identified by a deep cul-de-sac that contains bowel, usually small intestine, and often omentum[1] (Figure 9.1, *A*). It is a consequence of failure of fusion or defusion of the peritoneal walls of the cul-de-sac, which in fetal life extends all the way to the perineal body. Fusion of the anterior and posterior layers of peritoneum produces a strong surgically useful layer of the fascia of Denonvilliers. This peritoneal fusion fascia is firmly attached to the underside of the posterior vaginal wall, the very nature of this adherence giving some strength one to the other.

True enterocele differs from the deep cul-de-sac in that the former has an intestinal content within the sac.[2-4] For this to occur, elongation of the small intestinal mesentery is required. It is likely that traction to this mesentery from the weight of content within the bowel gives rise to the backache and feeling of pelvic fullness that is so characteristic of enterocele. The length of the mesentery of the small intestine is usually about 15 cm, not long enough to permit a loop of small intestine to descend far into the pelvis.[5] When the sac of peritoneum in this area includes small intestine, we do not know whether the elongation of the intestinal mesentery is the cause or the result of the enterocele. If it is the cause, the weight of the small bowel with its contents on the floor of the pelvic cavity may, in some people, push the cul-de-sac downwards, becoming an enterocele. This has significance in the results of surgery for enterocele, because although we may remove the sac of the enterocele and occlude the neck, we do nothing per se to the mesentery of the small intestine, which is just as long postoperatively as it was preoperatively. The weight and pressure of the bowel with this long mesentery may be one of the more common causes for recurrence of enterocele. Thus there is a difference between enterocele and a deep cul-de-sac. The two are not synonymous. A deep cul-de-sac provides an opportunity for development of a future enterocele and therefore should be obliterated.

The symptoms of backache and pulling are worse in the erect position and intensify as the day goes on, the consequence of the pull of gravity on the bowel and its elongated mesentery. Filling of the sac may produce a coincident sensation of vaginal fullness. These symptoms are relieved by lying down, when gravity pulls the intestine and its contents in a different direction, relieving the painful pull on the mesentery. A deep cul-de-sac without bowel content is itself not necessarily an enterocele, but it is a potential one. For there to be bowel

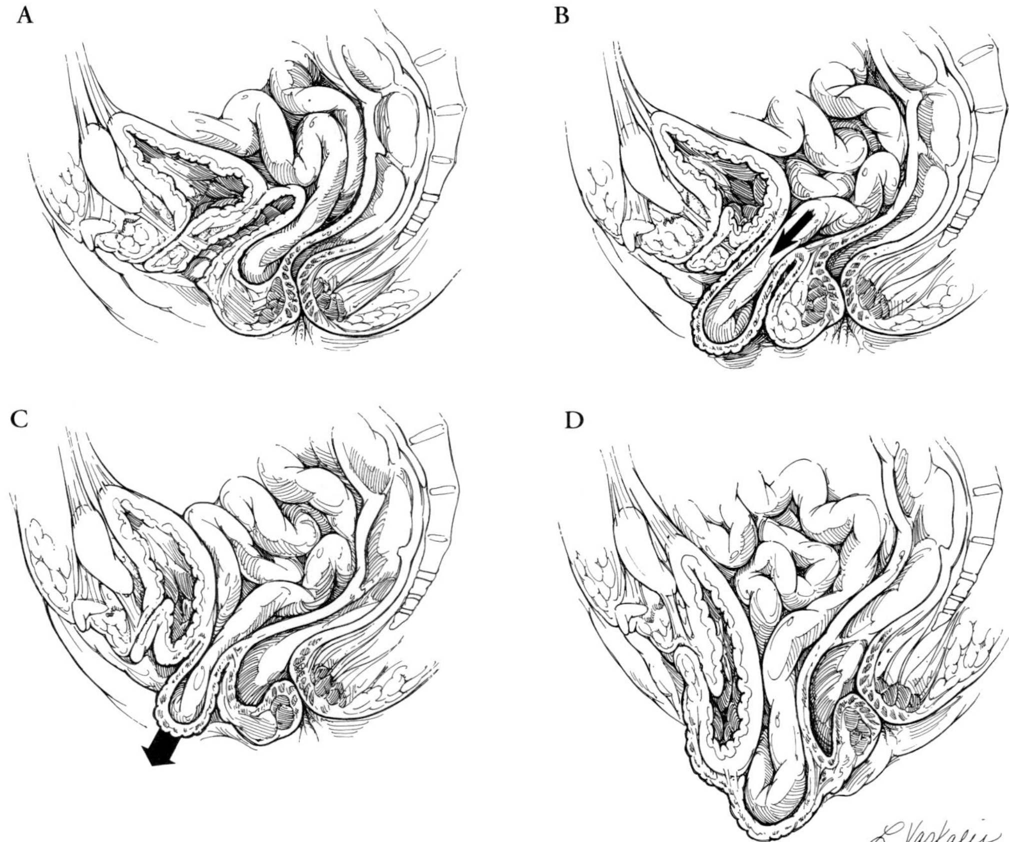

FIGURE 9.1 Examples of enterocele. **A**, Posterior "congenital" enterocele without eversion of the vagina. **B**, Pulsion enterocele; the upper vagina is everted and the enterocele sac follows the everted vault. Cystocele and rectocele are minimal. **C**, Traction enterocele; there is eversion of the upper two thirds of the vagina with enterocele, cystocele, and rectocele. **D**, Eversion of the entire vagina, including the tissues distal to the urogenital diaphragm. Notice the change in the urethral axis. (Redrawn from Nichols DH and Randall CL: Vaginal surgery, ed 4, Baltimore, 1996, Williams & Wilkins.)

within the sac, the intestinal mesentery must be pathologically long. It is not clear whether this mesenteric elongation is the cause or the result of the deep cul-de-sac. It is certain, however, that once this elongation develops, whatever the cause, it will remain permanently and serve to make persistent pressure against the site of an enterocele repair. It is therefore necessary that the repair be firm and strong enough to effectively resist this pressure if the chance of recurrence of enterocele is to be minimized.

Physical findings of the congenital type of enterocele include the presence of a deep cul-de-sac of Douglas and palpation of the bowel within the sac, best appreciated when a rectovaginal examination is performed when the patient is standing and bearing down, as by a Valsalva maneuver. There need be no prolapse of the vaginal vault nor coincident cystocele and rectocele.

Spinal anesthesia reduces the postoperative strain against the fresh repair that is more common coincident with nausea and vomiting following recovery from a general anesthetic. Intrathecal or epidural anesthesia further ensures surgical success of the reoperation by removing or minimizing this unnecessary postoperative strain.

The surgical treatment of the usual enterocele is by exposure and opening of the peritoneal sac, high purse-string ligation of its neck using a synthetic permanent or long-lasting suture, usually accompanied by a second ligation 1 cm distal to the first (Figure 9.2)[6] followed by resection of the sac. This will

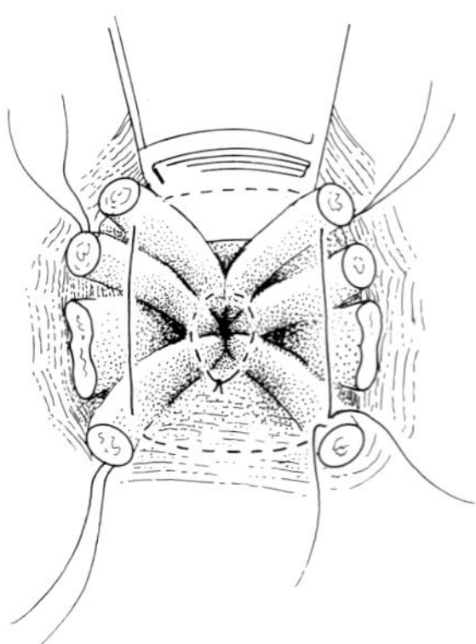

FIGURE 9.2 The enterocele has been resected and the peritoneal cavity closed by a purse-string suture that starts on the peritoneal side of the left uterosacral ligament, reefs the posterior peritoneum, the right uterosacral ligament, right round ligament, anterior peritoneum, and left round ligament. After this has been tied, a second purse-string suture is placed 1 cm distal to the first, reinforcing the closure. (Redrawn from Nichols DH and Randall CL: Vaginal surgery, ed 4, Baltimore, 1996, Williams & Wilkins.)

increase the thickness and firmness of the scar and provide suture reinforcement, one for the other. This can be accomplished alternatively in the patient with a very wide enterocele by obliterating the sac with a series of sagittally placed sutures. After all of the sutures have been tied, a reinforcing purse-string suture is placed, the excess peritoneum is excised, and the vaginal wall closed, preferably in a vertical direction.

The incidence of recurrent enterocele may be reduced by strengthening the scar through the use of nonabsorbable suture material in its repair and by closing and obliterating the peritoneal sac with more than one layer of suture.

A large neck enterocele is occasionally encountered during transvaginal surgery (Figure 9.3). Two rows of running, synthetic, absorbable suture are placed transversely in the peritoneum and subperitoneal retinaculum from the 3 o'clock to the 9 o'clock position. The knot is tied and the suture returned by a separate layer .5 cm distal to the first using a running stitch to the 3 o'clock position, where it is tied again, then followed by a purse-string suture a few millimeters distal to the transverse closure.[7] This effectively creates a three-layered stronger scar (Figure 9.4).

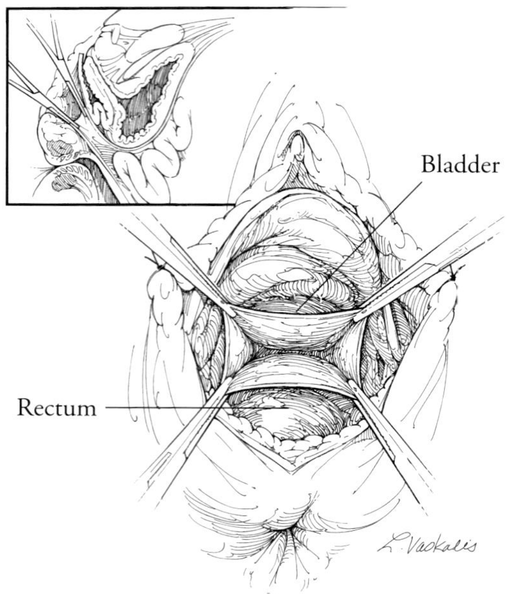

FIGURE 9.3 Transvaginal demonstration of enterocele. An incision has been made through the perineum and into the rectovaginal space. The posterior vaginal wall has been incised in the midline, reaching an enterocele sac that is identified as a double fold of peritoneum attached to the undersurface of the vagina. The sac has been opened, mobilized, and the edges held in hemostats as shown, preparatory to its resection. This is shown in sagittal section in the *inset.*

The reverse of this may be applied to the large enterocele. An effective, fast, and safe transabdominal method of repair that does not involve much peritoneal resection is to obliterate a wide pouch of Douglas by sewing a purse-string closure at the deepest part of the cul-de-sac. Then a layer is sewn from the front peritoneal surface to the back surface, a transversely placed continuous suture that begins at the bottom of the remaining cavity. By alternate bites 1 cm apart between the anterior and the posterior cul-de-sac surfaces, the suture is continued back and forth from one side of the pelvis to the other by using a running stitch. This is continued by additional rows each 1 cm or so cranial to its predecessor until the brim of the pelvis is reached, when the suture is tied. A final row of interrupted sutures 1 cm apart can be placed at the pelvic brim (Figure 9.5). When the surgeon wishes not to shorten a very deep cul-de-sac by conventional "Halban" stitches,[8] an alternate stitch shown in Figure 9.6 may be used.

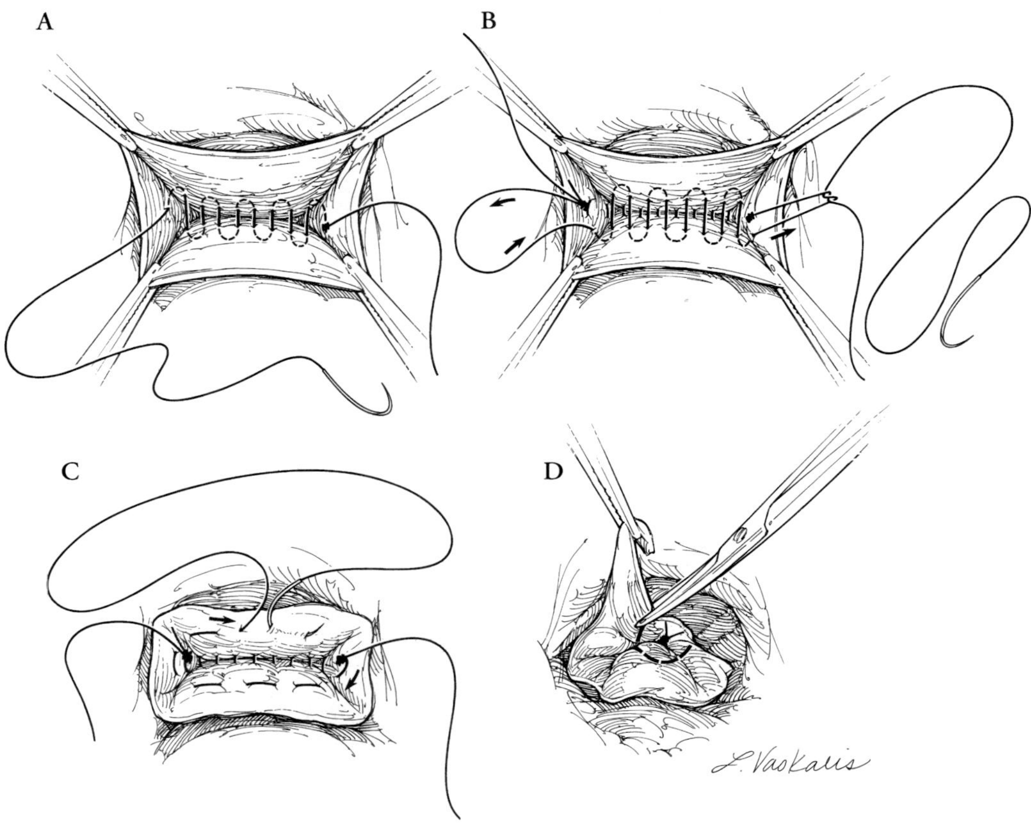

Figure 9.4 Three-layered transvaginal closure of the neck of a large enterocele. A synthetic monofilament nonabsorbable suture closes the neck of the sac from front to back (**A**). The knot is tied at the 9 o'clock position, the suture loop cut open, and the free end returned as a second slightly distal layer to the starting point, where it is tied to the original stitch end (**B**). A third distal layer is placed as a purse string (**C**), tied, and the edges of the sac trimmed (**D**).

Pulsion Enterocele

Enterocele may exist with or without coincident prolapse of the vaginal vault; just a prolapse of the vault may occur with or without enterocele, though most frequently with (Figure 9.7). Chronically increased intraabdominal pressure seems etiologically significant, especially when the vault is poorly supported, the vault is short (ending anterior to the margin of the levator plate), or there is an anteriorly inclined vaginal axis.

The condition, which may produce feelings of pelvic fullness, backache, and falling out, all made worse when the patient is in the erect position, can be best demonstrated when the vagina is examined while the patient is standing and straining (Figure 9.8). Because the primary weakness is in the supporting tissues of the upper portion of the vagina. coincident cystocele and rectocele may be absent (see Figure 9.1, *B*). Treatment requires opening and high ligation of the neck, then excision of the sac, followed by appropriate colpopexy, which will restore a normal vaginal axis. Colpopexy can be accomplished by either the transvaginal route (sacrospinous ligament fixation) or the transabdominal route (sacral colpopexy). Unless there are coincident cystocele and rectocele, simultaneous colporrhaphy is unnecessary.

Traction Enterocele

Traction enterocele is the consequence of downward pulling of a poorly supported vaginal vault by progressively enlarging cystocele and rectocele, which are invariably present (see Figure 9.1, *C*) and may or may not be symp-

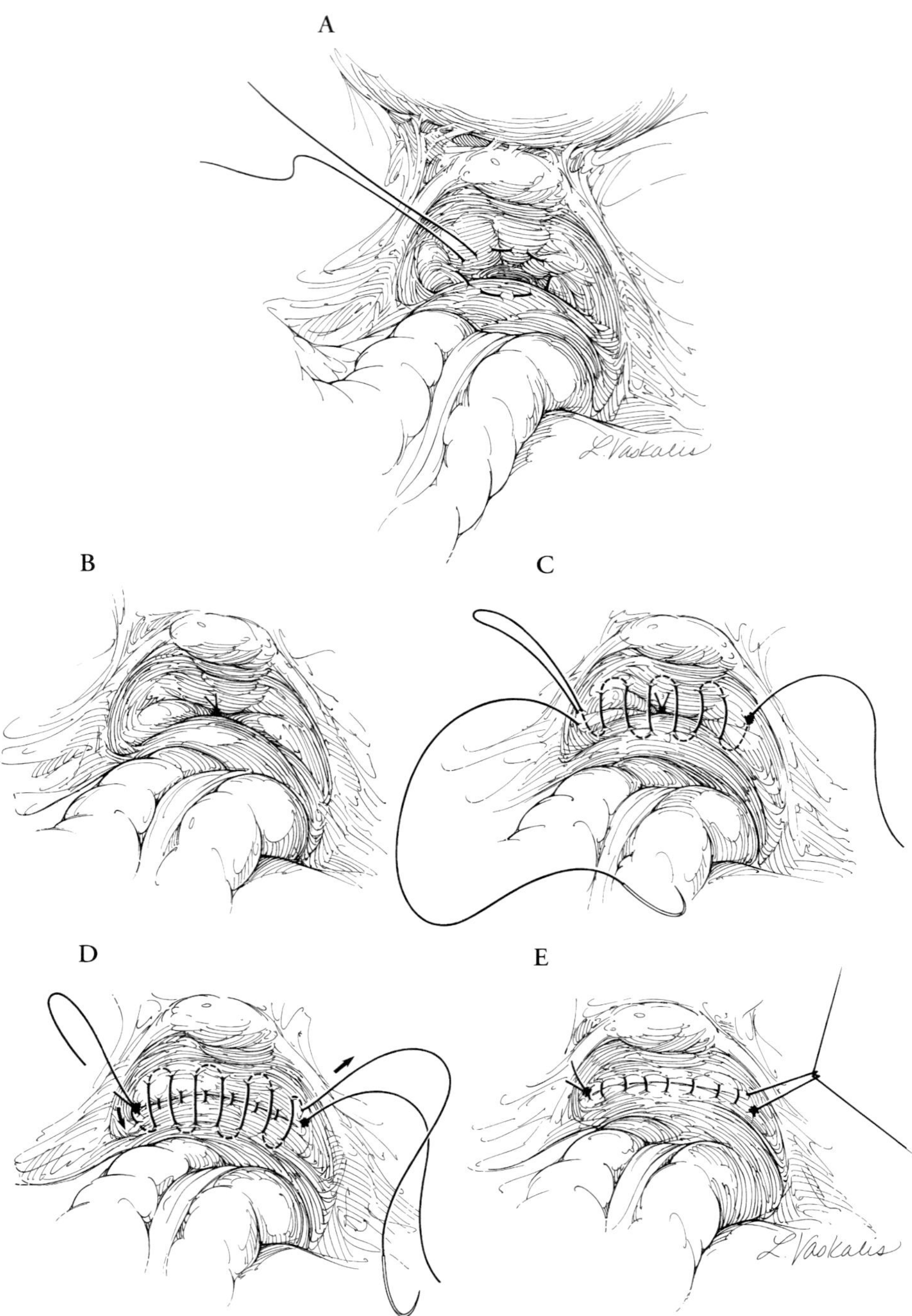

FIGURE 9.5 Three-layered transabdominal closure of the cul-de-sac. The steps are the same but in the reverse order of those described for the transvaginal closure. A purse string of synthetic monofilament nonabsorbable suture is placed at the bottom of the cul-de-sac (**A**). The suture is tied (**B**), and a second proximal layer placed from front to back (**C**), tied, and returned to the opposite side as a third proximal layer (**D**), and tied again. A fourth layer can be placed proximal to the third if necessary to completely obliterate the cul-de-sac (**E**).

tomatic. Again, the pathologic condition of pelvic support here is best demonstrated by pelvic examination of the erect patient who is straining. Vault descent with enterocele, cystocele, and rectocele are readily demonstrated.

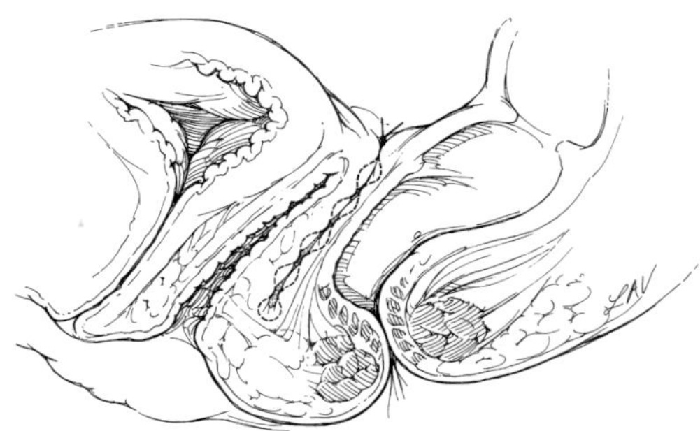

FIGURE 9.6 Alternate method of closing the cul-de-sac from front to back. For the especially deep enterocele a modification of the Halban sagittal closure that will shorten the cul-de-sac less is shown. Starting at the pelvic brim, stitches are taken alternately in the anterior then posterior wall of the full depth of the cul-de-sac peritoneum, the direction reversed at the bottom, and the suture returned to the site of origin, where it is tied to the free end. Several of these stitches are placed in a sagittal plane.

Surgical treatment is by dissection and opening of the enterocele, high double purse-string ligation of its neck, excision of the redundant peritoneum, colpopexy, and colporrhaphy, restoring both vaginal depth and caliber, and axis. This combination of procedures will not only relieve the patient's symptoms but also aid in restoring the normal anatomic relationships and organ functions.

Iatrogenic Enterocele

Iatrogenic enterocele is the consequence of a surgical change in the normal vaginal axis, thus leaving the cul-de-sac of Douglas unprotected and exposing it to the full range of changes in intraabdominal pressure that occur daily. The most common surgery that produces this change in vaginal axis are the Marshall-Marchetti-Krantz[9] and Burch[10] procedures, or the needle suspensions of the vesicourethral junction. Each of these pulls the vagina in an abnormal anterior direction, exposing the cul-de-sac, unless specific intraperitoneal surgical steps are taken to obliterate the cul-de-sac.

Ventral suspension of the vagina or uterus incurs the same risk, in addition to limiting the

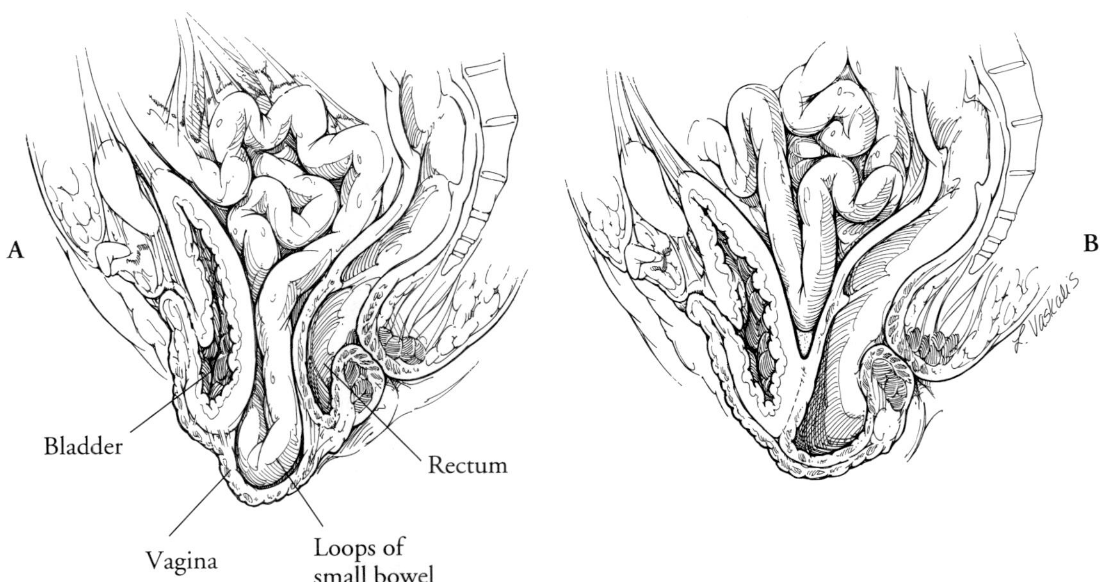

FIGURE 9.7 Massive eversion of the vagina. **A,** Massive posthysterectomy eversion of the vagina with enterocele. **B,** The less-frequent massive eversion without enterocele. In this case, the connective tissue capsule of the bladder is fused with that of the anterior rectal wall. (Redrawn from Nichols DH and Randall CL: Vaginal surgery, ed 4, Baltimore, 1996, Williams & Wilkins.)

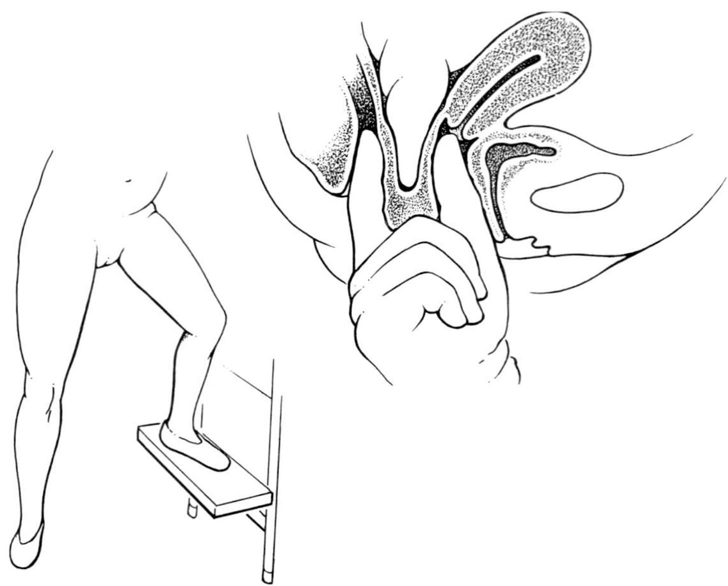

FIGURE 9.8 Examination of the patient in a standing position permits the thumb in the vagina to note and replace any descent of the vaginal vault, while the index finger introduced into the rectum permits evaluation of any possible rectocele. When the patient strains, any enterocele present is evidenced by palpation of a bowel-filled sac prolapse dissecting the rectovaginal septum. (Redrawn from Nichols DH: Repair of enterocele and prolapse of the vaginal vault. In Barber H, editor: Goldsmith's practice of surgery, Woodbury, CN, 1981, Cine-Med.)

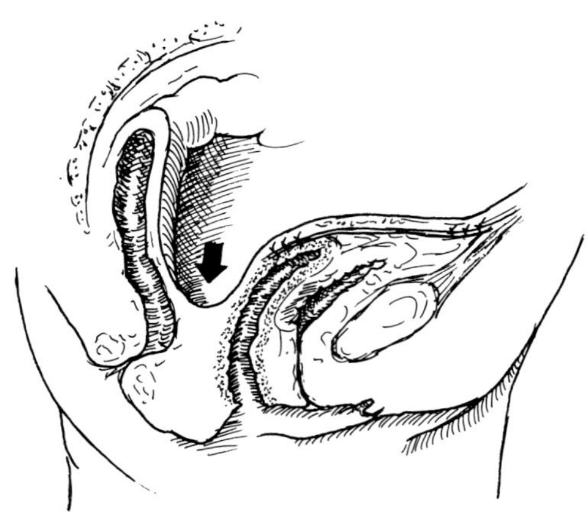

FIGURE 9.9 Change in the vaginal axis, as by ventral fixation, will expose an otherwise unprotected cul-de-sac *(arrow),* risking progressive enterocele and prolapse of the posterior vaginal vault. (Redrawn from Nichols DH: Repair of enterocele and prolapse of the vaginal vault. In Barber H, editor: Goldsmith's practice of surgery, Woodbury, CN, 1981, Cine-Med.)

volume of bladder filling, which may give rise to overflow incontinence (Figure 9.9). A pathologically wide vaginal vault is especially vulnerable to future prolapse and enterocele formation. Intraperitoneal obliteration may be produced by the sagitally placed sutures (Figure 9.10) described by Halban,[8] which cannot pull on the path of the ureter as might happen occasionally when sequential purse-string obliterative Moschcowitz's sutures[11] are used, originally but ineffectually introduced to treat rectal prolapse.

Our objection to the transabdominal Moschcowitz procedure for enterocele is that the original operation had been intended for a prolapsed or sliding rectum that was then attached by concentric purse-string sutures to a fairly strong vagina and cervix. Gynecologists, however, appropriated this operation, reversing the principle, by attaching a sliding vagina to the anterior wall of the rectum. The latter has rather poor structural support.

Halban's or Moschcowitz's obliteration of the cul-de-sac is for this purpose alone. It will help prevent an enterocele, although it will not treat a vault prolapse effectively. Neither the Halban nor the Moschcowitz stitch is able per se to provide support for the vaginal vault. Both obliterate the cul-de-sac, and neither requires skinning out or removal of excess peritoneum.

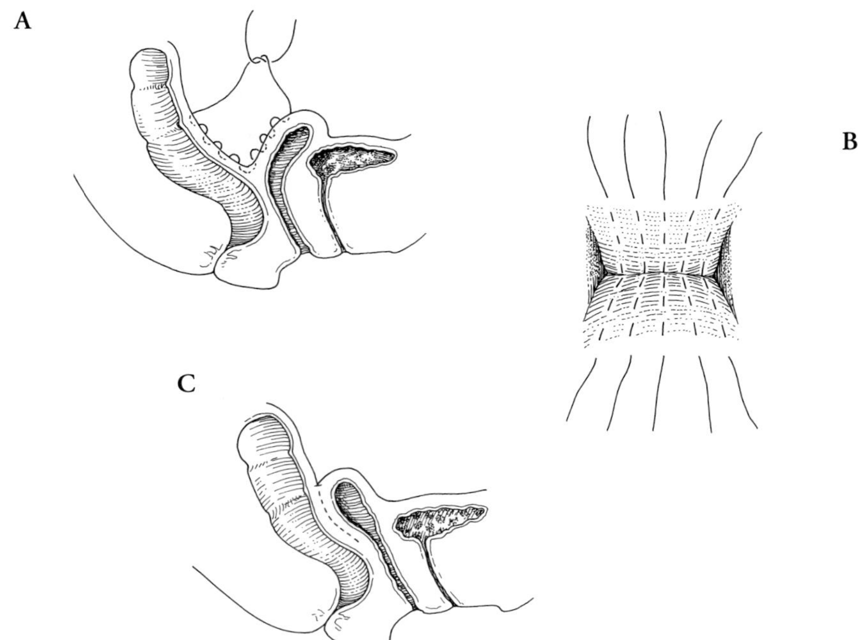

FIGURE 9.10 A, The cul-de-sac of Douglas may be obliterated by a series of sutures placed in the sagittal plane. After all of them have been placed, they are tied sequentially (**B**), fusing the posterior vaginal wall and vaginal vault to the anterior surface of the rectum (**C**). Stitches placed in this sagittal fashion do not disturb the course of the ureter. (Redrawn from Nichols DH and Randall CL: Vaginal surgery, ed 4, Baltimore, 1996, Williams & Wilkins.)

This postsurgical abnormal vaginal axis is readily demonstrable during pelvic examination.

Treatment includes high ligation of the neck of the sac, with resection of excess peritoneum, and restoration of a normal horizontally inclined vaginal axis. If there is coincident vault prolapse, colpopexy is required, whereas, if there are strong but long uterosacral ligaments, the New Orleans or McCall[12] type of cul-de-plasty may be used effectively (Figures 9.11 to 9.13). If strong and surgically useful ligaments are absent, transvaginal sacrospinous or transabdominal sacral colpopexy is useful. Correction of an abnormal pelvic tilt from a patient's poor posture is helpful.

ANTERIOR ENTEROCELE

When a surgeon has experienced difficulty finding the anterior peritoneal fold during vaginal hysterectomy and has dissected for some distance beneath the uterine peritoneum before opening it (Figure 9.14), an excess of anterior peritoneal flap remains that should be removed before peritonealization. Failure to recognize this redundancy in the anterior peritoneum is as troublesome as it is in the posterior peritoneum. The redundant peritoneum is not always obvious during hysterectomy when the patient is anesthetized and in the usual Trendelenburg position. Failure to recognize and resect to this redundant peritoneum is frequently followed by enterocele, in the former instance, anterior to the vagina (Figure 9.15). Preoperatively, it resembles the appearance of recurrent cystocele, but the distinction becomes obvious during reoperation when the peritoneum-lined sac is opened. Treatment is by high ligation and excision of the sac.

MISCELLANEOUS TYPES OF ENTEROCELE

Obturator Hernia

Recurrent obturator hernia is a rare occurrence.[6,13,14] The hernia is one in which the sac penetrates the pelvic diaphragm (Figure 9.16)

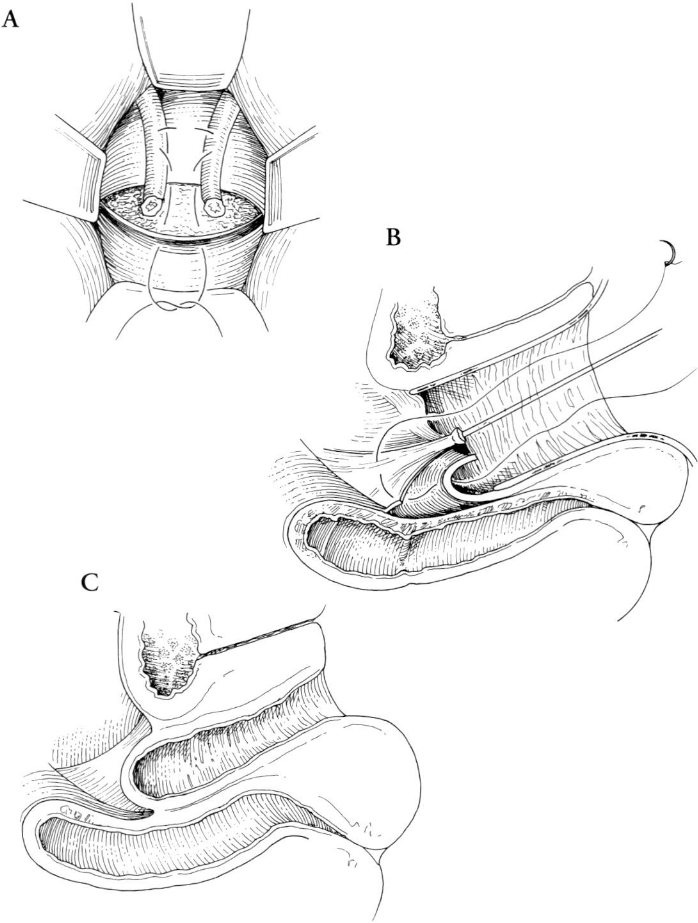

FIGURE 9.11 Modified cul-de-plasty. **A,** The enterocele sac has been resected, and a long-lasting synthetic absorbable suture has been placed through the vault of the vagina and cut edge of peritoneum. Traction on the stumps of the strong but long ureterosacral ligaments permits a deep bite into the substance of the left uterosacral ligament, then through the peritoneum covering the anterior surface of the rectum and the same structures on the opposite side. **B,** Suture placement in the sagittal section. **C,** Effects of tying and subsequent closure of the peritoneal cavity. The apex of the vagina is now cranial and posterior to the new peritoneal closure. (Redrawn from Nichols DH and Randall CL: Vaginal surgery, ed 4, Baltimore, 1996, Williams & Wilkins.)

and may recur if the suture line holding the neck shut becomes disrupted. The pain, often of sudden onset, may be bizarre. It may run down the medial thigh and knee, particularly when the patient is standing. Pressure on the obturator nerve by the hernia may elicit the Howship-Romberg sign, characterized by intermittent leg pain often associated with abdominal discomfort.[15] The hernia may be of the Richter type (partial herniation only), although if bowel is trapped within the hernia the condition may produce an intestinal obstruction. More commonly, there is an acute intestinal obstruction, partial or complete, manifested by the usual nausea, vomiting, and abdominal distention, because a loop of small bowel becomes trapped in the neck of the sac. The diagnosis is suspected by a history of previous obturator hernia. There may or may not be a precipitating incidence of sudden increase in intraperitoneal pressure, as during a fit of coughing, which disrupts the previous repair. Examination of a flat plate or GI series may show a loop of bowel identified as outside

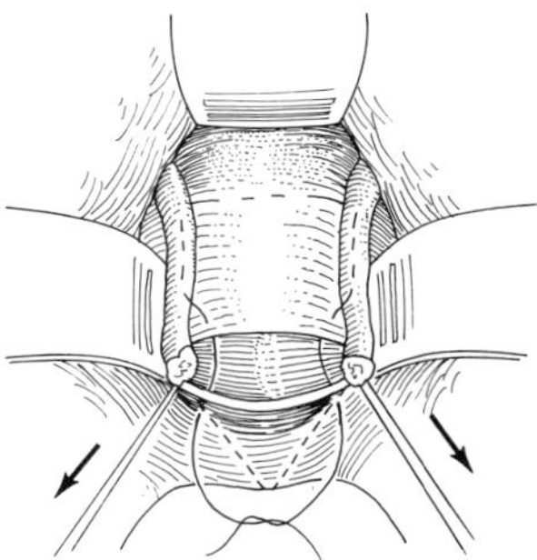

FIGURE 9.12 A pathologically wide vaginal vault should be narrowed by excision of a V-shaped wedge *(dashed line)*. (Redrawn from Nichols DH and Randall CL: Vaginal surgery, ed 4, Baltimore, 1996, Williams & Wilkins.)

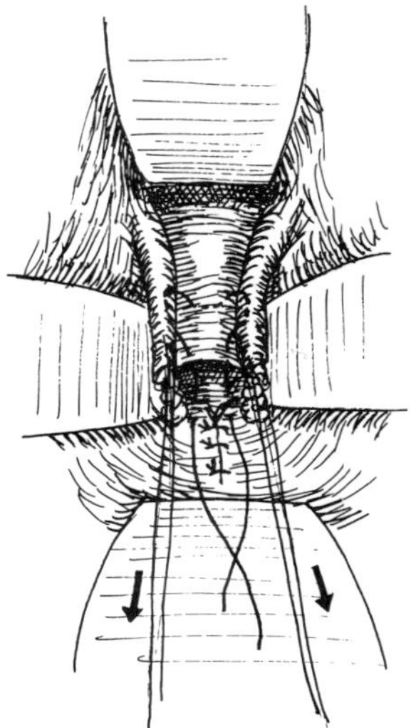

FIGURE 9.13 The edges of the V are sewn together, thus narrowing a pathologically wide vaginal vault.

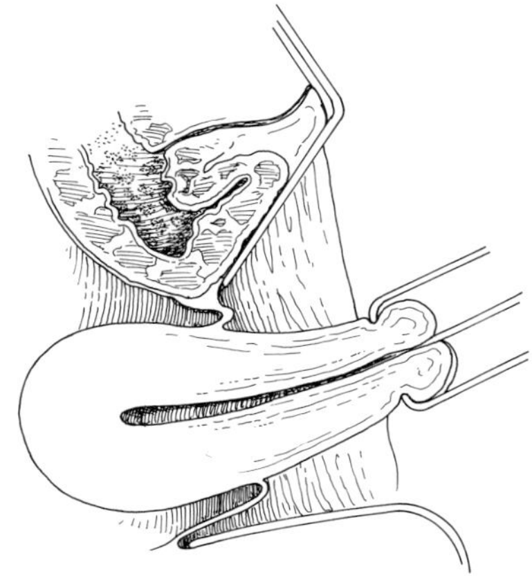

FIGURE 9.14 During vaginal hysterectomy, the bladder has been separated by sharp dissection from the lower uterine segment and held out of the way by an appropriate retractor. If the anterior peritoneum is dissected and opened far cranially, failure to resect this redundant peritoneum before peritonealization will risk subsequent anterior enterocele. (Redrawn from Nichols DH and Randall CL: Vaginal surgery, ed 4, Baltimore, 1996, Williams & Wilkins.)

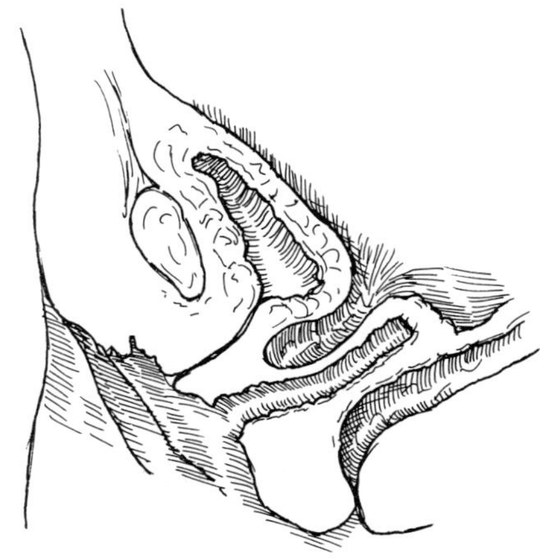

FIGURE 9.15 Sagittal view of an anterior enterocele located between the bladder and the anterior vaginal wall of a posthysterectomy patient. (Redrawn from Nichols DH: Obstet Gynecol 40:257, 1972.)

the pelvis. It will, of course, be in the hernial sac.[2,16,17] The patient has lower abdominal tenderness and distention, and if the hernia extends low in the pelvis, it may occasionally be palpated as a tender mass beneath the lateral wall of the vagina. If it should follow the canal of Nuck, it may be palpable within a labium majora.

Abdominal Hernias

Recurrent umbilical, femoral, or inguinal hernia is in a sense enterocele. The last of these usually refers generically to pudendal hernia, but it is a cumbersome term not often used. These miscellaneous hernias are represented by the reappearance of a soft mass at the site of the previous herniation and repair. The content of the sac is usually reducible. However, if

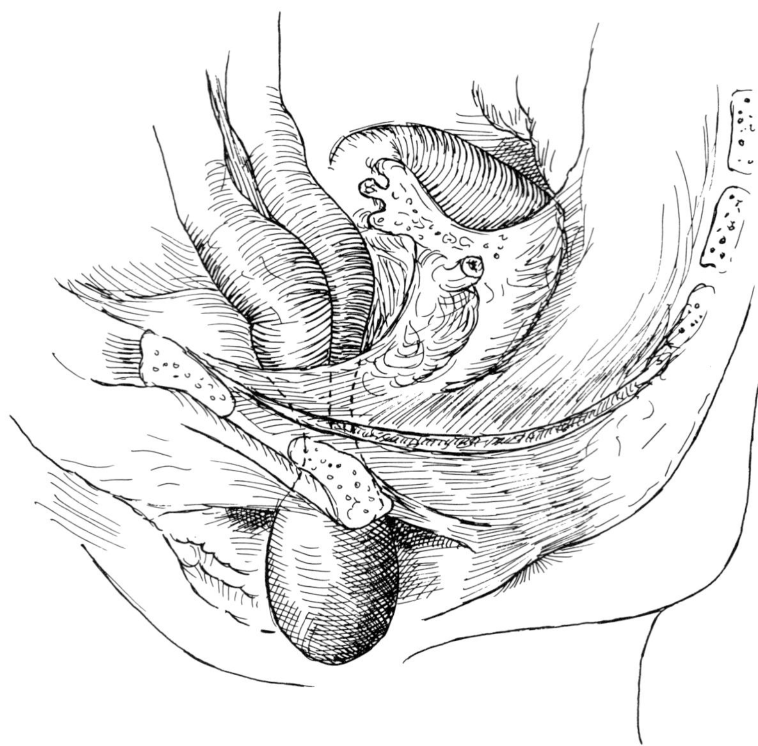

Figure 9.16 Lateral or pudendal enterocele projecting through a pathologic opening in the pelvic diaphragm or into the obturator canal. Notice the constriction of the bowel that may favor intestinal obstruction. (Redrawn from Nichols DH: Obstet Gynecol 40:257, 1972.)

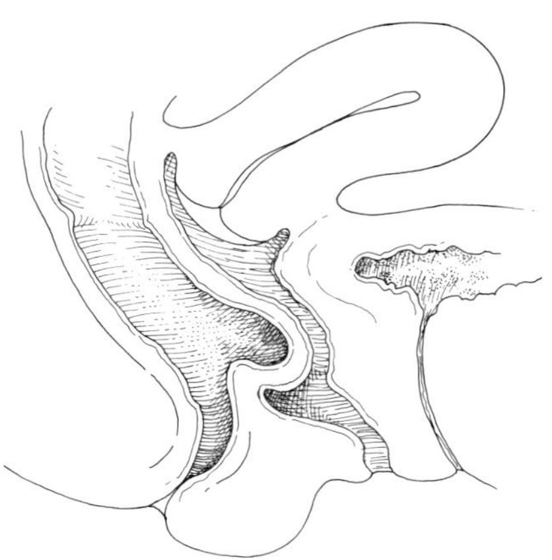

Figure 9.17 Perineorrhaphy may hide an unrepaired midvaginal rectocele, which may masquerade as a pseudoenterocele. Effective repair must always begin proximal to the weakness. (Redrawn from Nichols DH and Randall CL: Vaginal surgery, ed 4, Baltimore, 1996, Williams & Wilkins.)

it becomes incarcerated, edema, swelling, and pain supervene, and an emergency re-repair, often using a layer or two of permanent-type suture material, is necessary.

Pseudoenterocele

Persistent unrepaired rectocele, as may be seen in a patient with rectocele who has received only a perineorrhaphy for repair, looks very much like an enterocele on superficial examination (Figure 9.17), but its true nature is revealed by vaginal examination, particularly in the standing patient. It may have all the symptoms of the original rectocele, incomplete bowel movements and postevacuation aching, and is treated by reoperation and more extensive posterior colporrhaphy to repair the entire rectocele.

Summary

We have seen how the cause of a specific enterocele can be correlated with its location, which, in turn, correlates with the recommended surgical treatment (Table 9.1). This can apply to both the common and the rare type of enterocele. Appropriate choice of suture and surgical operation, correctly per-

Table 9.1 Correlation between etiology, location, and treatment of enterocele

Cause	Location	Treatment
Congenital	Sac between posterior vaginal wall and anterior rectal wall	Excision of the sac with high ligation of its neck; approximation of uterosacral ligaments
Pulsion (pushed)	With eversion of vaginal vault	Restoration of vault depth by shortening cardinal-uterosacral ligaments or cul-de-plasty if ligaments are strong
Traction (pulled)	Lower eversion (cystocele and rectocele) pulling vault into eversion	Same procedure as for pulsion plus anterior and posterior colporrhaphy
Iatrogenic	Anterior to vagina or posterior from change in vaginal axis	Excision or obliteration of sac and restoration of normal vaginal axis if it is defective

formed, and usually using synthetic long-acting or permanent suture material, will result in effective relief of symptoms and restoration of normal anatomic relationships and function. Appropriate choice of specific treatment, reducing the chance for reoccurrence and its attendant risks, discomforts, and expense, is well worth the trouble.

References

1. Nichols DH: Types of enterocele and principles underlying the choice of operation for repair, Obstet Gynecol 40:257, 1972.
2. Lenzi E: L'Ernia vaginale del Douglas O elitrocele, Pisa, 1959, Edizioni Omnia Medica.
3. Lenzi E and others: Per una migliore nosografia dell'ernia del Douglas: elitrocele o enterocele? Riv Ost Gin Perin 3:273, 1990.
4. Zacharin RF: Pelvic floor anatomy and the surgery of pulsion enterocele, New York, 1985, Springer-Verlag New York, Inc.
5. Warwick R and Williams PL: Gray's anatomy, Br ed 35, Philadelphia, 1993, WB Saunders Co.
6. Nichols DH and Randall CL: Vaginal surgery, ed 4, Baltimore, 1996, Williams & Wilkins Co.
7. Nichols DH, editor: Gynecologic and obstetric surgery, St Louis, 1993, Mosby.
8. Halban J: Gynäkologische Operationslehre, Berlin, 1932, Urban & Schwarzenberg.
9. Marshall VF, Marchetti AA, and Krantz KE: The correction of stress incontinence by simple vesicourethral suspension, Surg Gynecol Obstet 88:509, 1949.
10. Burch JC: Urethrovaginal fixation to Cooper's ligament for correction of stress incontinence, cystocele, and prolapse, Am J Obstet Gynecol 81:281, 1961.
11. Moschcowitz AV: The pathogenesis, anatomy, and cure of prolapse of the rectum, Surg Gynecol Obstet 15:7, 1912.
12. McCall ML: Posterior culdeplasty: surgical correction of enterocele during vaginal hysterectomy, a preliminary report, Obstet Gynecol 10:595, 1957.
13. Anderson WR: Pudendal hernia, Obstet Gynecol 32:802, 1968.
14. Cali RL and others: Rare pelvic floor hernia: report of a case and review of the literature, Dis Colon Rectum 35:604, 1992.
15. Wilson JM: Pelvic relaxations and herniations, Springfield, Ill, 1954, Charles C Thomas, Publisher.
16. Lash AF and Levin B: Roentgenographic diagnosis of vaginal vault hernia, Obstet Gynecol 20:427, 1962.
17. Chase HC: Levator hernia (pudendal hernia), Surg Gynecol Obstet 35:717, 1992.

10

Reoperation of the Tubes and Ovaries

J.F. HULKA
LYNDA WOLF

Pelvic pain and infertility are the two major indications for patients undergoing procedures, often multiple times, on their fallopian tubes and ovaries. The persistent and recurrent nature of infertility and pelvic pain after primary surgery, combined with the relative ease and safety of diagnostic laparoscopy, has led to an increase in reoperation for these conditions. In recent years the explosive emergence of operative laparoscopy for tubal and ovarian disease has created new questions. When we find recurrent or persistent disease, what is the efficacy of reoperation (by laparoscopy or laparotomy) of adnexal conditions? (Endometriosis is discussed in Chapter 11 and will not be reviewed here.) These questions can be outlined as follows:

I. Efficacy of reoperation
  1. Infertility
    A. Relysis of adhesions—tubal and ovarian
    B. Salpingostomy
  2. Recurrent pelvic pain
    A. Relysis of adhesions, including bowel
    B. Removal of adnexal masses
II. Recurrence or persistence: need to reoperate
  1. Recurrence of ovarian cysts
    A. Functional cysts
    B. Endometriomas
  2. Persistent ectopic pregnancy after salpingotomy
III. Sterilization by tubocclusion
  1. Reversal of sterilization (for desired fertility)
  2. Reoperation of tubal occlusion (after a pregnancy)

This chapter presents the existing data concerning the need for and efficacy of reoperation in these conditions. Since efficacy is dependent on basic biologic factors such as wound healing, natural history of diseases, and surgical techniques, comments on these factors will be offered to illustrate an approach to minimizing the need for reoperation.

EFFICACY OF REOPERATION

Infertility

With in vitro fertilization now widely available and having an overall birth rate of 18.3%,[1] patients who have undergone surgery for infertility without success have a reasonable alternative route to achieve pregnancy rather than reoperation. However, the expense and the inherent artificiality necessary for conception motivates many patients to seek repeat surgical efforts to achieve natural conception.

Surgery for restoration of fertility has shifted from microsurgery by laparotomy to operative laparoscopy, and there is active current debate as to which technique should be used. Throughout this review, efficacy is measured by the live birth (take-home baby [THB]) rate. This rate is influenced by the following factors:

- Extent of disease
- Coexistence of adhesions and tubocclusion
- Degree of tubal damage
- Concomitant ovulatory dysfunction and male factor
- Age of the patient
- Skill of the surgeon

Relysis of Adhesions. Recent studies have indicated that adhesions tend to re-form less frequently when lysed by laparoscopy than open laparotomy.[2-4] This is probably due to less direct trauma from swabbing during laparotomy, which results in mechanical abrasion and desiccation of serosal surfaces. Recent studies of wound healing and adhesion reformation have been reviewed in detail.[5,6] Peritoneal surfaces tend to heal from the "bottom up," by a process of peritoneal regeneration from underlying vasculature. Damage to this underlying vasculature during laparotomy results in cytokine release and alterations in plasminogen activator activity that is necessary for endogenous lysis of excess fibrinous attachments.[6]

In contrast, the ovarian surface is protected by loose cells derived from the peritoneal fluid, and damage to these cells stimulates tubal, bowel, and omental adhesions as the hypoxic cells on the ovary secrete angiogenic factors promoting "vascular grafts" from nearby viable tissue.[7] As a result of this process, the ovary is the pelvic structure most likely to re-form adhesions after attempts at lysis.[8] Further, the percentage of ovarian surface covered by adhesions is a major prognostic factor after adheseolysis for infertility.[9] Most recent animal and human observations suggest that the ovary heals best (with minimal adhesions) without attempts at reapproximation by suturing.[10-12] The role of chemical and mechanical adjuvants to prevent adhesion reformation such as Hyskon, corticosteroid, Interceed, or Gore-Tex have yielded mixed results in clinical experience. Thus the following four points are currently recommended in adheseolysis by laparoscopy or laparotomy to minimize recurrence:

1. Minimal use of absorbable sutures (which provoke an inflammatory and adhesive response)
2. Sharp dissection to cause minimal cell destruction
3. Less meticulous microhemostasis to allow normal clotting and vasoconstriction rather than tissue destruction by excess electrodesiccation or fulguration
4. Dilution of the angiogenic factors by leaving 1000 to 2000 ml of lactated Ringer's solution in the peritoneal cavity after surgery[13,14]

Second-look laparoscopy studies[8,15,16] reveal a surprising amount of adhesion reformation despite good surgical technique. Data studying the efficacy of relysis of adhesions for restoration of fertility[16] reveal reduction in adhesions without improvement in pregnancy rates, making efficacy of relysis for infertility questionable at this point.

Salpingostomy. The THB rate following salpingostomy is dependent on a number of factors:

Degree of tubal endothelial damage
Thickness of the tubal wall
Coexistent adhesions, specially ovarian
Age of the patient
Concomitant ovulatory dysfunction and male factor

Schlaff and others found that with mild disease, defined as an absent or small hydrosalpinx (less than 15 mm in diameter), inverted fimbria that are easily recognized, a normal rugae pattern, and the absence of structurally significant peritubal or periovarian adhesions, the success rate of microsurgery can be 80%.[17] Unfortunately, these favorable conditions occur in a small minority of patients with tubal occlusive disease.

In Europe studies using salpingoscopy[18] document that these optimal conditions are infrequent. The absence of ovarian adhesions with an occluded tube results in a THB rate of 30%.[9] The presence of adhesions in the pelvis markedly diminishes success to 10% to 15%.[19-22]

Laparoscopic reoperation will achieve tubal patency in up to 95% of patients.[9,21] However, in a total of 55 reoperations by microsurgical salpingostomy[19-22] the successful THB rate was 15%—similar to the rate achieved with in vitro fertilization. Verhoeven, Berry, and Frantzen reported greater success in reoperation among younger patients with less concomitant disease.[21] Winston's and Margara's report on the efficacy of microsurgical reoperation documented 25% and 40% delivery rates in patients with stage I and II disease, respectively. Winston's and Margara's classifi-

TABLE 10.1 Prognostic classification of distal occlusion

Stage I	Normal rugae, no ovarian adhesions Prognosis: 30%-70% take home baby (THB) rate Plan: microsurgery
Stage II	Damaged rugae, some ovarian adhesions Prognosis: 0%-30% THB, increased risk of ectopic pregnancy Plan: laparoscopic therapeutic salpingostomy
Stage III	Thick wall, denuded and agglutinated rugae, adhesions covering ovary Prognosis: 0% THB, increased risk of ectopic pregnancy Plan: In vitro fertilization

From Hulka JF and Reich H: Textbook of laparoscopy, ed 2. Philadelphia, 1994, WB Saunders.

cation of stage I and II disease is similar to mild and moderate tubal disease as defined by Schlaff and others.[23] The assumption by operative laparoscopists that reoperation by laparoscopy is as effective as microsurgery is disputed by Winston's and Margara's data. Recurrence of hydrosalpinx was 37% with laparoscopic procedures, compared to only 12% after microsurgical procedures.

Careful selection of patients for salpingostomy, both for operative management and reoperation, is therefore critical in determining outcome. Table 10.1 summarizes a patient's prognosis depending on the appearance of the adnexa and the recommended management.[24]

Recurrent Pelvic Pain

Relysis of Adhesions. The field of chronic pelvic pain is in its infancy as a clinical science. The clinical diagnosis most often made for which surgery is performed includes endometriosis, pelvic adhesions, chronic pelvic inflammatory disease (PID), and ovarian cysts. The relative ease of laparoscopic surgery has encouraged compassionate physicians to reoperate in order to relieve recurrent pain.[25] Although reoperative laparoscopy for relief of pelvic pain has been extensively reported in the literature, documentation of its efficacy is scant.

In a report of 30 reoperations for relief of chronic pelvic pain (defined as 6 months' or more duration) due to adhesions,[26] previous surgery included 25 laparotomies and 10 laparoscopies. No correlation between the severity of adhesions and pain was found. Pain was localized to the area of adhesions in 90% of patients. Although immediate postoperative pain relief was frequent, symptoms tended to recur in 6 to 12 months after surgery. (This observation, consistent with others, makes a follow-up period of observation of at least 6 months necessary to evaluate efficacy of treatment for pain.) Reoperative adhesiolysis resulted in long-term improvement of daily pain in 63%, with no improvement in 37%. Among patients with the chronic pain syndrome (see the discussion later in this section), dyspareunia was unchanged or worse in 4 out of 6 patients. Among these chronic pain patients with either pain and/or dyspareunia, 6 out of 10 showed no long-term improvement.

In contrast to restoring fertility, the relysis of adhesions for relief of recurrent pelvic pain appears somewhat more successful and may emerge as a legitimate indication for operative laparoscopy. Most recently, Steege has explored the use of small-diameter office laparoscopy for relysis on four occasions during the first 2 postoperative weeks.[27] The average interval between reoperation was 3 to 4 days. This interval was chosen to optimize outcome by lysing adhesions that were still filmy and had not been vascularized or collagenized. This study confirmed the feasibility and safety of relysis, but appropriate applications of this procedure remain to be defined.

Evaluation of the efficacy of reoperation for chronic pelvic pain is confounded by the occurrence of important associated psychologic conditions, termed by Steege "the chronic pain syndrome," with symptoms similar to those of chronic depression. This syndrome includes the following[28]:

Pelvic pain of 6 months or more that lacks apparent physical cause
Significantly altered physical activity, including work, recreation, sexual life
Disturbance of mood, mostly depression

Again, careful preoperative selection, including duration of symptoms, recurrence of symptoms after previous surgery, and psychologic and behavioral assessment are all important prognostic factors for both primary and reoperation for chronic pelvic pain. In a prospective study by Peters and others,[29] patients with chronic pelvic pain were divided into a group receiving routine laparoscopy and a group receiving an integrated approach giving attention to somatic psychologic conditions. In the second group, laparoscopy was not routinely performed. The integrated approach appeared to improve pelvic pain significantly more than the standard laparoscopic approach.

The importance of evaluation of the emotional component in patients with chronic pain was summed up well by a gynecologist trained later on as a psychiatrist who ruefully commented: "I have done many laparoscopies for depression."[30]

Removal of Adnexal Mass. Ovarian cysts are often found in patients with acute or chronic pelvic pain. Although the cause-and-effect relationship between adnexal masses and acute pain is clear, this relationship is questionable in chronic pain. Nevertheless, cystectomies and oophorectomies are often performed for relief of pain, particularly if there are adhesions on the ovarian surface. Although the relief of acute pain with removal of adnexal masses has been well documented, there are no data concerning the efficacy of adnexal mass removal for chronic pelvic pain.

Recurrence of Ovarian Cysts

Recurrence of ovarian cysts after cystectomy has been studied. Hasson[31] found that endometriomas recur 50% of the time if not completely excised. Fayez and Vogel[32] compared recurrence rates and adhesion formation for different laparoscopic treatments of endometriomas. They found stripping of the lining, laser ablation of the lining, and drainage with irrigation, all had a recurrence rate of 20%. When complete excision was accomplished, there were no recurrences but there was 100% adhesion formation compared to 30% with the other three methods. In contrast, more recent studies have indicated a rate as low as 2% for the recurrence of functional cysts after laparoscopic fenestration. However, when pelvic adhesions were seen at the time of laparoscopy, the recurrence rate increased to 11%. Postoperative hormonal therapy with a progestin or combined oral contraceptive pill demonstrated no protective effect. Follicular cysts had a recurrence rate of 2%, while corpus luteum cysts recurred in 14%. With both functional cysts and endometriomas, caution must be exercised weighing the significance of the finding of an ovarian cyst and contemplating its removal for relief of chronic pelvic pain.[33]

Persistent Ectopic Pregnancy

There is growing acceptance of laparoscopic salpingotomy for removal of an ampullary or fimbrial ectopic pregnancy while attempting to preserve the use of the involved tube to achieve future pregnancies. Whether by laparoscopy or laparotomy, the incidence of persistent ectopic as defined by incomplete removal of trophoblast tissue is between 5% and 20%.[34] The highest persistent rate occurs after fimbrial abortion. Persistent ectopic rates are not statistically different following laparotomy compared to laparoscopy. Repeat surgery is being replaced by medical management employing a 50 mg single IM methotrexate injection.[34] Stovall and Ling have documented the safety and efficacy of this therapy in the primary medical management of ectopic pregnancy.[35] Many centers have subsequently confirmed a similar efficacy and safety of this management of persistent ectopic pregnancy following conservative surgical management.

Sterilization

It is a curious coincidence that both sterilization reversal and sterilization failure occur at about the same incidence (about 1 such event per 100 procedures performed.) With an estimated 400,000 tubal sterilizations performed yearly, this problem becomes a relatively frequent one.

Reversal of Sterilization

The success of a sterilization reversal is almost entirely dependent on the nature of damage initially done to the tube. In the simplest terms, the total tubal length possible after anastomosis should be over 4 cm to anticipate pregnancies that are consistently intrauterine.[36] Lengths shorter than this carry increasing risks of pregnancies that end as ectopics or abortions. In terms of the previous sterilization procedure performed, the procedure with the least damage seems to have the best prognosis.[37] The range is from poorest prognosis (THB rate of less than 30%) after unipolar coagulation requiring ampullary implantation, to the best prognosis with the clip (85%) reversed with an isthmic-isthmic anastomosis. These operations are almost universally performed by microsurgery at laparotomy, though most recently reports of microsurgery via laparoscopy have been presented at meetings.

Reoperation on Failed Tubal Occlusion

In the United States, more than 8 million women have undergone tubal sterilization and are continuing to be sterilized at the rate of about 400,000 per year. The incidence of failure of these sterilizations is low, estimated to be 2 to 12 per 1,000 sterilizations per year, but with a cumulative 5- to 10-year pregnancy rate of at least 1%. Thus, with 400,000 women undergoing sterilization every year for the past 20 years, at least 4,000 each year will experience pregnancy after sterilization. These events can bring personal distress to the couple and can raise medicolegal problems in this litigious era. In addition, the physician managing the pregnancy is eventually faced with the problem of how to deal with sterilization failure to prevent reoccurrence, or how to resterilize the patient. This chapter reviews the known causes for these pregnancies and suggests management based on these causes.

Anatomy and Physiology of Tubal Division

Both the uterus and ampulla secrete fluid, mostly during the follicular phase. This fluid is constantly exchanged in minute amounts as a result of the pumping action of uterine contractions throughout the cycle. Both the amount of fluid and the pressure of the contractions vary considerably from individual to individual. When tubes are occluded in some women, the pressure and amount of fluid normally generated by the uterus will be sufficient to pump fluid by force through the healing process at the occlusive site, with resultant fistula formation. In 1973 Courey, Cunanan, and Taefi demonstrated these uteroperitoneal fistulas by performing hysterosalpingograms in women 3 or more months after unipolar electrocoagulation.[38] More than 10% of these sterilized women had demonstrable fistulas. Histologically, these fistulas were carefully documented by Stock in 1983 in both proximal and distal segments with tubal endothelium everted at the peritoneal surface of the fistula.[39] These fistulas allow the passage of sperm from the uterine cavity (where they are normally distributed after unprotected intercourse) into the peritoneal cavity. Some sperm will be swept in peritoneal fluid into the distal ampullary stump by fimbria, where they can fertilize an egg brought into the ampulla during normal ovulation (Figure 10.1).

Metz and Mastroianni[40] and Stock and Nelson[41] hypothesize that a fertilized egg can then implant in the ampulla and present itself clinically as an ectopic pregnancy. More remarkably, the fertilized egg can pass through a fistula in the ampullary stump, back into the uteroperitoneal fistula, and present itself clinically as a normal intrauterine pregnancy. These are rare events, but they do occur and account for some pregnancies occurring after properly occluded tubes.

In the description of the different techniques of sterilization and the subsequent healing process, a number of anatomic terms will be used, which are summarized for clarity in Figure 10.2.

Techniques of Sterilization

The Pomeroy Procedure

This procedure is the most common operation in the United States, performed postpartum or at the time of cesarean section. A knuckle of tube is brought up by a Babcock's clamp, an o plain catgut ligature occludes the base of the loop, the loop is excised, and the specimen is then sent to the pathology laboratory for confirmation of the correct structure being occluded. Six months after the procedure the

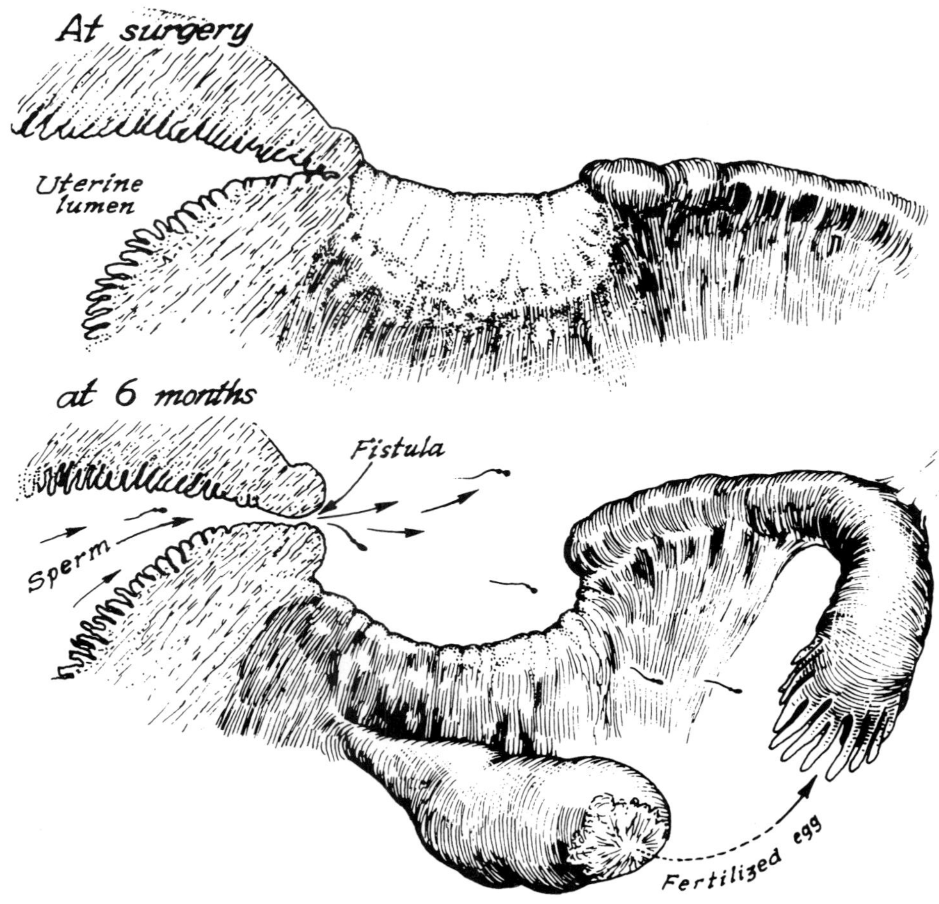

Figure 10.1 After electrocoagulation near the uterus, the isthmic segment is absorbed, allowing uterine fluid under pressure from uterine contractions to create a fistula to the peritoneum. Subsequent unprotected intercourse allows sperm to enter the peritoneum, reach the fimbria, and fertilize an egg. (From Hulka J: Textbook of laparoscopy, Orlando, Fla, 1985, Grune & Stratton.)

necrotic stumps have been absorbed, and the patient is left with a proximal segment (usually greater than 2 cm) consisting of isthmus next to the uterus, a gap of about 3 cm where the loop of tube was excised, and a distal segment consisting of varying lengths of ampulla. Sutures tight enough to achieve hemostasis may still allow fistula formation and recanalization of both segments.[41] After Pomeroy ligation, pregnancies are estimated to be primarily intrauterine.

Bipolar Coagulation (Electrodesiccation)

Electrodesiccation with bipolar forceps is the most common method of laparoscopic tubal sterilization in the United States. The term *electrodesiccation* correctly describes the heating of tissue to the point of driving all water out of cells. This is emphasized because the correct end point of destroying the tube is evidenced by the stopping of current flow as the tubal tissue essentially turns to leather and no longer conducts the current. In this method the fallopian tube is grasped by a forceps, and an electric current is passed between the prongs of the forceps through the tube. In serial laparoscopies following bipolar coagulation, Fishburne and Hulka observed that hypervascularization occurs around the dead coagulated tissue, which then is slowly reabsorbed.[42] When the absorption is complete 6 months later, the remaining segments fall apart, and the end stage of healing is similar to that seen after a Pomeroy: a segment of isthmus next to the uterus, a gap of varying length depending

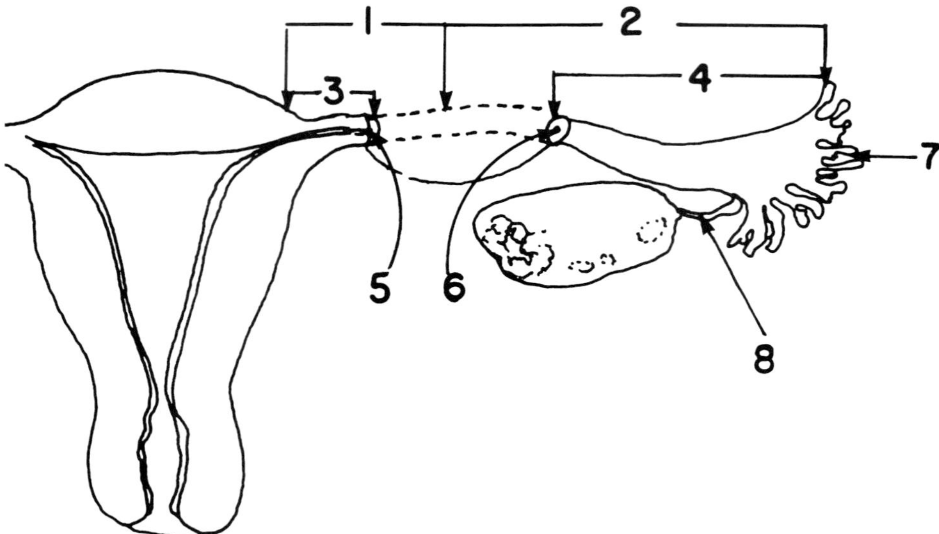

Figure 10.2 Fallopian tube. *1,* Isthmus; *2,* ampulla; *3,* proximal segment; *4,* distal segment; *5,* proximal (tuboperitoneal, uteroperitoneal) fistula; *6,* distal fistula; *7,* fimbria; *8,* fimbrica ovarica.

on the extent of coagulation, and a distal ampullary segment with varying incidence of fistula.

The incidence of pregnancy subsequent to properly performed bipolar sterilization techniques is about 2 to 4 of 1,000 sterilizations, with pregnancies tending to be ectopic as well as intrauterine. Pregnancy is believed to result from a short proximal segment leading to a uteroperitoneal fistula (see Figure 10.1). Pregnancies associated with operator error often involve a mismatch between forceps and the electrodesiccation current designed for that forcep, with the result that tubes are incompletely coagulated.[43] Pregnancy rates with incomplete coagulation have been as high as 20 per 1,000, the majority intrauterine. Since the bipolar method has been the one most frequently performed, it has received the best statistical scrutiny as to long-term efficacy. The combined 10-year cumulative pregnancy rate observed with bipolar electrodesiccation as performed in the United States is around 28 per 1,000, mostly ectopic.[44] Techniques to minimize the risk of these pregnancies will be presented later in this chapter.

Unipolar Electrocoagulation

In the 1970s the most popular method of laparoscopic sterilization was unipolar; a current flowed from a metal forcep on the tube to a ground plate on the patient's body. The end result was variable, from damage similar to that after a Pomeroy procedure to extensive destruction of the tube, with no proximal segment and with minimal ampulla and fimbria remaining. Pregnancies are both ectopic and intrauterine after this procedure.

As concern about the immediate and late complication (ectopic pregnancy) of electrocoagulation emerges, the mechanical methods of laparoscopic tubal occlusion are steadily increasing in popularity. Both mechanical techniques were introduced in the 1970s as alternatives to electrocoagulation to minimize the hazard of bowel damage due to burns.

The Band Procedure

The band is essentially a type of Pomeroy procedure, where a knuckle of tube is lifted up and constricted by an elastic band at its base and the loop allowed to necrose. The healing process is also similar to the Pomeroy; about 6 months later, the segments have been separated, and the band is enclosed in the peritoneum of one of the segments. A 3- to 4-cm segment of tube is missing with a fairly healthy proximal isthmic portion and a variable distal ampullary segment. The majority of subsequent pregnancies are intrauterine. Pregnancies attributable to operator error result from failure to completely occlude the lumen with

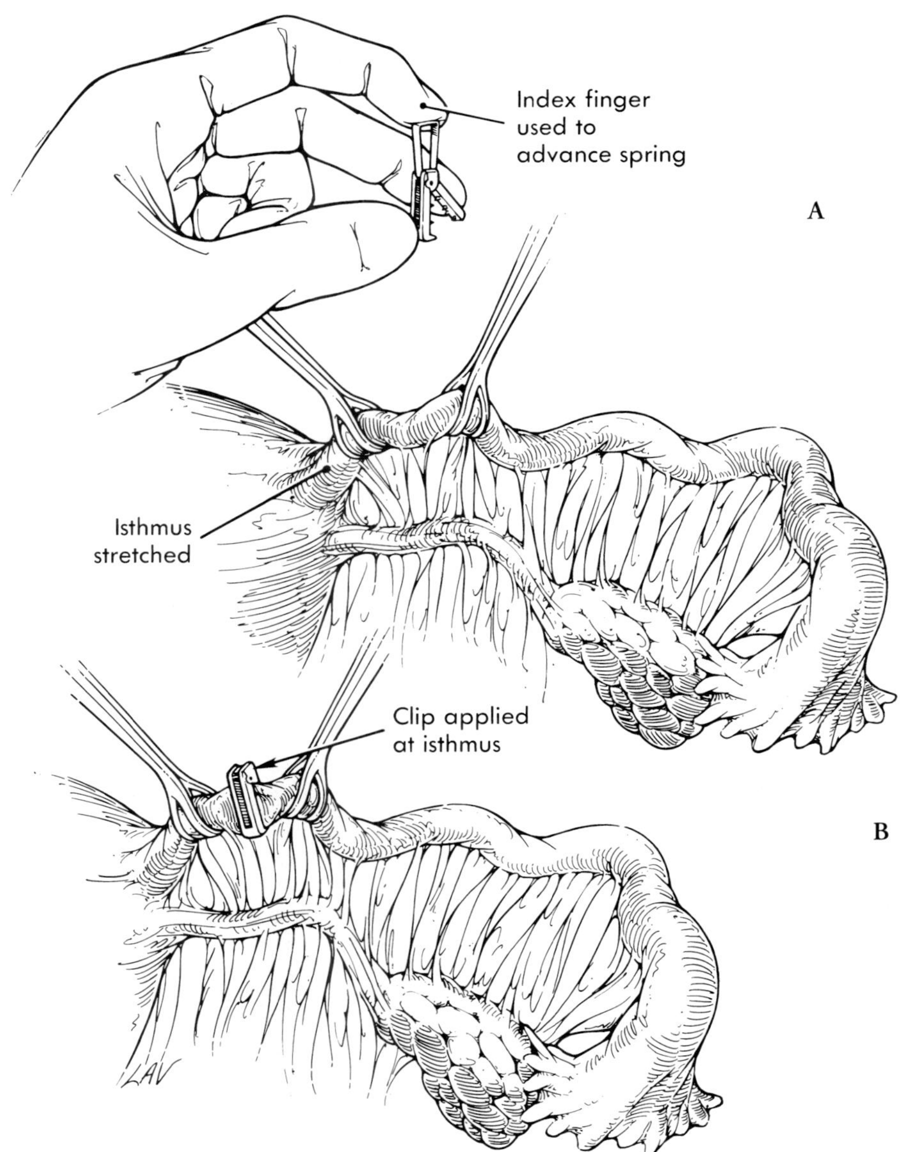

Figure 10.3 Clip at laparotomy. Two Babcock's clamps, one close to the uterus, put a segment of isthmus on the stretch. **A,** A spring clip is held between thumb and second finger and is placed on the stretched segment like a clothespin on a clothesline. **B,** The index finger pushes the metal spring over the plastic jaws to lock the clip on the isthmus. (From Hulka JF: Methods of female sterilization, In Nichols DH, editor: Gynecologic and obstetric surgery, St Louis, 1993, Mosby.)

the band, from incorrect application of the band onto the wrong structure, and even from slippage of the band off the tube.

The Spring Clip

The spring clip is designed to go across the isthmic portion of the tube. Although it was designed for laparoscopic application, it can be applied postpartum at minilaparotomy, using fingers only (no applicator) instead of a Pomeroy (Figure 10.3) for more reversibility and low postsurgical comfort.[45]

At the end of the healing process, in about 6 weeks, the clip remains where it was placed and is covered by epithelium. Both proximal and distal segments of the endothelium of the tube form blind pouches, and about 0.5 cm of the tube is destroyed. Incidence of proximal and distal fistula after this procedure is quite rare. Pregnancies occurring after this procedure are mostly intrauterine. Pregnancies result almost entirely from operator error in applying the clip incompletely across the isthmus or onto the ampullary segment.[43]

The Irving Procedure

The isthmus of a tube is divided and the proximal isthmic segment buried into the peritoneum of the uterus so that a proximal uteroperitoneal fistula is prevented. This procedure is usually done for sterilization at the time of elective cesarean section, when the tube and entire fundus can be easily visualized. An extensive review of the literature by Garb failed to reveal any pregnancies after this procedure.[46]

Cornual Resection

Excising the tube and performing a cornual resection were occasionally recommended as part of the management of ectopic pregnancy. A critical review of its efficacy revealed a variable incidence of ectopic and interstitial pregnancies subsequent to cornual resection.[47] In 1995 Rotten reported 5 such pregnancies after 105 cornual resections, for a subsequent pregnancy rate of 4.7%,[47] probably resulting from the formation of uteroperitoneal fistula.

Fimbriectomy

In 1969 Kroener described his father's successful technique of bilateral fimbriectomy by colpotomy.[48] He emphasized the importance of recognizing the fimbrica ovarica, a variable structure connecting the ovary and the fimbria. Although he described separate ligation of the structure to remove the fimbria completely, subsequent reports of failures did not mention this important detail; this omission led to remnants of fimbria when clamps and sutures did not get completely between the fimbria and the ovary. Though the vaginal approach has been abandoned, some physicians do fimbriectomies postpartum or at cesarean section. Pregnancies following fimbriectomies are usually intrauterine, because the egg is brought into a normal tube through a remnant of fimbrial opening.

Summary

Most techniques of sterilization have their failures. Failures can result from technical error at the time of sterilization or from the normal healing process after sterilization. It is mandatory for the total management of a pregnancy after sterilization to determine the exact anatomic cause of the pregnancy to choose the most effective technique of resterilization.

MANAGEMENT OF SUBSEQUENT PREGNANCY

Intrauterine Pregnancy

Although the majority of patients are upset or distraught by a pregnancy after sterilization, some patients consider the event a gift or a blessing. Depending on the patient's reaction, a therapeutic abortion or a term delivery is chosen.

If abortion is chosen, the patient should be urged to consider laparoscopy during the procedure or soon after the procedure to determine the cause of failure and to allow resterilization. At the time of resterilization, careful note should be made as to whether or not both tubes are, in fact, properly divided or occluded or whether an operator error has occurred. Sensitivity to the medicolegal implications of operator error while dictating operative notes and while describing the findings to the patient is urged in the spirit of "There, but by the grace of God, go I." It is our experience and that of others[41,43] that many intrauterine pregnancies result from technical errors. The proper management of this situation is to perform a correct sterilization at the time of laparoscopy by electrocoagulation, clip, or band as the patient and physician believe appropriate. If both tubes are properly occluded or divided but the intrauterine pregnancy has occurred anyway, the procedure should be a diagnostic laparoscopy only, and the patient should be involved in the next step of management. Vasectomy for the husband is a simple solution in a monogamous marriage. Resterilization of a technically successful sterilization would involve a laparotomy and an Irving procedure to bury the proximal isthmic stumps (if isthmic stumps are available). A hysterectomy may be an option if the patient feels the risks are worth the freedom from concern over subsequent pregnancy.

If the pregnancy goes to term, the patient should again be offered a postpartum tubal ligation with a larger incision to evaluate the cause of the pregnancy. If at this point a technical error is discovered, a repeat standard Pomeroy procedure (using a strongly ligated O plain catgut suture) could be carried out. If the tubes were properly divided or occluded and intrauterine pregnancy nevertheless occurred, an Irving procedure should be performed at this time. If there are insufficient tubal stumps to bury the tube, the patient should be so advised and should consider vasectomy of the husband or hysterectomy.

Ectopic Pregnancy

Ectopic pregnancy is a moderate to acute emergency where cool decisions and informed consent may not be reasonably expected. If the situation is elective (vasomotor stability, 1 or 2 days of observation of β-human chorionic gonadotropin titers, or ultrasound changes), the patient may have had an adequate chance to consider alternatives of management. The physician should use judgment to determine if the patient can make an informed consent as to the alternatives of management available.

Early Unruptured Pregnancy. Early unruptured pregnancies in the ampulla are increasingly managed by laparoscopy. In this technique, a salpingostomy is performed, and the ampullary ectopic pregnancy is aspirated. A laparoscopy then gives the opportunity to review the cause of the ectopic pregnancy. In a patient who has already agreed to a bilateral distal salpingectomy for prevention of further ectopic pregnancies, a judgment can be made whether the ampullary stumps could be excised by laparoscopic electrodesiccation and excision of the base. If this is judged not to be feasible, a laparotomy can be performed and bilateral ampullary removal performed. Some physicians may not be comfortable with the laparoscopic management of ectopic pregnancy. There are no animal or human data to suggest that such surgery has any effect on subsequent endocrine function such as menstrual regularity.

Acute Ectopic Pregnancy. In the acute ectopic pregnancy with vasomotor instability, an emergency laparotomy is the usual method of management. After the ectopic pregnancy is excised and bleeding is controlled, a decision can be made, based on the patient's degree of informed consent, as to whether the remaining distal ampullae should be removed as well.

Cornual Resection. Although cornual resection has been recommended by some as an additional step in the management of ectopic pregnancies, the rather high incidence of intrauterine or interstitial pregnancy after cornual resection[47] would seem to make this approach inappropriate. If no proximal fistula is found and a proximal isthmic stump is present, a performance of a cornual resection rather than an Irving procedure may actually increase the risk of a repeat ectopic pregnancy.

Prevention of the Need for Resterilization

The choice of techniques in the performance of sterilizations should reflect the lessons learned in management of pregnancies subsequent to sterilization failures. As this chapter indicates, uteroperitoneal fistulas are a common factor in pregnancies after sterilization procedures where a segment of tube is destroyed or excised. Current recommendations at the time of the initial sterilization are to leave at least 1 or 2 cm of isthmic tube as a stump at the uterine end. The musculature of the isthmus will then absorb the pressure of a uterine contraction expelling fluid into the tube and will minimize the risk of fistula formation. Putting the following recommendations into practice will minimize the need for resterilization.

The Irving Procedure

The Irving procedure should be recommended at elective cesarean section. This technique has good reversal potential in that no tubal tissue is destroyed. It is relatively easy to perform when the uterus is exposed after cesarean delivery. Since the proximal stump is buried in the myometrium, fistula formation is not a problem.

The Pomeroy Procedure

The Pomeroy procedure is a good technique in the early postpartum period after spontaneous vaginal delivery. Pomeroy used O plain catgut suture tied strongly. A good portion (1 to 2 cm) of proximal isthmic stump should be left to minimize the chance of proximal fistula and subsequent ectopic pregnancy.

Bipolar Electrodesiccation

Bipolar electrodesiccation should be performed at laparoscopy by starting at least 2 cm away from the uterus (Figure 10.4) and desiccating three times, going distally along the tube.[24,42,49] In addition, proper matching of forceps and generator has been stressed by Kleppinger,[49] Soderstrom,[43] and Hulka and Reich.[24] The end point for bipolar desiccation should be the disappearance of electric flow (as measured by a flowmeter) between the tips of the forceps during the process. Other clinical end points such as "turning white" or "popping" may represent superficial coagulation that allows lumen between the forceps to remain viable.

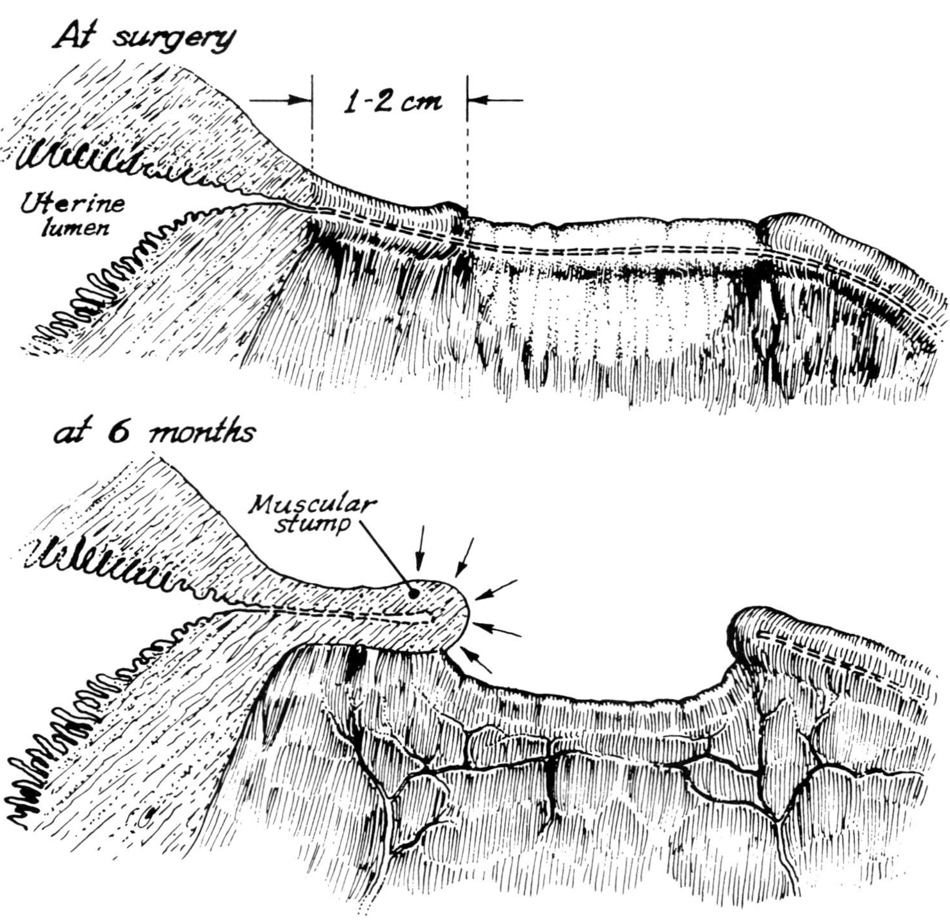

FIGURE 10.4 Electrocoagulation of a tube at least 2 cm from the uterus allows an isthmic segment to remain, which should minimize the chance of fistula formation by allowing a greater distribution and absorbtion of the pressure of uterine fluid. (From Hulka J: Textbook of laparoscopy, Orlando, 1985, Grune & Stratton.)

Bands and Clips

Bands and clips should be meticulously placed on the structures with correct technique: the band on the isthmic-ampullary junction where the tube is most mobile and the clips completely across the isthmus about 2 to 3 cm away from the uterus. Mechanical laparoscopic techniques require strict attention to surgical detail.

References

1. ASRM/SART: Assisted reproductive technology in the United States and Canada: 1993 results generated from the American Society for Reproductive Medicine/Society for Assisted Reproductive Technology Registry, Fertil Steril 64:13, 1995.
2. Luciano AA, Maier DB, and Koch EI: A comparative study of postoperative adhesions following laser surgery by laparoscopy versus laparotomy in the rabbit model, Obstet Gynecol 74:220, 1989.
3. Lundorff P, Hahlin M, and Kallfelt B: Adhesion formation after laparoscopic surgery in tubal pregnancy: a randomized trial versus laparotomy, Fertil Steril 55:911, 1991.
4. Operative Laparoscopy Study Group: Postoperative adhesion development after operative laparoscopy: evaluation at early second-look procedures, Fertil Steril 55:700, 1991.
5. diZerega GS: The peritoneum and its response to surgical injury. In diZerega GS and others, editors: Treatment of post surgical adhesions: proceedings of the First International Symposium for the Treatment of Post Surgical Adhesions, New York, 1990, Wiley-Liss.
6. Drollette CM and Badawy SZ: A pathophysiology of pelvic adhesions: modern trends in preventing infertility, J Reprod Med 37:107, 1992.
7. Ellis H: Internal overhealing: the problem of intraperitoneal adhesions, World J Surg 4:303, 1980.
8. Trimbos-Kemper TCM, Trimbos JB, and van Hall EV: Adhesion formation after tubal surgery: results of the eighth day laparoscopy in 188 patients, Fertil Steril 43:395, 1985.
9. Hulka JF. Adnexal adhesions: a prognostic staging and classification system based on a five year survey of fertility surgery results at Chapel Hill, North Carolina, Am J Obstet Gynecol 144:141, 1982.
10. Brumsted JR and others: Post operative adhesion formation after ovarian wedge resection with and without ovarian reconstruction in the rabbit, Fertil Steril 53:723, 1990.
11. Wiskind AK and others: Adhesion formation after ovarian wound repair in New Zealand white rabbits: a comparison of ovarian microsurgical closure with ovarian nonclosure, Am J Obstet Gynecol 163:1674, 1990.
12. Meyer WR and others: Ovarian surgery: the effect of cortex closure on adhesion formation and fertility in the rabbit, J Reprod Med 36:639, 1991.
13. Pagidas K and Tulandi T: Effects of Ringer's lactate, Interceed (TC7) and Gore-Tex surgical membrane on post surgical adhesion formation. Fertil Steril 57:199, 1992.
14. Sahakian V and others: Normal saline versus lactated Ringer's as irrigation with carbon dioxide insufflation: effect on adhesion formation, Obstet Gynecol 82:851, 1993.
15. Raj SG and Hulka JF: Second look laparoscopy in infertility surgery: therapeutic and prognostic value, Fertil Steril 38:325, 1982.
16. Tulandi T, Falcone T, and Kafka I: Second-look operative laparoscopy 1 year following reproductive surgery, Fertil Steril 52:421, 1989.
17. Schlaff WD and others: Neosalpingostomy for distal tubal obstruction: prognostic factors and impact of surgical technique, Fertil Steril 54:984, 1990.
18. DeBruyne F and others: The clinical value of salpingoscopy in tubal infertility, Fertil Steril 51:339, 1989.
19. Chartier M, Dubost M, and Cornu C: Notre experience des interventions iteratives dans la chirurgie tubularie: a propos de 15 observations, Rev Fr Gynecol Obstet 67:209, 1972.
20. Lauritsen JG, Pagel JD, and Vangsted P: Results of repeated tuboplasties, Fertil Steril 37:68, 1992.
21. Verhoeven HC, Berry H, and Frantzen C: Surgical treatment for distal tubal occlusion: a review of 167 cases, J Reprod Med 28:293, 1983.
22. Thie JL, Williams TJ, and Coulam CB: Repeat tuboplasty compared with primary mi-

crosurgery for postinflammatory tubal disease, Fertil Steril 45:784, 1986.

23. Winston RML and Margara RA: Microsurgical salpingostomy is not an obsolete procedure, Br J Obstet Gynaecol 98:637, 1991.

24. Hulka JF and Reich H: Textbook of laparoscopy, ed 2, Philadelphia, 1994, WB Saunders Co.

25. Howard FM: The role of laparoscopy in chronic pelvic pain: promise and pitfalls, Obstet Gynecol Surv 48:357, 1993.

26. Steege JF and Stout AL: Resolution of chronic pelvic pain after laparoscopic lysis of adhesions, Am J Obstet Gynecol 165:278, 1991.

27. Steege JF: Repeated clinic laparoscopy for the treatment of pelvic adhesions: a pilot study, Obstet Gynecol 83:276, 1994.

28. Steege JF, Stout AL, and Somkuti SG: Chronic pelvic pain in women: toward an integrative model, Obstet Gynecol Surv 48:95, 1993.

29. Peters AAW and others: A randomized clinical trial to compare two different approaches in women with chronic pelvic pain, Obstet Gynecol 77:740, 1991.

30. Bashford RA: Diagnosing depression in the OB/GYN office. Lecture presented at North Carolina OB/GYN Society Meeting, Asheville, NC, April 28-30, 1995.

31. Hasson HA: Laparoscopic management of ovarian cysts, J Reprod Med 35:863, 1990.

32. Fayez JA and Vogel MF: Comparison of different treatment methods of endometriomas by laparoscopy, Obstet Gynecol 78:660, 1991.

33. DeWilde RL: Recurrence of functional ovarian cysts after laparoscopic fenestration, Am J Obstet Gynecol 161:839, 1989.

34. Hoppe DE, Bekkar BE, and Nager CW: Single dose systemic methotrexate for the treatment of persistent ectopic pregnancy after conservative surgery, Obstet Gynecol 83:41, 1994.

35. Stovall TG and Ling FW: Single dose methotrexate: an expanded clinical trial, Am J Obstet Gynecol 168:1759, 1993.

36. Hulka JF and Halme J: Sterilization reversal: results of 101 attempts, Am J Obstet Gynecol 159:767, 1988.

37. Siegler AM, Hulka JF, and Peretz A: Reversibility of female sterilization, Fertil Steril 43:499, 1985.

38. Courey NG, Cunanan RG JR, and Taefi P: Sterilization via laparoscopy, NY State J Med 73:539, 1973.

39. Stock RJ: Histopathologic changes in fallopian tubes subsequent to sterilization procedures, Int J Gynecol Pathol 2:13, 1983.

40. Metz KGP and Mastroianni L: Tubal pregnancy subsequent to transperitoneal migration of spermatozoa, Obstet Gynecol Surv 34:554, 1979.

41. Stock RJ and Nelson KJ: Ectopic pregnancy subsequent to sterilization: histologic evaluation and clinical implications, Fertil Steril 42:211, 1984.

42. Fishburne JI and Hulka JF: Tubal healing following laparoscopic coagulation, J Reprod Med 16:129, 1976.

43. Soderstrom RM: Sterilization failures and their causes, Am J Obstet Gynecol 152:395, 1985.

44. Wilcox LD and others: Ten-year pregnancy rates after unipolar and bipolar sterilization, Fertil Steril 56:S12, 1991 (abstract).

45. Lee SH and Jones JS: Postpartum tubal sterilization: a comparative study of Hulka clip application and the modified Pomeroy technique, J Reprod Med 36:703, 1991.

46. Garb AE: A review of tubal sterilization failures, Obstet Gynecol Surv 34:554, 1979.

47. Rotten GN: Failure in sterilization, West J Surg 63:146, 1955.

48. Kroener WF Jr: Surgical sterilization by fimbriectomy, Am J Obstet Gynecol 104:247, 1969.

49. Kleppinger RK: Female outpatient sterilization using bipolar coagulation, Bull Postgrad Comm Med Univ Sydney, p 144, November 1977.

11

Recurrent Endometriosis

L. Russell Malinak

Endometriosis is the common name of a disease with a wide clinical spectrum. The mild form with superficial peritoneal implants is so common, and often asymptomatic, that it may not actually represent disease but a normal variation in pelvic anatomy. Mild disease, however, may cause significant pain and may be associated with infertility. The more severe forms of endometriosis are unquestionably pathologic, distorting anatomy with fibrosis and adhesions; commonly, pain and infertility are associated with this form of disease. To borrow an infectious disease model, mild endometriosis may behave like microbial colonization, living symbiotically with the host tissues, whereas severe endometriosis is akin to overt infection, with its destruction of normal tissue structure and function. Unfortunately, the natural history of endometriosis is yet to be clearly understood; which women will have the mild forms of endometriosis and which will have the destructive forms cannot be predicted. Until the natural history of endometriosis is better defined, clinicians must rely on their observations in the treatment of this disease.

Incidence of Recurrence

One aspect of the natural history of endometriosis is clear: both medical and surgical treatments are associated with all-too-frequent cases of recurrent disease.

A number of studies document the recurrence of endometriosis after medical therapy. Following danocrine (danazol) treatment, representative publications have found that (1) 5% to 20% of patients per year developed symptomatic recurrence,[1] (2) 40% of women treated with danazol alone had recurrent endometriosis after 3 years,[2] and (3) 33% of patients had recurrent symptoms or positive physical findings after 5 years.[3]

The recurrence rates after treatment with gonadotropin-releasing hormone agonists (GnRH-a) are similar to those after danazol therapy,[4] although exact comparison is difficult because crude recurrence rates of older publications are compared with more recent studies citing cumulative recurrence rates.[5] Waller and Shaw in a study of long-term follow-up after GnRH-a treatment noted a 53.4% cumulative recurrence rate for the fifth year after treatment ended. Of interest, they observed higher recurrence rates when initial disease was severe versus when initial disease was minimal.[5]

The incidence of recurrence following conservative surgery for endometriosis has been extensively documented.[6-8] The cumulative recurrence rate is 19.5% at 5 years and 31.6% for the seventh postoperative year, based on a study of 423 patients treated primarily at laparotomy as the index surgical procedure[9] (Figure 11.1). In a series of 359 patients who had excision of endometriosis at laparoscopy, the cumulative recurrence rate was 19% by the fifth postoperative year.[10]

Thus endometriosis is more likely to recur and earlier following medical therapy than following conservative surgery. The recurrence is more likely when the initial disease is severe rather than minimal or mild.

Diagnosis

One obvious difficulty with the current methods of diagnosing recurrent endometriosis is the reliance on reoperation; only those women with persistent infertility or recurrent pain will repeat operations. Therefore the incidence of recurrence after surgery may be higher than

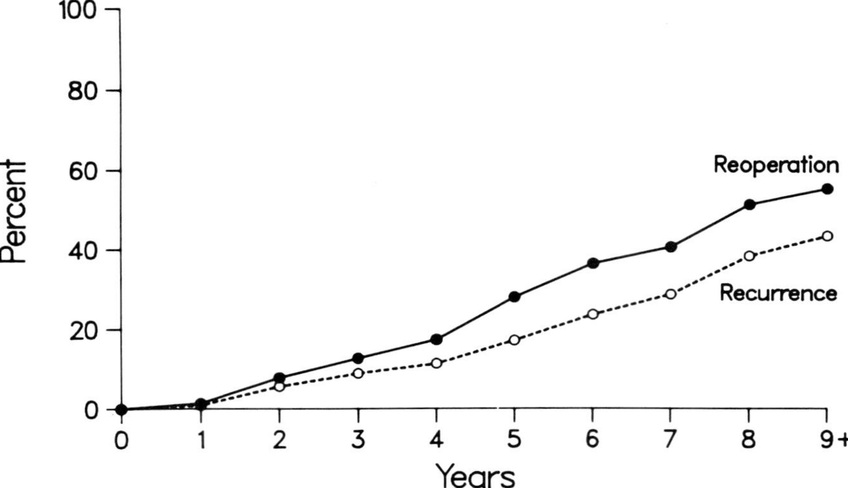

FIGURE 11.1 Cumulative rates of reoperation and recurrent endometriosis in 423 infertile women treated by conservative laparotomy. (From Olive D. In Schenken RB, editor: Endometriosis: contemporary concepts in clinical management, Philadelphia, 1989, JB Lippincott Co.)

that reported from clinical case series. Until noninvasive techniques allow diagnosis of recurrence without resorting to surgery, accurate knowledge of the incidence of recurrent endometriosis is impossible.[11]

One of the inherent problems with estimating the incidence of recurrent endometriosis after surgery is distinguishing recurrence, the growth of new lesions, from persistence, the growth of lesions inadequately treated or overlooked at initial surgery. A schematic representation of the pelvis (Figure 11.2) based on careful recording of findings might allow recurrent lesions to be distinguished from persistent endometriosis lesions. At short-interval second-look laparoscopy, patients who have implants most likely have persistent disease (i.e., lesions at a site of dissection, cautery, or vaporization at primary surgery).[12] Only by adopting accurate record keeping will knowledge of the course of endometriosis following surgical treatment be acquired.

MORPHOLOGY OF ENDOMETRIOSIS IMPLANTS

The many visual appearances of endometriosis present a problem not only for treatment, but also for estimating recurrence. In addition to the classic black or blue-black blebs, endometriosis has been histologically confirmed in flat, red to pink, subperitoneal, or even clear and vesicular lesions.[13] The surgeon must be alert to the many visual appearances of endometriosis at the time of diagnosis; awareness combined with magnification will likely improve the completeness of treating or removing subtle forms of the disease.

Stripling and others[13] and Batt and Smith[14] described peritoneal pockets (Figure 11.3) that often contain endometriosis implants; these pockets may be everted and excised either laparoscopically or at laparotomy, or the implants discovered in the pockets may be vaporized or cauterized.

Microscopic endometriosis cannot be identified by the surgeon's eye; using electron microscopy 20% of biopsy specimens of grossly normal peritoneum were found to harbor endometriosis.[15] Again, lack of knowledge of the natural history of endometriosis prevents determination of whether microscopic disease is clinically relevant to the treatment of women with recurrence of endometriosis.[16]

The problem of persistent microscopic endometriosis prompted several investigators to study combination medical and surgical therapy.[17] The concept inspiring combination therapy has parallels with the treatment of epithelial tumors of the ovary—initial surgery should be debulking, removing as much disease as possible, with chemotherapy used to treat residual implants or microscopic disease.

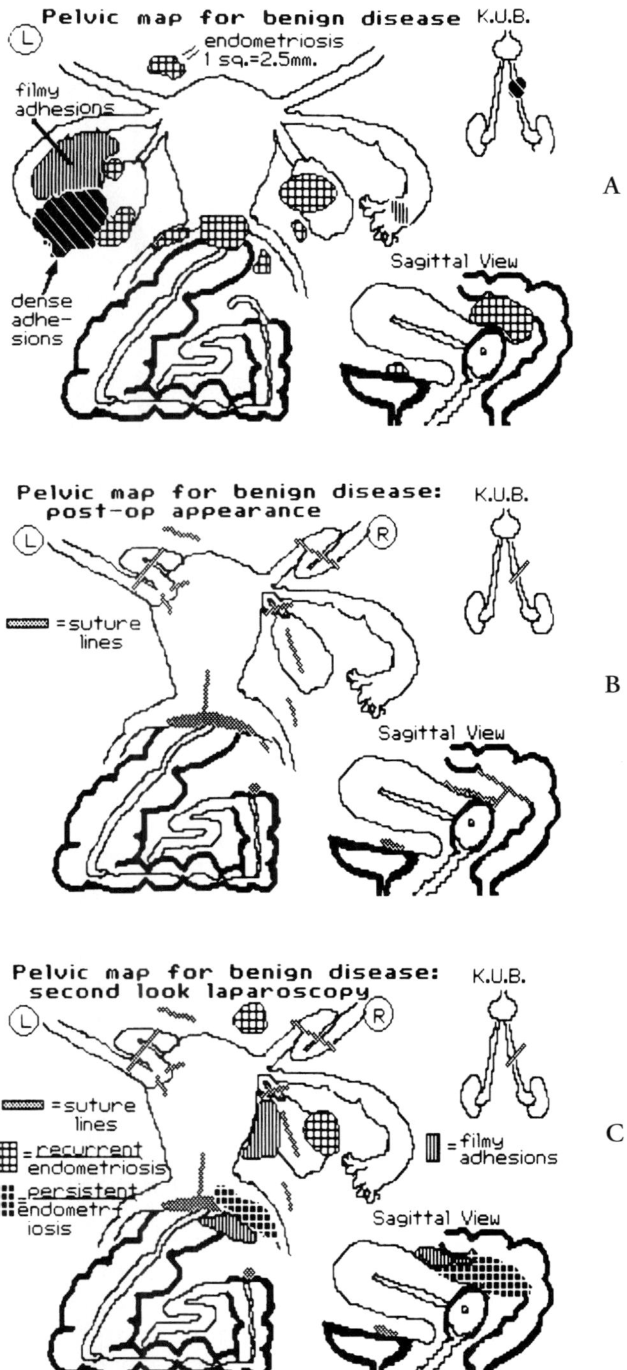

Figure 11.2 Pelvic mapping to distinguish recurrent from persistent endometriosis after conservative laparotomy. **A**, Extent and size (each square = 0.25 cm) of endometriosis and adhesions found at laparotomy. **B**, Postoperative appearance of the pelvis, including suture lines. **C**, Appearance of second-look laparoscopy 4 weeks after laparotomy. *Recurrent* lesions are de novo implants, whereas *persistent* lesions are at sites of previous dissection and represent incomplete excision.

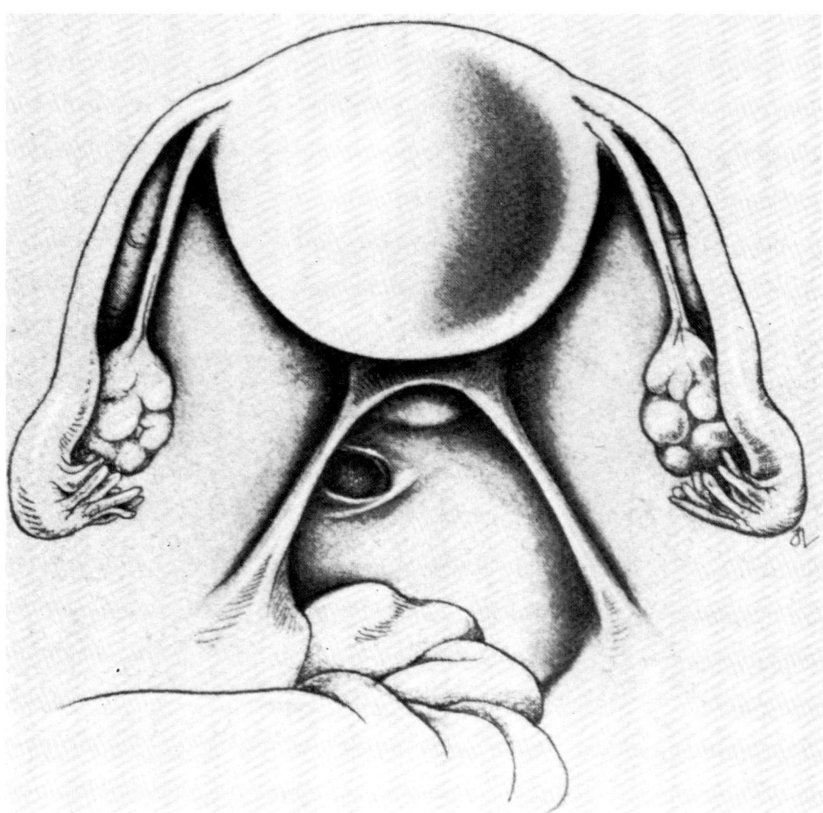

FIGURE 11.3 Posterior cul-de-sac peritoneal pocket under left uterosacral ligament; excision demonstrated endometriosis foci. (From Batt RE and Smith RA: Obstet Gynecol Clin North Am 16:15, 1989.)

This approach has included preoperative, postoperative, or both preoperative and postoperative medical treatment. Because the menstrual cycle is suppressed, preoperative medical therapy has the advantages of decreasing blood supply in the pelvis, suppressing functional cysts that might be confused with endometriomas, and allowing the patient and surgeon to schedule the operation without the limitation of erratic menses. In women with moderate and severe endometriosis, 3 to 6 months of postoperative Danazol produced lower long-term recurrence rates than did surgery alone.[18] This retrospective observational study still needs to be confirmed with the experience of other authors and other medications such as gonadotropin-releasing hormone (GnRH) agonists. Longitudinal prospective comparative trials should be conducted to determine the benefit, or lack thereof, of perioperative medical therapy. Until that is known, it is appropriate to utilize adjunctive perioperative medical treatment in advanced cases of endometriosis or when pelvic pain is a prominent preoperative symptom. However, because of ovulation suppression, perioperative medical therapy is usually not indicated in infertility patients.

NATURE OF RECURRENT ENDOMETRIOSIS

Studies by Koninckx and associates,[19] among others, suggest that endometriosis is a progressive disease. Superficial peritoneal lesions tend to "burn out" over time, decrease with age, and may or may not be associated with pain. In contrast, deeply infiltrating lesions, including ovarian endometriomas, tend to increase with age and are more likely to be associated with pelvic pain.[19] Severely symptomatic women usually have progressive or recurrent disease.[20] Corroboration that endometriosis is a progressive disease is suggested by the work of Redwine who found an age-related color appearance of endometriotic lesions.[21]

There are little data regarding biochemical differences between recurrent and primary endometriosis. A study by Bergqvist and Ferno demonstrated that progesterone receptor (PR) levels were significantly higher in recurrent than in primary lesions.[22] Their results indicate that two types of endocrine-regulated endometriotic lesions may exist; one may be hormonally more sensitive than the other, or a change in hormonal regulation may occur with time in endometriotic tissue, depending on different surrounding factors, degrees of invasiveness, and location of lesions.[22] Others have reported on estrogen receptor (ER) and PR in recurrent endometriosis.[23]

More clinical and basic investigation is necessary to determine the precise nature of recurrent endometriosis.

RECURRENCE AFTER SURGICAL EXCISION

It is likely that the multifocal nature of endometriosis, with missed lesions during surgery, is responsible for most cases of persistent/recurrent disease. Because of the common presence of microscopic disease adjacent to macroscopic lesions, surgeons have emphasized the importance of en bloc dissection of juxtaposed endometriosis implants.[24] As shown in Figure 11.4, the many implants in the posterior cul-de-sac were considered a "field," and the entire field was completely removed. It is unknown whether sharp dissection of all implants is associated with lower recurrence rates. One could safely assume that complete removal of the involved peritoneum, including the entire depth of the lesions, would certainly not increase the risk of recurrence.

Because the depth of infiltration of endometriotic implants is so variable, more superficial treatments might fail to remove deeper depths of disease. Martin, Hubert, and Levy found that one fourth of patients had lesions that penetrated the peritoneum more than 5 mm.[25] Because one pass of the carbon dioxide (CO_2) laser vaporizes tissue to a depth of 0.1 to 0.5 mm, even several passes of the laser could leave disease behind. Endometriosis has been histologically confirmed adjacent to carbon particles from previous laser surgery, suggesting incomplete treatment.[26] Whenever possible, fields of endometriosis should be excised, whether the surgeon is using scissors, knife, or laser. Figure 11.5 depicts this principle using the CO_2 laser; note the peritoneum is removed completely to the depth of retroperitoneal fat. Whether surgery is performed by laparoscopy or laparotomy, the ureter must be clearly identified throughout the case to avoid injury.

REPEAT CONSERVATIVE SURGERY

When persistent infertility, recurrent symptoms, or pelvic examination findings warrant evaluation for recurrent endometriosis, laparoscopy is performed. The pelvis is systematically inspected for implants; care must be taken not to confuse suture materials previously used for uterine suspension, presacral neurectomy, or peritoneal closure with implants of endometriosis. If recurrent disease is present, many cases can be managed laparoscopically, adapting the same microsurgical principles used during laparotomy. Tissues are manipulated bluntly to provide traction and countertraction for lysis of adhesions. If grasping instruments are used, the adnexa are manipulated only by the utero-ovarian ligament; the tube and ovarian cortex are not grasped. Adhesions are incised or excised; all visible endometriosis is excised or completely vaporized or cauterized. Ample irrigation and meticulous hemostasis complete the laparoscopic procedure. If significant areas of denuded peritoneum are present, Interceed is applied to reduce adhesion formation, after complete hemostasis is obtained.[27]

If the disease is not amenable to laparoscopic treatment, the patient is prepared for laparotomy. Moistened laparotomy sponges are placed around the wound edges and the self-retaining retractor is positioned; the procedure is performed very much like primary conservative surgery for endometriosis.[28] However, repeat presacral neurectomy is not attempted due to difficulty in dissection and bleeding caused by retroperitoneal scarring. Magnification in the form of 2.5 or 4× loupes

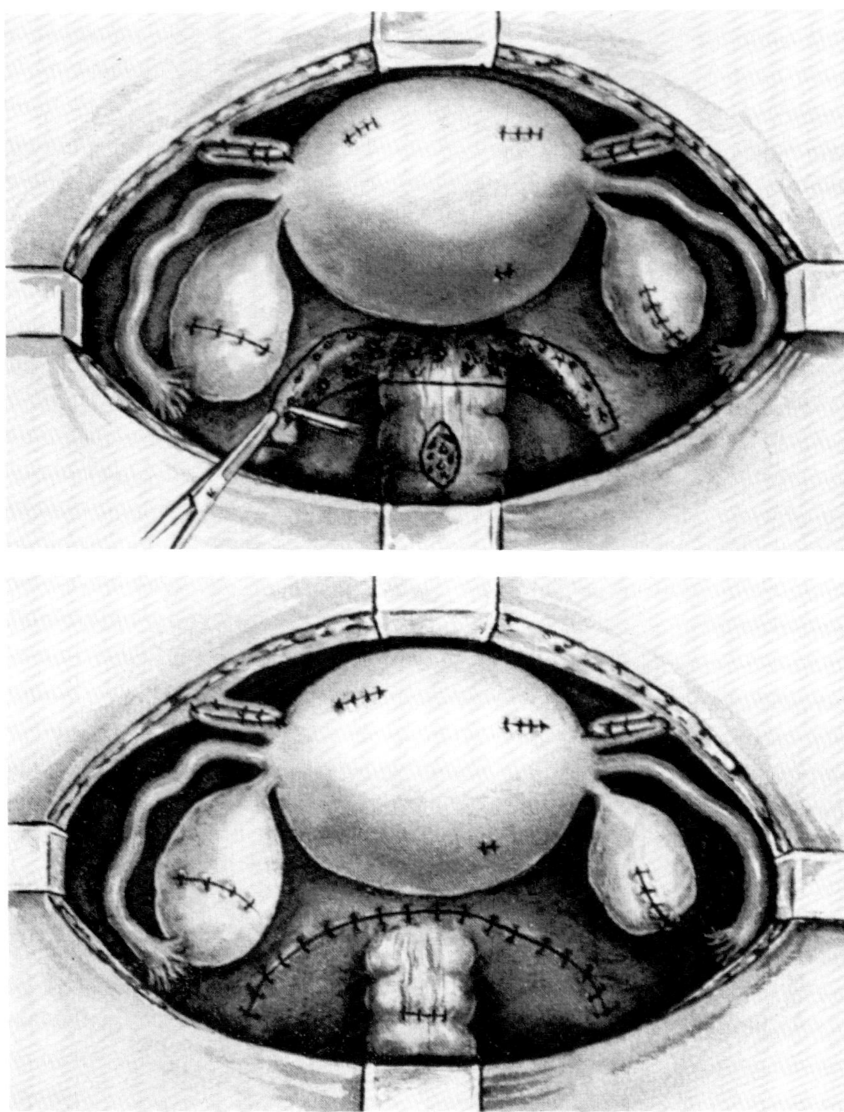

FIGURE 11.4 Management of posterior cul-de-sac with numerous endometriotic implants after closure of ovarian and uterine lesions. The entire field is excised en bloc and the peritoneum closed with continuous absorbable suture. (From Rogers SF and Jacobs WM: Fertil Steril 19:529, 1968.)

is useful in removing as much disease as possible. Tissues are handled minimally and kept continually moistened with a solution of warmed lactated Ringer's solution with 5,000 units of heparin per liter. The procedure is conducted anatomically to effect complete removal of disease. Special attention is paid to the GI tract,[29] including the appendix, which may be involved.[30]

After all areas of endometriosis and adhesions are excised, there are several options in the management of the peritoneal defects. If the peritoneum can be reapproximated with 4-0 to 6-0 absorbable suture without tension, primary closure is indicated. Peritoneal defects and/or suture lines may be covered with Interceed or Gore-Tex after complete hemostasis is achieved to reduce adhesion formation.[31,32]

Second-look laparoscopy 2 to 12 weeks after conservative laparotomy is useful in lysing new adhesions but has unknown effect on recurrence of endometriosis.

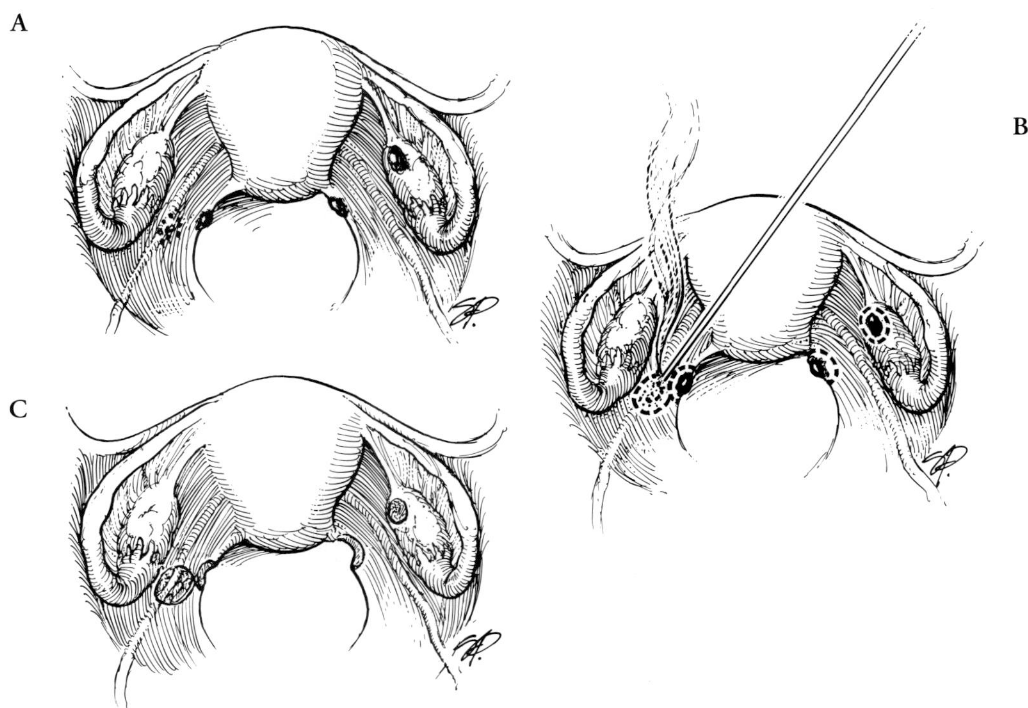

FIGURE 11.5 Management of diffuse endometriotic lesions with laser. **A,** Group of lesions, to be removed with 2- to 4-mm margins of normal tissue through the full thickness of the peritoneum. **B,** Lesions are circumscribed with CO_2 laser highly focused with 16 to 20 watts of power, preferably with superpulse mode. Once the lesion is circumscribed, the edge is lifted, and the laser is passed to and fro under the peritoneum to separate it from underlying adventitia and fat. Carbonization is minimized. **C,** Retroperitoneal fat as it appears after excision of the lesion; the same effect is possible with sharp dissection. The position of the ureter must be known to the surgeon operating via laparoscopy or laparotomy. (Copyright © Baylor College of Medicine, 1989.)

REOPERATION AND RECURRENCE AFTER CONSERVATIVE SURGERY

Of 117 patients followed for up to 3 years after conservative surgery, 28 (24%) required relaparotomy after diagnostic laparoscopy for recurrent pain and/or persistent infertility. The reoperation rate was 40.6% in those patients who remained infertile, whereas this rate was only 3.7% in those who conceived following initial operation. After a second laparotomy 12% of patients conceived, and 12% required hysterectomy as a third procedure.[6] Another study revealed a 47% (7:15) pregnancy rate after a second conservative laparotomy in patients followed 18 months.[7]

A larger series of 78 patients with recurrent endometriosis revealed that 42 (54%) had conservative reoperation, 17 (22%) received medical therapy, and 19 (24%) had hysterectomy and/or bilateral oophorectomy. Eight of 28 (28.6%) women who attempted to conceive achieved 13 pregnancies. A third operation was necessary in 6 patients (14%); 4 had a third conservative operation, and 2 had TAH and BSO.[33] The data on recurrence after a second reoperation are very limited.

There is a tendency toward more reoperations in patients whose initial surgery was for more advanced disease. A majority of available data on reoperation and recurrence describe laparotomy rather than laparoscopic surgery as the index operation. Long-term follow-up data on laparoscopic surgery is unavailable.

A third conservative operation is performed only rarely; this is usually in the form of an operative laparoscopy. If, on the third operation, the endometriosis is severe beyond laparoscopic surgical bounds, hysterectomy is advocated. The conscientious pelvic surgeon should be well versed in medical treatment of endometriosis, including perioperative adjunctive use. Preoperative and occasionally postoperative medical treatments are utilized in women with severe endometriosis and those with known residua that could not be dissected free at surgery.

Recurrence after Laparoscopic Surgery

Improved technology has allowed laparoscopic surgeons to approach more advanced endometriosis, particularly ovarian endometriomas, with increasing frequency. Several laparoscopic techniques have been ineffective, however. High recurrence rates of endometriomas (21% in 2 months) have been associated with laparoscopic drainage through a wide opening in the dependent part of the cyst cavity,[34] and endometriotic cysts aspirated at laparoscopy followed by GnRH agonist therapy recurred in all 29 patients (100%) who were followed for 6 months.[35] Other studies of laparoscopic aspiration reveal similar results.[36] The most appropriate method of laparoscopic management of endometriosis is resection or destruction of the epithelial lining.[37-39] Long-term data on recurrence following this technique are lacking. Persistence of endometriomas following laparoscopic surgery has been observed; since ovarian endometriomas may be multifocal, some may be missed at laparoscopy because the opportunity to palpate the ovary is absent. Disagreement persists whether to leave the ovarian cortex open following laparoscopic endometrial cystectomy or to close the cortex with sutures.[37,38,40] Small bowel obstruction has occurred secondary to adherence of the ileum deep in an ovary previously left open after laparoscopic surgery.[41]

Complete Operations

All treatises on surgical management of endometriosis include a section on complete or definitive operations such as hysterectomy and BSO. Unfortunately, endometriosis may recur following hysterectomy and oophorectomy. Such recurrence is more likely if special care was not taken to remove completely all areas involved with disease and all ovarian tissue.[42] Particular attention should be directed toward the surgical management of bowel disease since there is a 33% frequency of intestinal involvement in patients with recurrent disease who were previously castrated for endometriosis.[43]

If a woman has completed her childbearing and recurrent endometriosis is suspected of causing pelvic pain, laparoscopic examination may demonstrate mild to moderate extent of disease. If the woman is otherwise a good candidate for vaginal hysterectomy, operative laparoscopic techniques may allow lysis of adhesions, oophorectomy, or destruction of endometriosis inaccessible to the vaginal surgeon. Certainly vaginal hysterectomy should be undertaken if the goal of complete removal of disease, including ovarian endometriosis, is attainable. Although laparoscopically assisted vaginal hysterectomy and oophorectomy has allowed more cases to be safely completed vaginally, hysterectomies for more severe forms of the disease are better accomplished by TAH.

Abdominal hysterectomy is usually performed via the previous incision, unless a separate indication warrants a different incision. Careful tissue handling at hysterectomy is similar to that of conservative laparotomy; the only tissues clamped or grasped are those that ultimately will be removed. As depicted in Figure 11.6, an en bloc dissection is made, and all contiguously involved peritoneal surfaces are removed. All lesions of endometriosis are removed with 2- to 4-mm circumferential margins to the depth of retroperitoneal fat. In more cases than not, the ureter has to be identified high on the pelvic brim and dissected free of diseased peritoneum, especially if abnormal adnexa are being removed. If the posterior cul-de-sac is obliterated, the rectum must be dissected free, leaving as much disease on the uterus and as little residua on the colon as possible. If dissection is not possible, segmental resection with anastomosis of prepared bowel probably decreases the likelihood of future long-term recurrence of endometriosis. Dissection of the pararectal spaces in cases of endometriosis, leaving only

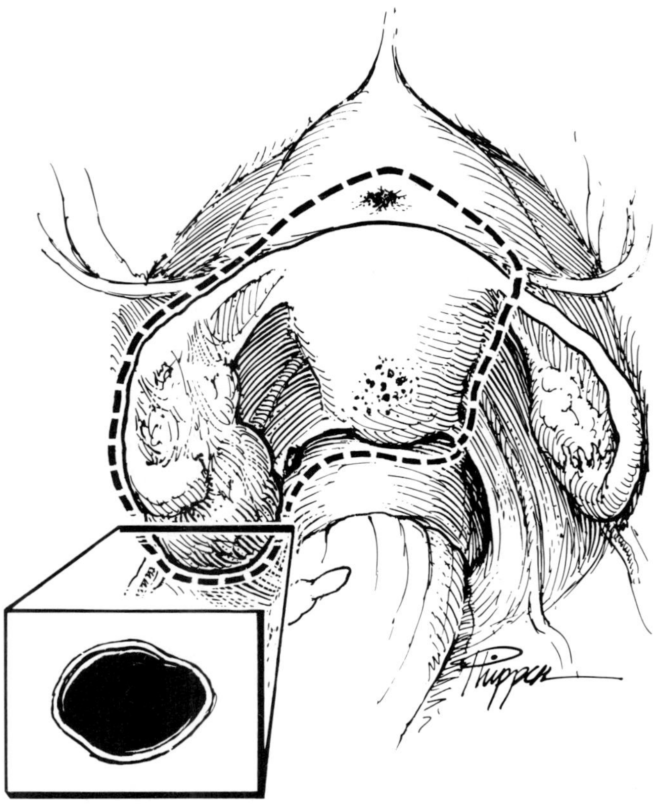

FIGURE 11.6 Hysterectomy for endometriosis. All endometriotic lesions are removed, preferably as an en bloc dissection *(dashed line)*. Any residual implants are removed or destroyed with laser or cautery. The left ovary containing a large endometrioma *(inset)* is removed. The normal right ovary can be preserved if the patient has no symptoms referrable to that adnexa. (Copyright © Baylor College of Medicine, 1989.)

healthy uninvolved tissues behind, is likely to lessen recurrence.[44] If cervical or vaginal endometriosis is suspected from preoperative speculum examination, the involved portion of the posterior vagina is included with the hysterectomy specimen. Otherwise, the cervix is removed completely, and the vaginal length is maximized.

In the most severe cases of endometriosis, the margins for dissection between the uterus, rectum, and bladder can be obliterated by active disease and fibrosis. Intrafascial hysterectomy is appropriate in these circumstances to avoid injury to the bowel, bladder, or ureters, if they cannot be easily dissected free. If fibrosis prevents safe intrafascial hysterectomy, supracervical hysterectomy is indicated in particularly severe cases.

Management of the ovaries at the time of hysterectomy for endometriosis is sometimes controversial. The decision to perform bilateral oophorectomy is simple if each ovary is significantly involved with endometriosis or compromised by adhesions. Bilateral oophorectomy should be performed if major bowel or urinary tract involvement exists, if invasive or recurrent disease is present, or if atypical epithelium has been noted. And, if the patient gives a history more of adnexal pain rather than the more classic central pain, removal of the ovaries is more likely to give complete pain relief in patients with uncomplicated stage I to III disease.

On the other hand, a normal-appearing ovary with only a superficial implant or two may be preserved. If the ovaries are suitable for preservation at the time of hysterectomy and are situated in proximity to the vaginal cuff, they should be suspended to reduce the likelihood of residual ovary syndrome. One tech-

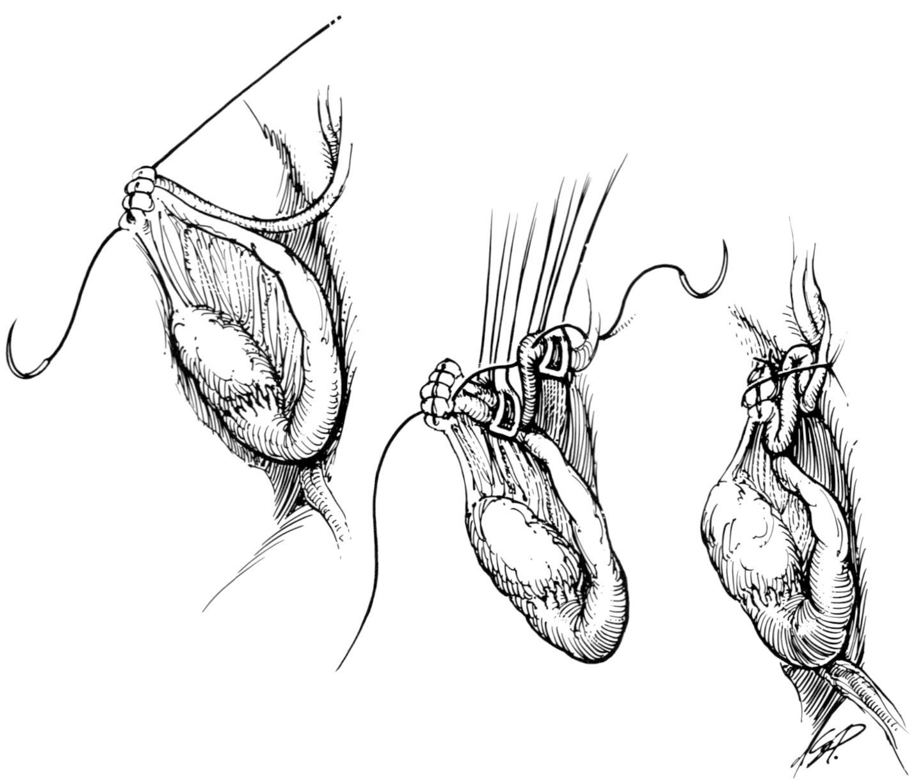

FIGURE 11.7 Management of the uninvolved adnexa at hysterectomy. The ovary is suspended from the proximal round ligament/utero-ovarian ligament stump high on the lateral abdominal wall. Care is taken not to distort the infundibulopelvic ligament with the suspension. (Copyright © Baylor College of Medicine, 1989.)

nique of ovarian suspension after hysterectomy is depicted in Figure 11.7. The interrupted round and utero-ovarian ligaments are sutured to the high lateral abdominal wall, without kinking the infundibulopelvic ligament.

Following hysterectomy, all areas are carefully checked for hemostasis; the vaginal cuff may be left open or can be closed if hemostasis is complete. The abdomen and pelvis are copiously irrigated. If the adnexa are preserved, they must not be near any raw areas because they may adhere and cause pain.

The appendix is removed if it is involved with endometriosis or if the cecum is redundant enough to allow the appendix to reach the pelvis and possibly adhere postoperatively. Cecopexy may be used to prevent descent of the cecum into the true pelvis.

HORMONE REPLACEMENT FOLLOWING HYSTERECTOMY AND OOPHORECTOMY FOR ENDOMETRIOSIS

The decision to initiate hormone replacement therapy (HRT) in patients who have undergone BSO for endometriosis may be problematic. If no macroscopic residual disease exists and the course of the disease has not been unusually complicated, the lowest effective dose of estrogen replacement therapy (ERT) that will control symptoms is prescribed beginning approximately the third postoperative day. A typical initial daily dose is 0.625 mg of conjugated estrogens or its equivalent; transdermal estrogen is an alternative. Estrogen implants are contraindicated.[45]

When the course of endometriosis has been complicated, unopposed ERT may not be appropriate. In patients whose disease is deeply invasive or incompletely resected, is a severe recurrence, or contains atypical epithelial changes, it seems prudent to withhold estrogen immediately following surgery.[46] Progestin therapy in the form of depo-medroxyprogesterone acetate 100 to 150 mg IM each month for 3 to 6 months may suppress residual disease and reduce the morbidity of hypoestrogenism until long-term HRT is introduced.[47] When estrogen replacement is initiated in these cases, concomitant progestin should be included,[45] since malignancy has been reported following long-term unopposed estrogen in patients previously operated for complicated endometriosis.[47] The usual regimen is 0.625 mg conjugated estrogen plus 2.5 mg medroxyprogesterone acetate daily or their equivalents.

Recurrence after Hysterectomy

Retrospective observational studies have estimated the incidence of symptomatic recurrence after hysterectomy with ovarian conservation to be 1% to 85%.[48-50] A recent historical prospective study compared symptom recurrence and/or reoperation after hysterectomy with or without ovarian preservation. Sixty-two percent of 29 patients with ovarian conservation had symptom recurrence, and half of them required reoperation. When compared with women who had oophorectomy with hysterectomy, these patients had a 6.1 times greater risk of developing recurrent pain and 8.1 times greater risk of reoperation.[51]

Occasionally a patient who has had hysterectomy and BSO will present with symptoms and signs suggestive of ovarian remnant syndrome (see Chapter 24). Laboratory findings of high-normal levels of follicle-stimulating hormone (FSH) or nearly normal estradiol levels suggest the presence of ovaries. However, ovarian remnants can cause pain and masses without biochemical evidence of ovarian function. These cases are managed surgically by careful dissection of the ureters and pararectal spaces, followed by removal of large areas of peritoneum containing the residual ovarian tissue.[52]

Serum Concentrations of CA-125 in Recurrent Endometriosis

CA-125 is a glycoprotein antigen that is expressed on the cell surface of some derivatives of embryonic coelomic epithelium. Since endometriotic lesions are likely to be derivatives of embryonic coelomic epithelium, extensive investigation of CA-125 as a tumor marker has been conducted in patients with this disease. Serum concentrations have been found to be elevated in over half of the patients with stage III and IV endometriosis and in some patients with lesser degrees of the disease.[53,54] Unfortunately, CA-125 levels lack sensitivity and specificity to serve as a screening test for the presence of endometriosis.[55,56] As a means of following patients after therapy, however, the test may have some utility.[57,58] Thus many patients with advanced disease and occasional patients with mild disease have elevated pretreatment CA-125 levels that decrease posttherapy. During follow-up, elevations in CA-125 might predict recurrence of disease. It is important to stress that this test is predictive of active endometriotic lesions but may be of no value for predicting adhesions.

Complications

If the endometriosis is amenable to laparoscopic surgery, care must be taken to avoid injury to the ureters and the GI tract. The largest blood vessels encountered by the careful operative laparoscopist are usually branches of the uterine artery during uterosacral ligament dissection, which can bleed severely unless grasped and coagulated or ligated. Laser laparoscopic injury to the ureters may occur; the incidence is unknown since many cases are unreported. Although the GI tract may be treated laparoscopically, the same precautions are taken as at laparotomy: prepared bowel, insertion of a finger into the rectum to assess mural depth of dissection, and endosuturing of large areas of excision.

Repeat conservative laparotomy is associated with rare complications. Ureteric injuries may be largely prevented if the ureter is identified high on the pelvic brim and the overlying peritoneum is dissected free. The ureter itself should never be stripped of its adventitial tissue, because vascular compromise may occur, promoting fistula formation. If the ureter is denuded due to direct invasion of endometriosis, a cystoscopically placed diversionary stent should be used until healing can be assured.

If endometriosis is mild enough to permit vaginal hysterectomy, no additional complications over the ordinary are likely. However, severe endometriosis treated by abdominal hysterectomy can be as difficult as cases of severe PID or ovarian carcinoma. Again, the ureters must be identified and dissected free under direct vision. The integrity of the bowel must also be protected; a preoperative bowel preparation is sorely missed should the colon be inadvertently entered.

If the blood supply to the adnexa (even if visually normal) is compromised by the surgery, oophorectomy is indicated. Otherwise the adnexa may be surgically suspended to the high lateral abdominal wall above the iliac vessels and far above the ureters and vaginal cuff.

SUMMARY

Many of the principles for treating endometriosis at initial operation hold true for treating recurrent disease. Surgical success is dependent on excision or vaporization of all gross disease; perioperative medical treatment may help with microscopic lesions or lesions incompletely removed at initial surgery. The infertile woman with endometriosis may be counseled that a second conservative procedure (at laparotomy or operative laparoscopy) has a reasonable chance of success; alternatives are in-vitro fertilization or hysterectomy. For the woman with pelvic pain, preferably having completed her family, hysterectomy offers the greatest chance of long-term freedom from the pain of her disease. At hysterectomy, the ovaries may be preserved if normal, and oophoropexy away from the cuff will lessen the chance for deep dyspareunia that otherwise might be attributed to recurrent disease.

The frequent recurrence of endometriosis, like its ability to invade contiguous structures and metastasize to distant sites, is another example of the "malignant" nature of this histologically benign disease. To the woman with endometriosis, risk of recurrence is a concern second only to likelihood of relief of pain or success of conception. More research is needed as to what factors and surgical techniques promote recurrence, as well as improved noninvasive methods of screening for recurrence. Until then, the most complete operation that is also the least damaging to remaining tissues is the method of choice, requiring case-by-case individualization by the gynecologic surgeon.

Acknowledgment

James M. Wheeler, MD, contributed significantly to the first edition of this chapter.

REFERENCES

1. Barbieri RL and Ryan KJ: Danazol: endocrine pharmacology and therapeutic applications, Am J Obstet Gynecol 141:453, 1981.
2. Buttram VC: Surgical treatment of endometriosis in the infertile female, a modified approach, Fertil Steril 32:635, 1979.
3. Barbieri RL, Evans S, and Kistner RW: Danazol in the treatment of endometriosis: analysis of 400 cases with 4 yr follow-up, Fertil Steril 37:737, 1982.
4. Metzger DA and Luciano AA: Hormonal therapy of endometriosis, Obstet Gynecol Clin North Am 16:105, 1989.
5. Waller KG and Shaw RW: GnRH analogues for the treatment of endometriosis: long-term follow-up, Fertil Steril 59:511, 1993.
6. Schenken RS and Malinak LR: Reoperation after initial treatment of endometriosis with conservative surgery, Am J Obstet Gynecol 131:416, 1978.
7. Wheeler JM and Malinak LR: Recurrent endometriosis: incidence, management and prognosis, Am J Obstet Gynecol 146:247, 1983.

8. Wheeler JM and Malinak LR: Recurrent endometriosis, Contrib Gynecol Obstet 16:13, 1987.
9. Olive D. In Schenken RB, editor: Endometriosis: contemporary concepts in clinical management, Philadelphia, 1989, JB Lippincott Co.
10. Redwine DB: Conservative laparoscopic excision of endometriosis by sharp dissection: life table analysis of reoperation and persistence of recurrent disease, Fertil Steril 56:629, 1991.
11. Redwine DB: Incidence of recurrent endometriosis remains unknown, Am J Obstet Gynecol 149:804, 1984, (letter).
12. Wheeler JM and Malinak LR: Computer graphic pelvic mapping, second-look laparoscopy, and the distinction of recurrent versus persistent endometriosis, Fertil Steril Abstracts (43rd annual meeting suppl):79 (Abstract 194), 1987.
13. Stripling MC and others: Subtle appearance of pelvic endometriosis, Fertil Steril 49:427, 1988.
14. Batt RE and Smith RA: Embryologic theory of histogenesis of endometriosis in peritoneal pockets, Obstet Gynecol Clin North Am 16:15, 1989.
15. Murphy AA and others: Unsuspected endometriosis documented by scanning electron microscopy in visually normal peritoneum, Fertil Steril 46:522, 1986.
16. Dmowski WP: Visual assessment of peritoneal implants for staging endometriosis: do number and cumulative size of lesions reflect the severity of a systemic disease? Fertil Steril 47:382, 1987.
17. Wheeler JM and Malinak LR: Postoperative danazol therapy in infertility patients with severe endometriosis, Fertil Steril 36:460, 1981.
18. Wheeler JM and Malinak LR: Danazol following conservative surgery for endometriosis at laparotomy significantly improves term pregnancy and recurrence rates in infertile women with moderate and severe endometriosis. Paper presented at the American Fertility Society Annual Meeting, Chicago, October 1985.
19. Koninckx PR and others: Suggestive evidence that pelvic endometriosis is a progressive disease, whereas deeply infiltrating endometriosis is associated with pelvic pain, Fertil Steril 55:759, 1991.
20. Rock JA and Moutos DM: Endometriosis: the present and the future—an overview of treatment options, Br J Obstet Gynaecol 99(suppl 7):1, 1992.
21. Redwine BD: Age-related evolution on color appearance of endometriosis, Fertil Steril 48:1062, 1987.
22. Bergqvist A and Ferno M. Estrogen and progesterone receptors in endometriotic tissue and endometrium: comparison according to localization and recurrence, Fertil Steril 60:63, 1993.
23. Metzger DA, Lessey BA, and Soper JT: Hormone resistant endometriosis following TAH and BSO: correlation with histology and steroid receptor content, Obstet Gynecol 78:946, 1991.
24. Rogers SF and Jacobs WM: Infertility and endometriosis: conservative surgical approach, Fertil Steril 19:529, 1968.
25. Martin DC, Hubert GD, and Levy BS: Depth of infiltration of endometriosis, J Gynecol Surg 5:55, 1989.
26. Martin DC and others: Laparoscopic appearances of peritoneal endometriosis, Fertil Steril 51:63, 1989.
27. Mais V, Ajossa S, and Marongiu D: Reduction of adhesion reformation after laparoscopic endometrosis surgery: a randomized trial with an oxidized regenerated cellulose absorbable barrier, Obstet Gynecol 86:512, 1995.
28. Wheeler JM and Malinak LR: The surgical management of endometriosis, Obstet Gynecol Clin North Am 16:147, 1989.
29. Prystowsky JB and others: Gastrointestinal endometriosis: incidence and indications for resection, Arch Surg 123:855, 1988.
30. Incidental appendectomy, ACOG Committee Opinion No 164, December 1995.
31. Sekiba K and others: Use of Interceed (TC7) absorbable adhesion barrier to reduce postoperative adhesion reformation in infertility and endometriosis surgery, Obstet Gynecol 79:518, 1992.
32. The Surgical Membrane Study Group: Prophylaxis of pelvic sidewall adhesions with Gore-Tex surgical membrane: a multicenter clinical investigation, Fertil Steril 57:921, 1991.
33. Candiani GB and others: Repetitive conservative surgery for recurrence of endometriosis, Obstet Gynecol 77:421, 1991.

34. Fayez JA and Vogel MF: Comparison of different treatment methods of endometriomas by laparoscopy, Obstet Gynecol 78:660, 1991.

35. Vercellini P and others: Laparoscopic aspiration of ovarian endometriomas, J Reprod Med 37:577, 1992.

36. Hasson HM: Laparoscopic management of ovarian cysts, J Reprod Med 35:863, 1990.

37. Bateman BG, Kolp LA, and Mills S: Endoscopic vs laparotomy management of endometriosis, Fertil Steril 62:690, 1994.

38. Adamson GD and others: Comparisons of CO_2 laser laparoscopy with laparotomy for treatment of endometrioma, Fertil Steril 57:965, 1992.

39. Daniell JF, Kuntz BR, and Gurley LD: Laser laparoscopy management of large endometriomas, Fertil Steril 55:692, 1991.

40. Mettler L and Semm K: Three step medical and surgical treatment of endometriosis, Fr J Med Sci 152:2, 1983.

41. Keckstein J: Adjuvants for clinical use: ovarian surgery. Paper presented at the Third International Congress on Pelvic Surgery and Adhesion Prevention, San Diego, March 2, 1996.

42. Dmowski WP, Radwanska E, and Rana N: Recurrent endometriosis following hysterectomy and oophorectomy: the role of residual ovarian fragments, Int J Gynaecol Obstet 26:93, 1988.

43. Redwine DB: Endometriosis persisting after castration: clinical characteristics and results of surgical management, Obstet Gynecol 83:405, 1994.

44. Knapp RC, Donahue VC, and Friedman EA: Dissection of paravesical and pararectal spaces in pelvic operations, Surg Gynecol Obstet 13:758, 1973.

45. Lam AM, French M, and Charnock FM: Bilateral ureteric obstruction due to recurrent endometriosis associated with hormone replacement therapy, Aust N Z J Obstet Gynaecol 32:83, 1992.

46. Endometiosis, ACOG Technical Bulletin No 183, September 1993.

47. Reimnitz C and others: Malignancy arising in endometriosis associated with unopposed estrogen replacement, Obstet Gynecol 71:444, 1988.

48. Ranney B: Discussion following Schenken RS and Malinak LR: Reoperation after initial treatment of endometriosis with conservative surgery, Am J Obstet Gynecol 131:416, 1978.

49. Sheets JL, Symmonds RE, and Banner EA: Conservative surgical management of endometriosis, Obstet Gynecol 23:625, 1963.

50. Hammond CB, Rock JA, and Parker RT: Conservative treatment of endometriosis: the effects of limited surgery and hormonal pseudopregnancy, Fertil Steril 27:756, 1996.

51. Nammoum AB and others: Incidence of symptom recurrence after hysterectomy for endometriosis, Fertil Steril 64:898, 1995.

52. Pettit PD and Lee RA: Ovarian remnant syndrome: diagnostic dilemma and surgical challenge, Obstet Gynecol 71:580, 1988.

53. Pittaway De and Fayez JA. The use of CA-125 in the diagnosis and management of endometriosis, Fertil Steril 46:790, 1986.

54. Patton PE and others: CA-125 levels in endometriosis, Fertil Steril 45:770, 1986.

55. Barbieri RL and others: Elevated serum concentrations of CA-125 in patients with advanced endometriosis, Fertil Steril 45:360, 1986.

56. Takahashi K and others: Serum CA-125 and 17-β estradiol in patients with external endometriosis, Gynecol Obstet Invest 29:101, 1990.

57. Fedele L and others: Serum CA-125 measurements in the diagnosis of endometriosis recurrence, Obstet Gynecol 72:19, 1988.

58. Nagamani M, Kelver ME, and Smith ER: CA-125 levels in monitoring therapy for endometriosis and in prediction of recurrence, Int J Fertil 37:227, 1992.

12

Myomectomy

SAMANTHA M. PFEIFER
CELSO-RAMÓN GARCÍA

Uterine myomas are among the most common tumors encountered in women. These smooth muscle uterine tumors also contain fibrous elements derived from the surrounding interstitial and vascular tissue. Uterine myomas vary considerably in size from small seedlings of millimeters in size to enormous tumors that have been reported reaching more than 100 pounds.[1] They can be present in various locations within the uterus and pelvis. The most common locations are subserosal, intramural, and submucosal. These myomas can have a broad base or a narrow stalk, as in the pedunculated myoma. Myomas also arise within the cervix (cervical) or become parasitic, deriving their blood supply and ultimately residing apart from the uterus, often a part of the omentum.

Uterine myomas can be particularly confusing since they often produce varied symptoms, depending on the number, size, location, and any associated pathologic condition that may accompany their presence. Among the wide array of symptoms are abnormal menstrual bleeding, abdominal and pelvic pain, abdominal enlargement, and GI tumor, leading to constipation and bloating. Moreover, these distortions can also produce dysfunction of the urinary bladder or, rarely, even obstruction of the ureter. Degenerating myomas can cause pain and on rare occasions can lead to abscess formation within the myoma. Myomas are also associated with infertility.[2-6] Although pregnancy can and does occur in their presence, the incidence is low. Some 41% of these pregnancies spontaneously abort, and about 13% are complicated by premature labor.[2] Moreover, the specific basis by which myomas interfere with achieving pregnancy often is not clearly understood. Some point to the effects on the endometrium, which may lead to hypermenorrhea. Compression of vascular flow to the adnexa could produce vascular changes leading to alterations affecting ovarian function. This could include anovulation and alterations of gamete transport. The pedunculated submucous myomas can produce an intrauterine device–like effect and prevent pregnancy. In addition, distortions of the cavity by intramural and submucosal myomas can affect the pregnancy, leading to pregnancy loss. The association of myomas and endometriosis has also been noted.

Generally myomas are simple insignificant pathologic tumors of the female reproductive system that have exceedingly low malignant potential (0.3%).[7] When the myomas are asymptomatic, and particularly if they are 3-months' gestational size or less, most physicians concur that nothing needs to be done. If, however, the woman is symptomatic, especially if the uterine mass is larger than a 3-month gestation, intervention would be strongly considered. The surgical approach depends on the number, the location, and the size of the myomas as well as the age and desires of the patient. In general, myomectomy is indicated in women who desire childbearing or who are determined to retain their reproductive organs. The procedure may be viewed as less appropriate for women who have reached an age of decreasing fertility.

Rapidly enlarging myomas often raise the concern of malignancy. Myomectomy or hysterectomy is often advised. Nonetheless, the incidence of malignancy is not higher in this group of women.[8] In all groups outlined the risk of myomectomy versus hysterectomy in the specific circumstances needs to be weighed and discussed with the patient and the details of the discussion documented.

MANAGEMENT CONSIDERATIONS

The American College of Obstetricians and Gynecologists (ACOG) has detailed the criteria for myomectomy and hysterectomy in women with a fibroid uterus.[9] In considering myomectomy in the infertile woman, there must be a probable indication of failure to conceive or, alternatively, recurrent pregnancy loss. Confirmation of the inability to reproduce successfully should be accompanied by the presence of a myoma of size or location that is the probable cause of reproductive failure in the absence of any other plausible explanation. The appropriate evaluation of other causes of infertility or pregnancy loss, including the endometrial cavity and fallopian tubes, must be detailed. In addition, it must be documented that there has been a discussion of the complexity of the disease process that could lead to hysterectomy during the myomectomy. Myomectomy is indicated in the noninfertile woman with myomas who is desirous of retaining her uterus when she has a palpable disturbing myoma that is otherwise asymptomatic. Myomectomy also is indicated for excessive uterine bleeding despite ovulatory cycles. Such profuse bleeding can be repetitive, last for more than 8 days, and anemia secondary to the blood loss may be present. In such cases the advantages and disadvantages of myomectomy versus hysterectomy must be discussed in detail and documented.

Myomectomy for infertility or a symptomatic myomatous distortion are the most compelling reasons to perform multiple myomectomy when the woman wants to preserve her reproductive function. However, the possible recurrence of myomas raises concerns regarding the appropriateness of myomectomy since under these circumstances the new tumor growth may lead to the possible need for reoperation. Even before the use of GnRH, 10% to 35% of postmyomectomy patients have required subsequent surgery because of myoma recurrence. Candiani and others[10] reported a cumulative 10-year recurrence rate of 27.9% in 622 patients. Malone and Ingersoll,[11] reporting on 75 cases, indicated a 29% recurrence. Babaknia, Rock, and Jones,[12] reporting on 46 cases, indicated a 28% recurrence, Buttram and Reiter,[2] reporting on 42 cases, indicated a 14% recurrence, and García,[13] reporting on 150 cases, indicated a 12% recurrence. Long ago Kelly warned readers about the performance of myomectomies: "When the growths are multiple and some of them small, the patient is likely to turn up again in a few years with another crop. It is wiser, therefore, generally speaking, to avoid multiple myomectomies!" However, Kelly did reflect: "The supreme result of a myomectomy lies in the pregnancy which may follow."[14]

In a randomized comparative study, Fedele and others confirmed that the use of GnRH preoperatively resulted in a higher frequency of myoma recurrence compared with patients who had not received pretreatment with the GnRH analogs before myomectomy.[14a,15] Others have not detected a difference.[16] Intuitively it is held that the more complete the excision of *all* myomas that are present, the lower the risk of recurrence. The use of GnRH agonist analogs as pretreatment for surgery makes the smaller myoma even smaller and more likely to be undetected, and as such unresected.

The feminist community argues for the preservation of reproductive organs and prefers myomectomy rather than hysterectomy at any age. They believe not only that hysterectomy is a reproductive loss but also that it seriously affects sexual feelings because of the loss of deep orgasm and that it can bring about premature estrogen deficiency secondary to ovarian failure. Much disagreement, however, still exists regarding the advisability of performing a myomectomy, especially in older women for whom reproductive needs may be unrealistic. Nevertheless, hysterectomy may severely affect some women who perceive it as a loss of their femininity, affecting their libido and sexual feelings. When discussing hysterectomy, women frequently challenge surgeons by asking whether they would be willing to have their reproductive organs removed. Aside from the psychosexual social considerations and the concern of not being able to preserve reproductive function, many women still fear blood loss and the recurrence of myomas. Myomectomy is categorized as having an increased risk of complications and the possible need for a future reoperation. The presence of coexisting pathologic conditions may make the surgery more prolonged and tedious. With the perception of so many confounding factors, many surgeons are less inclined to perform a myomectomy and advise hysterectomy instead. Most serious, albeit rare, is the difficulty associated with making the diagnosis of a leiomyosarcoma. The malignant transformation of myomas is of less concern since this occurs in less than one tenth of 1% of cases. Solitary or rapidly enlarging myomas, however, are more suspect. Nonetheless, this remote possibility must always be discussed with the patient. When encountered, these tumors also require more aggressive surgical attention and treatment.

Preoperative Evaluation

Preoperative considerations include the evaluation of the whole patient. For the woman desiring a myomectomy for the preservation of the uterus, it is essential that her cervical cytologic findings be followed to assure the absence of cervical malignancy. In the presence of abnormal uterine bleeding, evaluation should include screening for anovulation as well as an evaluation of the uterine cavity by either endometrial biopsy, dilatation and curettage (D & C), or hysteroscopy.

The selection of the more appropriate surgical management of uterine myoma has been significantly improved with the advent of diagnostic laparoscopy and hysteroscopy and the imaging technologies of ultrasonography and magnetic resonance imaging (MRI). Laparoscopy may prove difficult or may even be contraindicated when the enlarged uterine myomatous mass reaches the region of the umbilicus. Hysterosalpingography can compliment the other imaging techniques in the assessment of intracavitary myoma. Ultrasonography and MRI are of inestimable value as noninvasive techniques. With good resolution, MRI images not only may offer the advantage of distinguishing between myoma and adenomyosis but also may alert the surgeon to a leiomyosarcomatous appearance.[17] An excretory urogram is also advisable relative to the renal status and location of the ureters. Thus the extent of the myomas and their relationship to the total clinical features can be detailed, and a truly informed consent can be obtained from the patient.

Anemia

Women with myomas who are severely anemic secondary to hypermenorrhea need aggressive management of their anemia prior to proceeding with myomectomy. Many recommend having the patient donate 2 units of her blood before surgery for autologous use. This approach may be sound for mildly anemic women. Truly severely anemic patients need all the blood they have since their menses are usually profuse. Fortunately most patients respond well to aggressive hematinic therapy. Although autologous blood may have been made available, transfusing patients may not be as innocuous as some believe and can lead to cardiac overload and other risks incumbent with transfusions in general.[18] These risks have been appreciated and addressed by plaintiffs and their attorneys. At the other extreme, the preoperatively collected autologous blood that is available at surgery still might not be adequate, in the rare circumstance when there is *severe* blood loss. Blood from a directed donor also could be collected prior to the procedure. Of course, this could carry similar risks to the patient as blood from the blood bank pool. With greater awareness and careful screening this risk has become small: the estimated risk of transmitting the HIV virus is about 1:450,000 to 1:660,000, but the probability estimate is now believed to have been lowered to 1 in 26 million due to the improvement in screening and the better sensitivity of the enzyme-linked immunosorbent assays.[19,20] Upward of 7 or 8 units may be needed when there is significant bleeding. The careful surgeon who is constantly aware of the need to use every technique to attain meticulous hemostasis and who is continually alert for bleeding can avoid excessive blood loss. With such care and by using speed, without compromising the woman's tissues, the need for transfusion can be virtually eliminated. Indeed, at the Hospital of the University of Pennsylvania on the service of C-R García from 1970 to 1990, in over 200 multiple myomectomies, there was no need to transfuse a patient because of blood loss.

To improve the anemia of the woman having significant uterine bleeding related to the myomatous uterus, the preoperative alternative may be the use of a short-term continuous estrogen and progestagen therapy to induce amenorrhea. Alternatively, GnRH therapy might be used to down-regulate the pituitary and create a pseudomenopause. It is well to remember that myomas arise from myometrial cells. Since these muscle cells are responsive to the ovarian estrogens, the effect of GnRH down-regulation of the gonadotropins is to reduce the size of the myoma unless the interstitial cells predominate. In some myomas the fibrous interstitial elements can exceed the myometrial ones. Since the interstitial elements do not respond to GnRH as well as the myometrial ones, the reduction in size of many myomas with GnRH agonists is not always as dramatic as expected. The effects are far greater on the myometrium than on the fibroleiomyomas.[21] Nonetheless, the exact mechanism of the growth of myomas is not known. It appears to be related not solely to estrogens but also to other factors such as platelet-derived growth factor, insulin-like growth factor, and epidermal growth factor.[22,23] Indeed, serial ultrasonographic monitoring of myomas during pregnancy does not support the level of myomatous growth that estrogens are generally believed to cause.[24] Nonetheless, if a myoma does not show a reduction in size after 2 to 3 months of treatment with GnRH agonists, the surgeon should think of the possibility of a leiomyosarcoma.

Although the Food and Drug Administration (FDA) has approved the use of these agents for myoma and such an approach may be very useful to stop the hypermenorrhea, we must emphasize the need to manage the anemia aggressively with iron replacement during the menopause-like amenorrhea. Moreover, in women with submucous myomas, hemorrhage and infection as life-threatening complications have been reported with the use of the GnRH agonists.[16,25,26]

Studies advocating GnRH agonists to simplify the myomectomy as well as reduce blood loss are very relative. The reported savings of blood are at the level of 200 ml or less. In one recent study[27] the comparative experience with myomectomy reflected that the blood loss was 235 ml with GnRH versus 350 ml without, a statistically significant saving of 115 ml. While statistically significant, clinically 115 ml is not very impressive in most surgical situations. In addition, there is cause for concern when taking into consideration the effects on other target organs and the complaints that are offered by these women. Moreover, the transfusion rates between the GnRH-treated and untreated myomectomy cases were the same.[25] In another randomized prospective study[28] evaluating the efficacy of a preoperative GnRH analog in women undergoing myomectomy, no difference in blood loss or postoperative morbidity was demonstrated. In reviewing the literature Davis and Schlatt[29] concluded that at this time, aside from the enormous costs of these agents, no evidence supports routine use of GnRH analogs prior to myomectomy when the uterus is less than 600 cc in volume. Using the tourniquet-Pitressin technique, the blood loss averages less than 150 ml. This represents the total blood loss, not the blood loss saved. Despite such concerns regarding blood loss in myomectomy, appropriate techniques and speed of surgery, with compression when needed, meaningfully address the problem. In no way should myomectomy blood loss be compared with what may happen when a vascular pedicle gets loose at the time of hysterectomy.

General Operative Considerations

Asymptomatic myomas allow for more of an attitude of watchful expectancy. However, the more symptomatic, the more pressing the need for intervention. Endotracheal controlled general inhalation anesthesia supplemented by relaxing agents and analgesics allows for excellent relaxation, which affords better exposure. A Foley catheter, placed in the bladder, assures an empty viscus and monitors urinary output. Control of blood loss should start with the initial skin incision. A transverse lower abdominal modified Pfannenstiel's incision in which the dissection is carried out with the Shaw hemostatic scalpel (Oximetric) assures careful hemostasis and good exposure even with a myoma extending to the umbilicus. When in doubt, the larger myomas may be better addressed by a midline incision.

When reoperating on a patient who has recurrent myomas, the abdominal incision probably should follow that of the prior surgery. If a repeat transverse lower abdominal modified Pfannenstiel's incision is to be carried out, the Shaw scalpel with its thermal-hemostatic capability is exceedingly valuable in dissecting the tissues. Careful, meticulous hemostasis can be supplemented with bipolar forceps for the larger vessels. Such careful hemostasis must be assured with each step. The midline incision is less time consuming, but it leaves the patient with a visible scar that constantly reminds her of the operation.

Good exposure, good assistance, and careful isolation of the tumor or tumors are essential to minimize blood loss. It is also important to be experienced in the effective modes of achieving hemostasis. Uterine hemostasis can be assured with myometrial injection of vasoconstrictors such as dilute oxytocin (Pitocin) or perhaps more preferably vasopressin (Pitressin).[30] The tourniquet should be applied at the level of the cervico-uterine junction (Figure 12.1). It should compress the infundibulopelvic and uterine vessels. No serious untoward effects of curtailing uterine and ovarian blood supply for up to 3 to 4 hours have been noted. Nonetheless, it is preferable to aim for completing the myomectomy and removing the tourniquet in some 2 hours. This gives optimal time for most dissections and repair. Although the crop of ovarian follicles in the current cycle is lost, the subsequent cycle generates a new crop from the primordial germ cells, which tolerate the ischemia well.

During the removal of multiple myoma, the tourniquet application may become loose. The surgeon should be continually aware of the possible need for application of a second tourniquet to assure continued compression of the vessels and thorough hemostasis. Continual hemostasis can be maintained through appropriate compression, appropriate suture, and repeat injection of dilute vasopressin as needed. In most institutions the anesthesiologists address these potential vascular blood loss concerns preoperatively through volume expanders and the like.[31] This is another important measure aimed at reducing the need for transfusion and its incumbent risks.[18]

Care should be exercised to avoid the intravascular injection of Pitressin. Pitressin injected into the myometrium several minutes before applying the tourniquet causes a vasoconstriction of the uterine corpus, reducing the blood volume within the organ. Although some report a histamine reaction with the

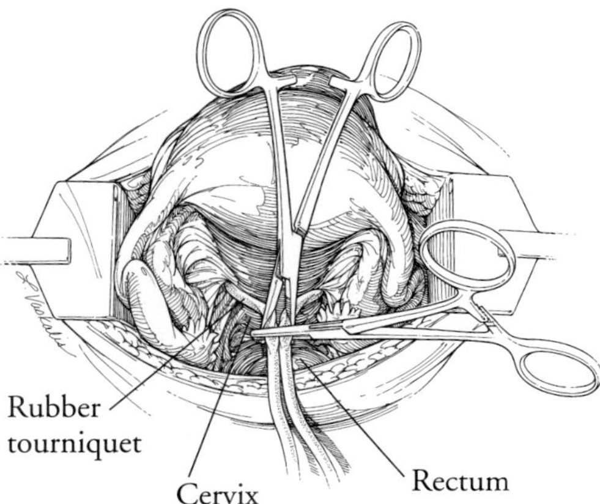

Figure 12.1 The rubber tourniquet is being applied to encompass the entire uterine mass. Note that the tourniquet application encompasses the adnexa and thus limits the flow of the uterine as well as the infundibulopelvic vessels. The rubber tourniquet is tightened in a stepwise application of Kelly' clamps. Although the initial clamp crosses both segments of rubber tubing, it is strongly recommended that the subsequent clamps grasp the tubing so that the two arms of the tubing are opposed when the clamp is crossed as is depicted in the more proximal application. This ensures that the rubber tubing does not slip through the clamp. It is not necessary to open a passage in the broad ligament to exclude the infundibulopelvic vessels. Avoiding this dissection reduces the potential of postoperative periadnexal adhesions to these dissected areas.

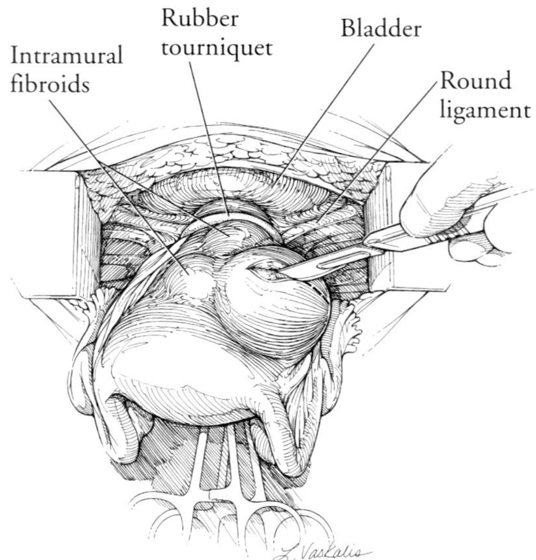

FIGURE 12.2 The site of the anterior uterine wall incision is selected as the thinnest area over the myoma. Dissection after the removal of the first myoma allows access to the other myomas. A transverse incision of the uterine wall over the myoma parallels the lateral uterine vascular distribution. This limits the potential of bleeding better than a vertical incision made in this lateral location, which would cut across the vascular distribution. By contrast, in the midline the relative avascularity would allow a vertical incision.

Pitressin,[32] this has not been the experience at the Hospital of the University of Pennsylvania, if not all centers in this country.

Abdominal Myomectomy Technique

Dissection of myomas should be carried out by incising the uterine wall starting at the thinnest locus over the myomas and by aiming to least disrupt the myometrial blood supply (Figures 12.2 to 12.4). The arterial blood supply at the locus of the myoma should dictate the direction of the incision: vertical at the midline of the uterus or transverse when lateral on the body of the uterus. After enucleation of the myoma through dissection in the pseudocapsule, permanent hemostasis can be assured by using a concentric spiraling stitch that obliterates the defect or defects while assuring anatomic restitution. This applies not only to an initial myomectomy but also to repeat surgery.

Meticulous technique with dedicated attention to containing blood loss is absolutely essential if the surgeon is to perform multiple myomectomy without significant blood loss. Appropriate selection of the site for the incisions and dissections of the pseudocapsules is needed while constantly assuring hemostasis. Uterine incisions should be placed parallel to the arterial supply and not across it. After each myoma is dissected, it is essential that its vascular pedicle be ligated while also progressing rapidly with the reconstructions. Although speed in enucleation, vascular pedicle ligation, and reconstruction of the uterine defects is essential, common sense in understanding the distorted vascular anatomy in the control of bleeding is paramount. Although myomectomy is based on simple surgical principles, the variations in location and size of the tumors require the ingenuity more often gained by experience.

Once the myoma is extirpated and its vascular pedicle ligated, the dissection should be turned to the adjacent myoma, extirpating it in a similar fashion. As many myomas as feasible should be excised through the same incision. Experience supports the view that it is not advisable to dissect through the endometrial cavity to excise myomas from the opposite wall. The opposing sites will become "kissing" operative sites that can fuse in repair, and adhesions within the endometrial cavity can occur, leading to Asherman's syndrome. Re-

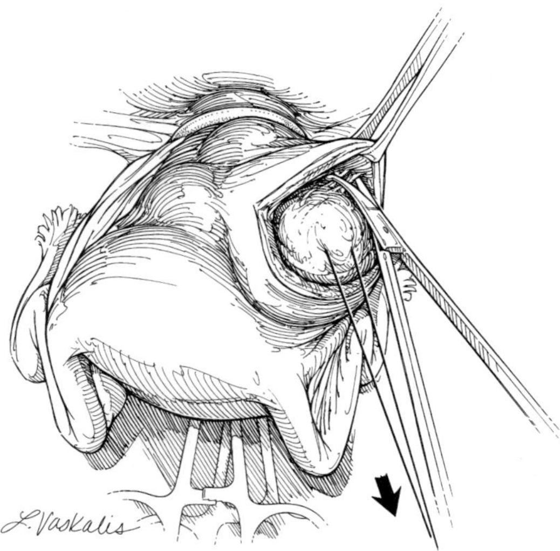

Figure 12.3 Using a traction stitch or a towel clamp can elevate the tumor to facilitate the dissection through the layers of pseudocapsule. This dissection can be carried out with blunt and sharp dissection. A Kelly's clamp, a periosteum elevator, and Strulli's scissors can be used for this dissection, but traction elevating the myoma is essential.

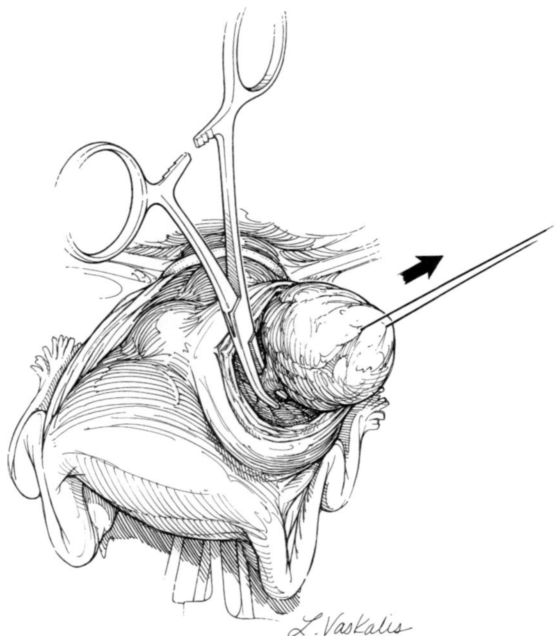

Figure 12.4 As the base of the myoma is reached, the vascular pedicle is clamped, the myoma extirpated, and the vascular pedicle is suture ligated. After the extirpation of the myoma shown in the figure, the remaining adjacent myomas can be reached by tunnelling dissection from the initial defect to avoid additional uteral incisions. The dead space from these distant myomectomies must be obliterated prior to closing the initial defect, as depicted in Figure 12.5.

pair of all defects created should reapproximate the tissues, preferably with a continuous spiraling stitch of no. 3-0 polyglactin suture material (Figure 12.5). Catgut should be avoided because of its reactivity and lower tensile strength. Posterior uterine wall incisional approaches raise concern because of the potential for postoperative peritoneal intestinal adhesions. Meticulous hemostasis and a subserosal approximation of the more superfi-

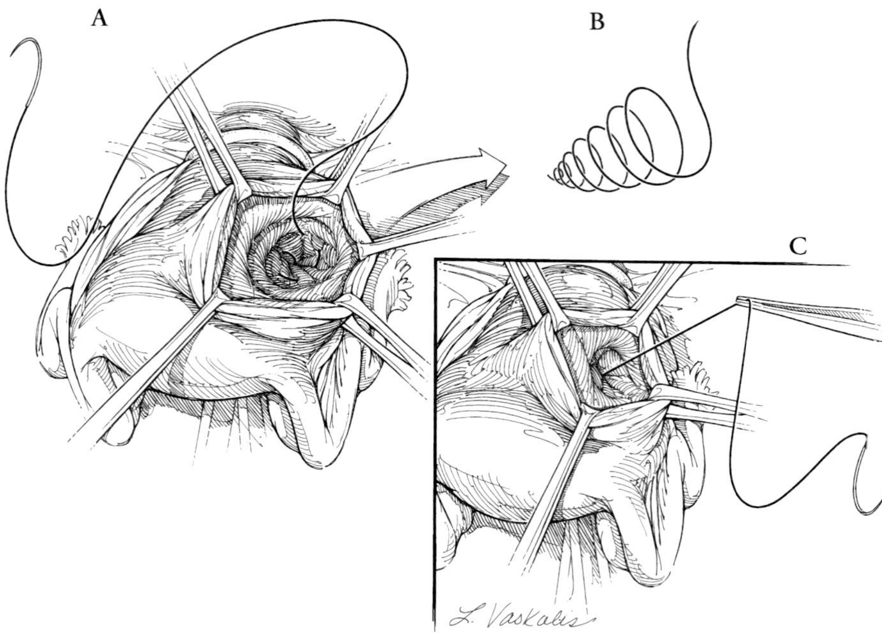

Figure 12.5 A, Application of a spiraling stitch, shown schematically, closes the defect after the myoma has been removed. Initial placement of several deep spiraling stitches in layers. B, Schematic of spiraling stitch. C, The spiraling stitch in lower layer has been cinched with firm pressure with diamond-tip forceps. The spiraling stitch is then continued to successively obliterate the remaining defect. This spiraling stitch not only repairs the defect but also is hemostatic.

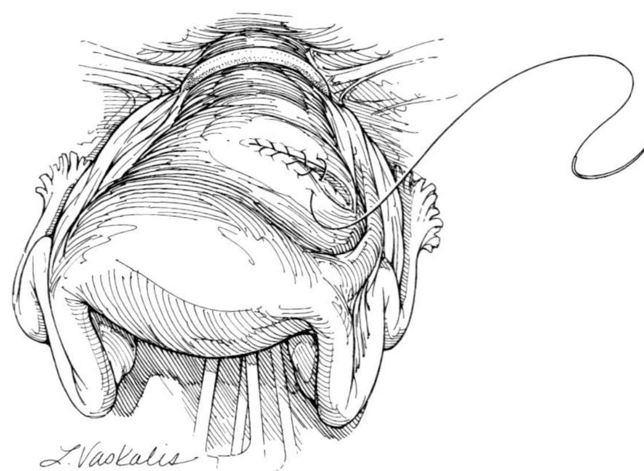

Figure 12.6 The superficial closure of the myomectomy defect can be accomplished with a subserosal, a Lembert, or, as illustrated, a baseball stitch, using a no. 4-0 polyglactin suture. The baseball stitch allows for a smooth approximation of the wound edges and also is hemostatic. Antiadhesion coverings have not been necessary.

cial area of the uterine wall with no. 6-0 polyglycolic acid–type suture (Vicryl or Dexon) (Figure 12.6) is recommended. Such a smooth approximation of the wound edges has reduced the occurrence of adhesions as is the case in cesarean sections. With meticulous repair the site of the prior surgery is often difficult to find later. Pedunculated submucous or intracavitary myomas are very difficult to assess at the time of abdominal surgery. These tumors should have been assessed during preoperative hysterosalpingography or hysteroscopy even before the surgery was scheduled. Such prior review allows the surgeon to discuss the options with the patient. Hysteroscopic resection of small submucous intrauterine myomas is often the preferable approach.

GnRH Agonist Analogs

Treatment of myomas with GnRH analogs has been hailed as a promising alternative to surgery. This medical approach has many disadvantages, and pregnancy rates are very low after cessation of therapy. In the older woman who does not want surgery, the use of the GnRH analogs with add-back therapy may have some advantage. Indeed the GnRH analogs may be of specific advantage, if not essential, when used preoperatively in preparation for hysteroscopic resection of myomas. The ability to resect the myomas is believed to be improved.

The cited regression in the size of myomas treated with GnRH agonists has been quite variable, from a slight increase in size to as much as 85% reduction in volume.[16,21,33,34,35] However, this reduction is maintained for only a limited duration after the use of GnRH analogs ceases.

Data support that the lumbar bone mineral content evaluated by dual photon absorptiometry is significantly affected by GnRH.[28] Although the mean values of bone mineral content in patients studied are believed to revert to almost normal levels after cessation of the GnRH suppression, it must be emphasized that these data are reported as mean values for the group. Mathematically this implies that the individual values included some that *did not* return to normal levels. It is of concern that use of these GnRH analogs may sustain and aggravate this undesirable adverse effect. Thus repeated courses of GnRH for reduction of uterine volume are not an acceptable approach. It has been advocated that the addition of estrogen and progestagen as add-back therapy to the GnRH can prevent the bone mineral content loss.[16] However, at the clinical seminar and workshop on the use of bisphosphonates presented during the 1995 annual meeting of the American Society of Reproductive Medicine, Drs. Charles H. Chestnut and Uwe Ulrich reported that even at 3 months of GnRH therapy, despite concomitant add-back therapy, biopsies of cancellous bone disclosed microfractures on scanning electron microscopy. Such degenerative changes are *not reversible.* The use of Alendronate additive therapy, which appears to be protective, along with calcium was suggested. Such adverse osseous effects produced by the preoperative use of GnRH to reduce the size of myomas to facilitate myomectomy need more careful randomized appraisal with oversight since the use of GnRH agonists has become so widespread. While the use of the GnRH agonists in women with large myomas appears to be more likely to be condoned, it has been stated that, after the review of the literature, there is no evidence to support the use of GnRH analog therapy prior to myomectomy in women whose uteri are smaller than 600 cm^3.

It should be recalled that the formula for volume of a sphere or a spheroid is proportional to the cube of the radius. Therefore changes in volume represent small changes in diameter. Clinical discussions regarding myoma size traditionally are described in terms of the diameter, measured in centimeters. The volume changes in myomas seen with the GnRH agonists represent smaller changes in diameter. For a 10-cm myoma a 50% reduction in volume represents only a 1.7 cm reduction in diameter. By contrast, the same percentage reduction in volume in a smaller myoma represents a far greater proportionate reduction in diameter in the seedling myomas. Thus this potentially reduces the very small myoma to an unrecognizable size at the time of surgery. After cessation of the suppressive therapy these seedlings will grow and increase the need for future reoperation.

While some advocate not removing the myomas that are close to the uterotubal junction, this is not a wise approach. These myomas could enlarge later and require attention. Abdominal laparotomy with microsurgical techniques may be required for the dissections of myomas in these areas. Pedunculated prolapsed submucous myomas should be treated vaginally. The smaller ones may lend themselves to resection with a snare or by hysteroscopy.

Alternative Surgical Approaches

Hysteroscopy

Resection of uterine myoma through the use of the hysteroscope for the submucous or the intrauterine pedunculated myoma is a satisfactory approach in the hands of the very experienced surgeon with monitored experience in these techniques.[36] Hemostasis is sought with Pitressin injected into the cervix or by pretreatment with the GnRH agonists. Although hysteroscopic resection, including the application of the resectoscope, laser, and other techniques, has been used with video monitoring for the removal of smaller submucous myomas, the hysteroscopic resection of larger myomas is probably preferably left for the more hysteroscopically skilled hands. The resections should probably be limited to myomas of less than 3 to 5 cm with at least 50% of the myoma projecting into the uterine cavity. Preferably the uterine cavity itself should be no greater than 10 cm in length (Figure 12.7). Moreover, the myomas should not impinge on the tubal ostia and if multiple, should not be at the same level as one on the opposing wall which tends to produce "kissing" adhesions. Simple perforations are often managed by expectant observation. Most often bleeding and sepsis are not a problem. Nonetheless, perforations with an active resectoscope can injure neighboring bowel, which if not recognized promptly, can develop into a significant concern. Bowel burns and its sequellae can become a very serious major problem. Meaningful observation is needed, and especially the patient must be very carefully counselled before discharge. Additionally, perforations that may not pose

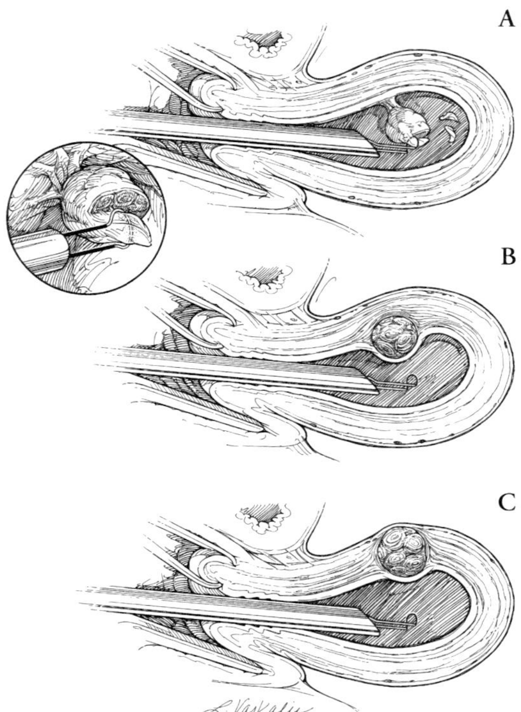

Figure 12.7 **A**, Hysteroscopic resection of a small intracavitary pedunculated myoma. *Inset* reveals close-up of resection technique. **B**, Hysteroscopic resection of an intracavitary uterine myoma that projects into the uterine cavity. **C**, Hysteroscopic resection of a myoma that involves the entire uterine muscularis and projects into the cavity. This is potentially a treacherous myoma to deal with hysteroscopically. Bleeding and perforation are a certainty if the entire myoma is removed. Some would advocate resecting perhaps one half and assessing the status several cycles later. If the remaining myoma mass projects into the cavity, a second phase resection could be contemplated. Alternatively, a transabdominal myomectomy could be done with an appropriate uterine wall repair.

an immediate problem may subsequently come to haunt since uterine rupture in those achieving pregnancy has occurred.[37]

The use of distention irrigating media also can be of concern, despite their utter utility. Dextran has been associated with acute hypervolemia, pulmonary edema, and severe coagulopathy.[38] It is now supplanted by glycine solution, but glycine also is not without the need for careful monitoring. Postoperative hyponatremia can occur with 1.5% glycine used to distend and irrigate the cavity.[39]

Laparoscopy

Laparoscopic resection is often used for pedunculated subserosal myomas with small pedicles. Larger myomas are laparoscopically resected by those with significant experience with the video laser laparoscopic operative techniques.[40] Resections of larger myomas can be very vexing because of bleeding, which not only is very common, even with GnRH pretreatment, but also at times can be very difficult to control. It is essential to have proper knowledge and ingenuity with the use of appropriate instrumentation and the Ultrapulse CO_2 laser as well as the high-voltage electrocoagulator for dissection and the low voltage for hemostasis. A pressure hydrodissector and suction are also essential. Vasopressin is not recommended during laparoscopic myomectomy since more often troublesome bleeding occurs from the uterine injection sites. Moreover, a high level of proficiency in the use of the varied instrumentation also requires an unusually high proficiency of motor-visual coordination ability and highly dedicated and skilled assistance. To achieve the best outcomes with the least complications requires a mastery of the technology along with a prior complete mastery of the fundamental surgical skills in the use of these varied approaches.

Laparoscopic myomectomy techniques appear crude when compared with the microsurgical laparotomy approaches. Broad myometrial defects following laparoscopic myomectomy can and often do lead to adhesions, whereas the laparotomy with microsurgical techniques allows for a more meticulous repair of the operative defects with far less likelihood of the occurrence of adhesions. Laparoscopic surgery offers tissue handling with large sutures and less-than-careful tissue repair. It is reminiscent of the surgical management and tissue repair with myomectomy that was extant in the 1930s and 1940s, when intestinal obstruction and its severe life-threatening complications beclouded the benefits of myomectomies carried out by the more tissue-respecting surgeons of that era such as Victor Bonney and Isidor Rubin. Indeed adhesions to the operative sites are seen with such frequency that the need for Gore-Tex and other adhesion preventive measures is advocated. With the microsurgical approaches, we have not seen the need for the adhesion preventive agents.[13]

Morcellation is often needed to remove the myoma through the operative laparoscopy portals unless a culdotomy incision is made through the pouch of Douglas or an enlargement of one of the abdominal portals. These portals need careful attention and closure since subsequent herniations have been noted.[41]

Laparoscopic myolysis[42] has been advocated with the laparoscopic application of the neodymium:yttrium-aluminum-garnet (Nd:YAG) laser or the bipolar needle for coagulation of the blood supply of the myoma. The intent is to cause atrophy and necrosis of the myoma by destroying its immediate blood supply. The most experienced advocate describes treating myomas up to 10 cm in diameter after GnRH pretreatment. The experience is based on 300 cases, but the complications are not fully detailed. The morbidity is said to be low. It is well known that necrosing myomas can and do produce pain, fever, and other symptoms and findings. Pyomyoma can also be expected, although it is rare.

Transcatheter embolization has been used to treat obstetric and gynecologic bleeding,[43] and fertility has been preserved after embolizing the uterine arteries before the termination of a 15-week cervical pregnancy; thus it is not surprising that arterial embolization has been applied to the treatment of uterine fibroids. Indeed recently a radiographically monitored catheterization of the uterine arterial branches has been utilized to embolize the nutritional source of the myomas, which resulted in the regression of the myomas.[44] Transient severe pelvic pain was a consequence. The experience is limited to 16 women so treated.

Supracervical Abdominal Hysterectomy

In a woman with recurrent symptomatic myomas the probability of successfully achieving pregnancy is less favorable than the 40% to 50% pregnancy rate seen with primary multiple myomectomy. The thought of a repeat myomectomy thus is less appealing. Although complications of myomectomy are infrequent, the overall risk is probably greater than that of supracervical hysterectomy with ovarian preservation when justified. The risks of myomectomy, including bleeding, infection, phlebitis, as well as the recurrence of myoma, are greater than those of supracervical hysterectomy; thus, the need and desire for preservation of the uterus has to be great enough to overcome the obvious disadvantages. Using a nondirective approach, one can usually guide the 40- to 45-year-old woman away from myomectomy.

In the woman who adheres to having frequent Pap smears and whose previous smears have not reflected changes suggesting risk for cervical carcinoma, preservation of the cervix and a supracervical hysterectomy could be an option. Of course, continued Pap smear surveillance would be needed. Supracervical hysterectomy offers less operative time and less risk than either multiple myomectomy or total hysterectomy. It also avoids shortening and scarring of the vaginal apex, which can occur with hysterectomy. Preservation of the cervix seems to be an acceptable alternative to total hysterectomy to those who believe that Kilkku's studies[45,46] of total versus supracervical abdominal hysterectomy show that the latter retains a higher incidence of patient acceptance than total hysterectomy from the standpoint of sexuality.

Postoperative Aspects

Following postoperative recovery from multiple myomectomy, women who had hypermenorrhea before the surgery report dramatically improved bleeding patterns and diminution of dysmenorrhea reported before surgery. Moreover, of those women with associated infertility, successful term pregnancies have been reported in more than 40% and as high as 87.5% of those individuals exposed to the possibility of pregnancy during the first 18 months after surgery.[13] Entering the uterine cavity during myomectomy supports a recommendation for subsequent cesarean section when pregnancy occurs. Generally speaking, there is less need for delay of attempted conception since the risk of potential immediate pregnancy is lower following myomectomy than following other infertility procedures. By the time that the earliest pregnancy occurs, which is not any sooner than 2 to 3 months after surgery and more often 6 months to 1 year, these patients experience no difficulty in safely carrying the pregnancy to term.

Reflections on the Alternative Approaches

The more recent popularity of the minimally invasive approaches has shown that, in selected situations, depending on the training and experience of the surgeon, endoscopic approaches both by video laser laparoscopy and by hysteroscopic resection of myomas may be feasible. Although enthusiastic advocates tout these approaches, they do admit that there is an increased complication rate, which is excused as related to the "learning curve." The analysis of the nitty-gritty of the case selection and of the extent of the complications is still forthcoming. Indeed, one of the leading advocates of laparoscopic surgery states: "It must be emphasized that the conversion to laparotomy when the surgeon becomes uncomfortable with the laparoscopic approach should never be considered a complication; rather it is a prudent decision that decreases patient risk profoundly."[32] Such expression may not be supported by the fact that the volume of gynecologic abdominal surgery cases is vastly decreasing. In some institutions the surgical experience and thus surgical dexterity and ability in abdominal cavity surgery is somewhat less than what it has been. Training has been emphasizing endoscopic approaches. Thus while the advice is given to turn to the abdominal approach when uncomfortable or unable to proceed with the laparoscopic one, such a recourse may offer a dilemma to some because of relative inexperience in both modalities. The general surgeons address this same concern in a review entitled "Is the

Laparoscopic Bubble Bursting?"[47] They also assert that there is a continuing need for controlled randomized trials to assess the relative merits and risks.

Myomectomy and Pregnancy

The incidence of myomas during pregnancy has been cited by Phelan to range from 0.09% to 3.9%.[48] Until recently, myomas during pregnancy were believed to enlarge secondary to endogenous hormonal tropism. More recently this has been challenged[24,49,50] since some 80% of uterine myomas followed by ultrasonography during pregnancy were unaltered or decreased in size.

The impact of myomas during pregnancy depends on the location and extent of the myoma. Complications of myomas arising during pregnancy include pain due to degeneration of the myoma or torsion of a pedunculated myoma. Other problems include pregnancy loss, premature labor, abruption, growth restriction, malpresentation, and sepsis. Myomas in the lower uterine segment increase the likelihood of malpresentation, cesarean section, and postpartum hemorrhage. In early pregnancy compression can be related to urinary retention. Other complications are radiculopathy and fetal deformities.

Degeneration of myomas during pregnancy occurs infrequently—in 5% to 8% of cases. The etiology is unclear, but such myomas can be symptomatic. Indeed, in some instances they can be exquisitely severely painful and tender with leukocytosis, and they can initiate premature labor requiring tocolytics. Ultrasonography[49] and/or MRI[51] of these painful myomas disclose characteristic cystic spaces in these tumors, which decreases the need for diagnostic exploratory surgery in these women. Medical management with analgesics, such as acetaminophen, nonsteroidal antiinflammatory medication (prior to 34 weeks) and narcotics, as well as bed rest and tocolytics, is usually successfully supportive.

Myomectomy has been advocated by some for the relief of pain in those women who do not respond to supportive medical management. The surgery is not without risk. Indeed, when at all possible it is probably better judgment to address the compelling complication medically. The problematic myoma(s) can then be addressed more reasonably following the pregnancy as an interim procedure prior to another pregnancy. There are a few, albeit small, studies reporting on myomectomy during pregnancy. Although Glavind and others[52] describe no surgical complications, they did indicate that 2 out of 11 pregnancies terminated as abortions following myomectomy. Burton and others[53] reported 6 antepartum myomectomies. All of the myomas were of the pedunculated variety with stalk size of 2 to 5 cm. All pregnancies progressed to term. Exacoustos and Rosati[54] performed 13 myomectomies prior to 26 weeks' gestation for subserous or pedunculated myomas. Five delivered prematurely between 32 weeks and term. There were no neonatal deaths. Although the complications reported appear minimal, selection of patients is paramount. There are no controlled studies to evaluate antepartum myomectomy. There are no reports of addressing this problem laparoscopically. This is probably wise given the uterine enlargement, which would make laparoscopy difficult. It is generally held that myomectomy during pregnancy should be limited to symptomatic pedunculated myomas with stalks of less than 5.0 cm.

Concerns have been raised regarding the advisability of myomectomy at the time of cesarean section (CS). As with resection of myoma during pregnancy, the resection at CS often leads to severe bleeding, which may not easily be controlled and may lead to hysterectomy. Obviously a small myoma in the incisional area may need to be resected and require meticulous attention and care to assure judicious speed and hemostasis. Burton and others[53] reported on 13 women who had incidental removal of myomas from submucosal, intramural, or subserosal locations. In 9 of these women the myomas were asymptomatic, but 1 of the cases was complicated by hemorrhage, which was controlled. Exacoustos and Rosati,[54] reported on 9 myomectomies at the time of CS, of which 3 women had severe hemorrhage that led to hysterectomy. It is probably wise to do what is essential, in keeping with the conservative adage that the less that is done without neglect of the patient, the better the patient is served.

CONCLUSIONS

Although myomas recur with some frequency, they more often tend to be asymptomatic. Thus the initial appropriate choice for dealing with the uterine myomas is paramount. Repeat myomectomy probably occurs less frequently since hysterectomy is accepted by a preponderant number of women requiring reoperation. The initial myomectomy requires a high degree of surgical ingenuity of the gynecologist. Choosing the incisional site over the myoma is of paramount importance, and there is need for an unusual dedication to the persistent retrieval of all the myomas, meticulous achievement of hemostasis, and a mastery in the reconstruction of the dissected uterus. Without attention to these specific details, myomas reccur with a higher frequency and/or disruption of the uterus with a subsequent pregnancy is more likely.

At this time it is difficult to compare the advantages of the various approaches to the management of uterine myoma. Assessment of the management by the alternative approaches through minimally invasive techniques still leaves many questions of the risks and true advantages of the so-called day surgery approaches. Reports of the degree of incapacitation of the patient after the procedures are biased since they do not take into account the competence of the surgeon. Patients having abdominal surgery, when appropriately screened, can and have gone home in 48 hours or less. The advantages claimed by the use of the minimally invasive approaches are indeed very attractive. However, the selection of subjects, the problems encountered, and the complications, as well as the assessment of not only the short-term but also the long-term outcomes, still escape us. They are not easily assessable. The attractiveness of the minimally invasive approaches, as presented by their enthusiasts, is so beguiling, when uncomplicated, that this euphoric aura tends to override the serious concerns that have been raised. Until better comparisons, preferably randomized and under strict oversight conditions, are available, surgeons will continue to assume the responsibility for selecting the therapeutic modality for their patients based on their own clinical appraisal of which approach is best suited for the level of the patient's pathologic condition and the surgeon's own assessment of personal competence.

> *Since cure without deformity or loss of function must ever be surgery's highest ideal, the general proposition that myomectomy is a greater surgical achievement than hysterectomy is incontestable.*[55]
>
> VICTOR BONNEY

REFERENCES

1. Singhabhandhu B and others: Giant leiomyoma of the uterus: report of a case and review of the literature, Am J Surg 146:391, 1973.
2. Buttram VC Jr and Reiter RC: Uterine leiomyomata: etiology, symptomatology, and management, Fertil Steril 36:433, 1981.
3. García C-R and Tureck RW: Submucosal leiomyomas and infertility, Fertil Steril 42(1):16, 1984.
4. Tulandi T, Murray C, and Guralnick M: Adhesion formation and reproductive outcome after myomectomy and second look laparoscopy, Fertil Steril 82(2):213, 1993.
5. Verkauf BS: Changing trends in treatment of leiomyomata uteri, Curr Opin Obstet Gynecol 5(3):301, 1993.
6. Wallach EE and Vu KK: Myomata uteri and infertility. In Uterine fibroids, Obstet Gynecal Clin North Am 22(4):791, 1995.
7. Leibsohn S and others: Leiomyosarcoma diagnosed in a series of hysterectomies performed for presumed uterine leiomyomas, Am J Obstet Gynecol 62(4):968, 1990.
8. Parker WH, Fu YS, and Berek JS: Uterine sarcoma in patients operated on for presumed leiomyoma and rapidly growing leiomyoma, Obstet Gynecol 83(3):414, 1994.
9. Uterine leiomyomata, ACOG Technical Bulletin No 192, 1994.
10. Candiani GB and others: Risk of recurrence after myomectomy, Br J Obstet Gynaecol 98(4):385, 1991.
11. Malone LJ and Ingersoll FM: Myomectomy in infertility. In Behrman SJ and Kistner RW, editors: Progress in infertility, Boston, 1975, Little, Brown & Co, Inc.
12. Babaknia A, Rock JA, Jones HW Jr: Pregnancy success following abdominal myomec-

tomy for infertility, Fertil Steril 30:644, 1978.

13. García C-R: The role of myomectomy in infertility and pelvic pain. Paper presented at FIGO World Congress, Rio de Janeiro, October, 1988.

14. Kelly HA: Benign tumors of the uterus. In Gynecology, New York, 1928, D Appleton & Co.

14a. Fedele L and others: Intranasal buserelin versus surgery in the treatment of uterine leiomyomata: long-term follow-up, Eur J Obstet Gynecol Reprod Biol 38:53, 1991.

15. Fedele L and others: Treatment with GnRH agonists before myomectomy and the risk of short term myoma recurrence, Br J Obstet Gynaecol 97:393, 1990.

16. Friedman AJ and others: Treatment of leiomyomata uteri with leuprolide acetate depot: a double-blind placebo-controlled, multicentered study. The Leuprolide Study Group, Obstet Gynecol 77:720, 1991.

17. Mayer DP and Shipilov V: Ultrasonography and magnetic resonance imaging, Obstet Gynecol Clin North Am 22(4):667, 1995.

18. Penner M and Sibrowski W: Benefits and risks of autologous blood donation, Infusionsther Transfusionsmed 21(suppl 1):64, 1994.

19. Lackritz EM and others: Estimated risk of transmission of the immunodeficiency virus by screened blood in the United States, N Engl J Med 333(26):1721, 1995.

20. Sloand EM and others: Safety of the blood supply, JAMA 274:1368, 1995.

21. Schlaff WD and others: A placebo-controlled trial of a depot gonadotropin-releasing hormone analogue (leuprolide) in the treatment of uterine leiomyomata, Obstet Gynecol 74(6):856, 1989.

22. Fayez Y and Schneider PJ: Prevention of pelvic adhesion formation by different modalities of treatment, Am J Obstet Gynecol 157(5):1184, 1987.

23. Tonmala P: Binding of epidermal growth factor in human endometrium and leiomyomata, Obstet Gynecol 74:658, 1989.

24. Aharoni A and others: Patterns of growth of uterine leiomyomas during pregnancy: a longitudinal study, Br J Obstet Gynaecol 95(5):510, 1988.

25. Friedman AJ and others: A randomized, placebo controlled, double-blind study evaluating leuprolide acetate depot treatment before myomectomy, Fertil Steril 52:728, 1989.

26. Thorp JM and Katz VL: Submucous myomas treated with gonadotropin releasing hormone agonist and resulting in vaginal hemorrhage: a case report, J Reprod Med 36:625, 1991.

27. Stovall TG and others: A randomized trial evaluating leuprolide acetate before hysterectomy as a treatment for leiomyomas, Am J Obstet Gynecol 164:1420, 1991.

28. Matta WHM and others: Doppler assessment of uterine blood flow changes in patients with fibroids receiving the gonadotropin-releasing hormone agonist Buserelin, Fertil Steril 49:1083, 1988.

29. Davis KM and Schlaff WD: Medical management of uterine fibromyomata, uterine fibroids, Obstet Gynecol Clin North Am 22(4):727, 1995.

30. Frederick J and others: Intramyometrial vasopressin as a hemostatic agent during myomectomy, Br J Obstet Gynaecol 101(5):435, 1994.

31. Trouwborst A and others: Acute hypervolemic haemodilution to avoid transfusion during major surgery, Lancet 336:1295, 1990.

32. Reich H: Laparoscopic myomectomy, Obstet Gynecol Clin North Am 22(4):757, 1995.

33. Andreyko JL and others: Use of an agonist analog of gonadotropin-releasing hormone (naferelin) to treat leiomyomas: assessment by magnetic resonance imaging, Am J Obstet Gynecol 158:903, 1988.

34. Letterie G and others: Efficacy of a gonadotropin releasing hormone agonist in the treatment of uterine myomata: long-term follow-up, Fertil Steril 51:951, 1989.

35. Matta WHM and others: Long term follow-up of patients with uterine fibroids after treatment with LHRH agonist buserelin, Br J Obstet Gynaecol 96(2):200, 1989.

36. Neuwirth RS: Hysteroscopic management of symptomatic submucous fibroids, Obstet Gynecol 62(4):509, 1983.

37. Yaron Y and others: Uterine rupture at 33 weeks' gestation subsequent to hysteroscopic perforation, Am J Obstet Gynecol 170(3): 786, 1994.

38. Vercellini P and others: Hypervolemic pulmonary edema and severe coagulopathy after

Dextran instillation, Obstet Gynecol 79(5): 838, 1992.

39. Gonzales R and others: Posthysteroscopic hyponatremia, Am J Kidney Dis 23(5):735, 1994.

40. Nezhat C and others: Laparoscopic myomectomy, Int J Fertil 36:275, 1991.

41. Boike GM et al: Incisional bowel herniations after operative laparoscopy: a series of 19 cases and review of the literature, Am J Obstet Gynecol 172(6):1726, 1995.

42. Goldberg HA: Laparoscopic coagulation of myoma (myolysis), Obstet Gynecol Clin North Am 22(4):807, 1995.

43. Yamashita Y and others: Transcatheter arterial embolization of obstetrical and gynecological bleeding: efficacy and clinical outcome, Br J Radiology 67(798):530, 1994.

44. Ravina JH and others: Arterial embolisation to treat uterine myomata, Lancet 346(8976): 671, 1995.

45. Kilkku PO: Total versus subtotal abdominal hysterectomy. In García C-R, Mikuta J, Rosenblum N, editors: Current therapy in surgical gynecology, Toronto, 1987, BC Decker.

46. Kilkku P, Lehtinen V, Hirvonen T, and Gronroos M: Abdominal hysterectomy versus supravaginal uterine amputation: psychic factors, Ann Clir Gynaecol Suppl (Finland) 202:62, 1987.

47. Treacy PJ and Johnson AJ: Is the laparoscopic bubble bursting? Lancet 346 (Supplement):23, 1995.

48. Phelan JP: Myomas and pregnancy, Obstet Gynecol Clin North Am 22(4):801, 1995.

49. Lev-Toaff AS and others: Leiomyomas in pregnancy: sonographic study, Radiology 164:375, 1987.

50. Muram D and others: Myomas of the uterus in pregnancy: ultrasonographic follow-up, Am J Obstet Gynecol 138:16, 1980.

51. Curtis M and others: Magnetic resonance imaging to avoid laparotomy in pregnancy, Obstet Gynecol 82(5):833, 1993.

52. Glavind K and others: Uterine myoma in pregnancy, Acta Obstet Gynecol Scand 69:617, 1990.

53. Burton CA and others: Surgical management of leiomyomata during pregnancy, Obstet Gynecol 74(5):707, 1989.

54. Exacoustos C and Rosati P: Ultrasound diagnosis of uterine myomas and complications in pregnancy, Obstet Gynecol 82(1):97, 1993.

55. Bonney V: A textbook of gynaecological surgery, ed 6, New York, 1953, Hoebel.

13

Operative Injuries to the Urinary Tract

JOHN D. THOMPSON
ANNE WISKIND

The bladder and pelvic ureters are directly adjacent to the reproductive tract. They may be involved in gynecologic disease and are always at risk of injury when gynecologic surgery is performed. In spite of this, injuries to the urinary tract are uncommon. This is testimony to the technical skill of gynecologic surgeons, the attention given to understanding the close relationship between the two organ systems, and the pride in doing surgery correctly to avoid injuries to adjacent organs and structures whenever possible. However, in spite of technical skill, surgeons' pride in their work, and attention to details, injuries to the urinary tract do still occur. They can cause enormous disability in patients and are the leading cause of malpractice suits against gynecologic surgeons.

In this chapter, the measures to prevent urinary tract injuries and to facilitate their early recognition will be emphasized. Some operative procedures to correct injuries when they occur will be discussed.

OPERATIVE INJURIES TO THE URETER

Injury to the ureter is one of the most serious complications of gynecologic surgery. Ureteral injuries are far more serious and troublesome than injury to either the bladder or rectum. Delay in the diagnosis is often associated with postoperative morbidity, ureterovaginal fistulas, and the potential loss of kidney function. For example, Lee and Symmonds reviewed 68 patients referred to the Mayo Clinic with a diagnosis of ureterovaginal fistula. In 34 (50%) a nephrectomy was necessary because delay in the diagnosis of ureteral injury had resulted in loss of kidney function.

Fortunately, ureteral injury is uncommon. Its prevalence varies between 0.1% to 1.5%, depending on a variety of factors, including the number of extensive hysterectomies and other difficult operations included in the series. However, ureteral injury may also occur unexpectedly even in the course of uncomplicated operations, clearly indicating the need to adopt a routine procedure to confirm ureteral integrity at the end of each major gynecologic operation, vaginal and abdominal.

This discussion will emphasize the prevention and early recognition of ureteral injury, hopefully at the operation of injury. Management of simple injuries by gynecologic surgeons will be discussed. More complicated injuries that require special skill and experience in pelvic surgery will be mentioned.

Anatomy

The reproductive tract and urinary tract develop embryologically in close proximity. Because of this close proximity, alterations in anatomy and physiology may occur in one system in the presence of disease in the other system. Diseases of the reproductive system may cause urinary tract signs or symptoms, and the opposite may also occur. Congenital anomalies of one system may be associated with anomalous development in the other system. When significant parts of the müllerian duct system are congenitally absent or obstructed, major anomalies of the upper urinary tract will be found in 35% to 40% of patients. Approximately 1% of females will have duplication of the ureters, more common unilaterally than bilaterally. Especially when difficult gynecologic surgery is performed, it is extremely helpful to know if ureteral duplication is present. If a ureteral catheter has been placed preoperatively in only one ureter of the duplicated system, the ureter without the catheter is more likely to be injured. The course of the ureter of a pelvic kidney may be tortuous and difficult to dissect. The commonly accepted explanation for duplication and other anomalies of the ureters is a variation in the origin of the ureteral bud or buds from the posterolateral wall of the mesonephric ducts at the fifth week of embryonic development.

The wall of the ureter is composed of smooth muscle with longitudinal, circular, and spiral fibers to produce regular peristaltic waves several times each minute. The lumen is lined with transitional epithelium. A condensation of connective tissue forms a pseudosheath that surrounds and protects the plexus of freely anastomosing vessels that course longitudinally up and down the ureter. Just before its entrance into the bladder, the lower ureter is surrounded by a layer of smooth muscle that extends a short distance upward from the bladder. This layer is called *Waldeyer's sheath.*

The ureter measures approximately 25 to 30 cm, depending on the person's height. The abdominal and pelvic components are approximately equal in length. In its course from the kidney to the bladder, the abdominal ureter rests on the medial border of the psoas muscle close to the vena cava on the right and the aorta on the left. The ureters enter the pelvis by crossing over the lower common iliac artery just at its point of bifurcation. At this point it is easily identified on the right beneath a thin peritoneal covering. Its entry into the pelvis on the left may be obscured by the sigmoid colon. The pelvic ureter courses beneath the peritoneum on the posterolateral pelvic wall, just above and lateral to the uterosacral ligaments and anterior and medial to the hypogastric artery. When the anatomy is normal and the peritoneum is not involved or thickened by disease, the ureter can usually be followed visually from the pelvic brim throughout its course beneath the peritoneum along the lateral wall of the pelvis until it disappears beneath the uterine vessels (Figure 13.1). Peristalsis can be seen in the ureter beneath the peritoneum on the lateral pelvic sidewall. Peristalsis can be stimulated by gently stroking the ureter through the peritoneum.

After crossing under the uterine vessels, the ureter enters a tunnel through the cardinal ligament. It is approximately 1 to 1.5 cm lateral to the cervix at the level of the internal cervical os (Figure 13.2). Just before entering the bladder wall, the ureter turns medially and anteriorly over the lateral vaginal fornix, where it can sometimes be palpated through the vaginal mucosa. It enters the bladder wall just above and lateral to the trigone. This angulation of the lower ureter is sometimes called the "knee" of the ureter.

It is important for gynecologic surgeons to realize that the course of the ureters may not be symmetric in their relation to the cervix. As shown by the classic studies of Sampson, the proximity of either ureter to the cervix may vary according to the position of the uterus in the pelvis even in the absence of a pathologic condition (Figure 13.3).

The ureter has the advantage of a rich blood supply from multiple sources along its course. The upper ureter receives blood supply from branches of the renal and ovarian arteries; the midureter receives arterial branches from the aorta and common iliac artery; and the pelvic ureter receives arterial branches from the hypogastric, uterine, vaginal, middle hemorrhoidal, and vesical arteries (Figure 13.4). There is a rich collateral anastomosis of vessels up and down the ureter beneath its pseudosheath. In mobilization of the ureter, these vessels will not be damaged as long as the dissection preserves the periureteral pseudosheath. This interconnecting network of vessels gives the ureter preferential healing capabilities in case of injury. Sampson described the importance of preservation of the periureteral arterial plexus, especially in extensive operations for gynecologic cancer. If these vessels are damaged by trauma or by excessive skeletonization of the ureter by removing its sheath, local ischemia of a segment of the ureter may be followed by necrosis and rupture of the ureteral wall. In addition, there may be fibrosis and scarring of the ureteral wall and periureteral tissues with subsequent stenosis of the lumen and proximal hydroureter. The

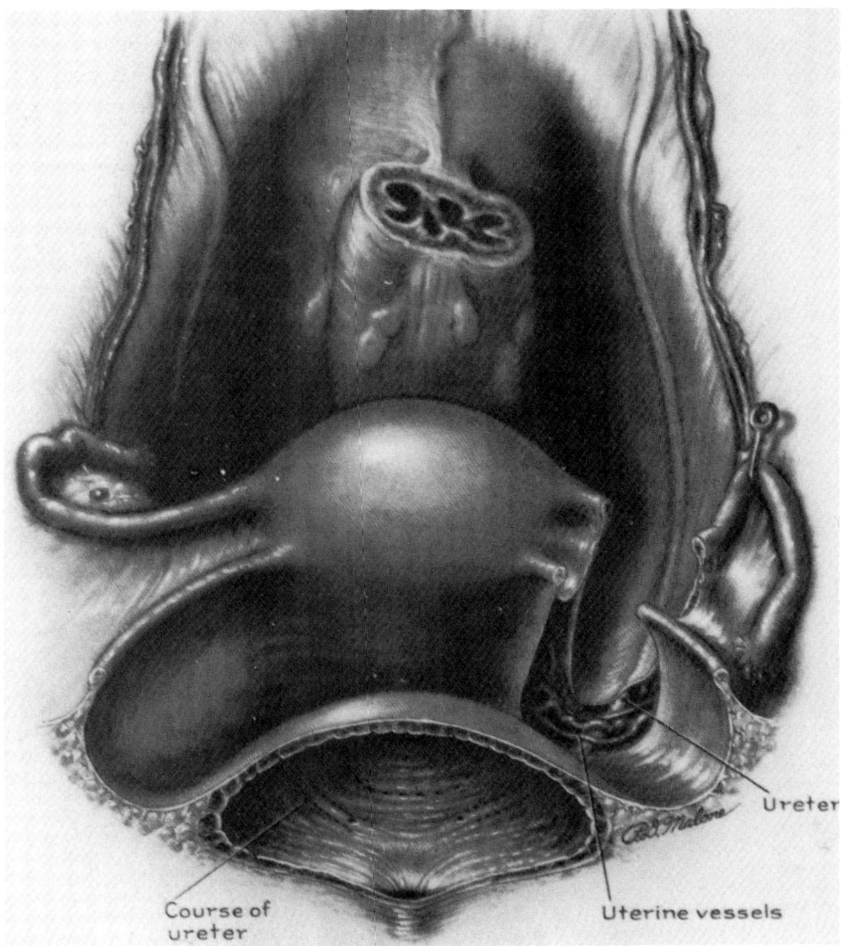

Figure 13.1 Dissection showing relation of ureters to pelvic viscera. (From Rock JA and Thompson JD: TeLinde's operative gynecology, ed 8, Philadelphia, 1996, Lippincott-Raven.)

resulting intraureteral pressure increase may cause kidney damage and permanent loss of kidney function if left uncorrected.

Ureteral Involvement by Gynecologic Diseases, Operations, and Other Conditions

In its course through the pelvis, the ureter is susceptible to involvement, distortion, and/or compression by a variety of normal and pathologic conditions of other pelvic organs and structures. Conditions such as the following may place one or both ureters at greater risk of injury.

Intrauterine Pregnancy. An enlarging and dextrorotated gravid uterus and distended vessels in the right infundibulopelvic ligament may compress the right ureter at the pelvic brim, causing ureteral dilatation above, whereas the sigmoid colon protects the left ureter against compression. High levels of progesterone in pregnancy also may cause ureteral ectasia, which promptly disappears following delivery. This physiologic dilatation of the ureters will be impressive but should not be troublesome should pelvic operations be required during pregnancy.

Large Pelvic Tumors. Large solid or cystic ovarian tumors or large uterine leiomyomas may compress the ureters against the pelvic brim. Ordinarily, simply lifting the tumor off the ureter will relieve the compression. Leiomyomas can also cause compression of the

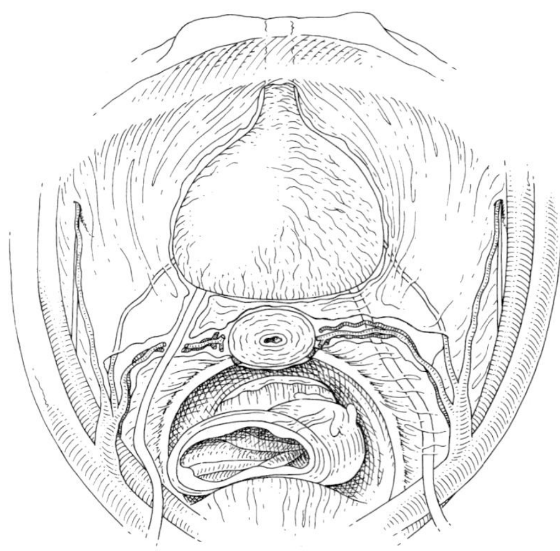

Figure 13.2 Pelvic portion of the ureter showing its course along the sidewall of the pelvis and its relationship to the common iliac vessels, the hypogastric vessels, the uterosacral ligaments, the uterine vessels, and the cervix.

lower ureter or ureters if they arise from the cervix or lower uterine segment.

Gynecologic Malignancies. Invasive carcinoma of the cervix may extend laterally into parametrial tissues and obstruct one or both ureters. Endometrial adenocarcinoma, uterine sarcomas, and ovarian malignancies can also involve the ureters but not as commonly as cervical cancer.

Endometriosis. In the presence of extensive endometriosis involving the ovaries, uterosacral ligaments, cul-de-sac, and/or rectosigmoid colon, the ureters may also be involved and obstructed. Involvement of the ureters may not be suspected preoperatively by clinically specific signs or symptoms. The fibrosis and scarring of endometriosis may draw the ureter closer to the infundibulopelvic ligament, the uterosacral ligament, the uterine vessels, and the rectosigmoid colon.

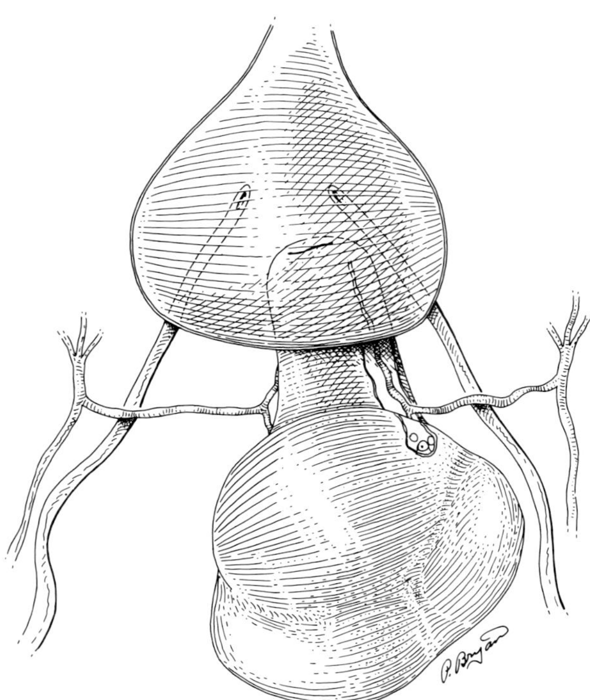

Figure 13.3 The cervix is closer to the right than the left ureter. During total abdominal hysterectomy (TAH), the right ureter is at greater risk of injury. (From Rock JA and Thompson JD: TeLinde's operative gynecology, ed 8, Philadelphia, 1996, Lippincott-Raven.)

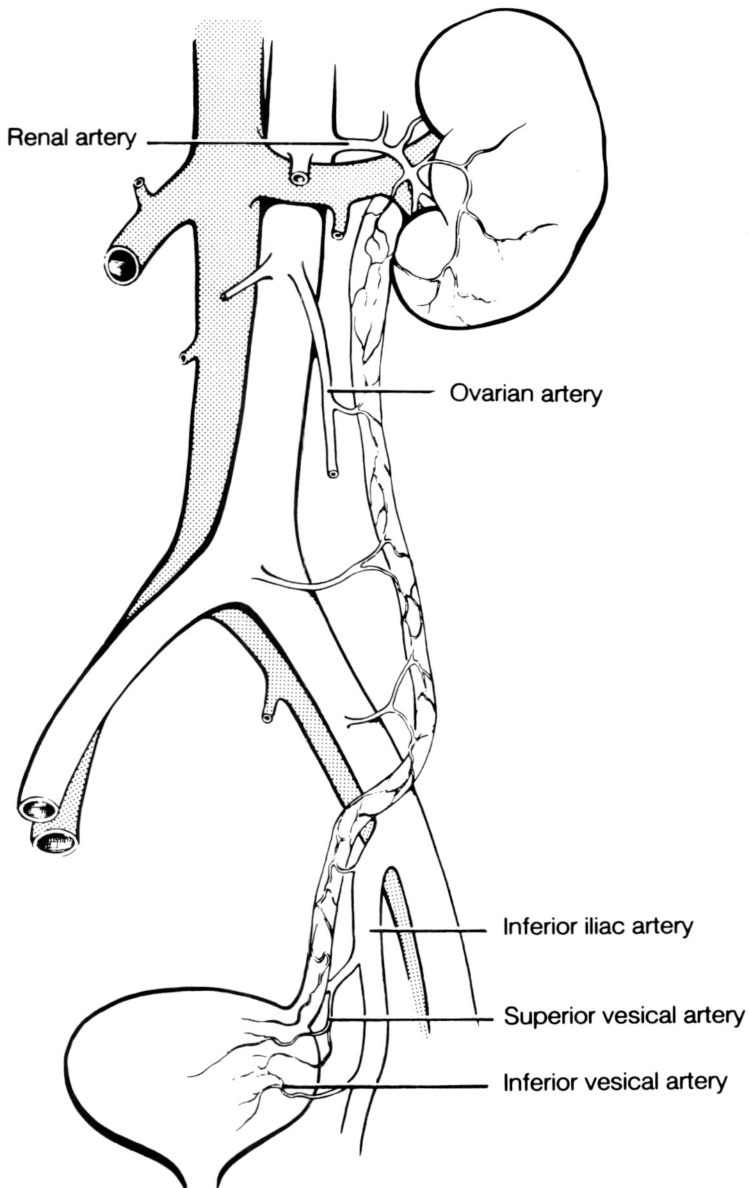

Figure 13.4 Blood supply of the ureter. (From Rock JA and Thompson JD: TeLinde's operative gynecology, ed 8, Philadelphia, 1996, Lippincott-Raven.)

Pelvic Infection. Although patients with acute and chronic PID usually will show no evidence of ureteral involvement, hydroureteronephrosis may be found in association with acute exacerbations of chronic PID with tubo-ovarian abscess or abscesses. The obstruction may be unilateral or bilateral. If the infection extends to retroperitoneal planes and spaces, ligneous pelvic cellulitis with ureteral obstruction may result. The obstruction usually will be relieved by antibiotic therapy plus removal of the abscess or abscesses when necessary. Skillful dissection will be required to prevent ureteral injury.

Retroperitoneal Tumors. Usually anterior and medial deviation of the ureter will be caused by a retroperitoneal tumor growing beneath the ureter and lifting it away from the pelvic sidewall. Smaller retroperitoneal masses, such as retroperitoneal lymph nodes containing metastatic tumor, will cause less dramatic deviation in the normal course of the ureter. If an excretory urogram is done to detect ureteral displacement, it is helpful to have oblique and lateral views of the abdomen and pelvis. Straight anteroposterior views may not show the displacement.

Uterine Procedentia. Hydroureter and even hydronephrosis may be marked and bilateral when complete uterine procidentia has been present over many months or years. The ureters are caught beneath the uterine arteries and surrounded by the parametrial tissues that compose the tunnel. As these structures descend, the ureters are brought with them to a location outside the body. The so-called knee of the ureter is exaggerated and acutely angulated and compressed against the medial borders of the urogenital hiatus, causing obstruction above. The obstruction is promptly relieved when the procidentia is relieved.

Miscellaneous Conditions. A variety of other conditions may involve the ureter. An ovarian remnant may cause hydroureter. A pelvic hematoma developing after delivery or after operation or a pelvic lymphocyst developing after pelvic lymphadenectomy may cause deviation, obstruction, or both of the ureter. Again, skillful dissection, possibly with the aid of surgical loupe magnification, will be needed to avoid injury. When a postpartum or postabortion patient develops septic pelvic thrombophlebitis that involves the ovarian vein with thrombophlebitis, the inflammatory process may extend to periureteral tissues and cause obstruction. However, the normal ovarian vessels in the infundibulopelvic ligament rarely, if ever, cause clinically significant symptoms from ureteral compression, and operations for the ovarian vein syndrome are rarely, if ever, justified.

Operative Procedures Involved in Ureteral Injury

About 75% of operative injuries to the ureter result from gynecologic operations. The remainder are the result of urologic, general surgical, and vascular surgical procedures. When only gynecologic procedures are considered, about 75% result from abdominal operations and about 25% from vaginal operations.

Almost all gynecologic operations have been implicated in ureteral injury. The incidence is highest with extensive abdominal hysterectomy and pelvic lymphadenectomy (1.0% to 2.0%). The incidence is higher for abdominal hysterectomy (0.4% to 0.6%) than for vaginal hysterectomy (0.1% to 0.3%). The risk is greater during abdominal operations since patients with extensive disease possibly involving the ureters are more likely to have abdominal operations. The incidence of ureteral injury with adnexal surgery or with retropubic colpourethropexy is approximately 0.1%. A partial vaginectomy done with either abdominal or vaginal hysterectomy is associated with a higher risk of injury, as is the extrafascial technique of abdominal hysterectomy. The posterior cul-de-plasty technique using the uterosacral ligament to support the posterior vaginal fornix and obliterate the cul-de-sac must be done carefully to avoid ureteral injury. The ureters are located just above and lateral to the uterosacral ligaments. If not done carefully, the Moschcowitz technique of closing the cul-de-sac can cause the same problem. In such cases, a suture placed in close proximity to the ureter may cause obstruction simply by kinking the ureter. The ureter can also be damaged during laser operations done through the laparoscope. Use of laser or electrocoagulation for ablation or removal of endometriosis, lysis of adhesions, transection of uterosacral ligaments, or tubal sterilization can cause ureteral injury.

Ureteral injuries are possible with obstetric operations. If deep lacerations of the lateral vaginal fornicies are caused by difficult forceps operations for obstetric delivery, the ureter may be involved. Plauche reports that the incidence of ureteral injuries was 0.44% and the incidence of ureterovaginal fistulas was 0.1% among 5,220 cesarean hysterectomies. The incidence may be higher if the cesarean hysterectomy is done as an emergency in the peripartum period. The risk of ureteral injury in such cases may be decreased if a subtotal hysterectomy can be performed.

Unfortunately, the incidence of ureteral

injury has improved only slightly in several decades. However, the fact that injury to the ureter occurs infrequently is a credit to the attention given the ureter by gynecologic surgeons and their technical skill at the operating table. Although ureteral injury may be almost unavoidable in some situations, even in the hands of the most skillful and experienced gynecologic surgeons, a continuing effort must be made to reduce the incidence of ureteral injury even further.

Measures to Prevent Ureteral Injury with Gynecologic Surgery

Preoperative Evaluation and Preparation. Primary prevention of ureteral injuries begins with a careful evaluation of the patient's gynecologic disease and recognition of the likelihood of ureteral involvement either by the disease or by the operative procedure planned. An experienced pelvic examiner will be able to tell whether or not the disease in the pelvis encroaches on the course of the ureter. In complicated cases, special diagnostic imaging techniques (ultrasonography, computed tomography (CT), and/or MRI) may be useful. Excretory urography has been the most useful special diagnostic procedure but certainly is not needed in the preoperative workup of every patient. It is possible to be selective and avoid unnecessary, expensive, time-consuming, and potentially hazardous preoperative studies by using sound clinical judgment. If disease in the pelvis is strategically located in an area that is likely to involve the ureter, preoperative excretory urography may be helpful. It should also be considered an appropriate part of the preoperative workup when an extensive operation is planned for benign or malignant disease (cancer of the uterus, endometriosis, etc.), when anomalous development of the müllerian ducts is present, and when there is a history of previous pelvic surgery (for medicolegal as well as other reasons). Although there is no proof that preoperative excretory urography can reduce the incidence of ureteral injury, many gynecologic surgeons do believe that prior knowledge of the anatomy of the lower urinary tract may help avoid such injury. When the films show an abnormality, they may be displayed for viewing in the OR to provide easy access should intraoperative review be needed.

Most experienced gynecologic surgeons prefer not to place ureteral catheters preoperatively, believing that they cause unnecessary trauma to the ureteral wall. In our experience, ureteral catheters have been helpful in only a small number of cases, perhaps 5% of pelvic laparotomies. They may be useful in operations for cervical leiomyomas, for ovarian remnant syndrome, when retroperitoneal fibrosis from endometriosis or infection is present, when dissecting around a retroperitoneal tumor, or when debulking an extensive ovarian malignancy. They are not used in extensive abdominal hysterectomy and bilateral pelvic lymphadenectomy. If a ureteral catheter is needed during the course of the operation and has not been placed preoperatively, it can always be placed intraoperatively through a cystotomy incision or through a cystoscope. Cystoscopy is more easily accomplished intraoperatively if the patient has been positioned for operation in Allen Universal stirrups.

Exposure. It is necessary to have proper exposure to prevent injury to important structures and organs in the field of operation. This is a basic principle in all of surgery. Certainly proper exposure is necessary to avoid injury to the ureter during gynecologic surgery. Proper exposure begins with an adequate incision. We believe that a Pfannenstiel's incision usually does not provide enough exposure for a safe abdominal hysterectomy or other major abdominal gynecologic procedures. The transverse Maylard incision is preferred because the structures on the lateral pelvic sidewalls are more easily visualized. Good illumination of the operative field, strategically placed retractors, willing assistants, and anesthesia sufficient for good muscle relaxation are also essential elements to provide proper exposure. But most important, the gynecologic surgeon must not allow exposure of important structures in the pelvis to be limited by a limited incision.

It is another cardinal axiom in surgery that the important structures in the operative field at risk of injury should be identified and visualized and, if necessary, dissected and mo-

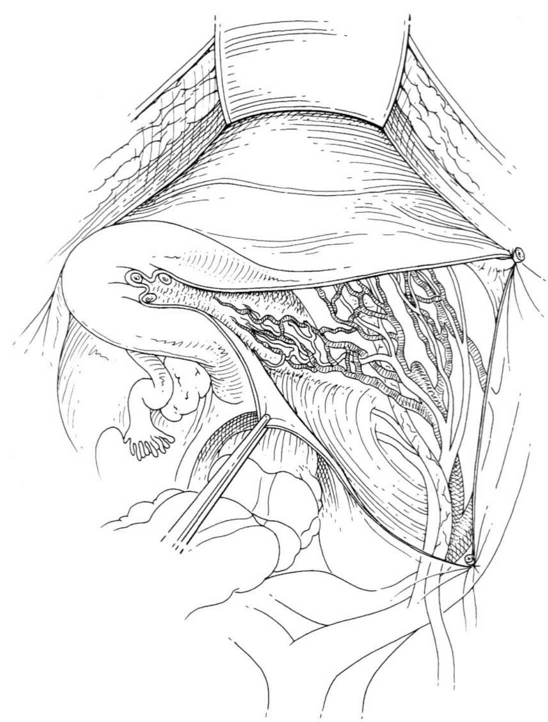

Figure 13.5 When the peritoneum is reflected medially, the ureter can be easily identified down to the point where it crosses beneath the uterine vessels and enters the tunnel in the cardinal ligament.

bilized to allow retraction out of harm's way throughout the procedure. This axiom has no better example than the ureter in gynecologic surgery. The ureters can be easily visualized along the pelvic sidewall in most abdominal operations. If visualization is difficult, an incision can be made in the peritoneum lateral to the infundibulopelvic ligament. If necessary, the round ligament may be clamped, cut, and ligated. As the peritoneum is dissected medially away from the lateral pelvic sidewall, the ureter comes away with it and can be traced fairly easily from the pelvic brim above down to its disappearance beneath the uterine vessels, where it enters its tunnel in the cardinal ligament (Figure 13.5). In most cases, the ureter can be palpated in normal cardinal ligament tissue and should be felt in every case when clamps are placed adjacent to the cervix in TAH (Figure 13.6). Dissection of the lowest 3 cm of ureter may be done but is more difficult than dissection of the upper ureter and could itself result in injury to the ureter if not done carefully. Dissection, palpation, and/or visualization of the pelvic ureter has been recommended as a routine in every abdominal gynecologic operation as the best way to prevent ureteral injury.

When intraoperative bleeding occurs, there is a tendency to place clamps blindly deep in the pelvis in a pool of blood attempting to clamp bleeding vessels. Ureters may be clamped and ligated by such desperate maneuvers. It is far better to control the hemorrhage with temporary measures using the pressure of the finger, a stick sponge, or a pack and then to suction away the blood, replace the blood lost if necessary, request appropriate instruments and sutures, and arrange for proper exposure. Then the bleeding vessel can be definitively ligated or clipped, hopefully without injuring adjacent structures such as the ureters.

Where the Ureter Is at Greatest Risk of Injury. Of course, the ureter may be injured at any point along its course in the pelvis. When the infundibulopelvic ligament is clamped, cut, and ligated, the ureter that has a normal relationship lies only 1 cm away. Distortion of anatomy by tubo-ovarian abscess, endometriosis, paraovarian cysts, or ovarian tumor may result in a shortened infundibu-

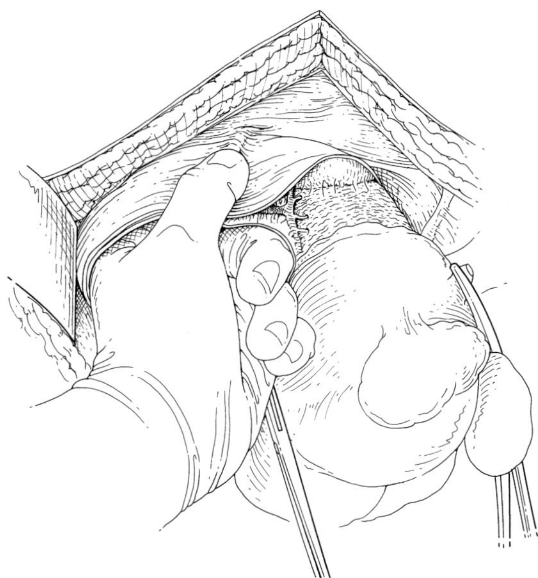

Figure 13.6 In normal paracervical cardinal ligament tissues, the ureter usually can be "snapped" between the thumb and index finger. This method of ureteral identification is not always possible nor reliable.

lopelvic ligament that may be even closer to the ureter. The location of this segment of the ureter should be verified by visualization, palpation, and/or dissection before the highest clamp is placed across the ovarian vessels. After the highest clamp has been safely placed, the other clamps can be placed medially and below it.

When an abdominal operation involves the lateral pelvic sidewall, the ureter is at risk of injury during removal of adherent residual adnexa or ovarian remnants, freeing adnexal structures adherent to the posterior broad ligament, suspending the posterior vaginal fornix to the uterosacral ligaments, closing the cul-de-sac with a Moschcowitz's operation, and reperitonizing the pelvis. In all of these procedures, the ureter must be identified before clamps and sutures are placed.

The ureters are in even greater danger of injury when the uterine vessels are clamped and ligated. Injury is avoided by first skeletonizing the vessels and then clamping them with three clamps after palpating the ureter in the cardinal ligament. The lowest clamp is placed first, at a right angle to the uterus, at the level of the internal cervical os. The other two clamps are placed above the lowest clamp. The uterine vessels are cut between the upper and middle clamps. The two lower clamps are replaced by suture ligatures that should contain only the uterine vessels. This technique is designed to ligate the uterine vessels securely while at the same time avoiding ureteral injury.

In our experience, the most common site of ureteral injury is in the lowest 3 to 4 cm, between the level of the uterine vessels and the entrance of the ureter into the bladder. This is the part of the dissection involved with removing the cervix. It is the removal of the cervix in performing a TAH that causes the largest number of ureteral injuries. As mentioned earlier, the ureters are less than 2 cm away from the cervix, but this distance is not always constant, as described by Sampson. Several maneuvers will help to avoid ureteral injury here. The bladder must be well mobilized inferiorly and laterally. The ureter should be palpated in the cardinal ligament and even pushed laterally if possible before clamps and sutures are placed in the cardinal ligament (Figure 13.6). When induration and fibrosis of paracervical tissue occur, the ureters may be drawn abnormally close to the cervix, may be difficult to palpate, and will not fall away from the cervix and vagina as the dissection proceeds. In these cases and in every TAH for benign disease, development of the pubovesicocervical fascia will be helpful. If clamps are placed beneath this fascia, as in the Richardson intrafascial technique, ureteral injury should not occur. Finally, if necessary, the ureter may be identified by dissecting it free and retracting it out of harm's way.

If one is uncertain of the location of the ureters when doing a suprapubic urethropexy, it may be helpful to open the lower anterior bladder wall and pass ureteral catheters up through the ureteral orifices. This is not often necessary as long as the urethropexy sutures are placed in anterior paravaginal fascia adjacent to the urethra and not higher up. Most ureteral injuries with retropubic colpourethropexy are probably due to acute augulation of the anterior vaginal wall with kinking rather than ligation of the ureter.

When the surgeon is operating vaginally, the ureter may be at risk of injury at several points. When anterior colporrhaphy is performed, the ureters may be only 0.9 cm away from sutures, as measured by Hofmeister using a special intraoperative cineradiographic fluoroscopic technique. It is difficult to explain why the ureters are not injured more fre-

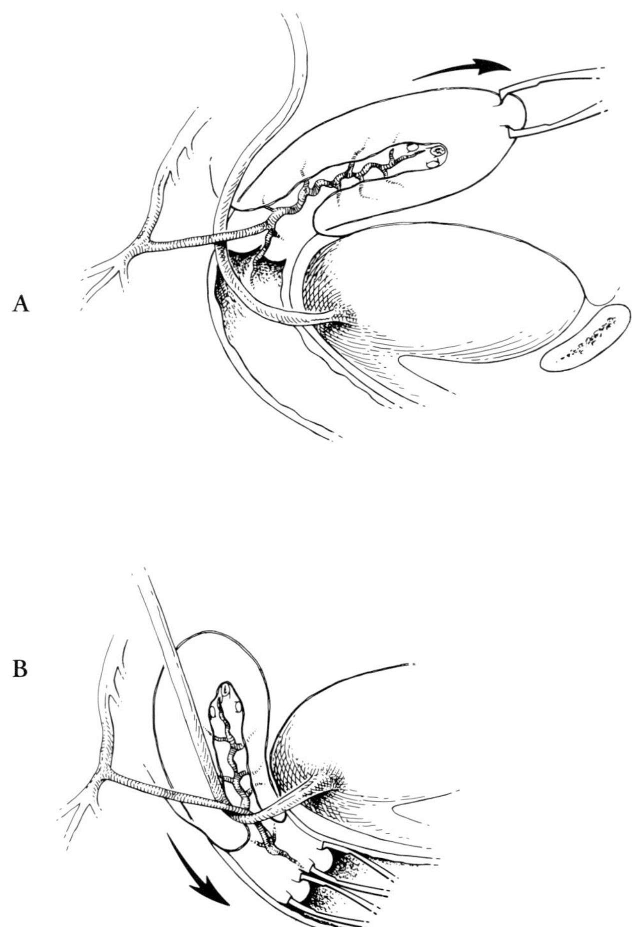

FIGURE 13.7 **A,** In abdominal operation, upward traction on the uterine fundus pulls the uterine vessels away from the ureters. **B,** In vaginal operation, downward traction on the cervix exaggerates the knee of the ureter and draws it into the operative field. (From Rock JA and Thompson JD: TeLinde's operative gynecology, ed 8, Philadelphia, 1996, Lippincott-Raven.)

quently with this operation. When downward traction is made on the cervix during vaginal hysterectomy, ureters are drawn further down into the operative field by exaggerating the knee of the ureter (Figure 13.7). Complete development of the vesicocervical space with retractor elevation of the bladder will help to lift the ureters away from clamps and sutures. This may be further facilitated by clamping the bladder pillars adjacent to the cervix on each side of the vesicocervical space. Locating the ureter by palpation in the cardinal ligament may also be helpful in avoiding ureteral injury (Figure 13.8). A method of identifying the ureter during vaginal hysterectomy also has been described by Lee and Cruikshank. Care must be exercised in the placement of clamps and sutures on the cardinal ligaments and uterine vessels. A single rather than double clamps technique should be used, taking only small bites of tissue. And again, when the posterior cul-de-plasty technique is used to support the posterior vaginal fornix after the uterus is removed vaginally, the sutures must be placed carefully and only in the uterosacral ligaments. If sutures are placed higher on the pelvic wall, the ureters may be incorporated or kinked. Clamping the infundibulopelvic ligament vaginally to remove the tubes and ovaries is hazardous since the ureter is only 1 cm away.

Proving Ureteral Integrity. In our series of ureteral injuries, when the injury was recognized and repaired at the operation of injury, no kidneys were lost, and only one reoperation was required. Immediate recognition and repair of injury to the ureter are extremely important in prevention of secondary serious postoperative morbidity and loss of kidney function. It is important to keep in mind the wise statement of many pelvic surgeons, to wit, "The venial sin is injury to the ureter; the mortal sin is failure of recognition." Emphasis is generally placed on prevention of ureteral injuries during difficult and complicated operations for extensive pelvic disease. However, ureteral injury may also occur during a standard uncomplicated operation. Symmonds

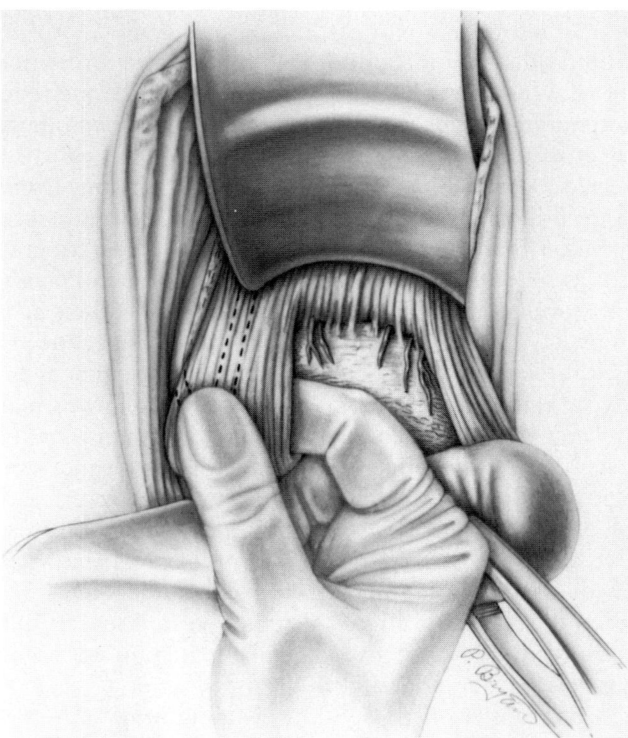

Figure 13.8 The ureter may be palpated in the bladder pillar during vaginal hysterectomy, thus allowing placement of clamps to avoid injury. (From Rock JA and Thompson JD: TeLinde's operative gynecology, ed 8, Philadelphia, 1996, Lippincott-Raven.)

believes that "the easy hysterectomy (or other straightforward gynecologic operation), not the hazardous or difficult dissection, is responsible for most of the genitourinary tract injuries (and fistulas) in this country."

Because of the importance of detecting ureteral injuries at the operation of injury, we recommend that gynecologic surgeons adopt a routine and effective method of accurately determining ureteral integrity before the operation is ended, whether this be by palpation, mobilization and inspection, ureteral catheterization, or some other means. We have adopted an intravenous dye test that we use routinely at the end of each major gynecologic operation, both abdominal and vaginal. Before the incision is closed in abdominal operations, ureteral integrity may be quickly ascertained by injecting 5 ml of indigo carmine intravenously, placing a cystoscope in the bladder, and observing efflux of the dye from each ureteral orifice in 3 to 5 minutes. This single procedure is facilitated by having placed the patient in Allen Universal stirrups for the laparotomy. Of course, for vaginal operations, this simple procedure is even easier to perform since the external urethral meatus is a part of the operative field. Should the dye not spurt from a ureteral orifice (even after adequate hydration), the corresponding ureter should be explored along its course and the problem identified and corrected. Ureteral catheter placement may help in localizing the site of injury. It is our contention that adoption of this simple procedure as a routine measure would result in discovery of all ureteral injuries at the operation of injury.

Our experience with routine cystoscopy and indigo carmine dye injection at the end of gynecologic operations has been reported by Wiskind and Thompson. During the course of 3597 major gynecologic operations (excluding laparoscopy) in which routine cystoscopy was done at the end, five unsuspected ureteral injuries were identified. Two injuries were found at the completion of total vaginal hysterectomy with posterior cul-de-plasty; two with total vaginal hysterectomy, anterior and posterior colporrhaphy and posterior cul-de-plasty; and one with TAH and BSO. Four of the five injuries were repaired at the operation of injury: two by removal of the posterior cul-de-plasty suture; one by removal of a hemostatic suture near the right bladder base, and one by the removal of the vaginal cuff angle suture. The fifth patient had a ureteroneocystostomy on postoperative day 1. In these five patients, routine cystoscopy at the end of the operation avoided a delay in the diagnosis and avoided an additional operation in four.

Pettit and Petrou have reported on the value of cystoscopy in major vaginal surgery. Among 236 patients who had cystoscopy as part of their major vaginal operation, five ureteral injuries were discovered, one with anterior colporrhaphy, three with McCall's cul-de-plasty, and one with a Pereyra bladder neck suspension. These authors state that cystoscopy with indigo carmine dye injection should be part of all pelvic surgery when the integrity of the lower urinary tract cannot be assessed at the completion of the procedure.

Even though the optimal time for diagnosis of ureteral injury is at the operation of injury, there is still an opportunity to prevent serious morbidity and permanent impairment of kidney function if the injury is diagnosed as soon as possible. In the first week after operation, signs of ureteral injury include flank pain, persistent ileus, unexplained fever, lower abdominal mass (urinoma), urinary discharge from the vagina, and reduced urinary output. Special diagnostic studies that may be useful in evaluating the integrity of the ureters include excretory urography (sometimes including delayed films), ultrasonography of the kidneys, cystoscopy with retrograde passage of a ureteral stent, and an IV indigo carmine dye test. Stanhope and others at the Mayo Clinic reported their experience with 18 patients who had suture entrapment and secondary ureteral obstruction following major pelvic operations for benign conditions. In none of these patients was the diagnosis made at the operation of injury. However, early diagnosis in the postoperative period was facilitated by comparison of preoperative and postoperative serum creatinine levels. The mean change in the serum creatinine level in patients with unilateral obstruction was an increase of 0.8 mg/dl.

Maintaining Ureteral Consciousness. The level of consciousness about the ureter in the mind of the gynecologic surgeon has much to do with primary prevention of ureteral injury. It begins preoperatively with a careful assessment of the extent of pelvic disease, preoperative cystoscopy and excretory urography when indicated, and preoperative ureteral catheterization in a few selected patients. It must continue with an appropriate level of consciousness throughout the entire pelvic dissection and especially at certain key points in the operation. A heightened level of ureteral consciousness is required to prove ureteral integrity at the end of each major gynecologic procedure, and it must continue in the postoperative period. Patients with persistent postoperative fever, persistent abdominal distention, costovertebral angle tenderness, hematuria, and, of course, urinary drainage from the vagina should be investigated with postoperative excretory urography and other appropriate studies to determine the presence of ureteral injury as early as possible in the postoperative period in case it was not recognized at operation. "Out of sight, out of mind" is unfortunately responsible for many ureteral injuries and the damage they can cause to the kidneys. "Taking a chance," either consciously or subconsciously, that the ureter is in its normal position anatomically, is uninvolved with the disease process, and will not or has not been injured at operation is not a wise course.

Types of Sequelae and Ureteral Surgical Injury

A ureter may be injured during the course of an easy, difficult, or careless pelvic dissection. It may be kinked or partially or completely ligated with a suture. It may be crushed with one or more clamps. It may be cut or partially or completely resected either unintentionally or sometimes intentionally, usually during the course of operations for gynecologic malignancy. Or it may undergo ischemic necrosis of the ureteral wall, usually from stripping the blood supply from around the ureter for several centimeters, especially in the presence of infection and irradiation. The injuries may be single or multiple, unilateral or bilateral.

Depending on many different circumstances, a variety of sequelae to ureteral injury may occur. When injury has been minor, spontaneous resolution and healing may occur with only temporary and minimal interference with function. A minor degree of kinking or obstruction may eventually disappear. Spontaneous healing of more serious injuries, such as ureterovaginal fistula, is possible but should not be expected and is unlikely to occur without impaired kidney function.

When it is not recognized that the ureter has been ligated completely, it is inevitable that the kidney function will gradually disappear. Silent atrophy of the kidney as a result of unrecognized ureteral ligation at gynecologic operations is very uncommon, although undoubted cases have been reported. More commonly, infection supervenes, and the patient may be seriously ill before the ureteral ligation is recognized. A silent renal atrophy is possible only in the absence of infection. There have been reports of ureteral obstruction lasting more than 100 days in which relatively normal kidney function returned after relief of the obstruction.

When the ureter is ligated, the pressure within the lumen of the ureter rapidly rises from a mean of approximately 6.5 mm Hg to 50 to 75 mm Hg within 1 hour. Patients experience flank pain at the higher pressures. The pressure gradually decreases over time, and the pain subsides. Atrophy in the distal renal nephron begins in the first week and extends to the cortical region in the second week. Protein casts are deposited in Bowman's space of glomeruli. Urine escapes by pyelocanalicular and pyelosinus backflow and by the lymphatic and venous systems. The afferent arterioles are constricted, and the glomerular filtration rates and total renal blood flow are reduced. Even incomplete obstruction can destroy kidney function given sufficient time. The recovery potential following release of obstruction is dependent on many factors, including the length of time the kidney has been obstructed, the completeness of the obstruction, the presence or absence of infection, the degree of backflow, and the degree of functional impairment of the opposite kidney. After the obstruction is relieved, most kidneys will continue to show some impairment of function. The longer the obstruction is allowed to exist, the more likely the function of the affected kidney will be severely or permanently impaired.

A ligated ureter usually will not stay ligated. As pressure distends the lumen and pushes the thinned ureteral wall more and more tightly against the suture, an ischemic area will rupture, allowing escape of urine. A urinoma will form that is sometimes palpable on pelvic or abdominal examination. If a fresh incision exists in the vaginal apex, urine will dissect there and escape, thus creating a ureterovaginal fistula. Sometimes an overzealous stripping of the blood vessels of the periureteral arterial plexus occurs during extensive hysterectomy for invasive cervical cancer. Necrosis of the ureteral wall with extravasation of urine can result.

Eventually, at the site of injury, a stenosis of the ureteral lumen will develop and will progressively cause more and more hydroureter and hydronephrosis above. When the stenosis is complete, the kidney function is in danger of being lost if the stenosis is not relieved.

Bilateral ureteral injury with obstruction will quickly result in uremia if not relieved. Ligation of the ureter of a solitary kidney will also result in uremia.

Surgical Repair of Ureteral Injuries

The ureter should be handled gently, preferably with the operator's fingers or with noncrushing clamps or forceps. The ureter should not be freed from its bed except as necessary for repair of the injury. However, mobilization of the ureter must always be sufficient to allow repair without tension on the suture line. Reanastomosis or reimplantation must always be done without tension.

The ureter is capable of regenerating uroepithelium and smooth muscle, thus bridging the site of repair. This will be facilitated by carefully approximating the ureteral muscularis and mucosa, by taking measures to avoid tension on the suture line, and by minimizing urinary leakage through the repair site. The success of repair will also depend on the health of the tissues that surround the ureters. If the periureteral tissue is rigid and fibrotic, there will be interference with healing of the repair site, but healing can be enhanced by wrapping the ureter in omental fat.

The controversy regarding use of ureteral stents in repairing ureteral injuries has not been resolved. We prefer to use stents across the repair site to stabilize and immobilize the ureter and to prevent angulation during healing, to encourage an orderly regeneration of uroepithelium and smooth muscle, to reduce urinary extravasation at the repair site, and to prevent stenosis of the lumen. The stent must fit the lumen size comfortably without distending the ureter. Single- or double-ended pigtail or J catheters are popular since they are not likely to be pushed into the bladder after placement. A Silastic tubing is well tolerated without causing inflammation but becomes soft and pliable at body temperature with a tendency to be expelled unless reinforced with stainless steel wire in the lumen. A plastic pediatric feeding tube of proper caliber may also be used as a stent.

The decision regarding urinary diversion above the repair site is critical to the success of the repair. Unless the repair is a simple one with no technical difficulty and minimal urinary extravasation, diversion of the urinary stream with percutaneous nephrostomy is required. A Jackson-Pratt drain should be placed extraperitoneally to suction extravasated urine from the repair site.

The repair should be made with a minimal number of fine delayed absorbable no. 4-0 sutures, either polyglycolic acid or polyglactin. Permanent nonabsorbable sutures should not be used. The lumen at the repair site should be enlarged by angulated incisions. The edges should be carefully approximated without strangulation. Magnification with surgical loupes may be helpful in suture placement.

As emphasized earlier, the best time to diagnose and repair ureteral injury is at the operation of injury. Should the diagnosis not be made until later, there is controversy regarding the correct timing of surgical repair. A number of different circumstances must be considered, including the patient's condition; the extent, location, and duration of the injury; and the condition of periureteral tissues. In general, it is now regarded as acceptable to attempt early repair of simple injuries in the immediate postoperative period should circumstances be ideal. Otherwise, percutaneous nephrostomy is the treatment of choice with definitive repair delayed until the induration of periureteral tissues has resolved. This may require a delay of 6 to 8 weeks, during which time a percutaneous nephrostomy may be required. Those situations in which extensive devascularization of the ureter has occurred, as with extensive hysterectomy, should not be repaired immediately. Definitive repair also should be delayed in the presence of significant pelvic infection, cellulitis, or postoperative abscess formation or in any patient with a chronic, debilitating disease in whom primary healing of the repaired ureter may be impaired.

Finally, one additional principle must be emphasized. If a suture is found tied around a ureter, it should, of course, be removed. Inspection may then reveal a fairly normal-appearing ureter. However, if the suture has been in place for any length of time (sometimes even less than 30 minutes), a defect will usually develop in the wall of the ureter after the suture has been removed. The defect may not be apparent at the time of disligation but may develop later. Simple disligation of a ureter is not usually sufficient for a ureter that has been ligated more than a few minutes. If possible, a stent may be placed above the site of injury through the cystoscope and left in place 10 to 14 days. Ureteroneocystostomy or ureteroureterostomy will be necessary in most cases. The same principle applies to a crushing injury to the ureter.

Ureterovaginal Fistula. Although mentioned earlier as a sequela of ureteral injury, ureterovaginal fistula deserves additional comment. Urine may drain from the vagina in the immediate postoperative period if the ureter has been cut and not ligated. This is unusual since the ureter is ordinarily included in a ligated pedicle. Usually after a febrile postoperative course that also may be complicated by persistent abdominal distention and costovertebral angle tenderness, urine may begin leaking from the vagina in 10 to 14 days as the suture loosens or the ureteral wall undergoes necrosis. When ureteral damage results from stripping the ureter of its blood supply as in extensive hysterectomy for cervical cancer, a longer period of time may elapse before ischemia has progressed to the point of necrosis of the ureteral wall and fistula formation. When urine begins draining through the vagina, the patient's clinical condition may improve temporarily and the fever may subside.

Excretory urography is one of the first studies indicated after appearance of urine from the vagina. Renal ultrasonography will also be useful. Hydroureteronephrosis will usually be present on the same side as the injured ureter. A concomitant vesicovaginal fistula can be ruled out by instilling methylene blue dye into the bladder through a transurethral catheter. If a tampon placed in the vagina is wet but unstained with methylene blue, a ureterovaginal fistula is suspected. The location of the fistula can be identified more precisely by cystoscopy, with inspection of ureteral orifices for efflux of indigo carmine dye injected intravenously, and by attempting passage of a ureteral catheter on the side suspected of injury by these previous tests. As a rule, the ureteral catheter will not pass above the point of injury. A retrograde pyelogram will confirm the point of obstruction. It may also demonstrate periureteral extravasation of dye and a fistula tract. If by chance a catheter can be passed beyond the point of obstruction, it should be left in place for 14 to 21 days, during which time the ureteral wall will hopefully heal. Before the catheter is removed a retrograde pyelogram should be done to demonstrate healing of the fistula.

Usually a ureteral catheter cannot be passed beyond the obstruction. In these patients, there is a tendency for progressive stenosis of the ureter to occur at the site of injury with the passage of time. If a repair operation is to be delayed, such patients must be followed by excretory urography or renal scan every 2 to 3 weeks to be certain that the kidney is still functioning well. A reasonable period of expectant management may be permissible without establishing kidney drainage with percutaneous nephrostomy. However, cessation of urinary leakage through the vagina usually associated with recurrent pyelitis is an ominous sign and an indication that the obstruction is complete. Urinary drainage by either percutaneous nephrostomy or ureteral reimplantation will be required to salvage kidney function. Cessation of urine flow through a ureterovaginal fistula is almost never a good sign that the ureter has healed without stenosis. Only when excretory urography is normal, demonstrating an intact ureter, can it be considered a good sign.

Whether done immediately or delayed, the preferred operation to correct a ureterovaginal fistula associated with injury to the lowest

3 to 4 cm of ureter is reimplantation of the ureter into the bladder. Fashioning a bladder flap may be necessary to bridge the gap if a direct ureteroneocystostomy cannot be done without tension.

Bilateral Ureteral Ligation. Bilateral ureteral ligation is a rare complication of gynecologic surgery but must be suspected when a patient is anuric in the first 24 to 48 hours following surgery. Soon thereafter the blood urea nitrogen (BUN) and creatinine levels begin to rise, and the patient may experience back pain and bilateral costovertebral angle tenderness. Failure to relieve the obstruction will result in progressive uremia and renal failure. Ureteral obstruction is easily demonstrated by excretory urogram, which will show evidence of bilateral faintly visible nephrograms and hydroureteronephrosis on delayed films. Before emergency surgery is undertaken, cystoscopy with attempt to pass catheters beyond the point of obstruction should be done but will usually be unsuccessful. When the diagnosis of bilateral ureteral ligation is certain, a decision must be made regarding the most appropriate management. If the diagnosis is made within the first 48 to 72 hours, before the patient is profoundly ill from uremia, and other circumstances are favorable, immediate operation to perform disligation and establish ureteral patency is the treatment of choice. Bilateral percutaneous nephrostomies are preferable to attempting disligation or anastomosis in a seriously ill patient who is not a candidate for surgery. After nephrostomy drainage is established, ureteral repair may be deferred for several weeks until the patient is a good surgical candidate. But before a definitive operation is done, another attempt at passing ureteral catheters beyond the point of obstruction should be made upward through the cystoscope or downward through the nephrostomy tube. Whether the problem is solved by operative or nonoperative means, the patient must have frequent excretory urograms to assess ureteral patency and kidney function.

Ureteroureterostomy. The ureteroureteral anastomosis may be done at the time of injury (always preferable) or at the time of subsequent delayed repair. The procedure is performed for injuries just above or below the pelvic brim. Ureteroureterostomy is technically difficult to do on the lowest 3 to 4 cm of ureter, and the results are not satisfactory. A transperitoneal approach is preferred. The site of injury is usually in the vicinity of the common iliac artery and vein and the hypogastric artery and vein, so dissection of the ureter must be done carefully. Locating the site of injury is facilitated by cystoscopic passage of a ureteral catheter as high up as possible. The peritoneum is incised and reflected along the lateral border of the ureter. The point of injury is identified, and the traumatized ureteral tissue is excised to the point of viability along with edematous, indurated, and/or infected periureteral tissue and suture fragments. The freshened ends of the ureter must have an adequate blood supply. If there is doubt about this, fluorescein dye and Wood's lamp may be used for confirmation. The ureter above and below the site of injury must be mobilized sufficiently to allow anastomosis without tension (Figure 13.9). The free ends of the ureter are cut obliquely and spatulated for 5 mm to ensure a wide lumen at the anastomotic site. A double-ended J or pigtail ureteral stent is passed upward to the renal pelvis and downward into the bladder. With the ureter splinted by a splint of proper caliber, the two ends of the ureter are brought together snugly by four to six interrupted no. 4-0 delayed absorbable sutures placed through the ureteral wall above and below. The sutures are tied securely but without strangulating the tissue. Before the abdomen is closed, extraperitoneal drainage of the operative site is established by placing a Jackson-Pratt drain through a small stab wound. The drain should not touch the site of anastomosis.

Silastic tubing may be used as an alternate method of splinting the ureter. It may be passed to the renal pelvis. A suture should be placed to identify the end that is passed into the bladder. If there is any question regarding whether or not the stent is patent and draining, the end in the bladder can be easily identified and withdrawn through the urethra with a cystoscope. It can then be irrigated whenever urinary drainage seems inadequate.

If the anastomosis is entirely satisfactory, we tend to use only the indwelling stent left in place for 14 to 21 days, depending on a variety of circumstances. However, in difficult cases

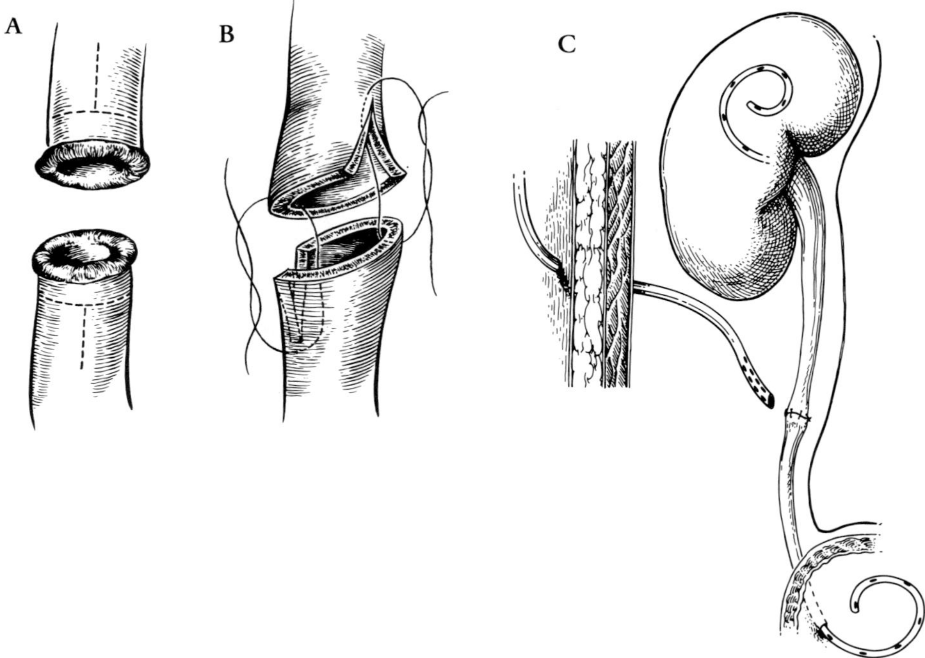

Figure 13.9 **A,** The ends of the ureters are trimmed and spatulated. **B,** Fine delayed absorbable sutures are used to approximate the ends of the ureter. **C,** The anastomosis is done over a double J or pigtail stent. A suction catheter is placed retroperitoneally to the side of the anastomosis. (From Rock JA and Thompson JD: TeLinde's operative gynecology, ed 8, Philadelphia, 1996, Lippincott-Raven.)

where the outcome is not as certain, we may also consider placing a percutaneous nephrostomy drainage tube for decompression of the anastomotic site until healing is secure. In addition, in cases where the anastomosis lies in a bed of indurated, infected, and unhealthy tissue, an omental pedicle should be mobilized and sutured beneath the ureter.

Ureteroneocystostomy. When injury has occurred in the lowest 4 to 5 cm of the ureter, implantation into the bladder gives better results than attempts to do a ureteroureterostomy. Again, a transperitoneal approach is usually preferred. The ureter may be directly implanted into the bladder through a small incision in the bladder wall. This operation is referred to as the "fish-mouth" procedure since the ends of the ureter are incised on each side for approximately 5 mm to produce ureteral flaps that are sutured to the bladder wall from inside out. The no. 4-0 delayed absorbable sutures are placed on each side of the incision in the bladder wall in such a way that the split ends of the ureter are held open. Any remaining defect in the bladder is closed with no. 3-0 delayed absorbable sutures. Adjacent peritoneum may be used to reinforce the anastomosis and to prevent tension on the suture line. A ureteral stent is usually employed (Figure 13.10).

Because of the high incidence and associated risk of vesicoureteral reflux, this simple direct implantation of the ureter into the bladder is not used often, although it has served gynecologic surgeons well on emergency occasions when more complicated operations are not appropriate. In the absence of UTI or chronic renal disease, ureteral reflux, if it occurs, has not usually produced serious problems such as chronic recurrent ascending infection with loss of renal function.

The preferred method of ureteral implantation is the submucosal tunnel technique, since it more nearly establishes the normal intramural anatomy of the ureter and avoids reflux. The distal ureter is carefully dissected from the site of traumatic injury. All devitalized tissue is debrided. Unhealthy tissue at the distal end of the ureter must be excised. Mo-

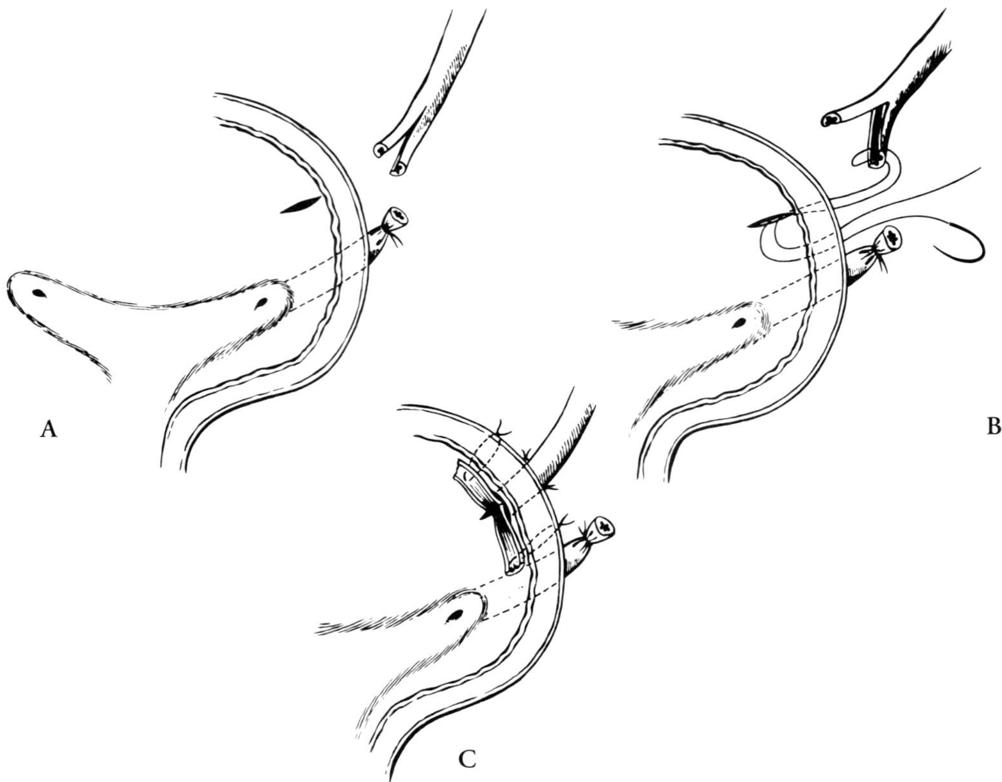

FIGURE 13.10 Ureterovesical implantation, fish-mouth technique. **A**, Excised free end of ureter is spatulated for 1 to 2 cm. New ureteral orifice has been made by scalpel above the trigone in position to reach excised ureter. **B**, Each end of ureteral flap is anchored with a mattress suture of no. 4-0 delayed absorbable suture and passed through new ureteral orifice and full thickness of bladder wall. **C**, Bladder flaps are tied on external surface of the bladder and reinforced with seromuscular sutures in bladder wall and ureter at site of implantation. (From Rock JA and Thompson JD: TeLinde's operative gynecology, ed 8, Philadelphia, 1996, Lippincott-Raven.)

bilization of the ureter and bladder base should help ensure that the anastomosis can be made without tension. The bladder dome is opened transversely. The most dependent portion of the posterior bladder wall that will allow a tension-free anastomosis is selected, and a submucosal tunnel 1 to 1.5 cm long is fashioned. The incision is extended through the entire thickness of the bladder wall at the superior margin of the tunnel. The ureter is drawn through and sutured to its new orifice at the lower end of the tunnel. Size 4-0 delayed absorbable sutures and an indwelling splinting catheter are used. The transverse incision in the anterior bladder wall is closed longitudinally in two layers. A Jackson-Pratt drain is placed extraperitoneally, and the operative site is peritonized. The splinting catheter is left in place for 14 to 21 days before removal (Figure 13.11).

An alternate method of using a submucosal tunnel for ureteroneocystostomy is shown in Figure 13.12.

When extensive trauma to the lower ureter results, after debridement, in a ureter that is too short for ureteroneocystostomy without tension, some special techniques of bridging the gap must be employed. The bladder base can be mobilized by incising the lateral peritoneal attachments of the bladder. The bladder base can be sharply dissected and mobilized from its fascial attachments to the vagina. The ureter can be mobilized for a greater distance above. If anastomosis without tension is still not possible, a transverse incision should be made in the anterior bladder wall. A finger

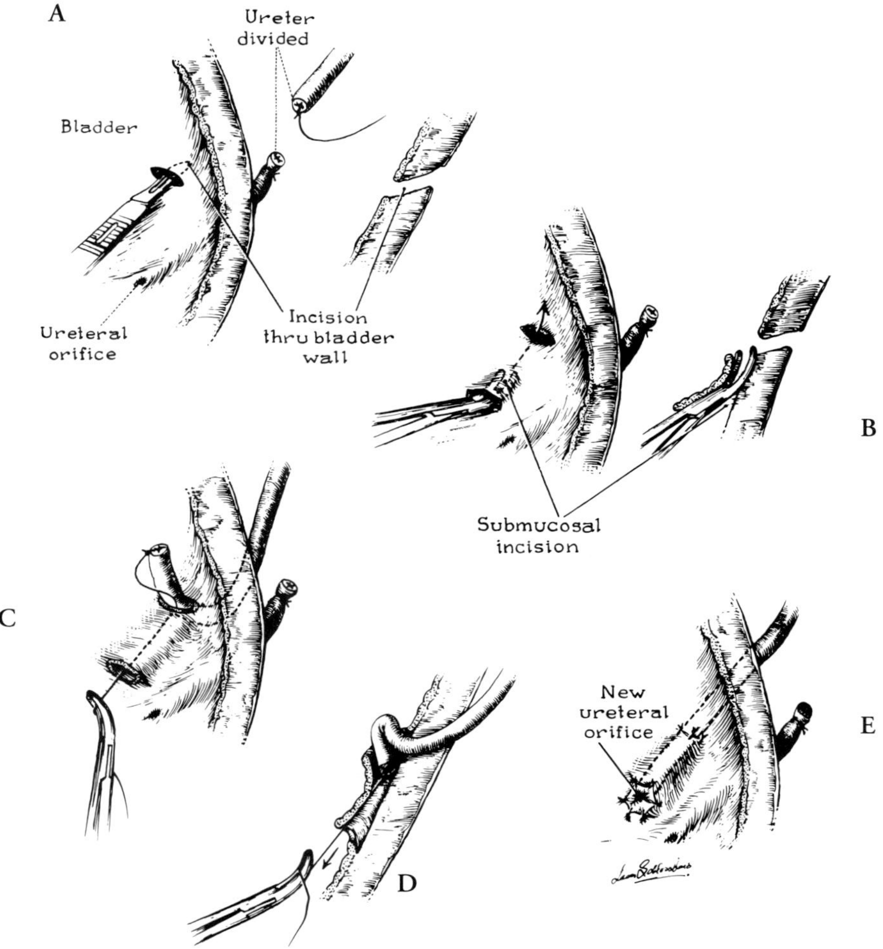

FIGURE 13.11 Submucosal tunnel technique of ureterovesical implantation. **A**, Bladder mucosa is incised above trigone at planned site of implantation; oblique incision through bladder wall is made from exterior. **B**, Adson's clamp is inserted through new orifice and tunneled beneath mucosa for 1.5 cm to upper mucosal incision. **C**, Ureter is guided through bladder wall and upper mucosal orifice and gently guided through submucosal tunnel. **D**, By traction suture. **E**, Mucosa-to-mucosa anastomosis of ureter to bladder; upper incision is closed with fine suture. (From Rock JA and Thompson JD: TeLinde's operative gynecology, ed 8, Philadelphia, 1996, Lippincott-Raven.)

is placed inside, and the cornu of the bladder is elevated and sutured to the psoas muscle tendon as high as possible. The transverse bladder incision then should be closed longitudinally. Following mobilization and elevation of the bladder to the psoas muscle, a ureteroneocystostomy usually can be done without tension according to the most appropriate technique (Figure 13.13).

This psoas muscle hitch method of bridging the gap between the bladder and a short ureter is superior to developing a Boari flap of bladder muscle. The flap procedure is frequently associated with reflux and may also become ischemic and stenotic. Ingenious techniques of developing bladder flaps should be used as a last resort to bridge the gap to a short ureter, especially if the pelvis has been irradiated.

Other Procedures. In special circumstances, transvaginal repair of simple injuries to the lower ureter may be possible and entirely satisfactory, especially if the injury was the result of a vaginal operation in which only the lowest 3 cm of ureter was involved. The surgeon must be familiar with the anatomy of the lower ureter as seen through the vagina. De-

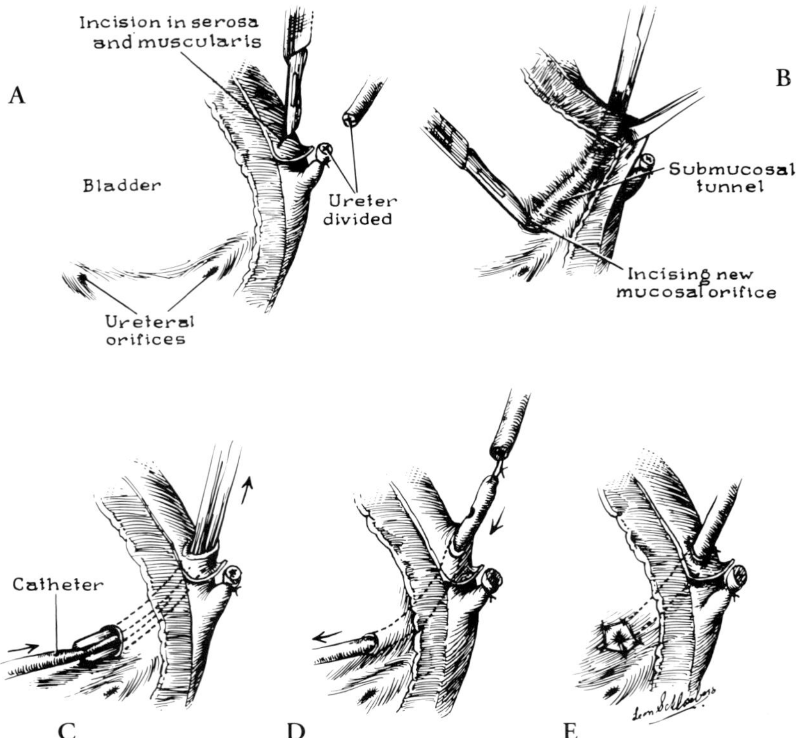

FIGURE 13.12 Submucosal tunnel procedure for ureterovesical anastomosis, external technique. **A**, Oblique incision through bladder wall initiated on external surface. **B**, Adson's clamp passed through muscular wall and beneath mucosa for 1.5 cm (tunnel formation); bladder mucosa incised over tip of clamp at site of new ureteral orifice. **C**, Small, straight rubber catheter drawn through tunnel and bladder wall. **D**, Catheter sutured to excised ureter; ureter guided through bladder wall and tunnel by traction on catheter. **E**, Mucosa-to-mucosa anastomosis of ureter to bladder. (From Rock JA and Thompson JD: TeLinde's operative gynecology, ed 8, Philadelphia, 1996, Lippincott-Raven.)

pending on the extent and location, the injury may be repaired with simple disligation or with ureteroneocystostomy. A simple technique of implanting the ureter into the bladder is used.

Other more complicated procedures, usually beyond the scope of most gynecologic surgeons, have been used in the management of patients with extensive ureteral injuries. Transureteroureterostomy (i.e., anastomosis of the upper ureter on one side to the intact ureter on the opposite side through a subperitoneal tunnel) can be successful in selected cases. However, this creates the potential for compromising the function of the kidney on the normal side.

Many ingenious techniques have been devised for substituting a segment of ilieum for a ureter that has been damaged too extensively to be repaired or implanted into the bladder. In fact, the ileum may be substituted for the entire course of the ureter on one or both sides. Of course, both ureters may be anastomosed to the ileum, which may then be anastomosed to the skin (Bricker's pouch) if the bladder is not present or is not suitable for implantation. Continent reservoirs may also be constructed. An anastomosis of the ureters to the intact colon or to the skin should be avoided.

Autotransplantation of the kidney to the pelvis may be considered in a patient who has no possibility of repair of the injured ureter and poor function of the opposite kidney. It has the potential for excellent results when done by an experienced renal transplant surgeon.

OPERATIVE INJURIES TO THE BLADDER

Currently throughout the world, injury to the bladder resulting from prolonged obstructed

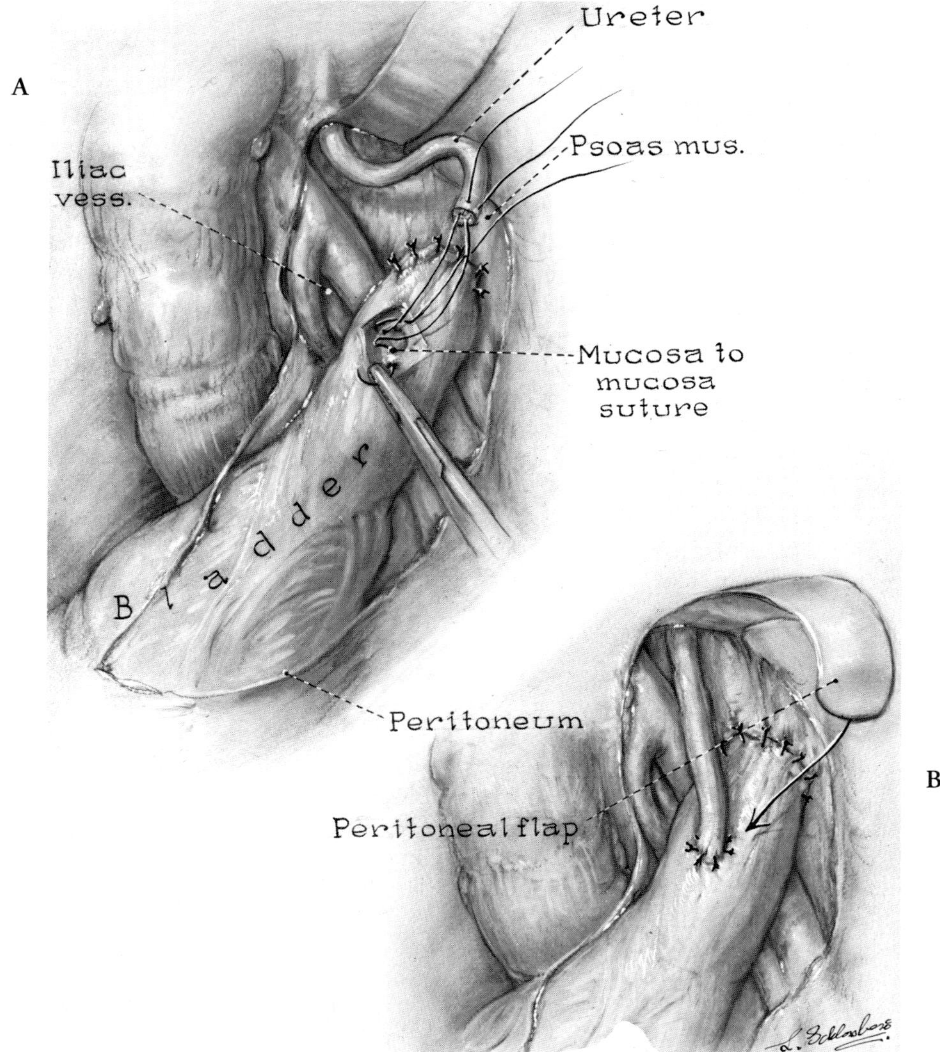

Figure 13.13 Ureterovesical anastomosis of the short ureter–psoas muscle hitch procedure. **A**, Bladder peritoneum is incised from lateral pelvic wall, and bladder is mobilized and anchored to psoas muscle at pelvic brim (psoas muscle hitch) near site of planned ureterovesical anastomosis. Mucosa-to-mucosa anastomosis of ureter to bladder is performed. **B**, Ureterovesical anastomosis is reinforced with fine serosal sutures, and peritoneum is advanced over anastomotic site. (From Rock JA and Thompson JD: TeLinde's operative gynecology, ed 8, Philadelphia, 1996, Lippincott-Raven.)

labor and producing vesicovaginal fistula causes tragic social and medical problems for many young women, especially in developing countries. Tahzib studied 1,443 patients with vesicovaginal fistulas between 1969 and 1980 in northern Nigeria, the largest series of vesicovaginal fistulas ever reported. Eighty-three percent were caused by prolonged obstructed labor. Thirteen percent resulted from gishiri cut, a traditional tribal practice of cutting the anterior vaginal wall with a razor blade to treat a variety of conditions, including backache, dyspareunia, goiter, infertility, and obstructed labor. In this series, only 1% of vesicovaginal fistulas resulted from operative injuries to the bladder. This major health problem for women in the world deserves greater attention. Measures for prevention must include not only improved and accessible medical services (including contraceptive services) but also universal education and improved status for women. For example, in Ethiopia young girls are frequently married by age 10 years. There are only 87 hospitals and 800 physicians for 45 million people. Under these circumstances, it is difficult to conceive of doing cesarean sections for all patients with obstructed labor and providing contraceptive services to teenagers.

In many countries in the world, including the United States, vesicovaginal fistulas of obstetric etiology are rare. In the last 35 years at Grady Memorial Hospital in Atlanta, no vesicovaginal fistulas have occurred during the course of 200,000 obstetric deliveries in a predominantly black and indigent population. Major contributors to prevention have been improved management of obstetric problems and techniques of delivery, especially the more liberal use of CS with a concomitant decrease in the number of difficult forceps operations, and improvements in the management of labor. Because of this, few American gynecologists have or need experience in the repair of vesicovaginal fistulas of obstetric origin.

In the United States today, the most important measures for reducing the incidence and morbidity of vesicovaginal fistulas must be directed to proper techniques of gynecologic surgery. Although a rare vesicovaginal fistula results from other causes (e.g., radiation therapy for cervical cancer), gynecologic surgery is the most common cause in the United States and in many other developed countries in the world. The principles of repair of vesicovaginal fistula of obstetric etiology established in the nineteenth century, although still applicable today for obstetric fistulas, must be modified for management of the postsurgical fistulas of the twentieth century. The modifications are necessary to recognize that the subject of vesicovaginal fistula is not a single subject but many different subjects depending on etiology, location, size, and so forth. This discussion will emphasize the subject of trauma to the bladder that results from the operative management of gynecologic disease and conditions.

Prevention

When gynecologic surgery is done properly, postoperative vesicovaginal fistula may be a very rare occurrence. Between 1970 and 1985, 24,883 patients underwent major gynecologic surgery at the Mayo Clinic. Only one patient developed a postoperative vesicovaginal fistula (after primary radical hysterectomy). In spite of this commendable record, the bladder is the most common site of injury to the urinary tract, and injury to the bladder occurs in approximately 1% of patients undergoing gynecologic surgery.

Bladder injury occurs most commonly during hysterectomy. Among 75 posthysterectomy vesicovaginal fistulas reported by Miller and George, 54 followed TAH, 18 followed total vaginal hysterectomy, and 3 followed radical hysterectomy. None followed subtotal abdominal hysterectomy. In the past several decades, total rather than subtotal abdominal hysterectomy has become the routine procedure. Thus injury to the base of the bladder occurs more frequently now than before and is reported in 0.5% to 1% of patients undergoing a TAH. To reduce the risk of vesicovaginal fistulas, Baker has suggested that the gynecologic surgeon consider leaving the cervix in place by doing a subtotal hysterectomy when the cervix is benign, when removing the uterine corpus will remove the patient's pathologic condition, and where conditions such as endometriosis or tubo-ovarian abscess may increase the risk of bladder injury when the cervix is removed. We subscribe to this principle of using good surgical judgment. No operation, even total hysterectomy, should be routine for every patient. However, it should be possible for the experienced gynecologic surgeon to remove the cervix without injury to the bladder in almost every patient. This is especially important in younger women who may be exposed to cervical carcinogens for many years to come. Certainly if in the judgment of the gynecologic surgeon the danger of removing the cervix is greater than the danger of leaving it in, a subtotal hysterectomy should be done. In addition, the danger of removing the cervix includes the possibility of injury not only to the bladder but also to the ureters and rectum as well.

The gynecologic surgeon must be thoroughly familiar with the anatomy of the bladder and especially its boundaries in relation to the lower uterine isthmus, the cervix, the anterior vaginal wall, and the anterior abdominal wall. The base of the bladder above the interureteric ridge rests on and is draped across the anterior lower uterine isthmus, the cervix, and the upper anterior vaginal wall. The bladder trigone is at a lower level below the cervix and rests on the middle third of the anterior vaginal wall. It is therefore less susceptible to injury when a total hysterectomy is done. If the bladder is injured during its dissection away from the cervix and vagina, the injury will fortunately be located above the interureteric ridge and trigone in almost all cases. This anatomic relationship is extremely important to keep in mind (Figure 13.14). If the surgeon places a cystoscope in the bladder and watches as an index finger pushes up along the anterior vaginal wall, it is easy to confirm this relationship.

Injury to the bladder base is more common with TAH than with vaginal hysterectomy. This is probably because patients with more extensive disease (e.g., endometriosis, large leiomyomas, tubo-ovarian abscess, and gynecologic malignancy) are usually operated on abdominally. Some injuries to the bladder base from TAH are caused by vigorous or blunt dissection in the wrong plane between the bladder base and the pubovesicocervical fascia covering the cervix. This dissection should be done precisely and sharply with scissors. Pushing down vigorously against the vesicovaginal and vesicocervical attachments with a stick sponge will weaken the bladder wall and should be discouraged. Injury may also result from inadequate mobilization of the bladder inferiorly and laterally so that clamps and sutures placed in the cardinal ligament and anterior vaginal cuff may "pinch" the bladder base (Figure 13.15). The vesicocervicovaginal space should be developed completely and the bladder thoroughly mobilized both inferiorly and laterally. Pulling the uterine corpus superiorly while retracting the bladder base anteriorly will facilitate the full development of the vesicocervicovaginal space and help prevent bladder injury. Also helpful is the utilization of the intrafascial technique of removing the cervix, described by Richardson of the Johns Hopkins Hospital in 1929. This technique employs an inverted V or T incision in the pubovesicocervical fascia covering the cervix. When the cervix is removed, the anterior arm of the cardinal ligament clamp is placed beneath the pubovesicocervical fascia and actually peels the fascia off the cervix as the clamp is closed. Clamps placed beneath the pubovesicocervical fascia will not include the bladder wall. But before clamps are placed across the cardinal ligaments and before an incision is made in the anterior vaginal wall, the vesicocervicovaginal space must be developed completely and the bladder thoroughly mobilized inferiorly and laterally. Some vesicovaginal

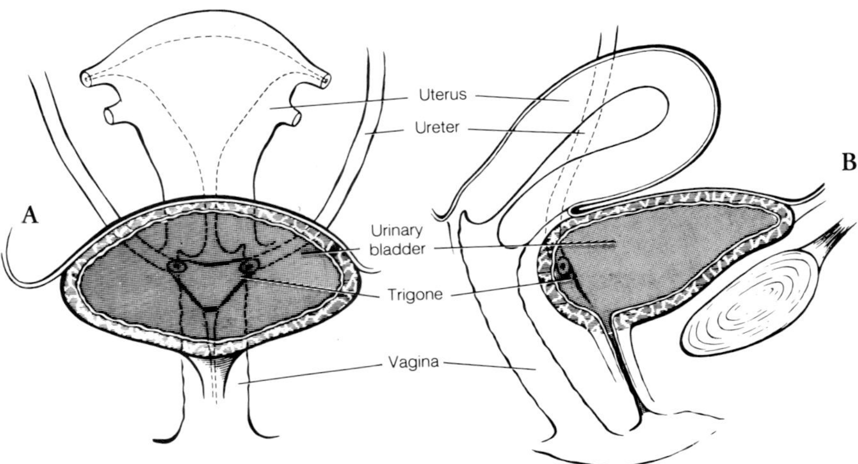

Figure 13.14 **A,** Anterior view of the normal anatomy of ureter and bladder. The terminal end of the ureter passes medially from the lateral pelvic wall and crosses over the anterior fornix, where it enters the trigone of the bladder, which rests on the upper one third of the anterior vaginal wall. **B,** Sagittal view of anatomic relationship of ureter and bladder base. Note that the ureter enters the trigone in the area of the upper one third of the vagina. (From Rock JA and Thompson JD: TeLinde's operative gynecology, ed 8, Philadelphia, 1996, Lippincott-Raven.)

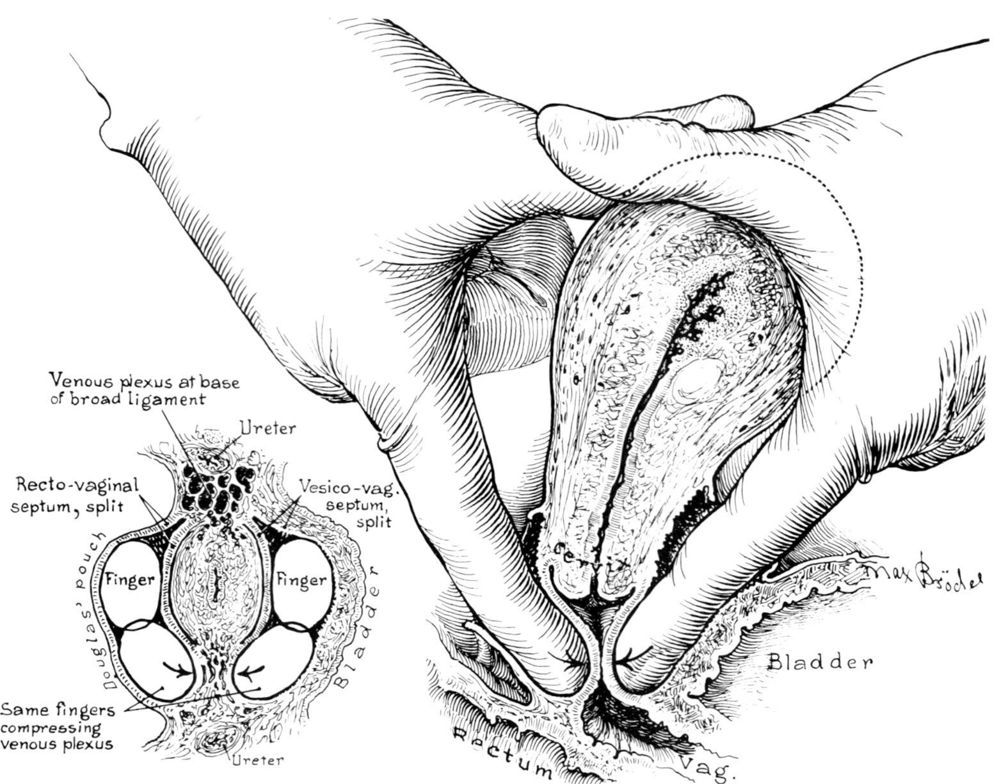

FIGURE 13.15 TAH. Testing the depth of the anterior and posterior dissections. The *inset* shows the method of segregating the vascular plexus on each side into a narrow zone adjacent to the basal segment of the broad ligament. (From Richardson EH: Surg Gynecol Obstet 48:248, 1929.)

fistulas are caused by placing sutures through the bladder base when the cuff is sutured. Again, this results from inadequate mobilization and retraction and inadequate exposure, possibly because of a limited incision in the abdominal wall. When a suture catches the bladder base, gradual necrosis of the bladder wall will lead to vesicovaginal fistula formation about 7 to 10 days after surgery.

As with TAH, the bladder is most frequently injured during total vaginal hysterectomy when the bladder is dissected away from the cervix and the lower anterior uterine isthmus. The location of the injury is the same as in TAH. Ordinarily the plane of dissection between the cervix and the bladder is easy to identify and relatively avascular. The dissection may be facilitated by injecting sterile saline beneath the vaginal mucosa. We prefer not to use a vasopressor in the injecting solution because of experimental and clinical evidence that vasopressors interfere with the local tissue resistance to infection, and vasopressors are not necessary to control bleeding. An incision is made through the vaginal mucosa at its point of attachment to the cervix just above the anterior lip. It is extended to the 3 and 9 o'clock positions laterally. The blade of the electrosurgical Bovie unit, slightly bent at the tip, can be used for this dissection. Strong traction is made downward with a tenaculum placed on the anterior cervical lip. Counteraction beneath the bladder above will expose the tissues that need to be cut. With the tip pointed downward toward the cervix, the operator uses the Bovie as an artist might use a brush on a canvas, taking brief short strokes and cutting tissue that is under stretch. Small bleeding vessels may be coagulated along the way. Scissor dissection with the handles elevated and the points against the uterus can also be used. However, dissection with a gauze-covered finger is too blunt and may injure the bladder wall. When the dense attachment of the bladder has been dissected through, the loose space above, covered only with the vesicouterine peritoneal reflection, can be felt with the finger. It should not be pushed away. With proper retraction and lighting, the peritoneum can be identified and incised. When one is able to see contents of the peritoneal cavity through this small incision, confirming that the peritoneal cavity and not the bladder has been entered, the incision in the peritoneum may be extended. After this, the bladder is held up and out of the way with a retractor.

Unfortunately, development of the vesicocervical space is not always easy. When the dissection is misdirected and difficult, or there is abnormal adherence between the bladder and cervix, troublesome bleeding may obscure the operative field. The dissection may be too deep in the muscle of the anterior lower uterine isthmus, the most frequent and understandable error since the operator may be trying to avoid bladder injury. Or the dissection may be too anterior, and the bladder wall may be weakened or the bladder actually entered. Hopefully, the operator will not extend the dissection into the bladder before recognizing the error. If there is a possibility that the dissection has been directed too far anteriorly, two helpful suggestions may prevent final entry into the bladder. First, one should place an instrument (a Kelly's clamp or uterine sound will do nicely) into the bladder through the urethra. The tip of the clamp can be felt and will identify the location of the bladder wall in relation to the plane of dissection. Second, 5 ml of methylene blue or indigo carmine can be instilled into the bladder through the urethra. The dye will stain the bladder mucosa, making it more visible to avoid an entry into the bladder. This simple measure can be adopted as a routine before every vaginal hysterectomy, since it is not possible to predict when the dissection will be difficult. It might be especially useful in patients who have had a previous CS and who can be expected to have an abnormal adherence between the bladder and the lower anterior uterine isthmus. Previous cesarean section or sections can cause this difficulty when total vaginal or total abdominal hysterectomy is done. As the number of CSs in the United States increases, the frequency with which the gynecologic surgeon encounters this problem will also increase. In our experience, the dissection is less difficult with vaginal hysterectomy because one is able to pass an instrument transurethrally to help identify a proper plane for dissection. Of course, transurethral passage of an instrument is also possible when one is operating abdominally if the patient has been positioned in Allen Universal stirrups for the operation.

Jaszczak and Evans have proposed an intrafascial technique for vaginal hysterectomy designed to avoid injury to the bladder. Although the idea may be sound, it has not been evaluated extensively. Bladder injury and vesicovaginal fistula resulting from vaginal hysterectomy are best prevented by finding the proper plane of dissection between the bladder base above and the cervix and anterior lower uterine isthmus below, by opening the vesicouterine fold of peritoneum carefully, by mobilizing the bladder laterally by clamping and cutting the bladder pillars on each side, by placing a retractor beneath the bladder for its protection, and by properly placing clamps and ligatures on small bites of paracervical and parametrial tissue as close to the uterus as possible.

Although much less common, there are several other situations in which bladder injury may occur. Finding a proper plane for dissection for repeat anterior colporrhaphy may be difficult. The operator will be well advised to inject sterile saline just beneath the vaginal mucosa and dissect carefully between the mucosa and the fascia beneath rather than trying to find a deeper plane for dissection. If a patient has had a previous suprapubic urethropexy, the space of Retzius may be difficult to develop in any subsequent operation because of adherence between the anterior bladder wall, the symphysis, and the pubic rami. Bleeding from large veins may obscure dissection in the proper plane. Sharp dissection will usually be required to release the dense fibrous adhesions. Blunt dissection is risky and may tear into the bladder. Repeat suprapubic urethropexy and Goebel-Stoeckel suburethral sling operations must be done with care to avoid injury to the anterior bladder wall.

When the bladder is mobilized away from the uterus to perform a CS (especially a repeat CS), abnormal adherence and dissection in the wrong plane may result in accidental bladder entry. This may be even more likely when the CS is done for emergency indications.

Distortion of the lower anterior uterine isthmus by leiomyomas can cause difficulty in finding the proper plane of dissection beneath the bladder (Figure 13.16, *A* to *C*). If uterine leiomyomas obstruct the vesical neck, considerable hypertrophy of the bladder muscle will result over time much the same as in men with benign prostatic hypertrophy. The bladder can become so large as to reach to the umbilicus and will definitely be encountered when an incision is made in the lower abdomen (Figure 13.16, *D*). In extreme cases, it may be necessary to begin a midline incision above the umbilicus, identify the top of the bladder, dissect it free laterally, and fold it down over the patient's thighs to gain access to the pelvis to remove the leiomyomas. Fortunately, such extreme cases are not as commonly seen in the United States today as in previous decades. Before a transverse Maylard or Cherney incision is made across the lower abdomen, the bladder must be completely empty. Otherwise, the incision may go through the dome of the bladder.

It is common practice in reperitonizing the pelvis following subtotal abdominal hysterectomy to pull the edge of the bladder peritoneum over the top of the cervix and suture it posteriorly. If removal of the cervix either vaginally or abdominally is indicated later, the operator will do well to recognize this abnormal position of the bladder. The exact boundaries of the bladder will be obscured by its abnormal adherence to the top and back of the cervix.

In patients with the Mayer-Rokitansky-Küster-Hauser syndrome (congenital absence of the uterus and vagina), the Abbe-Wharton-

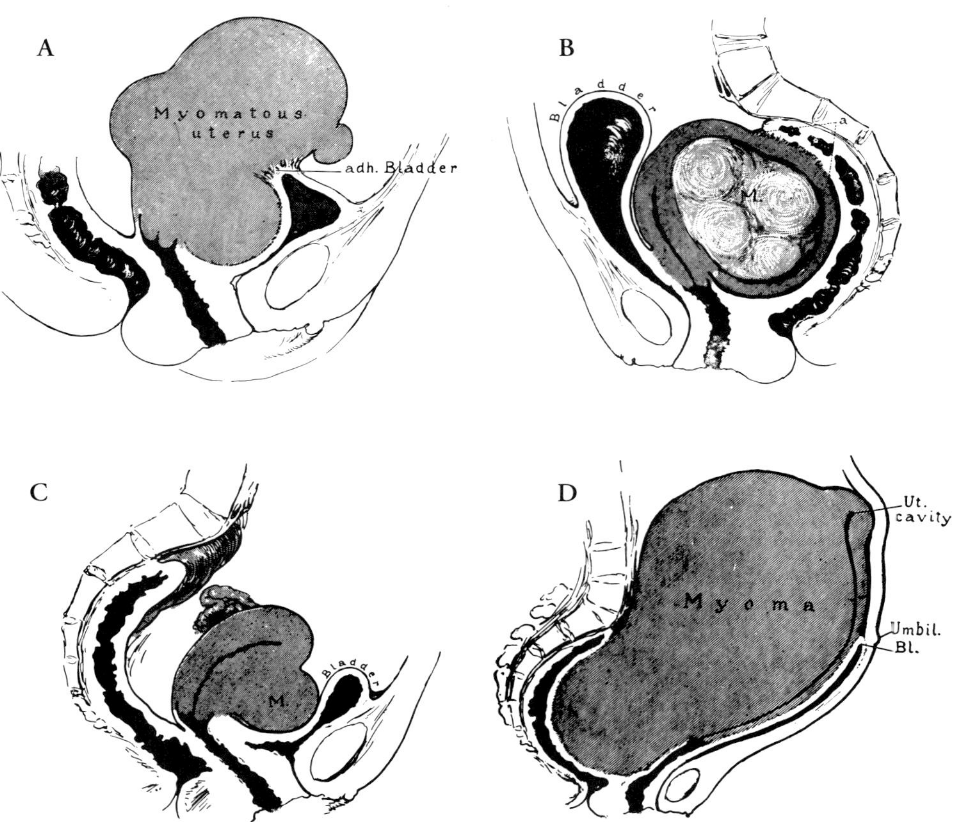

FIGURE 13.16 Abnormal relationships of the uterus and bladder caused by uterine leiomyomas. **A,** The uterus is abnormally adherent to the bladder. **B,** A large posterior myoma pushes the bladder against the symphysis. **C,** An anterior myoma pushes the bladder against the symphysis. **D,** A large myoma causes obstruction of the vesical neck with bladder hypertrophy extending to the umbilicus. (From Kelly HA and Cullen TS: Myomata of the uterus, Philadelphia, 1909, WB Saunders Co.)

McIndoe operation attempts to develop a space for sexual intercourse between the urethra and bladder anteriorly and the rectum posteriorly. Definition of the correct plane for dissection can be easy or difficult. A difficult dissection can be facilitated by placing an instrument in the urethra and double-gloved finger in the rectum to avoid injury to the bladder and rectum.

One percent to 3% of patients will develop vesicovaginal fistulas following extensive hysterectomy as primary treatment for invasive cancer of the cervix. If such an extensive operation is done after previous pelvic irradiation, the incidence is higher. Boronow and Rutledge found a fourfold increase in vesicovaginal fistula formation even when simple hysterectomy was performed on patients who had been previously irradiated. Hysterectomy, especially extensive hysterectomy, further compromises the blood supply to the base of the bladder already compromised by the obliterative endarteritis caused by radiation treatment. Since postirradiation fistulas are the most difficult to close, every precaution should be taken to prevent their formation. For example, Petty, Lowy, and Oyama reported five patients who developed new cervical or uterine neoplasms 1 to 27 years after initial radiation therapy for cervical cancer. All underwent abdominal hysterectomy without postoperative vesicovaginal fistula formation. Success was attributed to cautious surgical technique and the use of an omental pedicle graft to bring new vascularity to the bladder base. Such a preventive measure makes good sense.

Operative Repair of Bladder Injury

If any injury to the bladder can be discovered at the time of operation and properly repaired, a vesicovaginal fistula is not likely to occur. Indeed, the gynecologic surgeon can even be encouraged to intentionally enter the bladder when it is necessary to define the anatomic limits of a pathologic condition or a proper plane for dissection. In an analysis of 77 cases of recognized bladder entry, Everett and Mattingly found no case that failed to heal when repaired at the time of initial entry. The unirradiated bladder is rich in collateral blood supply. Defects will heal when closed correctly. Healing is not dependent on the placement of large numbers of sutures. Accurate placement of a correct number of sutures is more important. Injury to the bladder should not be considered a dreaded and serious complication when recognized and closed correctly.

One of the most frequent sites of injury is the dome of the bladder, especially when an incision is made in a patient who has had a previous incision or in a patient in advanced pregnancy. Fortunately, entry into the bladder dome is easy to recognize and repair. A double-layered closure should be used. An initial continuous no. 3-0 delayed absorbable suture in the bladder mucosa is reinforced by another layer of continuous suture in the bladder muscle. In closing the abdominal incision later after the operation is completed, the site of repair of the bladder should be extraperitonized if possible. An indwelling transurethral catheter should be left for 7 to 10 days postoperatively, depending on the extent of injury, security of repair, and whether the repair site in the dome is intraperitoneal or extraperitoneal.

Injuries to the base of the bladder are more likely to result in fistula formation if they are not recognized and repaired correctly, probably because the bladder base is the most dependent portion. Injury in this site is usually the result of removal of the cervix in total hysterectomy, either abdominal or vaginal. Once the bladder has been entered, the dissection can be redirected into the proper plane and the operation completed before the defect is repaired. Then the extent of the injury should be carefully determined, especially its proximity to the ureteral orifices inside the bladder. Ordinarily, the defect will be above the interureteric ridges. If one cannot be certain of the location of the ureteral orifices, injection of 5 ml of indigo carmine dye IV will cause blue urine to spurt from the orifices in 3 to 5 minutes. Ureteral catheters can be passed, but this is not often necessary. After careful assessment of the limits of the defect in all directions, the first layer of closure is usually a continuous no. 3-0 delayed absorbable suture that carefully approximates and inverts the bladder mucosa, making certain that the closure goes beyond the limits of the defect (Figure 13.17). The security of this first layer of closure should be tested by instilling 200 ml of sterile milk or dilute methylene blue into the

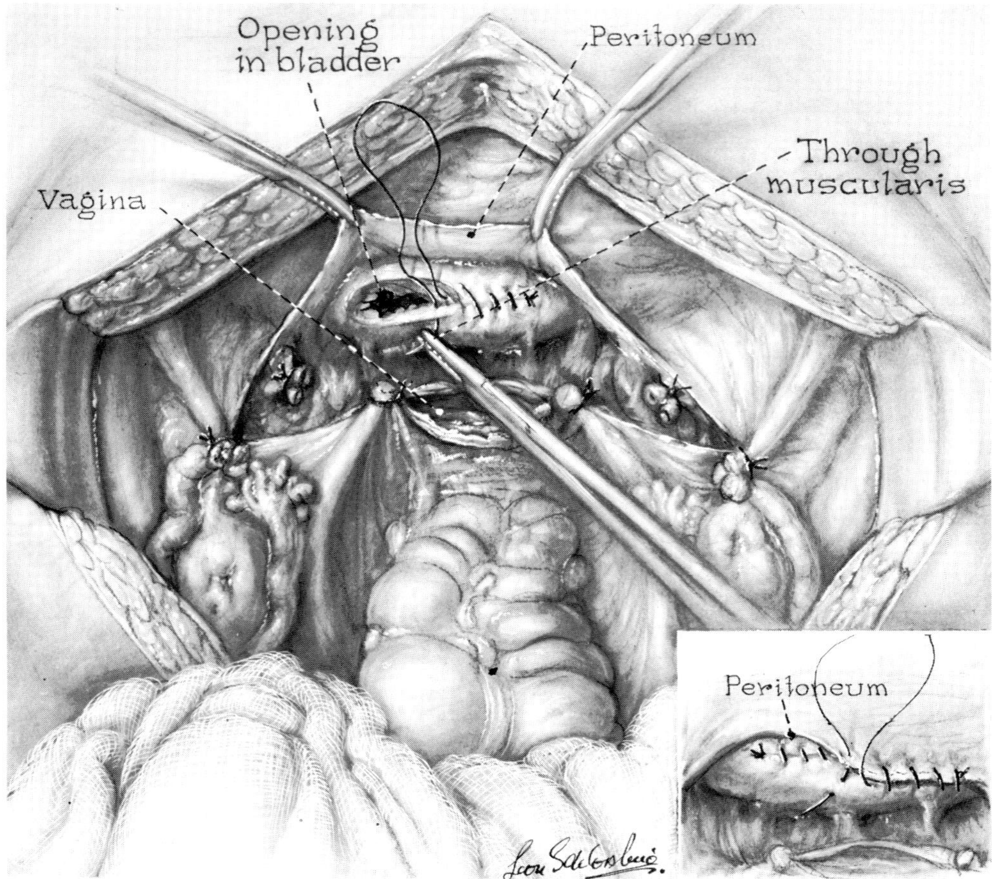

FIGURE 13.17 Closure of accidental opening of bladder during TAH. The bladder is closed with a continuous no. 3-0 delayed absorbable suture, inverting mucosa into the bladder. A second muscular layer of interrupted sutures should support the initial layer. The suture line is then reinforced by bringing the peritoneum over the operative defect and suturing it in place. *Inset,* Advancement of the bladder peritoneum over the suture line will protect it from postoperative pelvic cellulitis and make certain that no leakage occurs into the vagina. (From Rock JA and Thompson JD: TeLinde's operative gynecology, ed 8, Philadelphia, 1996, Lippincott-Raven.)

bladder. Any point of leakage should be reinforced with additional sutures. The closure must be without tension. There usually will have been sufficient mobilization of the bladder base to accomplish closure without tension, especially if the suture line is horizontal. A second and possibly third layer of sutures is placed in the bladder muscle. These may be interrupted vertical mattress sutures or continuous sutures.

The next step is most important. The edge of the vesical peritoneum is sutured to the anterior vaginal cuff. This superimposes another layer between the bladder mucosa and the vaginal vault and also helps to relieve tension on the suture line. This is a very useful maneuver and should be used to reinforce any suspected area of weakness in the bladder wall, even if the bladder has not actually been entered. The peritoneum is interposed between the vaginal apex and the bladder defect.

Finally, at the end of the operation, cystoscopy should be performed. Indigo carmine is injected IV. Dye spurting from each ureteral orifice assures ureteral integrity. The bladder side of the repair should be inspected for bleeding. The bladder should be kept as empty as possible with an indwelling suprapubic or transurethral catheter. A suprapubic catheter is preferred if the repair of the defect involves the bladder trigone. The catheter may be removed in 7 to 14 days depending on the extent of the defect, the security of the closure, the condition of the tissues, and the condition of the patient.

This technique of repairing a defect in the bladder base may be used whether the defect results from abdominal or vaginal hysterectomy.

Whenever there is a suspicion of bladder weakness or injury but the problem is not clearly determined by examination, 200 to 300 ml of sterile saline should be instilled to distend the bladder wall. A careful inspection for leakage of fluid or weakness in the muscle should be carried out. If there is any concern that the bladder wall is too thin at a particular point, several sutures should be placed for reinforcement.

Vesicovaginal Fistula

Diagnosis. When a patient develops a vesicovaginal fistula, review of the operative and postoperative record may show nothing to suspect that such a complication would occur. On the other hand, such a review will often show that the patient had serious and extensive pelvic disease (e.g., adhesions, pelvic infection, malignancy, or endometriosis) at operation or a history of previous irradiation or gynecologic surgery. In addition, the operation may have been difficult because of obesity, difficulty with anesthesia, or poor exposure. The postoperative recovery may have been complicated by persistent fever, unusual discomfort, prolonged ileus, or hematuria. When the index of suspicion that a vesicovaginal fistula is developing is high, sterile saline stained with methylene blue may be instilled into the bladder through a urethral catheter for confirmation.

When definite leakage of urine from the vagina does begin sometime during the first 3 weeks of the postoperative period, successful treatment depends on an exact diagnosis. Leakage may come through the urethra, through a vesicovaginal fistula, through a ureterovaginal fistula on one or both sides, or through various combinations of any and all of these. A fistula opening may or may not be found by speculum examination of the vaginal apex. Regardless, a dilute solution of indigo carmine should be instilled in the bladder. If the fistula is small and cannot be demonstrated with the patient in the dorsal lithotomy or knee-chest position, the three-tampon test of Moir should be used. In this test, three dry cotton tampons are placed in the vagina in tandem. Dilute indigo carmine (200 ml) is instilled into the bladder. The patient is asked to walk about for 10 to 15 minutes and the tampons are then removed and inspected. If the lowest tampon is wet and stained blue, the patient is presumed to have transurethral incontinence. If the upper tampon in the vaginal apex is wet and blue, a vesicovaginal fistula is indicated. If the upper tampon is wet but not stained blue, a ureterovaginal fistula is indicated. The vaginal orifice of the fistula may be located by noting the position of the staining or wetness on the tampon in relation to its position in the vaginal apex.

These simple tests require confirmation by excretory urography and cystoscopy. If the vesicovaginal fistula is so large that the bladder cannot be distended with running sterile water, air cystoscopy may be done using a regular cystoscopy with the patient in the knee-chest position. The bladder orifice of a small fistula can be demonstrated more easily if a probe is passed into the bladder through the vaginal orifice of the fistula. Cystoscopy is necessary to confirm the diagnosis of vesicovaginal fistula, to look for other fistula sites, and to determine the size of the fistula and its proximity to the ureteral orifices and the internal urethral meatus. Intravenous indigo carmine spurting from the ureteral orifices will rule out ureterovaginal fistula or fistulas.

There may be very little incontinence of urine when the vesicovaginal fistula is very small, and the amount may depend on the position of the patient. Voiding in large quantities may still be possible. More often with larger fistulas, the incontinence is total and voiding is absent. With such marked incontinence, the patient will become depressed and reclusive. Some patients will become frankly psychotic with despair if the incontinence remains for an extended period. The vulva becomes excoriated, reddened, and tender from the constant wetness of urine and the irritation of perineal pads, diapers, and rubber pants. The odor of urea is offensive and embarrassing to the point of precluding social interaction.

Except for vulvar irritation, most traumatic fistulas are painless. However, fistulas caused by radiation may be painful and surrounded by encrustations and necrotic tissue.

Management and Repair. For this discussion of management, vesicovaginal fistulas will be divided into two categories: simple and complicated. Simple vesicovaginal fistulas are small fistulas that develop as a result of relatively minor trauma to an otherwise healthy bladder during the course of total hysterectomy, abdominal or vaginal. Complicated fistulas are those that are large, develop in irradiated tissue, involve a ureteral orifice, follow extensive hysterectomy, are associated with other fistulas (rectovaginal, ureterovaginal, urethrovaginal, etc.), or have had previous unsuccessful attempts at repair. The major emphasis in this discussion will be given to the management of patients with simple vesicovaginal fistula, by far the largest group.

Simple Fistulas

Preoperative Management. Very little can be done to help patients stay comfortable before the fistula repair is done. A vulvar cream containing lanolin may relieve some discomfort. Some patients prefer to spend long periods of time in the water (tub, swimming pool, etc.). A variety of collecting devices have been tried, but none is satisfactory because of the difficulty in maintaining a tight seal. Some patients prefer to wear a transurethral catheter in the bladder with a leg bag, and some do not. Some patients require tranquilizers, and some do not. Antibiotics are not required since cystitis and pyelitis are uncommon in patients with vesicovaginal fistulas. Patients who are postmenopausal or young patients who have had both ovaries removed should be placed on oral estrogen therapy. The patient will always need the encouragement and support of her family and friends and her physician during this trying time.

In our experience, spontaneous healing of a simple vesicovaginal fistula is a rare occurrence. However, it has been reported to occur in 15% to 20% of patients. The fistula must be very small, and there must be no extenuating circumstances. Spontaneous healing may be facilitated by inserting a large-caliber indwelling transurethral catheter. If the transvaginal urinary leakage stops, there is a better chance of spontaneous healing. In 3 weeks, the catheter is removed and the outcome determined. Fistulas that heal spontaneously have been known to break apart at some later time. Superficial fulguration of the epithelium of the fistula tract has been successful in closing some minute vesicovaginal fistulas according to some reports. Most experts do not recommend fulguration since it may increase rather than decrease the caliber of the opening. Prolonged catheter drainage with or without fulguration is only occasionally successful and is usually just another disappointment for a patient who desperately wants the urine leakage to stop now!

Timing of repair. Simple vesicovaginal fistulas, that is, those small fistulas that develop from relatively minor trauma to an otherwise healthy bladder during the course of total hysterectomy (abdominal or vaginal), usually can be repaired soon after the diagnosis is made. The concept of early repair began with the report of Collins and Prent in 1960. In 15 cases, all were operated on within 8 weeks and most within 4 weeks of the diagnosis; successful closure was achieved in 13 cases on the first attempt. The fistulas resulted from operations for benign disease. All repairs were done transvaginally. In another report in 1971, Collins and others achieved a 72.4% success rate on the first attempt in 29 patients without malignancy when the operation was done in the first 2 weeks after fistula discovery. The most recent Tulane University experience with early repair was reported by O'Quinn and others in 1984. Fifty-four patients with acute fistulas were operated on within 8 weeks of the discovery of the fistula; 43 of the 54 patients were operated on within 4 weeks. Of the 54 patients, 48 had successful first-attempt closures; 4 patients were reoperated on 12 days later with successful closure on the second attempt. The remaining 2 patients had a successful second attempt at closure 5 and 6 weeks later. All patients had a simple transvaginal operation for repair of the fistula.

Cruikshank reported his experience with early repair of posthysterectomy vesicovaginal fistulas. A simple transvaginal repair was used in nine patients who had a simple, small, noncomplicated fistula. All of the repairs were done between 13 and 19 days following diagnosis, which was made between 6 and 15 days following hysterectomy. The repair was successful in all nine patients on the first attempt. Our experience at Emory University in a small series of patients has been similar.

The Tulane University group has always advised preoperative administration of cortisone to bring about "resolution of inflammatory reaction" around the fistula. However, our experience and that of others suggest that success can be regularly achieved without using steroids. We no longer recommend their use. Also, based on our experience and that of others, we have no hesitation in recommending repair of simple posthysterectomy vesicovaginal fistula shortly after the diagnosis is made. A simple transvaginal Latzko's partial colpocleisis will be successful in more than 90% of cases.

Some experienced gynecologists prefer to wait 3 to 4 months to repair a vesicovaginal fistula, believing that the tissue should be completely normal and without edema, infection, or induration so that dissection, suturing, and healing will result in the best possibility of successful closure. Of course, in the meantime the patient is terribly uncomfortable, irritated, embarrassed, depressed, and restricted in social and marital activities. During this long period of delay, not having been completely convinced that she should be required to remain in this unpleasant state for months, she is likely to seek other advice. Much unpleasantness can be avoided by offering an early repair with a reasonable chance of success.

Consider the following description of two hypothetical groups of patients. In the first group, 100 patients with simple posthysterectomy vesicovaginal fistulas have a repair after 3 months with a 95% success. The remaining 5 patients are repaired successfully with a second attempt 3 months later. The calculated total number of "wet days" in this group is 9,450. Contrast this with 100 patients in the second group who have a repair within 1 month with an 80% success. The remaining 20 patients have a successful attempt at repair 3 months later. The calculated total number of wet days in this group is 4,800. In other words, in this hypothetical comparison, the total number of wet days is reduced by almost 50% by early repair. Certainly it is always important to think in terms of a successful repair. However, it is also important to do everything possible to relieve the patient's misery. If given the facts and an opportunity to choose, most patients will opt for early repair.

The Operation. All simple posthysterectomy vesicovaginal fistulas should be closed with a transvaginal Latzko's partial colpocleisis. The operation is simple and rapid, and recovery is prompt with few postoperative problems. Extensive transperitoneal-transvesical operations are not needed for these simple fistulas. Many complicated vesicovaginal fistulas also can be closed with a transvaginal operation.

Our preference is to place all patients in the dorsal lithotomy position for transvaginal vesicovaginal fistula repair. We never use the Sims' lateral or knee-chest position.

Cystoscopy should be available to examine the bladder orifice of the fistula just before the repair is done and at the end of the operation. If necessary, ureteral catheters may be inserted.

Most fistulas can be repaired with a basic instrument set with a few additions such as a long-handled, fine-pointed scissors; long delicate needle holders; an assortment of long scalpel handles and blades; the extender for the needle point Bovie; and an assortment of vaginal retractors.

Some of the technical difficulties in performing transvaginal fistula repair may be solved by innovations in the use of special instruments. However, it is more likely that the technical difficulties will be solved by improved exposure and accessibility of the fistula itself. In the ordinary case, sufficient exposure is achieved simply by retracting the vaginal walls. On the other hand, if there is a narrow subpubic arch, a rigid vagina scarred from recent operations, a tight vaginal outlet, or a well-supported deep vaginal vault, an episiotomy or Schuchardt's incision may be needed and should be made without hesitation. Such a simple maneuver can convert a technically difficult and possibly unsuccessful operation into an easy operation with a successful result. Sometimes exposure can be improved by placing traction sutures in the vaginal wall at several points around the fistula or by placing a pediatric Foley catheter into the bladder through the fistula. When the bulb is distended in the bladder and downward traction is made on the catheter, the fistula is more accessible to repair.

If the fistula is fresh and the tissue is still indurated, the entire tract, including the vaginal and bladder orifices, should be excised (Figure 13.18, *A*). Excision of the tract will inevitably result in a larger hole in the bladder, and this is as it should be. For the repair of a fresh fistula to be successful, all of the indurated tissue surrounding the tract must be removed so that normal tissue can be approximated for better healing (Figure 13.18, *B* and *C*).

If the fistula is mature and the tissue is no longer indurated but completely epithelialized with fibrotic scar tissue, the tract may not need to be excised. Instead, when sufficient mobilization has been achieved, the tract may simply be entropionized by the first layer of sutures.

The vaginal mucosa must be widely mobilized for several centimeters around the fistula in all directions. If the fistula is fresh, wide mobilization will also include an extensive debridement of all infected and indurated tissue back to healthy bleeding tissue. Success in closing a fresh fistula depends on the willingness of the operator to remove all the unhealthy tissue.

The correct plane of dissection is just beneath the vaginal mucosa. All fascia and muscle should be left intact on the bladder side. Dissection in the proper plane is facilitated by injecting sterile saline just beneath the vaginal mucosa. The vaginal mucosa must be excised for several centimeters around the fistula, leaving the vaginal vault denuded. Care should be taken not to enter the peritoneal cavity. Any entry should be closed.

The vaginal orifice of the fistula will always sit on the transverse scar across the top of the vagina where the anterior and posterior vaginal cuff were approximated at the time of hysterectomy or were allowed to heal together in case the vagina was left open.

Our suture preference for closure of vesicovaginal fistula is no. 3-0 delayed absorbable polyglactin or polyglycolic acid suture. This suture retains its tensile strength longer and causes less tissue reaction than catgut and may be partly responsible for better results with early repair. The suture is swaged onto a fine, semimalleable, round needle of small caliber. This suture can be used for all layers and does not need to be removed. Permanent sutures should not be used.

The bladder orifice of the fistula is carefully closed by approximating the bladder mucosa with a horizontal line of no. 3-0 delayed absorbable interrupted mattress sutures (Figure 13.18, *D*). This first row of sutures is most important to the success of the closure. Good bites should be taken in healthy tissue to close the hole securely. This first layer of closure should be tested by instillation of 200 ml of dilute methylene blue or sterile milk into the bladder. Any point of leakage is noted and reinforced with additional sutures. If the first layer of closure is watertight, the chance of success is good. A vesicovaginal fistula repair is not likely to be successful unless the bladder orifice of the fistula is closed securely.

After the bladder orifice of the fistula is closed securely, the closure is reinforced by two or three additional lines of no. 3-0 delayed absorbable horizontal mattress sutures to approximate the anterior and posterior vaginal walls (Figure 13.18, *E*). This approximation of broad surface to broad surface without tension is another important axiom in fistula repair. If the layers do not come together without tension, a wider dissection of the bladder base is required. The excess vaginal mucosa is trimmed, but generous flaps are left for approximation without tension. All suture lines should be transverse to the longitudinal axis of the vagina (Figure 13.18, *F*).

At the end of the operation, cystoscopy is performed to confirm hemostasis in the bladder and to test for ureteral integrity. Five milliliters of indigo carmine dye is injected IV. In 3 to 5 minutes, the dye will spurt from each ureteral orifice, proving that the intramural portion of the ureter has not been incorporated in the repair.

There is no hard and fast rule about postoperative bladder drainage after initial repair of simple vesicovaginal fistulas. The determination regarding the type and duration of bladder drainage should be made at the end of the operation and will depend on a number of factors, including the operator's impression of the security of the closure and the location of the repair site inside the bladder. When the operation has gone extremely well and there is every reason to expect a successful result, we have left an indwelling transurethral catheter

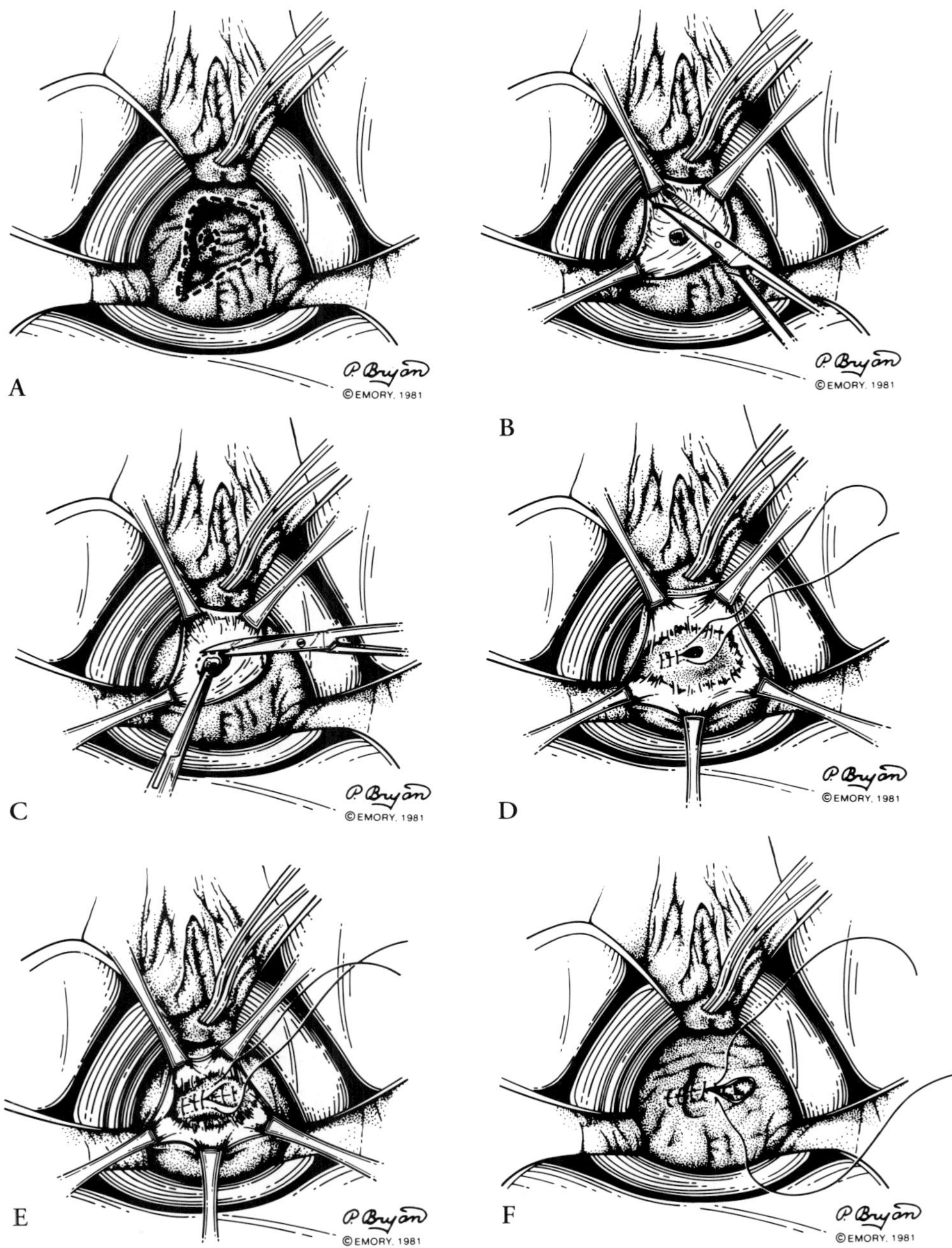

Figure 13.18 Operation for a closure of a simple posthysterectomy vesicovaginal fistula by the Latzko technique. **A,** Ureters have been catheterized to prevent encirclement of a ureter by a suture. Incisions about the fistula opening and about the indurated vaginal mucosa margin are marked by the dotted lines. **B,** The vaginal mucosa is dissected back from the fistula opening for a sufficient distance to mobilize the bladder wall about the fistula. **C,** The fistula tract is sharply and completely excised. **D,** No. 3-0 delayed absorbable interrupted mattress sutures taken parallel to the edge of the fistula tract are used as the initial suture line, inverting tissue into the bladder. The security of the closure should be tested by instillation of 100 to 200 ml of dilute methylene blue or sterile milk into the bladder. **E,** Two or three additional layers should approximate the bladder muscularis broad surface to broad surface without tension. Size 3-0 delayed absorbable interrupted mattress sutures should be used. **F,** The vaginal mucosa is closed transversely with interrupted no. 3-0 delayed absorbable sutures. (Copyright, Emory University, 1981.)

in overnight and removed it the next morning. The patient is discharged after demonstrating a satisfactory voiding pattern with instructions to void frequently and not allow the bladder to become distended. On other occasions, the catheter has been left in for 7 to 14 days. Suprapubic catheters are very seldom used after initial repair of a simple posthysterectomy vesicovaginal fistula.

Care must be taken to make certain that the catheter does not become obstructed. Many good vesicovaginal fistula repairs have been ruined by an obstructed catheter and an overdistended bladder. Patients who are discharged with a catheter should be instructed to cut the catheter with scissors and remove it immediately if there is any sign of inadequate drainage and bladder distention and then to report for assessment of the situation. The best way to keep the catheter open and to avoid UTI is to ensure an adequate intake of fluids sufficient to produce output of a large quantity of dilute urine, preferably at least 100 ml/hour.

Complicated Fistulas

Again, complicated vesicovaginal fistulas are those that are large; those that have had previous unsuccessful attempts at repair; those that involve one or both ureters, vesical neck, or urethra; those that are associated with intestinal fistulas; and those that result from extensive surgery or radiation therapy (or both) for gynecologic malignancy. Many complicated fistulas can still be closed using a transvaginal Latzko's partial colpocleisis. The basic principles of fistula repair just described for simple fistulas will apply when complicated fistulas are repaired and perhaps should be applied even more strictly. For very difficult fistulas, the repair may need to be done in stages. For example, if a patient has a radiation-induced vesicovaginal and rectovaginal fistula associated with bilateral ureteral stenosis and hydroureter, such a complicated problem may require three operations for solution. The first operation would include bilateral ureteroileocutaneous anastomosis and colostomy; the second operation would be closure of the fistula; and the third operation would be closure of the colostomy and anastomosis of the ileal conduit to the bladder if the second operation is successful.

Special techniques and management principles may be needed to achieve continence in a patient with a complicated vesicovaginal fistula. Although early repair of simple posthysterectomy vesicovaginal fistula is appropriate, the repair of a complicated fistula should be delayed until the tissue around the fistula is healed and healthy. This may take 3 to 6 months. In the case of a radiation-induced fistula, it may take much longer, and one must wait until the effects of the acute irradiation injury have subsided and the fistula has finally achieved its ultimate size. This may take many months, during which ERT may be useful.

Very complicated vesicovaginal fistulas may require a combined transvaginal-transvesical-transperitoneal approach for final closure. A dissection from below might mobilize the vaginal mucosa and possibly bring in a bulbocavernosus fat flap. The vaginal mucosa is closed before making an abdominal incision to open the bladder. Ureteral catheters can be passed and the bladder mucosa mobilized and closed. Then a peritoneal flap and/or omental flap can also be mobilized to be interposed between the bladder and vagina. A technique of abdominal closure of vesicovaginal fistula using bisection of the bladder and wide mobilization of the bladder from the vagina, allowing for closure of the vaginal and bladder in separate layers, described by O'Connor, is illustrated in Figure 13.19.

When local tissue healing is impaired by radiation, diabetes, chronic infection, or other factors, hard sclerotic and fibrotic tissue with occluded arterioles may extend a considerable distance beyond the fistula margins. Neovascularization from fresh, well-vascularized tissue pedicles brought to the fistula site will support the repair and promote healing. Small arterioles migrate from the normal tissue pedicles into the ischemic tissues at the repair site.

Various techniques of autografting have been described by Zacharin. The most common techniques are the bulbocavernosus labial fat pad, the omental pedicle grafts, and the gracilis muscle graft. These techniques may be extremely useful in surgical closure of complicated vesicovaginal fistulas since the key to successful closure of these fistulas is to bring in a new blood supply to devitalized vaginal and bladder tissues.

After repair of a complicated vesicovaginal

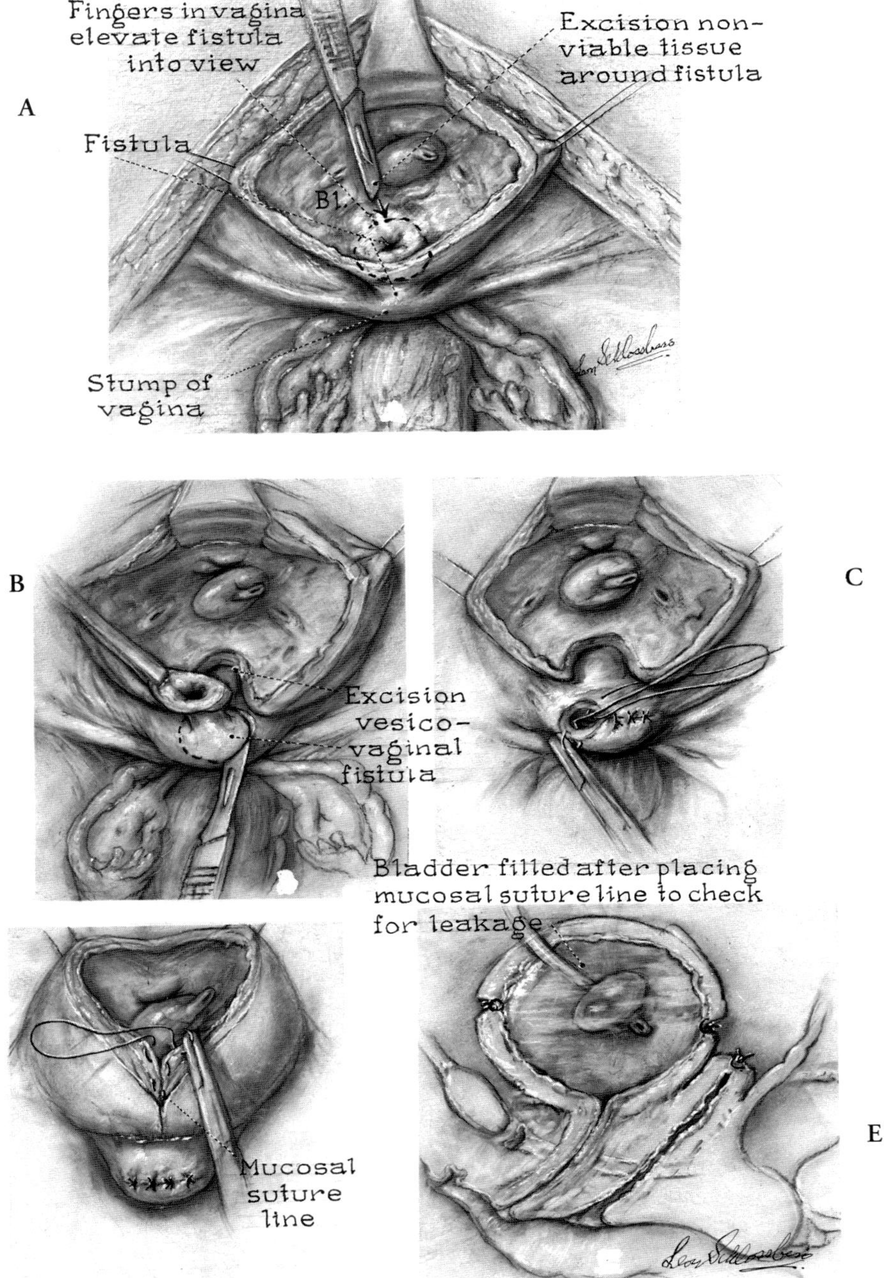

FIGURE 13.19 Transabdominal, transvesical closure of vesicovaginal fistula. **A**, A longitudinal incision in the bladder dome illustrates the vesical opening of the fistula and its relationship to the vagina and the ureteral orifices. **B**, The incision in the bladder wall is extended around the orifice of the fistula. The fistulous tract and its vaginal orifice are completely excised. **C**, Interrupted no. 3-0 delayed absorbable sutures are used to close the vaginal opening in one or two layers. **D**, A continuous no. 3-0 delayed absorbable suture closes the bladder mucosa longitudinally. **E**, A suprapubic catheter is placed through the bladder dome in an extraperitoneal location. The bladder is distended to check for security of closure.

Continued.

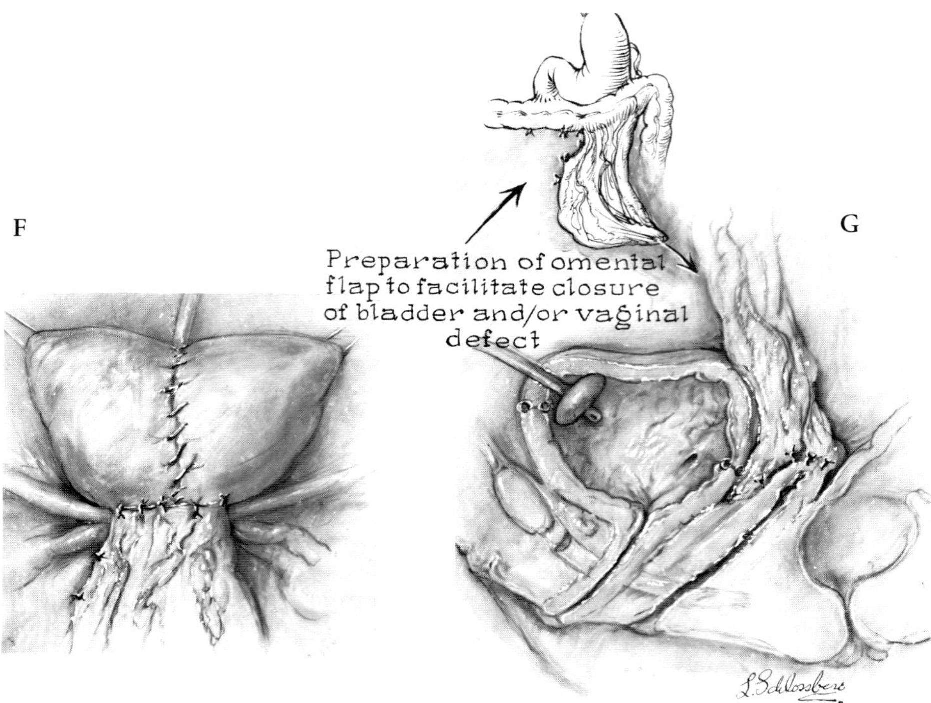

FIGURE 13.19, cont'd. F, The bladder muscularis is closed with no. 3-0 delayed absorbable continuous or interrupted sutures. G, In complicated fistulas, an omental flap may be developed and sutured between the bladder closure and the vaginal closure. (From Rock JA and Thompson JD: TeLinde's operative gynecology, ed 8, Philadelphia, 1996, Lippincott-Raven.)

fistula, prolonged drainage of the bladder is usually required. Depending on a variety of circumstances, suprapubic or transurethral drainage (or both) is used. On rare occasions, for very complicated fistulas, patients are asked to lie on their abdomen with a suprapubic catheter draining directly into a bottle on the floor through the mattress.

Only when the closure of the vesicovaginal fistula is considered technically impossible should urinary diversion above the bladder be advised. This is most often necessary for painful postirradiation fistulas. Ureteral anastomosis to the intact functioning sigmoid colon is not an appropriate operation because of the attendant metabolic and electrolyte problem of hyperchloremic acidosis, because of chronic hydroureteronephrosis with pyelonephritis, and because of the development of colon malignancies at the anastomotic site. Anastomosis of the ureters to an ileal conduit is our preferred procedure. Newer procedures using intestinal segments in ingenious but complicated ways to provide urinary continence on the abdominal wall are available.

Unusual Fistulas. In the United States, serious urethral damage causing fistula is uncommon from any cause. Urethral damage from prolonged obstructed labor or difficult forceps operations caused urethral injuries many years ago. A urethrovaginal fistula may be seen after suburethral diverticulectomy or anterior colporrhaphy or radiation therapy for carcinoma involving the anterior vaginal wall or urethra. The uretha may be damaged if the bulb of an indwelling catheter is accidentally inflated in the urethral lumen, but this does not ordinarily result in fistula formation. Lymphogranuloma may destroy the urethra. Operations to repair urethral injuries are technically tedious and difficult. An operation to repair urethral damage, first described by Symmonds, is shown in Figure 13.20.

Vesicouterine and vesicocervical fistulas are uncommon and today will usually result from injury and necrosis of the bladder wall directly over the dehiscence of a lower uterine segment cesarean section incision. The patient may complain of some involuntary loss of urine through the vagina, or she may re-

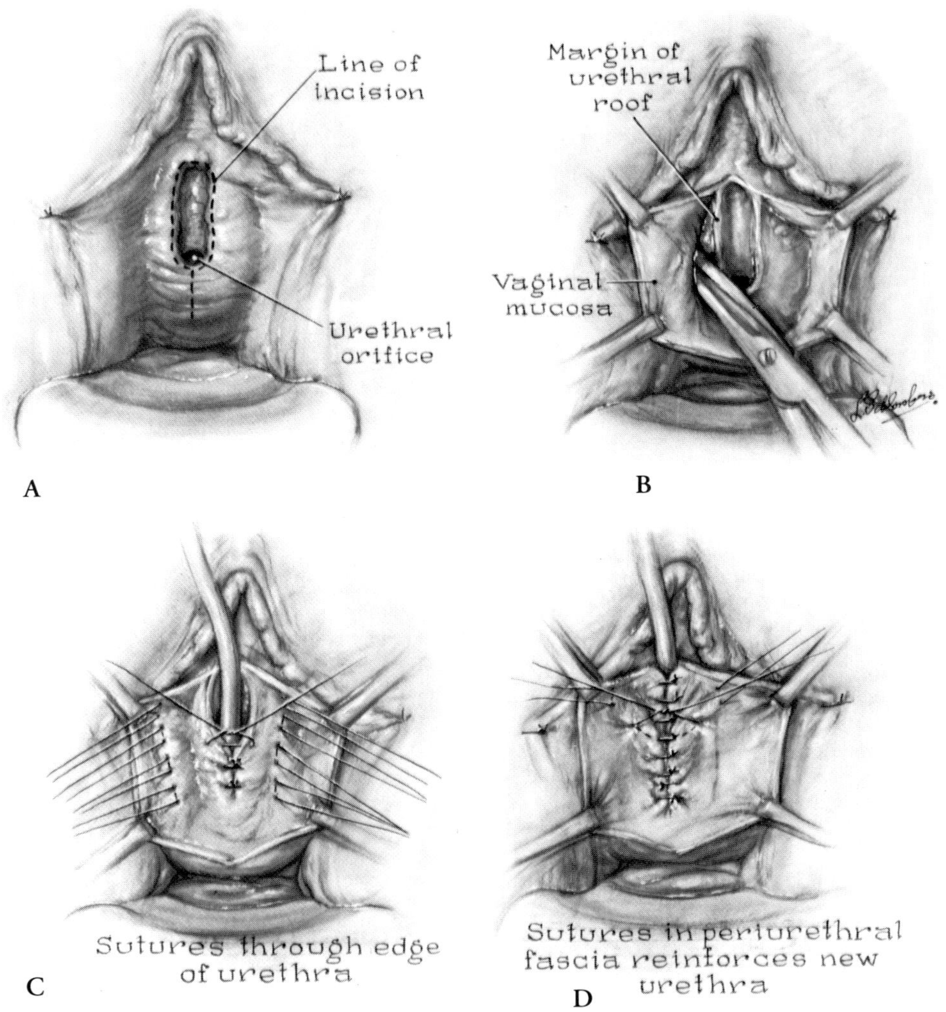

FIGURE 13.20 Reconstruction of total or partial loss of urethral floor. **A,** Line of incision along lateral margin of roof of urethra and beneath bladder base. **B,** Enough of the urethral margins and fascia are freed from the vagina to permit approximation of the urethral mucosa in the midline. **C,** Urethral edges are approximated in the midline over a no. 12 French catheter with interrupted no. 3-0 delayed absorbable sutures. Mobilized urethral fascia is sutured on each side of the total length of the urethra. The lower strand of each suture is tied beneath the urethral floor, **D,** and the upper strands of the two sutures are used to pull the fascia beneath the urethra, where they are tied.

Continued.

main continent of urine. Instead, she may experience cyclic hematuria (menouria) and amenorrhea. Cystoscopy, cystogram, and hysterogram are useful diagnostic procedures. The fistula will always be supratrigonal. The operation to repair the fistula can be done abdominally or vaginally depending on a variety of circumstances. The bladder is dissected free from the lower anterior uterine isthmus. Following identification of the fistula tract, the bladder and uterine orifices are closed separately. A layer of peritoneum should be mobilized and sutured between the repair sites. A hysterectomy is not required for successful repair. If a hysterectomy is done, it should be indicated for some other reason, including the presence of a large defect in the uterine wall, repair of which appears to be technically unsatisfactory.

Complications of Fistula Repair. Except for breakdown of the repair, there are few

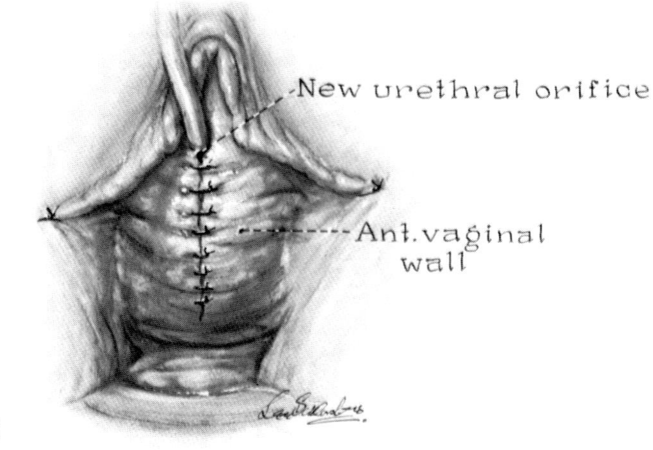

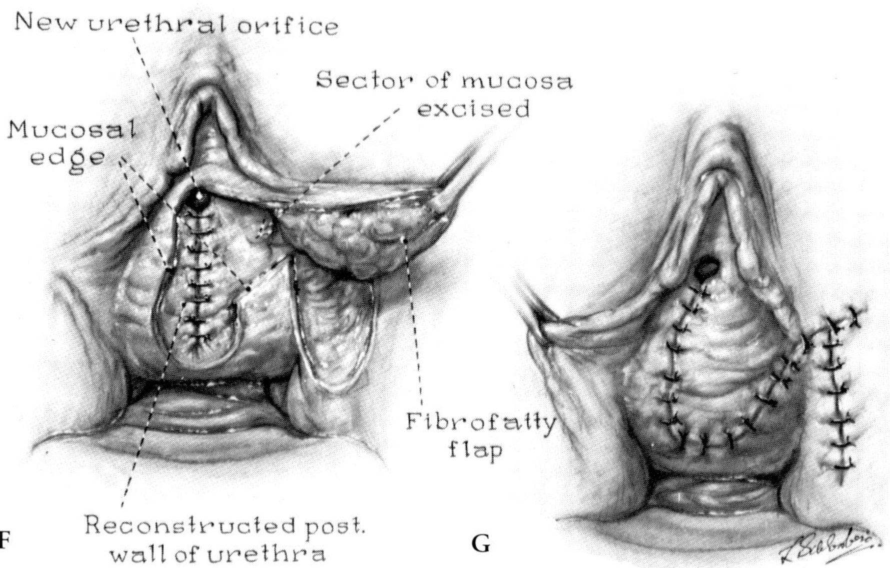

FIGURE 13.20, cont'd. **E,** The vaginal mucosa is closed without tension. The bladder is filled with sterile water before the catheter is removed, and a suprapubic tube is inserted. **F,** Alternatively for additional reinforcement, a labial fat pad is developed by a U-shaped incision along the lateral and medial aspects of the labia, leaving a broad pedicle superiorly. The lateral vaginal mucosa is resected between the urethral operative site and the labial graft. **G,** The skin margins of the labial graft are sutured to the vaginal margins with no. 3-0 interrupted delayed absorbable suture. The labial skin margins are closed so as to produce a flat vulvar surface. (From Rock JA and Thompson JD: TeLinde's operative gynecology, ed 8, Philadelphia, 1996, Lippincott-Raven.)

complications of fistula repair. Injury to the intramural portion of the ureter can be diagnosed and corrected if cystoscopy with the indigo carmine dye test is performed at the end of the repair. Cystoscopy will also diagnose intravesical bleeding, providing an opportunity for control before clot formation inside the bladder with bladder distention and obstruction of catheter drainage damaging the repair site.

The most dreaded complication of all is, of course, failure of the fistula repair to heal. This is usually evident 7 to 10 days after the operation. If the repair breaks down, a large-bore catheter should be placed in the bladder and allowed to remain for several weeks. This will provide an opportunity for the fistula to heal spontaneously or, if not, to heal with the smallest defect possible so that the next attempt at repair will have the best chance of success. During this time, the gynecologic surgeon will need to make the best possible effort to provide emotional support to the patient. Fortunately, almost all fistulas can be closed eventually, even complicated ones.

Bibliography

Baker HW: Selective indications for subtotal hysterectomy, J Ky Med Assoc 83:355, 1985.

Beland G: Early treatment of ureteral injuries found after gynecological surgery, J Urol 118:25, 1977.

Bergman H, editor: The ureter, New York, 1981, Springer-Verlag New York, Inc.

Betson JR: Bulbocavernosus fat pad transplant, Obstet Gynecol 9:303, 1980.

Blandy JP and others: Early repair of iatrogenic injury to the ureter or bladder after gynecologic surgery, J Urol 146:761, 1991.

Boronow RC: Repair of radiation-induced vaginal fistula utilizing the Martius technique, World J Surg 10:237, 1986.

Boronow RC and Rutledge F: Vesicovaginal fistula, radiation, and gynecologic cancer, Am J Obstet Gynecol 111:85, 1971.

Boyce WH: Use of the internal ureteral stent in surgery of the kidney and ureter. In Boyarksy S and others, editors: Urodynamics: hydrodynamics of the ureter and renal pelvis, New York, 1971, Academic Press, Inc.

Clarke DH and Holland JB: Repair of vesicovaginal fistulas: simultaneous transvaginal-transvesical approach, South Med J 68:1410, 1975.

Collins CG and Prent D: Results of early repair of vesicovaginal fistula with preliminary cortisone treatment, Am J Obstet Gynecol 80:1005, 1960.

Collins CG and others: Early repair of vesicovaginal fistula, Am J Obstet Gynecol 111:524, 1971.

Cruikshank SH: Surgical method of identifying the ureters during total vaginal hysterectomy, Obstet Gynecol 67:277, 1986.

Cruikshank SH: Early closure of posthysterectomy vesicovaginal fistulas, South Med J 81:1525, 1988.

Davits RJAM and Miranda SI: Conservative treatment of vesicovaginal fistulas by bladder drainage alone, Br J Urol 68:155, 1991.

Dotters DJ and Droegemueller W: Diaphragm catheters for vesicovaginal fistula management, Contemp Ob Gyn 36:45, 1992.

Ehrlich RM, Melman A, and Skinner DG: The use of vesicopsoas hitch in urologic surgery, J Urol 119:322, 1978.

Elkins TE: Surgery for the obstetric vesicovaginal fistula: a review of 100 operations in 82 patients, Am J Obstet Gynecol 170:1108, 1994.

Elkins TE and others: Vesicovaginal fistula revisited, Obstet Gynecol 72:307, 1988.

Everett HS and Mattingly RF: Urinary tract injuries resulting from pelvic surgery, Am J Obstet Gynecol 71:502, 1956.

Falk HC and Orkin LA: Nonsurgical closure of vesicovaginal fistulas, Obstet Gynecol 9:538, 1957.

Fearl CL and Keizur LW: Optimum time interval from occurrence to repair of vesicovaginal fistula, Am J Obstet Gynecol 104:205, 1968.

Flynn JT and others: The early and aggressive repair of iatrogenic ureteric injuries, Br J Urol 51:454, 1979.

Fry DE, Milholen L, and Harbrecht PJ: Iatrogenic ureteral injury: options in management, Arch Surg 118:454, 1983.

Garlock JH: The cure of an intractable vesicovaginal fistula by the use of a pedicled muscle flap, Surg Gynecol Obstet 47:225, 1928.

Gillenwater JY: The pathophysiology of urinary tract obstruction. In Walsh PC and others, editors: Campbell's urology, ed 6, Philadelphia, 1992, WB Saunders Co.

Gomel V and James C: Intraoperative management of ureteral injury during operative laparoscopy, Fertil Steril 55:416, 1991.

Graham JB: Painful syndrome of postradiation urinary vaginal fistula, Surg Gynecol Obstet 124:1260, 1964.

Hache L, Pratt JH, and Cook EN: Vesicouterine fistula, Mayo Clin Proc 41:150, 1966.

Harrow BR: A neglected maneuver for ureterovesical implantation following injury at gynecologic operation, J Urol 100:280, 1968.

Hatch KD, and others: Ureteral strictures and fistulae following radical hysterectomy, Gynecol Oncol 19:17, 1984.

Hedgegaard CK and Wallace D: Percutaneous nephrostomy: current indications and potential uses in obstetrics and gynecology—literature review and report of a case, Obstet Gynecol Surv 42:671, 1987.

Hofmeister FJ: Pelvic anatomy of the ureter in relation to surgery performed through the vagina, Clin Obstet Gynecol 25:821, 1982.

Hyman RM: Coagulation therapy for small vesicovaginal fistulas, Clin Obstet Gynecol 8:465, 1968.

Iloabachie GC and Njoku O: Vesicouterine fistula, Br J Urol 57:438, 1985.

Jaszczak SE and Evans TN: Intrafascial abdominal and vaginal hysterectomy: a reappraisal, Obstet Gynecol 59:435, 1982.

Kaplan JO and others: Dilatation of a surgically ligated ureter through percutaneous nephrostomy, AJR 39:188, 1982.

Kiricuta I and Goldstein AMB: The repair of extensive vesicovaginal fistulas with pedicled omentum: a review of 27 cases, J Urol 108:724, 1972.

Krupp P, Hoffman M, and Roeling W: Terminal ileum as ureteral substitute, Obstet Gynecol 35:416, 1970.

Kursh EC and others: Prevention of the development of a vesicovaginal fistula, Surg Gynecol Obstet 166:490, 1988.

Larson DM and others: Ureteral assessment after radical hysterectomy, Obstet Gynecol 69:612, 1987.

Latzko W: Postoperative vesicovaginal fistulas, Am J Surg 58:211, 1942.

Lee RA: Atlas of gynecologic surgery, Philadelphia, 1992, WB Saunders Co.

Lee RA and Symmonds RE: Ureterovaginal fistula, Am J Obstet Gynecol 109:1032, 1971.

Lee RA, Symmonds RE, and Williams TJ: Current status of genitourinary fistula, Obstet Gynecol 72:313, 1988.

Mann WJ and others: Ureteral injuries in an obstetrics and gynecology training program: etiology and management, Obstet Gynecol 72:82, 1988.

Margolis T and Mercer LJ: Vesicovaginal fistula, Obstet Gynecol Surv 49:840, 1994.

Martius H: Vesicovaginal therapy especially by plastic transplantation of flaps, Z Geburtshilfe Gynakol 103:22, 1932.

Miller NF and George H: Lower urinary tract fistulas in women: a study based on 292 cases, Am J Obstet Gynecol 68:436, 1954.

Moir JC: Vesicovaginal fistula, Proc R Soc Med 59:1019, 1966.

Moriel EZ and others: Experience with the immediate treatment of iatrogenic bladder injuries and the repair of complex vesicovaginal fistulae by the transvesical approach, Arch Gynecol Obstet 253:127, 1993.

Murphy M: Social consequences of vesicovaginal fistula in Northern Nigeria, J Biosoc Sci 13:139, 1981.

Nezhat C and others: Injuries associated with the use of a linear stapler during operative laparoscopy: review, diagnosis, management, and prevention, J Gynecologic Surg 9:145, 1993.

O'Connor VJ Jr: Repair of vesicovaginal fistula with associated urethral loss, Surg Gynecol Obstet 146:251, 1978.

O'Quinn AG and others: Early repair of vesicovaginal fistula following preliminary corticosteroid treatment. Paper presented at the Society of Pelvic Surgeons, New Orleans, November 1984.

Patil V, Waterhourse K, and Laungani G: Management of 18 difficult vesicovaginal and urethrovaginal fistulas with modified Ingelman-Sundberg and Martius operations, J Urol 123:653, 1980.

Persky L, Herman G, and Geurrier K: Non-delay in vesicovaginal fistula repair, Urology 13:273, 1970.

Pettit PD and Lee RA: Ovarian remnant syndrome: diagnostic dilemma and surgical challenge, Obstet Gynecol 71:580, 1988.

Pettit PO and Petrou SP: The value of cystoscopy in major vaginal surgery, Obstet Gynecol 84:318, 1994.

Petty WM, Lowy RO, and Oyama AA: Total abdominal hysterectomy after radiation therapy for cervical cancer: use of omental graft for fistula prevention, Am J Obstet Gynecol 154:1222, 1986.

Piscitelli JT, Simel DL, and Addison WA: Who should have intravenous pyelograms before hysterectomy for benign disease? Obstet Gynecol 69:541, 1987.

Plauche WC: Cesarean hysterectomy: indications, technique, and complications, Clin Obstet Gynecol 29:318, 1986.

Podratz K, Symmonds RE, and Hagen JV: Vesicovaginal fistulae, Baillieres Clin Obstet Gynaecol 1:4124, 1987.

Ponig BF Jr: Microsurgical ureteroureterostomy in ureteral injuries, J Urol 128:594, 1982.

Richardson EH: A simplified technic for abdominal panhysterectomy, Surg Gynecol Obstet 48:248, 1929.

Ridley JH: Indirect air cystoscopy, South Med J 44:114, 1951.

Rock JA and Thompson JD: TeLinde's operative gynecology, ed 8, Philadelphia, 1996, Lippincott-Raven.

Sampson JA: Ligation and clamping of the ureter as complications of surgical operations, Am Med 4:693, 1902.

Sampson JA: The relations between carcinoma cervicis uteri and the ureters and its significance in the more radical operations for that disease, Johns Hopkins Med Bull 156:72, 1904.

Sampson JA: Ureteral fistulae as sequelae of pelvic operations, Surg Gynecol Obstet 8:479, 1909.

Shapiro SR and Bennett AH: Recovery of renal function after prolonged unilateral ureteral obstruction, J Urol 115:136, 1976.

Shoenwald MB and Orkin LA: Bilateral intravesical ureteral ligation: complication of Cooper's ligament suspension, J Urol 3:787, 1974.

Stanhope CR and others: Suture entrapment and secondary ureteral obstruction, Am J Obstet Gynecol 164:1513, 1991.

Symmonds RE: Ureteral injuries associated with gynecologic surgery: prevention and management, Clin Obstet Gynecol 19:623, 1976.

Symmonds RE: Incontinence: vesical and urethral fistulas, Clin Obstet Gynecol 27:499, 1984.

Symmonds RE and Hill M: Loss of the urethra: a report on 50 patients, Am J Obstet Gynecol 130:130, 1978.

Tahzib F: Epidemiological determinants of vesicovaginal fistulas, Br J Obstet Gynecol 90:387, 1983.

Tancer ML: The post total hysterectomy (vault) vesicovaginal fistula, J Urol 123:839, 1980.

Taylor JS, Hewson AD, and Rachow P: Synchronous combined transvaginal transvesical repair of vesicovaginal fistulas, Aust N Z J Surg 50:23, 1980.

Thompson JD and Benigno BB: Vaginal repair of ureteral injuries, Am J Obstet Gynecol 3:601, 1971.

Turner-Warwick R: The use of pedicle grafts in the repair of urinary tract fistulae, Br J Urol 44:644, 1972.

Turner-Warwick R: The use of the omental pedicle graft in urinary tract reconstruction, J Urol 116:341, 1976.

Turner-Warwick R and Worth PH: The psoas bladder hitch procedure for the replacement of the lower third of the ureter, Br J Urol 41:701, 1969.

Wiskind AK and Thompson JD: Should cystoscopy be performed after every gynecological operation to diagnose unsuspected ureteral injury? J Pelv Surg 1(3):134, 1995.

Witters S, Cornelissen J, and Vereecken R: Iatrogenic ureteral injury: aggressive or conservative treatment, Am J Obstet Gynecol 155:582, 1986.

Youssef AF: "Menouria" following lower segment cesarean section: a syndrome, Am J Obstet Gynecol 73:759, 1957.

Zacharin RF: Grafting as a principle in the surgical management of vesicovaginal and rectovaginal fistulae, Aust N Z J Obstet Gynaecol 20:10, 1980.

Zacharin RF: Obstetric fistula, New York, 1988, Springer-Verlag New York, Inc.

14

Recurrent Anal and Rectal Fistula

David H. Nichols

The majority of rectovaginal fistulas are asymptomatic. The presence of fistula can be suspected from incontinence of rectal gas or of liquid or solid stool even in the presence of an intact perineum and functional external anal sphincter. When these contaminants are passed through the vagina, the bacterial concentration may precipitate a chronic, recurrent vaginitis. There may be dyspareunia when infection and fibrosis are present.

In the evaluation of a patient with recurrent rectal fistula, the surgeon must first rule out active inflammatory bowel disease, such as Crohn's disease, tuberculosis (TB), or lymphopathia venerea, which may be suspected by a patient history of frequent bowel movements, weight loss, passage of mucus, and on physical examination of the fistula, finding pain to touch, induration and edema, and granulations. The surgeon must further exclude by history and biopsy the presence of invasive neoplastic disease at the site of fistula formation. (Biopsies should be performed on areas suspected of neoplasia, including ulceration with palpably hard margins that often are whitish and occasionally are bloody.)

Intestinal diverticulosis may be recognized from the patient's history, and perforation through the internal genitalia may lead to fistula formation at the vault of the vagina; however, this is usually colovaginal and not rectovaginal, because diverticulosis does not involve the rectum. The diagnosis is confirmed by barium enema and sigmoidoscopy or colonoscopy or by retrograde vaginal fistulogram using water-soluble dye.

The diagnosis of most cases of rectovaginal or rectoperineal fistula should be preceded and accompanied by suitable proctoscopy. Occasionally the rectal opening of the fistula is difficult to demonstrate except by gentle probing under anesthesia. When it is still not demonstrable with certainty, traction by an Allis' clamp on the external secondary opening, as described by Bacon and Ross, usually produces dimpling at the primary opening, which is often found in an anal crypt.

When the patient's history includes previous pelvic radiation, often in the distant past, the presence of a degree of endarteritis obliterans can be assumed or suspected. In the previously irradiated patient, a history of prior vaginal or rectal biopsy of some reddish or granular area on the surface of the posterior vaginal wall of the vagina may be the cause of the fistula. Although such an area is usually not malignant, the biopsy site may not heal well, and due to the local devascularization, a rectovaginal fistula may develop. A better primary approach to the evaluation of such a postradiation redness would be the use of cytology from a surface smear and colposcopy, with careful biopsy only of a site found likely to be malignant. Repair of such a postradiation rectovaginal fistula from which malignancy has been excluded should not be attempted until the patient has experienced at least 1 year of intravaginal estrogen supplementation, and the technique of repair must include meticulous dissection with a layered closure and interposition between the rectum and vagina of a Martius bulbocavernosus graft between the two layers. If the tissues and layers can be closed without tension, hemostasis is adequate, and the surgery is carried out precisely and with the most gentle handling of tissue, a complementary diverting colostomy may not be necessary.

Most recurrent lower intestinal fistulas in women are either anoperineal or rectovaginal. There is as large a world of pathologic and surgical difference between a recurrent anal fistula and a recurrent rectovaginal fistula as there is between their previously unrepaired counterparts. In most instances both etiology and treatment of the two conditions are quite distinctively different.

Anal Fistula

Anal fistula is frequently associated with anal abscess but may follow trauma to anal tissue and may be associated with inflammatory bowel disease such as Crohn's disease. Parks has demonstrated that anal glands may penetrate the internal anal sphincter at the base of the anal crypt and theorizes that infection of such a glandular duct can result in an abscess that can spread in various directions, not infrequently leading to subsequent development of anal fistula. Some of these sites of abscess formation with fistula are shown in Figure 14.1. Although incision and drainage are critical to resolution of the abscess, it is essential to determine by gentle probing the relationship between the abscess, a fistula, and the internal or external anal sphincter and whether or not the abscess is above or below the patient's levator ani. It must be remembered that supralevator abscess may be associated with inflammatory bowel disease. Ischiorectal abscess should be drained through an incision close to the anal canal and usually under hospital OR anesthesia. If by examination an opening into an anal crypt is identified, often by noting the escape of pus from the abscess into the crypt, this should be noted in the operative report for a reference during subsequent search and surgery. Culture of a perianal abscess should be taken. If it shows predominantly *Escherichia coli,* recurrence is more likely than if it shows *Staphylococcus aureus,* because the former suggests fistulous communication with the rectum. Search for a probable fistula should be undertaken anoscopically about 2 weeks after evacuation of the abscess cavity.

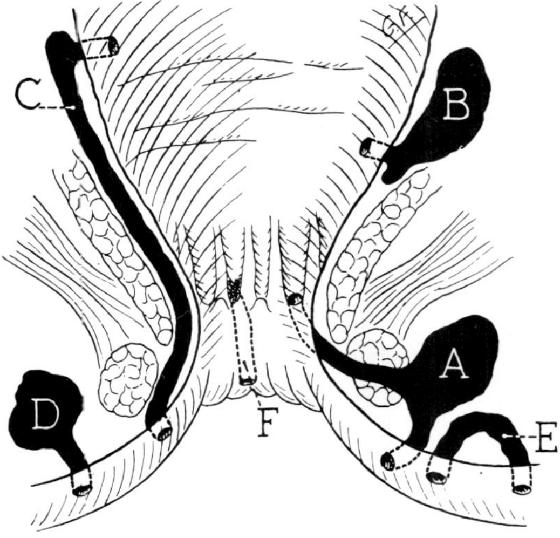

Figure 14.1 Various locations of anorectal fistulas and sinuses. *A*, Complete fistula between an internal opening in an anal crypt, tunneling through the external sphincter, and external opening on the perineum. *B*, Internal rectal sinus. *C*, Complete rectal fistula. *D*, Perianal sinus. *E*, Complete external perianal fistula. *F*, Complete submucocutaneous fistula. (From Hirschman LJ: Synopsis of ano-rectal diseases, ed 2, St Louis, 1942, Mosby.)

Abscess between the internal and external anal sphincters (in contrast to a submucosal abscess between the internal sphincter and the rectal mucosa) should be excised transrectally, including the crypt-bearing area, leaving the wound open for subsequent healing by granulation.

Most anal fistulas are preceded by a history of an abscess that either ruptured spontaneously or was drained. The surgery to correct anal fistula may be far more difficult than that for a rectovaginal fistula, because severe anal incontinence may develop postoperatively consequent to disruption in fibrosis of the anal sphincter mechanism. Goodsall's rule describes the relationship between the fistulous tract and the two ends of the fistula, which is important because the lining of the tract should be exposed and curetted or excised due to its probable glandular content. The rule states that when the external fistulous opening lies anterior to a horizontal plane drawn through the center of the anal canal, the internal opening tends to be located radially at the end of a straight line from the external opening. When the external opening lies posterior to this plane, the tract is usually curved, and the internal opening is located in the posterior midline. Application of this rule is a great help in locating and probing a fistulous tract. Fistulas of the intersphincteric plane most commonly have a single external opening, but transsphincteric fistulas may have multiple openings arising from the ischiorectal fossa and postanal space, producing the horseshoe-type fistula, each tract of which must be separately exposed and curetted. Failure to expose all of this gland-bearing tissue in the tract will cause a recurrence first of an abscess, then of a fistula. Injections of milk, which is nonstaining, or of a solution of indigo carmine, which stains the tissues very deeply, using a short blunt or Marx needle may help demonstrate the tract. Probing of the tract should precede excision of each of its segments. This will cure most intrasphincteric and transsphincteric fistulas, but the supralevator extension should not be drained into the rectum. Probably the advice of a surgeon with special experience in this area should be obtained, because there is a great chance of fecal incontinence developing from division of the puborectalis sling.

When it is difficult to demonstrate a suspected pinhole-sized rectovaginal fistula, its specific site may be determined by filling the vagina of the recumbent patient with warm water or soapy water sufficient to cover the expected site of the fistula, placing a Foley catheter with a 10-ml bulb into the rectum, and instilling air through the catheter. A stream of air bubbles coming through the vaginal water pool indicates the site of the fistula through which a blunt probe can be placed.

If the vagina will not contain the soapy water, the site of the fistula can be determined by instilling milk or a concentrated solution containing methylene blue or indigo carmine into the rectal Foley catheter and watching where it appears on the posterior vaginal wall.

In seeking radiographic demonstration of the tract of a small rectovaginal fistula, the surgeon can inject a mixture of barium, mashed potato mix, and water into the rectum using a caulking gun. A lateral radiograph is taken while the patient bears down.

Surgical repair should be considered when a fistula has caused troublesome symptoms and when local edema and inflammation have subsided (usually coincident with relief of pain).

When a lower fistula transgresses the external sphincter, the surgeon during excision of the tract may incise a part of the sphincter, anticipating its reunion by scar tissue during the healing phase. If this appears to risk sphincter integrity, a seton of no. 2 polyglycolic acid (Dexon) or silk may be used (Figure 14.2). Its use, as Corman suggests, is similar to the principle of a weighted wire cutting progressively through a block of ice, which, if the sides are in continuous contact, will readhere after division by the wire. After the skin between the anal canal and the perineum is excised, the seton of doubled no. 2 Dexon or silk is placed around the sphincter and tied very tightly, and the ends are cut long. It is retightened in about 2 weeks, by which time the muscle and tract will have been cut through and the latter reunited by scar tissue. One week later, the retightened seton will have cut through the remainder of the muscle; the suture is removed and the wound permitted to heal. This can be used through the puborectalis sling during treatment of the extrasphincteric fistula, par-

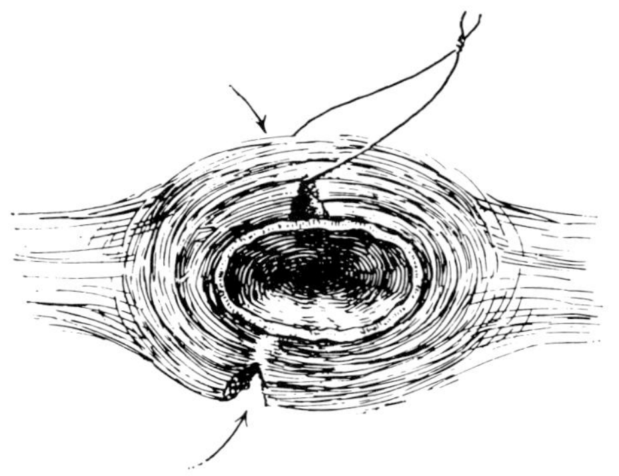

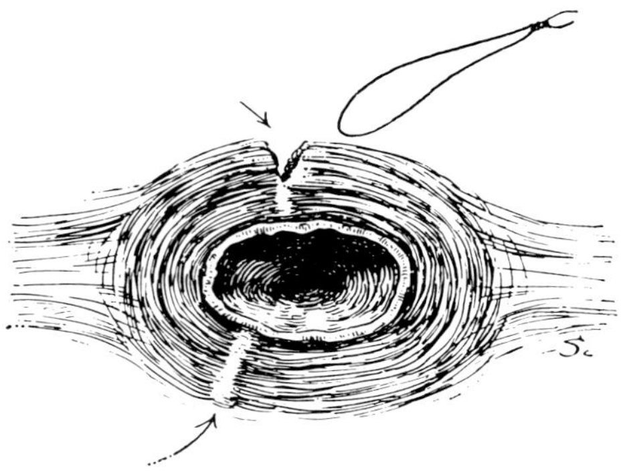

FIGURE 14.2 Details of division of sphincter by seton *(arrows)*. (From Hirschman LJ: Synopsis of ano-rectal diseases, ed 2, St Louis, 1942, Mosby.)

ticularly when the internal opening of the fistula is above the levator ani. Complete excision of an extrasphincteric fistula risks postoperative wound breakdown of any sphincter repair with subsequent incontinence, which may be difficult to repair.

Rectovaginal Fistula

A genital fistula has a high-pressure side and a low-pressure side, and material flows from the high-pressure side to and through the low-pressure side and not the other way around. With rectovaginal fistula, the high-pressure side is the rectum, and the low-pressure side is the vagina. For this reason symptomatic material does not flow from the vagina into the rectum but flows from the rectum into the vagina; therefore the effective closure or removal of the *rectal* opening (the high-pressure side of the equation) is the primary goal. If the rectal opening of the fistula is removed and the opening closed, the vaginal opening generally requires little or no attention, because it will granulate in and become reepithelialized. This may occur a little faster if the epithelialized edges have been trimmed, but the vaginal opening need be approximated only by one or two loosely placed sutures.

The surgeon must determine that a suspected recurrence of fistula is not, in fact, a previously undiagnosed second rectovaginal fistula, because the surgical prognosis is considerably more favorable for the latter.

When recurrent rectovaginal fistula follows previous surgical repair, the surgeon must consider that the initial repair may have been surgically satisfactory from a mechanical and technical standpoint and therefore consider and exclude or treat any previously undiagnosed inflammatory bowel disease that may be a significant etiologic factor. Characteristically such recurrent and usually larger fistulas will be unexpectedly evident several weeks or months following the initial repair. When a patient with Crohn's disease requests surgical repair, she should be made fully aware of the risks and prognosis. The repair should be performed during the period of remission of the disease and following 1 month's preparation using 1000 mg of metronidazole daily and 20 mg of prednisone daily in divided doses. The transperineal rectal flap operation, shown in Figure 14.3, is most useful for such fistulas in the lower third of the vagina. It exteriorizes the rectal fistula, which will be removed with the resection of the anterior rectal wall.

Layered Closure

Recurrent rectovaginal fistula in the midvagina may be repaired by a layered technique in which the rectal wall containing the fistula is carefully mobilized about 2 cm in each direction lateral to the fistula's opening, which is then excised (Figure 14.4). The rectal muscularis is approximated by transversely applied interrupted mattress sutures of fine polyglycolic acid or chromic suture material, inverting the cut mucosal edge into the rectal lumen. A second layer of mattress stitches inverts and reinforces the first layer, from which it removes much of the tension, which otherwise might tend to draw the suture layer apart. A layer of intervening tissue, often by a bulbocavernosus fat pad transplant, must be inserted between the rectum and vagina if the blood supply here is poor and the full thickness of the vagina approximated in a direction at right angles to the suture line in the rectal wall. If the external anal sphincter is not intact, it should be repaired by appropriate transvaginal sphincterplasty and perineorrhaphy. Occasionally so little tissue will be present that the technique is much like that of freshening the edges and repairing a fourth-degree perineal laceration.

Because the external anal sphincter is usually competent with recurrent rectovaginal fistula, easily assessed by asking the patient to contract her perineal muscles during preoperative examination, it is often functional and intact. It is neither necessary nor desirable to cut it to facilitate repair of a fistula cranial to this site.

For recurrent rectovaginal fistulas in the lower third of the vagina, the most common site, a transperineal rectal flap sliding operation is most satisfactory. For all operations involving the voluntary muscle sphincter repair, a light general anesthetic without muscle relaxants is preferable so that skeletal muscle remnants can be easily recognized for incorporation in the repair.

Text continued on p. 238.

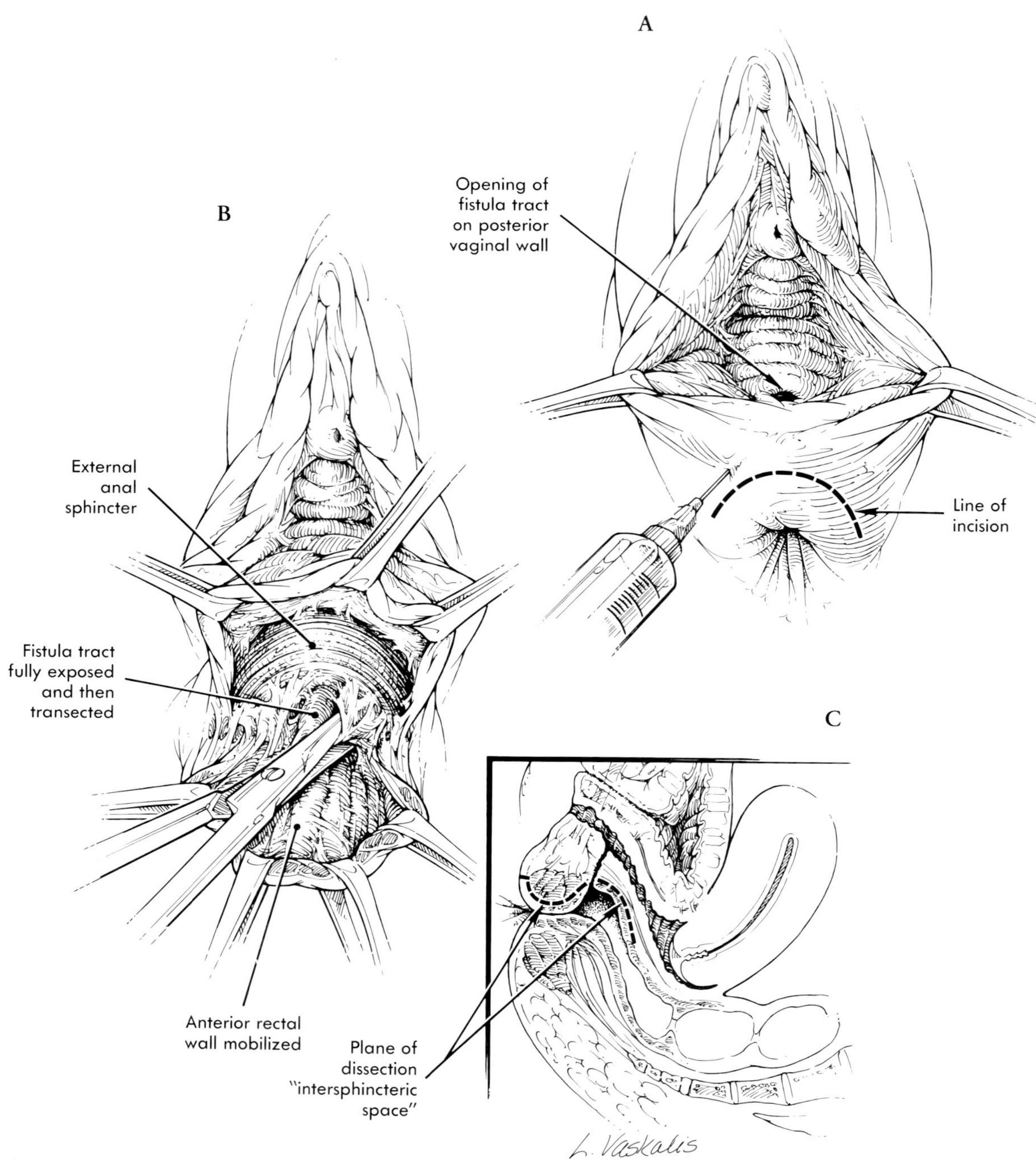

FIGURE 14.3 Transperineal rectal flap sliding technique for repair of rectovaginal fistula. **A,** The site of the fistula is noted, and the perineum and perineal body thoroughly infiltrated by 1:200,000 epinephrine in 0.5% lidocaine. A semilunar incision is made around the anus posterior to the external anal sphincter along the course of the dashed line. **B,** Allis' clamps grasp the edges of the incision, and, by gentle traction to those placed on the anterior portion of the anus, the dissection proceeds beneath the capsule of the external anal sphincter into the intersphincteric space. The fistula tract is fully exposed as the anterior rectal wall is mobilized, and the tract is then transected. **C,** Sagittal view of the path of dissection beneath the external anal sphincter and into the intersphincteric space.

Continued.

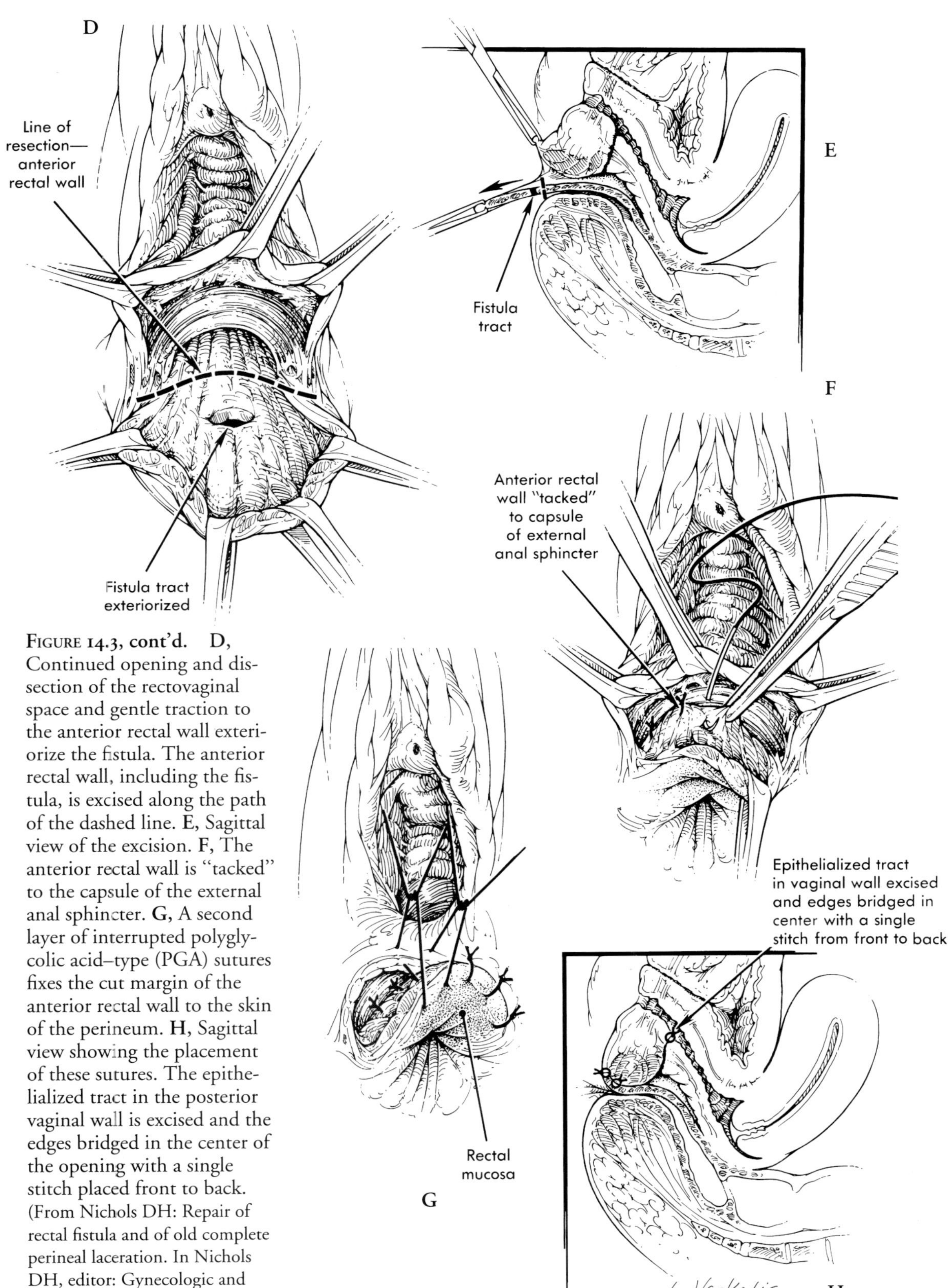

Figure 14.3, cont'd. D, Continued opening and dissection of the rectovaginal space and gentle traction to the anterior rectal wall exteriorize the fistula. The anterior rectal wall, including the fistula, is excised along the path of the dashed line. **E,** Sagittal view of the excision. **F,** The anterior rectal wall is "tacked" to the capsule of the external anal sphincter. **G,** A second layer of interrupted polyglycolic acid–type (PGA) sutures fixes the cut margin of the anterior rectal wall to the skin of the perineum. **H,** Sagittal view showing the placement of these sutures. The epithelialized tract in the posterior vaginal wall is excised and the edges bridged in the center of the opening with a single stitch placed front to back. (From Nichols DH: Repair of rectal fistula and of old complete perineal laceration. In Nichols DH, editor: Gynecologic and obstetric surgery, St Louis, 1993, Mosby.)

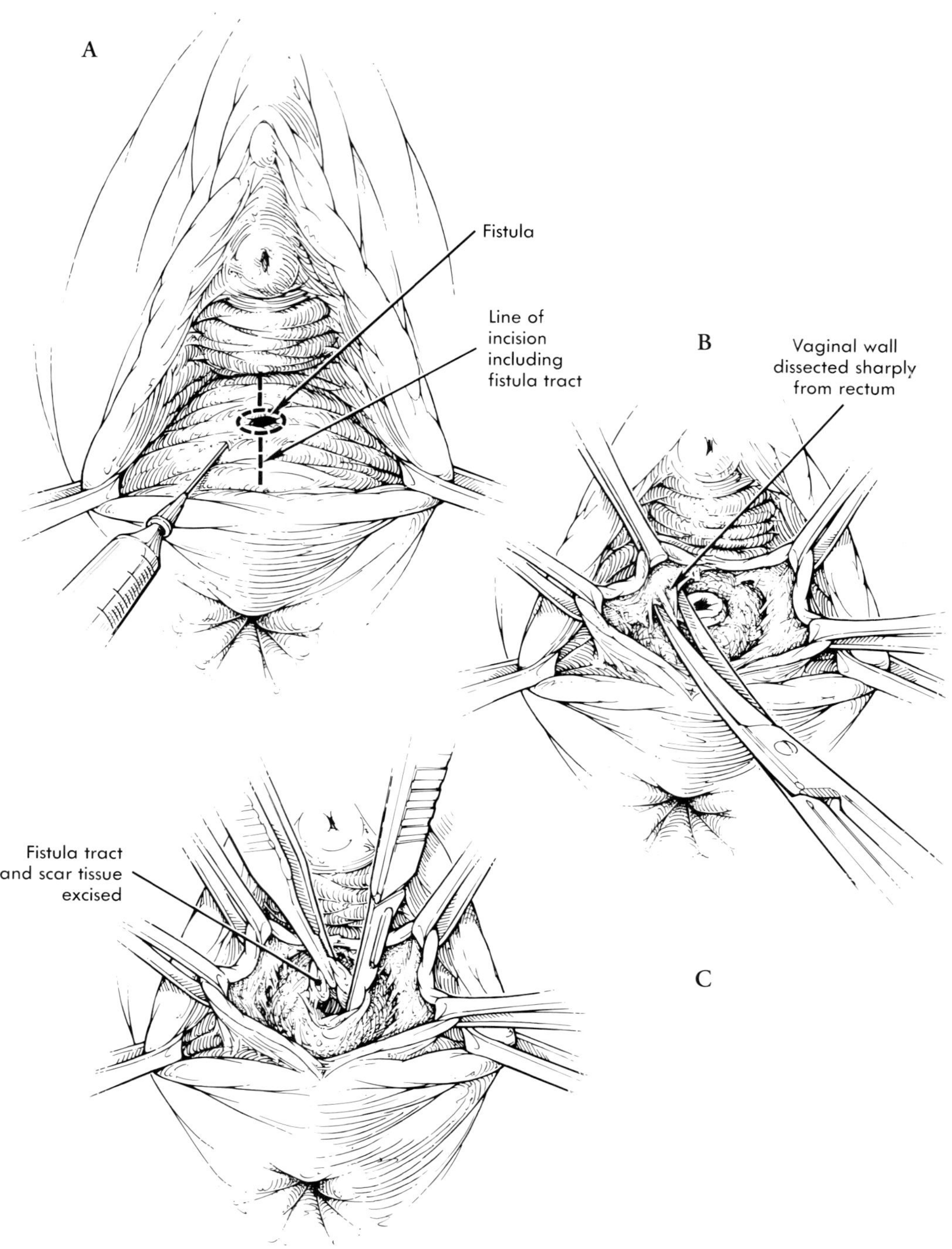

FIGURE 14.4 Layered closure of a midvaginal rectovaginal fistula. **A,** The tissues around the site of the fistula are thoroughly infiltrated by 1:200,000 epinephrine in 0.5% lidocaine, and an incision is made along the path indicated by the *dashed line*; the incision also circumscribes the tract of the fistula. **B,** The cut edges of the vagina are grasped by Allis' clamps and sharply dissected from the anterior rectal wall. **C,** The fistula tract in its entirety is excised along with its surrounding scar tissue.

Continued.

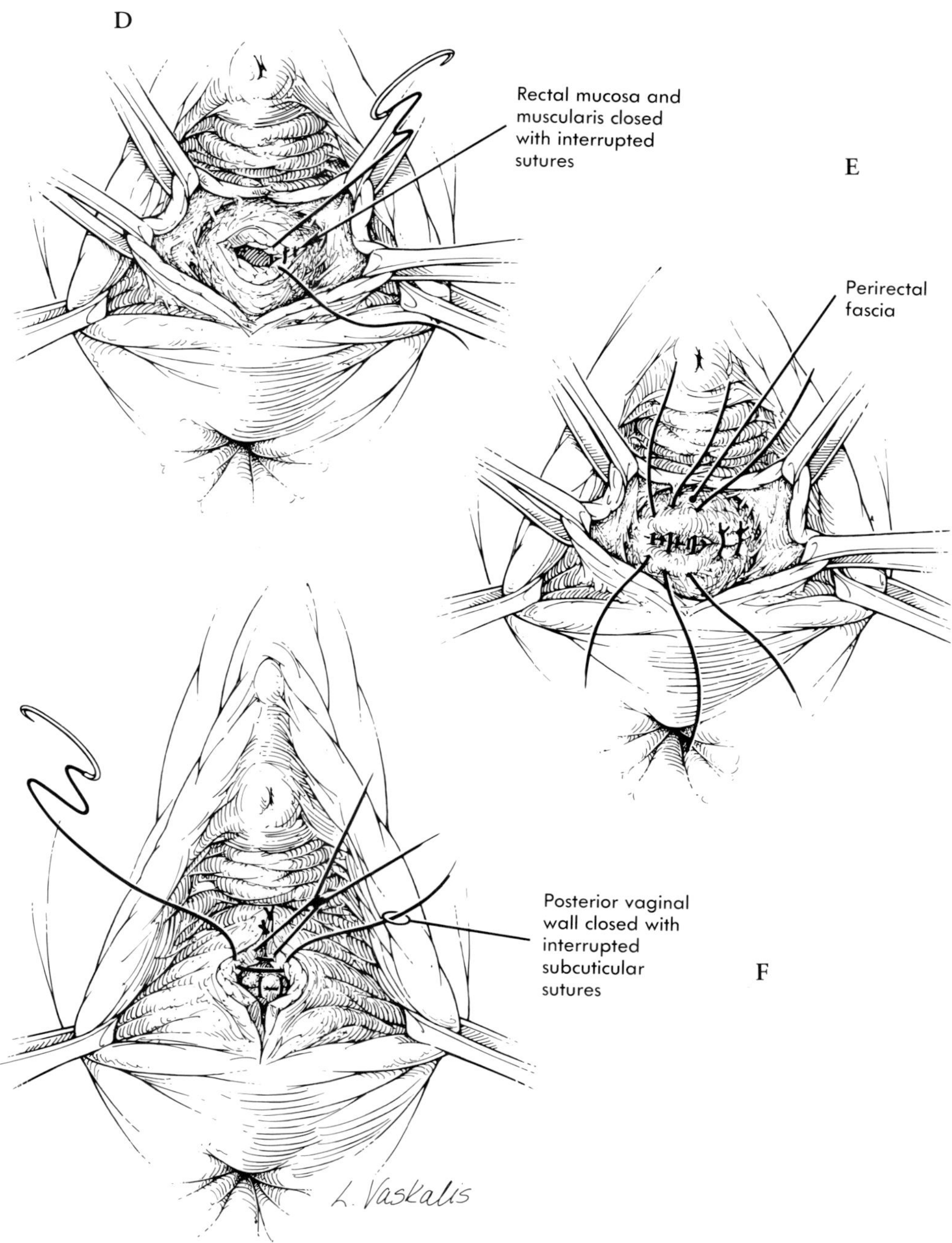

Figure 14.4, cont'd **D,** The rectal submucosa and muscularis are closed with interrupted sutures. **E,** The suture line is buried by a second layer of interrupted sutures in the muscularis and perirectal fascia. **F,** The wound may be thoroughly irrigated with sterile saline solution, and the posterior vaginal wall closed longitudinally and at right angles to the repair in the rectal wall using interrupted subcuticular sutures in the fibromuscular wall of the vagina. (From Nichols DH: Repair of rectal fistula and of old complete perineal laceration. In Nichols DH, editor: Gynecologic and obstetric surgery, St Louis, 1993, Mosby.)

Transperineal Flap Sliding Operation

I usually perform this operation by thoroughly infiltrating the prerectal area of the perineum with a 1:200,000 epinephrine in 0.5% lidocaine solution. Then a semicircular incision is made through the anal skin beneath the external anal sphincter (Figure 14.4) sharply dissecting the full thickness of the anterior rectal wall from the perineum. If scarring is extensive, I may choose an alternative dissection directly beneath the vaginal wall, over the perineal body, and into the rectovaginal space. The latter is opened widely. Traction to the rectal wall exteriorizes the portion including the fistula, and the wall is transected. A deep layer of interrupted stitches attaches the undersurface of the remaining anterior rectal wall to the external anal sphincter. The cut edge of rectum is sewn to the perineal skin by a series of interrupted polyglycolic acid sutures.

In rare instances, as with a very large recurrent fistula in a patient with previous massive pelvic radiation, the fistula may be closed by a modified colpocleisis, in which the anterior vaginal wall is sewn to cover the defect in the anterior rectal wall.

PRINCIPLES OF REPAIR

The following guidelines should be observed for optimal surgical success in rectovaginal fistula closure:

1. A time for fistula repair should be chosen when granulation tissue, infection, edema, and pain are minimal.
2. The repair must interrupt the continuity of the fistula.
3. The epithelialized fistulous tract should be excised.
4. Unless the anterior rectal flap sliding operation has been performed and the exteriorized rectal wall, including the fistula, excised, the rectal side of the fistula should be closed with a layer of interrupted mattress stitches placed in the muscularis in such a fashion that the cut edge of rectal mucosa will be everted into the rectal lumen. A second layer of sutures should be placed, inverting the first layer.

Preoperative Preparation

A clear liquid diet is begun 2 days before admission to the hospital, and one-half bottle of citrate of magnesia or two bisacodyl (Dulcolax) tablets are given the afternoon before admission.

Although mechanical cleansing of the bowel lumen reduces the total fecal mass, it does not significantly reduce the number of bacteria present on the intestinal epithelium. The patient is given a whole-gut lavage with an electrolyte cleanser such as polyethylene glycol (PEG) 3350 with electrolytes (NuLYTELY) by mouth, as much of the solution as can be rapidly swallowed, beginning the morning of the day before surgery.

One-half hour before surgery, 2 gm of a broad-spectrum antibiotic such as cefoxitin (Mefoxin) is administered IV. This may be repeated 2 hours later.

If whole-gut lavage is not used, the patient may be given two Fleet enemas 1 hour apart the evening before admission and plain water or saline enemas the morning of surgery until the return is clear. Preliminary diversion of the fecal stream by colostomy is not recommended in the majority of cases.

Postoperative Care

A clear liquid diet is advised for the first 3 postoperative days, followed by a low-residue diet for the next 3 weeks.

A stool softener, such as docusate sodium (Colace), should be given for 5 weeks to keep the stool on the soft side. If intestinal cramps are troublesome, the patient may be given 10 drops of tincture of opium in water 3 times daily for 5 days.

There should be a bowel movement between the fifth and seventh day postoperatively. If none has occurred spontaneously, a small oral dose of NuLYTELY is preferable to an enema.

No coitus is permitted for 3 months postoperatively.

BIBLIOGRAPHY

Bacon HE and Ross ST: Atlas of operative technique: anus, rectum, and colon, St Louis, 1954, Mosby.

Ball TL: Gynecologic surgery and urology, ed 2, St Louis, 1963, Mosby.

Beecham CT: Recurring rectovaginal fistulas, Obstet Gynecol 40:323, 1972.

Boronow RC: Management of radiation induced vaginal fistulas, Am J Obstet Gynecol 110:1, 1971.

Corman ML: Colon and rectal surgery, Philadelphia, 1984, JB Lippincott Co.

Goligher JC: Surgery of the anus, rectum, and colon, ed 3, Springfield, Ill, 1975, Charles C Thomas, Publisher.

Goodsall DH: Anorectal fistula. In Goodsall DH and Miles WE, editors: Diseases of the anus and rectum: part I, London, 1900, Longmans, Green and Co.

Hirschman LJ: Synopsis of ano-rectal diseases, ed 2, St Louis, 1942, Mosby.

Mengert WF and Fish SA: Anterior rectal wall advancement, Obstet Gynecol 5:262, 1955.

Nichols DH, editor: Gynecologic and obstetric surgery, St Louis, 1993, Mosby.

Nichols DH and Randall CL: Vaginal surgery, ed 4, Baltimore, 1996, Williams & Wilkins.

Nichols RL: Bowel preparation: perioperative care. In Wilmore DW and others, editors: Care of the surgical patient, New York, 1989, Scientific American.

Noble GH: A new operation for complete laceration of the perineum designed for the purpose of eliminating danger of infection from the rectum, Trans Am Gynecol Soc 27:357, 1902.

Parks AG: Fistula-in-ano. In Morson BC, editor: Diseases of the colon, rectum, and anus, New York, 1969, Appleton-Century-Croft.

Rosenshein NB, Genadry RR, and Woodruff JD: An anatomic classification of rectovaginal septal defect, Am J Obstet Gynecol 137:439, 1980.

Rothman D and Dedick P: Vaginography for colovaginal fistula, NJ Med 85:227, 1988.

Solla JA and Rothenberger DA: Preoperative bowel preparation, Dis Colon Rectum 33:154, 1990.

Tancer ML and Veridiano NP: Genital fistulas caused by diverticular disease of the sigmoid colon, Am J Obstet Gynecol 174:1547, 1996.

Tancer ML and Veridiano NP: Genital fistulas secondary to diverticular disease of the colon: a review, Obstet Gynecol Surv 51:67, 1995.

Wiskind AK and Thompson JD: Transverse transperineal repair of rectovaginal fistulas in the lower vagina, Am J Obstet Gynecol 167:694, 1992.

15

Recurrent Anal Incontinence

Rene R. Genadry
David H. Nichols

Anal incontinence is a condition truly devastating to the afflicted patient's lifestyle at a personal and social level, both in public and in her immediate family. The inability to control and retain rectal gas and liquid or solid stool becomes a source of embarrassment to the patient who has already undergone often numerous yet unsuccessful external anal sphincter plication procedures with or without perineorrhaphy. Ill-equipped to deal with such persistent loss of control in the most inappropriate circumstances, the family of an elderly member is inclined to search for an alternative environment where such accidents are more or less expected and can be better handled: the nursing home. This prospect, however, generally fosters a certain reluctance within the patient herself to admit the problem and thus seek proper care, preferring rather to deal with it in a progressively self-ostracizing setting until it finally manifests itself through despair or indifference. The rapid aging of the population calls for an urgent and persistent effort towards prevention, evaluation, and correction of the detrimental effects of this condition. In such patients a distinction must be made between frequent bowel movements as might occur with irritable bowel or diverticulosis and anorectal incontinence characterized additionally by involuntary rectal soiling.

The prevalence of persistent fecal incontinence has been reported to be in the range of 2% to 3% in the United States.[1] Careful and complete evaluation to determine the reason for the failure of prior therapy and to establish the most appropriate approach for the condition's management is required. In essence, the goal of such evaluation is to identify the nature of the incontinence as resulting from one of the following:

1. An anatomic defect of the external anal sphincter, usually of traumatic obstetric origin, often unrecognized or imprecisely repaired
2. An anal sphincter dysfunction, as seen in patients in whom the external anal sphincter is intact but suffers a faulty innervation
3. A mixed anatomic and neurologic dysfunction, each of which should be properly addressed
4. An irritable or hyperactive bowel

It is important to review briefly the normal mechanism for rectal continence and its possible disorders in order to properly evaluate and treat them. Particular attention thus should be paid to the most common factors leading to persistence or recurrence of incontinence, such as those resulting from inappropriate indication or choice of procedure, insufficient diagnosis, less-than-optimal surgical technique or healing, or a different etiology for the recurrence.

Physiopathology

The Continence Mechanism

Anorectal continence requires the coordinated function of many factors, such as:

1. Stool of normal consistency
2. A compliant rectal reservoir
3. A normal anorectal sensation of fullness, urge to defecate, and differentiation between gas, liquid and solid stool
4. A normal anorectal angulation maintained by the action of the puborectal muscle

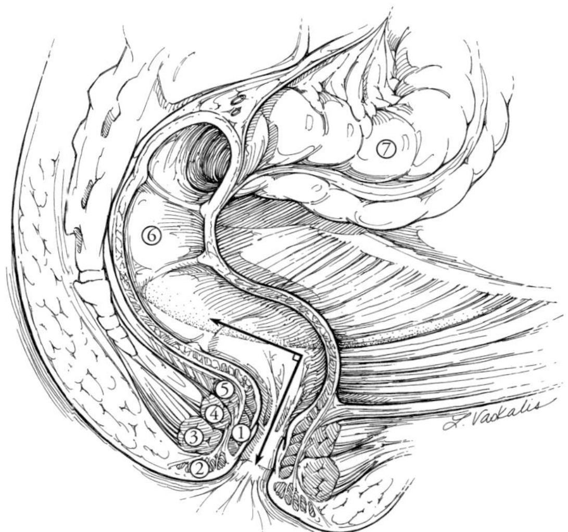

Structure	*Function*
1. Internal Anal Sphincter	*Tonic contraction (passive barrier)*
2. Subcutaneous Portion of External Anal Sphincter	*Active contraction (active barrier)*
3. Superficial Portion of External Anal Sphincter	
4. Deep Portion of External Anal Sphincter	
5. Puborectalis Portion of Levator Ani	*Maintains anorectal angle and active contraction (active barrier)*
6. Rectum	*Compliant reservoir*
7. Sigmoid	*Delays stool progression via contraction*

FIGURE 15.1 Functional anatomy of anorectal canal.

5. A high-pressure barrier maintained by the complementary function of both the internal and external anal sphincters

These conditions should allow the anorectum to perform its function of fecal storage and fecal emptying at a socially opportune and acceptable time. Rectal emptying (defecation) also requires a well-orchestrated series of events resulting in the appropriate relaxation of the anal sphincter and the pelvic floor muscles to allow the proper expulsion of stool. Indeed the perception of rectal distension leads to a reflex relaxation of the external and internal anal sphincters and a voluntary relaxation of the pelvic floor muscles. Their voluntary contraction is an acquired response to social circumstances. This function requires a normal anatomic continence system controlled by a normal physiologic apparatus to ensure the proper coordination of its elements and their potential adaptation to the required response (Figure 15.1). Disorders in emptying and storage function of the anorectum are listed in Table 15.1.

Thus normal anorectal functioning relies upon intact external and internal anal sphincters and puborectal muscle, responsible for effective anorectal angulation, and an adequate rectal compliance and perception not unlike the urinary continence mechanism. The latter also requires an adequate reservoir, capable of normal sensory perception, backed up by an appropriately responsive sphincteric mechanism of contraction and relaxation, including the pubourethral component of the levator ani, as well as the internal and external urethral sphincteric components.

There is a network of neuromuscular receptors within the levator ani that not only can detect rectal fullness but also can discriminate between gas, liquid, and stool content of the bowel. Stimulation of these receptors by increasing rectal content is followed by an increase in the tone of these muscles, which are never entirely at rest. The levator ani muscles are innervated by branches of the pudendal nerve, which similarly innervate the external anal sphincter. These muscles contract simultaneously and synergistically. They differ from the other voluntary muscles of the body in that they maintain, via this network of neuromuscular receptors, a constant state of tone proportional to the quantity of the rectal contents. Their unique capacity for discrimination can permit the slow escape of rectal gas while retaining solid content even during sleep. Because intestinal peristalsis continues during sleep, it is the reflex contraction of these voluntary muscles that maintains continence. The ability of these muscles to contract effectively depends therefore on both their integrity and that of their nerve supply, primarily the pudendal or the accessory pudendal nerves. Disruption of either nerve through congenital weakness, as might be noted with spina bifida or from acquired trauma from a pathologic

Table 15.1 Disorders in emptying and storage function

Disorders in emptying and storage function
Storage disorders
Rectum
Prolapse
Proctitis and colpoproctitis
Congenital anomalies
Fistulas
Anal sphincter
Anatomic
Focal—obstetric trauma
Global—perineal descent syndrome (late)
Neurologic
Peripheral—obstetric, surgical
Central—multiple sclerosis, cerebrovascular accident, sacral cord lesion
Emptying disorders
Rectum
Hirschprung's disease, megacolon, obstruction
Anal sphincter
Neuro-anatomic
Focal—obstetric
Global—perineal descent syndrome (early stage)
Neuropsychologic
Peripheral—levator spasm
Central—psychogenic

degree of stretching during childbirth or from chronic straining at stool, may result in a loss of this major component of rectal continence.

Thus the rectum acts as a reservoir through its elastic properties due to the thinner longitudinal muscle layer as compared to that of the colon. It is able to accommodate over 400 ml of a substantial amount of feces to allow for a more socially convenient defecation. Any decrease in compliance, caused by irritation, inflammation, scarring, or ischemia, may lead to incontinence.

Ordinarily, the gastrocolic reflex regularly assists defecation by providing large intestinal peristalsis, which becomes part of the habit pattern of normal defecation. If, however, this reflex is consistently inhibited by voluntary postponement of this cleansing process, constipation may occur. In chronic constipation, rectal compliance may be increased, resulting in the development of a megarectum. Progressive impaction can lead to overflow incontinence due to increased rectal secretion around a hard fecal mass that is difficult to move. In addition, the reflex contraction of the intact pubococcygei creates an anorectal valve that can be identified by the angulation of the anorectal junction, the anterior wall of the rectum covering the central lumen when the pubococcygei are contracted. This valve effect adds an additional mechanical mechanism to the maintenance of continence. It is reflexively relaxed during defecation, allowing the funneling of the lower rectum into the upper anal canal. Weakness or poor innervation of the pubococcygei leads to perineal descent and the perineal descent syndrome. Its persistent contraction, on the other hand, may be the source of pain and bowel dysfunction seen in proctalgia, whereas its paradoxical contraction during defecation may be a cause of functional constipation (pelvic floor dyssynergia). It is directly innervated via S3, S4 branches of the spinal cord. Its activity is normally synchronous with that of the external anal sphincter.

A backup system of continence occurs through the internal anal sphincter, which is an involuntary smooth muscle continuous with the inner circular layer of the rectum below the anal rectal junction. It is innervated by the enteric nerves and is responsible for 50% to 75% of the tonic resting anal canal pressure. It provides a barrier for the leakage of liquid and gas. By complex interaction, the internal sphincter reflexively relaxes preceding and during the act of defecation to permit the unimpeded transit of stool. When the levator ani or external anal sphincter or its nerve supply have been effectively compromised, the internal anal sphincter may remain as the sole barrier to rectal incontinence.

A voluntary component of this high-pressure barrier is provided by the external anal sphincter, which although divided into three distinct bundles—subcutaneous, superficial, and deep—functions synchronously as a unit including tonic and phasic contractions. It contributes 30% to 50% of the reported anal canal pressure via its tonic contractions, its voluntary contractions raising twofold to threefold the closing pressure in the anal canal. It is reflexively inhibited during defecation as a result of rectal distension and the perception of fullness. Its innervation is mediated by the pudendal nerves and an intact spinal cord.

Patients with disruption of the external anal sphincter may secondarily develop a state of continence consequent to hypertrophy of the pelvic diaphragm through long-standing exercise of habitual voluntary isometric pubococcygeal contractions. A generation ago, Kelly described such acquired continence among Pennsylvania farm women whom he had seen with unrepaired fourth-degree lacerations sustained many years previously. If the levator ani is intact, voluntary overdevelopment and hypertrophy may produce an almost sphincter-like action that can be most effective. There is an indirect role of the levator ani in providing a similar mechanism assisting urinary continence. When this mechanism has been disrupted, there may be associated SUI as well as anorectal incontinence. A sudden onset of both urinary and anal incontinence following a fall leads one to consider the possibility of acute herniation of an intervertebral disk, which may interfere with the pudendal nerves at their origin between S3 and S4. Careful neurologic examination is important in establishing this diagnosis since disk herniation into the cauda equina may be present though not demonstrated by myelography.

Thus, the mechanism of continence relies upon the sensation of rectal distension resulting in a contraction of the sphincteric barrier, including an external anal sphincter and puborectalis and an adequate rectal reservoir capacity that allows within 5 seconds the accommodation of the rectum to the volume of stool. An impairment at any level of the continence mechanism may result in incontinence.

The Factors of Recurrence

The causes of anorectal incontinence include a variety of insults affecting the reservoir capacity, the sphincteric barrier, or bypassing the continence mechanism altogether, as summarized in Table 15.2. Each etiologic factor should be considered in the differential diagnosis of persistent or recurrent anorectal incontinence.

The major etiologic event in the development of anal incontinence in healthy women results from childbirth trauma.[2-4] The mechanism of action of such trauma remains unclear as both neural and musculofascial components of pelvic support can be affected.[5-7] Indeed, anorectal incontinence is more common in women. Furthermore, pudendal nerve damage has resulted from vaginal delivery, particularly following the use of forceps.[3,5,8] Is the neurologic dysfunction secondary to muscular trauma and subsequent traction injury at straining to defecate, or is the initial neural traction and compression injury the cause of subsequent muscular dysfunction and further neural damage and poor sphincteric function? Although the degree of contribution of each factor must vary with each clinical circumstance, knowing the etiologic role is critical to the choice of therapy. It is important to keep such interaction in mind in the evaluation and management of these unfortunate patients and to tailor the therapeutic options to the predominant etiologic component without neglecting all other factors contributing to the problem of incontinence.

Table 15.2 Etiologic classification of anal incontinence

Congenital
Anatomic
Neurologic
Traumatic
Obstetric
Surgical
Neurogenic
Central
Peripheral
Neurovascular insult
Neoplastic
Ischemic
Radiation
Inflammatory
Degenerative/aging
Fistulas

In patients previously treated surgically for anal incontinence, recurrence or persistence can be the result of a multitude of contributory and additive factors, including persistence of the anatomic defect[5,7,9,10] and less-than-optimal circumstances,[11,12] techniques, or healing.[13] In addition, an incomplete evaluation that fails to recognize the contribution of the neural component and/or fails to address it may lead to persistent incontinence although the severity of the denervation of the anal striated sphincter has not been commensurate with the severity of the incontinence.[14] Furthermore, this multifactorial aspect of incontinence may lead to less-than-optimal results even if an appropriate surgical procedure restoring normal anatomy is carried out.[11] Finally, the cause of the recurrence may be altogether unrelated to that which led to the original surgical approach, thus emphasizing the need for a full and complete evaluation of the patient with recurrence and/or persistent incontinence.

Physiopathologically, anorectal incontinence can be simple or complex (Table 15.3). Simple anatomic incontinence falls into one of four types:

Type I—Anatomic incontinence due to a traumatic disruption of the anal sphincter
Type II—Dysfunctional incontinence due to a noncompliant reservoir (rectum unable to distend because of endometriosis, tumor, radiation, scarring, etc.)
Type III—Intrinsic sphincteric incompetence due to a functionally damaged anal sphincter of neurogenic or traumatic origin
Type IV—Fistulas

Complex incontinence results from any combination of the above categories.

Double incontinence refers to urinary and anal incontinence in patients with a significantly weakened pelvic floor.[15] It is important

Table 15.3 Anatomic classification of anorectal incontinence

Simple
Type 1—External sphincter defect
Traumatic—obstetric, surgical
Neurogenic
Type 2—Rectal reservoir disorder
Inflammatory
Neoplastic
Systemic
Degenerative
Type 3—Intrinsic sphincter defect
Neurogenic—motor or sensory
Traumatic—obstetric, surgical
Type 4—Bypass of continence mechanism—fistulas
Inflammatory
Traumatic
Complex
Any combinaton of above

to realize that functionally incontinence is subjectively relative in its severity and various degrees exist. In borderline continence, one additional factor such as diarrhea or surgical trauma may lead to incontinence. It is the functional impairment of the patient that dictates the degree of incontinence. Nonetheless, such degrees also can be objectified by anorectal function studies. The perineal descent syndrome has been cited as the most typical example of the interaction between anatomy and innervation that should be recognized in order to prevent its progression, which could lead to fecal incontinence. However, such correlation between perineal descent and pudendal neuropathy has been recently questioned.[16]

Evaluation

The evaluation of anorectal incontinence, particularly when recurrent, should rely on a comparison of the patient's history before and after the repair procedure and a careful physical examination complemented by manometric and dynamic imaging studies of the continence mechanism.

Although the details of the history are limited to its aspects pertinent to the pelvic floor and anorectum, a general history of the patient, as well as the chronologic details of the events surrounding the incontinence, is of critical importance in understanding the current situation to adequately plan the future evaluation and correction of the disorder.

More specifically, the presence of pain or bleeding with defecation is an important element that usually motivates patients to seek advice without much delay. More significantly, a discharge, particularly when not related to bowel function, may alert the surgeon to the possible bypass of the continence mechanism, as seen in inflammatory fistulizing disease or any circumstance leading to fistula formation, and/or may be indicative of some degree of incontinence. Such mucoid discharge may be responsible for itching, irritation, and soiling and could be related to any of the following

1. An overproduction of mucus from goblet cells, as seen in internal hemorrhoids, villous tumors, irritable co-

lon, or inflammatory disease of the bowel
2. An eversion of the rectal mucosa, as seen in rectal prolapse, prolapsed hemorrhoids, or ectropion
3. An incontinence due to sphincter injury, weakness, or paralysis

Incontinence should induce the evaluation of the sphincteric mechanism, as well as the bowel, which could contribute to abnormal stool consistency. Indeed, a history of trauma should focus the attention on muscular defects resulting from childbirth or surgery. A history of explosive and loose bowel movements, along with frequency and urgency, may be related to irritable bowel disease. In addition, age is a factor that may relate to the weakening of the sphincteric mechanism.

Associated medical conditions should be sought, including the presence of uncontrolled diabetes with neuropathy, which can result in constipation secondary to dismotility, osmotic diuresis, and dehydration. A low-output cardiac condition can result in ischemic changes. A history of pelvic irradiation could cause tenesmus, sphincteric dysfunction, blood loss, and diarrhea. The surgeon should also recognize the importance of relative physical immobility in the geriatric population.

The history should include an accurate account of the patient's medication intake. Finally, a family history of familial cancer, inherited polyposis, Crohn's disease, or ulcerative colitis may be of significance.

The physical examination should assess the general status of the patient but should be directed primarily to the abdomen and pelvis. During the abdominal palpation the surgeon looks for left lower quadrant tenderness, indicative of irritable bowel disease or diverticular disease, and checks for a full sigmoid colon as a sign of chronic constipation.

The pelvic examination should establish the depth and axis of the vagina and rectum. Normally the upper part of the vagina rests on the rectum, which rests on an intact levator plate. The anorectal angle is established as the rectum bends over the edge of this intact levator plate. When the vaginal or rectal axis is vertical in the resting position, there is damage to the levator plate, either structural or neurologic.

Inspection starts with the examination of the anus and perineum. The examiner should be looking for dynamic and static abnormalities. Dynamic maneuvers, including Valsalva and the squeeze maneuver, will reveal the presence of prolapse, muscular disorder, neurologic deficit, or regional deficits, including a cystocele and/or a rectocele. When the patient is asked to contract voluntarily her pubococcygei, her ability to perform this action is noted carefully. When the patient cannot demonstrate effective contraction of these muscles, a neuropathy may be present. One should similarly test the integrity of the external anal sphincter by asking the patient to voluntary contract it. Its reflex contraction may be noted by the insertion of a finger into the rectum. When the reflex is found wanting, the surgeon must seek to determine whether the failure is the consequence of disruption of the external anal sphincter from unrepaired trauma or the consequence of a neuropathy. An intact but patulous external anal sphincter suggests the latter, although that condition may be temporarily induced by a coincident rectal prolapse. In the latter, intussusception of the rectum causes the rectal mucosa to protrude through the external anal sphincter and acts as a dilating wedge, disturbing the reflex contraction of the muscle. The shape and location of the anus can provide information regarding the site of muscular injury as an anterior displacement results from a posterior muscular disruption, whereas a posterior displacement is commonly seen with an anterior muscular injury. The presence of perianal wetness or fecal soilage documents the effective presence of sphincter incontinence. The presence of scars should be noted, particularly in association with swelling or skin lesions indicative of deeper infections or neoplastic lesions.

If both pubococcygeal and external anal sphincter muscles appear to be nonfunctional, a primary pudendal neuropathy is likely. If only one component is nonfunctional, usually the external anal sphincter, traumatic disruption of the sphincter is likely.

On palpation, the examination of the vaginal introitus, the perineal body, and the ischiorectal fossa and anal space are investigated. Any area of induration or fluctuance is noted, along with the presence of muscular defects in the anorectal ring. The presence or absence of mucosal or extramucosal masses should be determined. The perirectal spaces are carefully investigated for the presence of abscess or tumor. A finger in the rectum while the patient is straining and then squeezing will assess the sphincteric function mechanism. It is important that the examiner determine that the patient is contracting only the internal muscles of the pelvis. Erroneous contraction of the gluteal and hip muscles will provide a false assumption of internal pelvic muscular efficacy. With the fingertip in the anus, a contraction of all four quadrants can assess their strength and symmetry. While hooking the finger over the rim of the rectum posteriorly and asking the patient to contract, the relative contribution of the puborectalis versus the external anal sphincter could be measured. With traction of the pelvic floor causing pain, the possibility of levator syndrome should be assessed. Palpation of involuntary pubococcygeal spasm and tenderness support this possibility. The presence and consistency of stool in the rectum should also be noted.

A brief neurologic examination may identify changes in sensitivity of the pelvic skin with or without demonstrable leg pain. When these are present, further examination of that portion of the nervous system is indicated, such as by selective electromyography of the pelvic diaphragm or external anal sphincter, and evaluation of function, as by defecogram and barium enema. Fasting blood glucose levels can be examined to determine more effectively the possibility of neuropathy secondary to an abnormality in carbohydrate metabolism. The examiner should look for the presence of the anal wink and the effect of commands such as squeezing, tightening, and straining as noted above. It is important to realize that the resting tone reflects the function of the internal anal sphincter, which normally should be contracted.

The pelvic examination of the integrity of the pelvic floor should be repeated by confirmation when the patient is standing with one foot resting on a shelf or stool at the end of the examining table. In this position, the patient first "holds" by voluntarily contracting her pelvic muscles to the best of her ability and then pushes using a Valsalva maneuver.

Physical examination at times may identify a perineal prolapse that is coexistent with a perineal descent syndrome, where there is pathologic stretching and funneling of the levator ani, usually as the result of obstetric damage or straining at stool. The defect may result from abnormality in the integrity of the pubococcygei themselves or in their nerve supply. The ability of the patient to contract these muscles voluntarily suggests which of the two abnormalities is present.

Any disruption of the perineal body should be noted, as its importance is that the puborectal muscle is deficient, rendering the anal canal vulnerable anteriorly. Its disruption results in a loss of the anterior angulation of the rectum on the anus. The descending perineum syndrome is suggested by the finding that the anus is the most dependent portion of the patient's perineum, a situation made worse by voluntary straining as the pathologic funneling of the muscles increases. Patients with recurrent or persistent anal incontinence and all patients with fecal incontinence should have the benefit of a complete preoperative evaluation with regard to the cause of their incontinence, including manometric and neurophysiologic studies and endoscopic and imaging techniques.[11,13,17-20]

It is important to emphasize that although these sophisticated tests have a distinct role in the evaluation of patients with persistent or recurrent anal incontinence, their interpretation should rely on a careful history and a detailed clinical examination. The tests include anal manometry, electrophysiologic studies, perineometry, defecography, and endosonography. For optimum evaluation, more than one test is required.

Manometry provides a quantifiable evaluation of the internal and external anal sphincter function. It has been demonstrated that digital examination can be as accurate as anal manometry in the assessment of pressure generated by the anal sphincter.[21] Such evaluation remains very subjective, and the need for an objective assessment and comparison is obvious. The physiologic requirements for continence[18] include the following:

1. The ability to perceive rectal distension of 10 ml or less

2. The ability to contract the external anal sphincter and puborectal muscles with enough strength to prevent incontinence for at least 3 seconds
3. The availability of a sufficient reservoir capacity in the rectum (over 100 ml)
4. A definite motivation to avoid incontinence

The anorectal manometric evaluation assesses the function of the internal and external anal sphincters as well as the sensory threshold of the rectal reservoir.[22] Its components include the following:

1. The resting and squeezing anal canal pressures. They are obtained by pulling a manometry catheter through the anal canal three times and averaging the peak pressures. At rest the average is 30 to 90 mm Hg. With maximum squeeze the pressure rise and duration reflect the strength of the phasic contraction of the external anal sphincter, whereas the resting pressure reflects the tonic contraction of the internal and external anal sphincters as well as that contributed by the levator muscle (Figure 15.2).
2. The vector volume study. A 6 to 8 radially oriented perfusion port catheter is pulled through the sphincter while the patient is resting and again while squeezing. A computer program can construct a three-dimensional image of the anal canal pressures (Figure 15.3). This represents a very sensitive method of screening for anatomic defects in the sphincter that correlates very well with more recently available anal endosonography.[9,23-25] Recently Goes, Simons, and Beart used vectograms to study the relative position of the highest mean resting pressure segment in the anal canal and suggested it is in a more proximal location in incontinent patients than in controls.[26]
3. The sensory threshold of the rectum. This can be assessed by distending a balloon with 30 ml of air. This maneuver is repeated with progressively reduced volumes down to 5 ml, and the lowest volume that is consciously detectable is noted as the sensory threshold. The study requires a standard anorectal manometry catheter, including a balloon in the rectum and perfusion ports in the anal canal.
4. Rectal compliance. The anorectal manometry catheter also allows the measurement of rectal compliance, which is the maximum tolerated volume (MTV) in the rectum. With gradual distension of the rectal balloon (20 ml of air per minute up to MTV or 500 ml), the examiner notes the minimum volume that results in sustained urge (over 60 seconds) to defecate, the minimum volume resulting in rectal contraction of over 5 mm Hg of amplitude, and the maximum tolerated volume (200 to 300 ml).
5. The response to straining to defecate or the rectoanal inhibitory reflex (RAIR). This reflex is normally mediated by local visceral nerve plexuses in the submucosal and myenteric layers.[27] With two perfusion ports in the anal canal, in normal individuals the straining to defecate results in a decrease in the anal canal resting pressures (Figure 15.4). In patients with pelvic floor dyssynergia, a paradoxical contraction is noted.[28]

Using a manovolumeteric method of simultaneous recording of anal pressures and rectal volumes in response to graded rectal distension pressures, Holmberg and others have suggested that in incontinent patients, sphincteric dysfunction represents the primary defect.[29]

The value of anal manometry in predicting the outcome of surgical procedures for fecal incontinence has been controversial. Increase in sphincter length and sphincter pressures have been shown in some studies[30] although not in others that have been successful.[31,32]

Resting pressures are lower in traumatic sphincter injury, rectal prolapse, pudendal nerve traction injuries, spinal caudal equina injury, chronic inflammatory bowel disease, proctitis, and increasing age. Although indicating lower than normal or normal anal

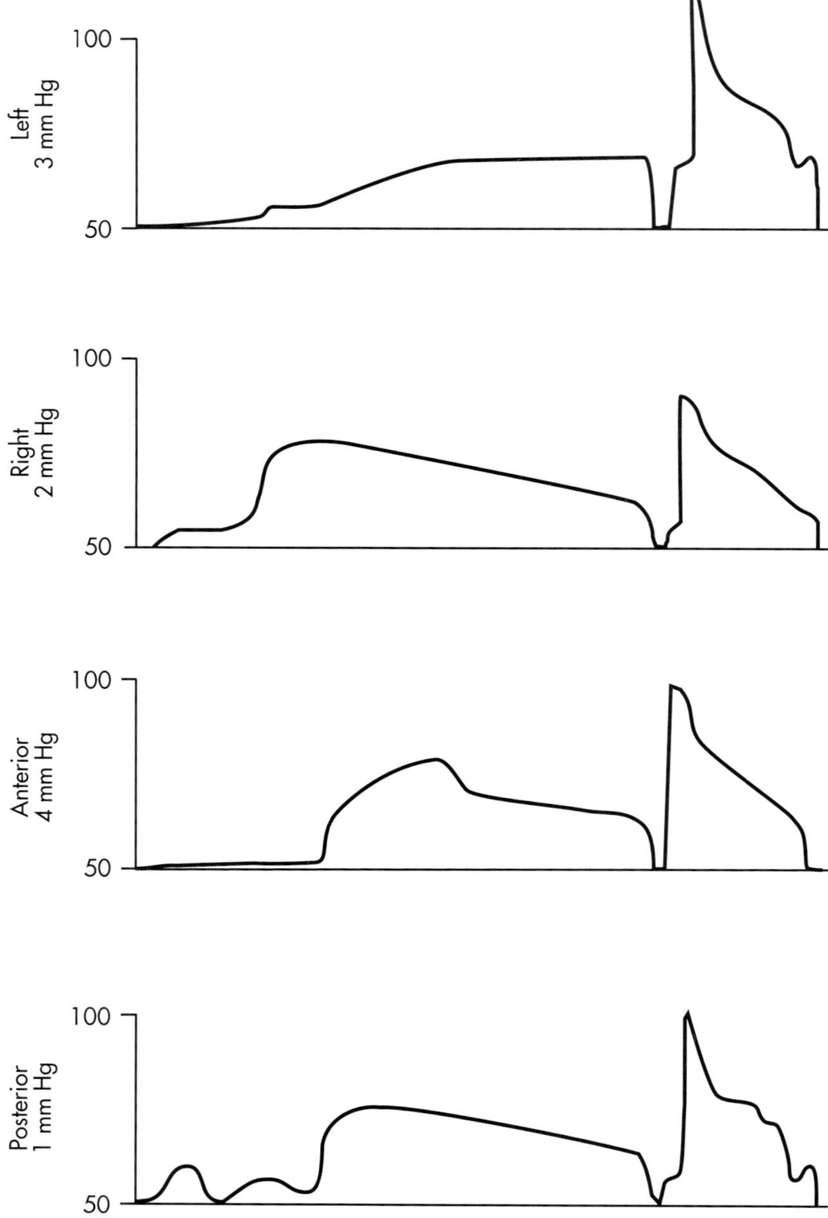

FIGURE 15.2 Resting and squeeze anal canal pressures with quadrant variations.

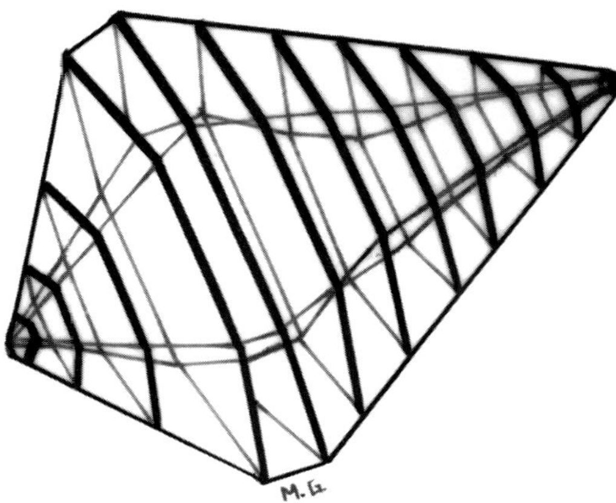

Figure 15.3 Three-dimensional representation of anal canal pressures.

pressures, anal manometry cannot by itself differentiate between the various causes of such diminished pressures, particularly anatomic versus neurogenic. More recently, ambulatory anorectal manometry seems to provide information emphasizing the concept that continence is dependent not simply on pressure but on the interrelationship of various factors involved in rectal continence, as spontaneous transient episodes of sphincter relaxation are demonstrable in normal subjects.[31,33]

Electrophysiologic studies for the assessment of the anal sphincter and the pelvic floor can be used to detect elements of denervation. These studies include surface electrode electromyography or single fiber electromyography, along with nerve stimulation techniques and testing of sensory function. Good correlation has been obtained between noninvasive surface electromyography using an intraanal plug electrode and anal manometry.[34] In pelvic floor electromyography a surface electrode acrylic plug is inserted in the anal canal after the catheter is removed. The resting level of the pelvic floor electromyogram (EMG less than 2 μv) along with the response to squeeze (greater than 30 μv) and strain to defecate are noted. A normal EMG with low squeeze pressure usually indicates sphincter muscle separation, whereas a slow squeeze pressure and low EMG squeeze is suggestive of a neural injury. The principle of surface electromyography is widely used in biofeedback retraining of pelvic floor and anal sphincter muscles.

Mapping of sphincter defects can be done by using concentric needle electrodes and is reasonably accurate. As improved resolution allows the definition of the external and internal anal sphincters, anal endosonography seems to provide adequate mapping with less discomfort.[35] Single fiber electromyography assesses the denervation and reinnervation of striated muscles as patients with pudendal nerve traction injury have increased fiber density consistent with reinnervation.[36] In those patients surgery is not as effective in improving function. The use of smooth muscle electromyography has demonstrated a reduction in the frequency of the ultraslow wave activity in patients with fecal incontinence.[31]

Nerve stimulation techniques can help assess the integrity of the motor supply to the pelvic floor. The pudendal nerve terminal motor latency is increased in fecal incontinence and perineal descent syndrome, reflecting local damage to the nerve. Transcutaneous spinal stimulation at L1 to L4 could help to test the integrity of the cauda equina.[37]

Sensory function testing at various levels of the anal canal demonstrates a significant difference in both mucosal electrosensitivity and thermal sensitivity in the upper anal canal between continent patients and patients who are incontinent with excessive perineal descent.[38,39] A saline infusion into the rectum to stress the anal sphincter mechanism assesses the volume at which fecal incontinence occurs. It has been shown that patients with idiopathic incontinence leak fluid at a lower volume than normal, demonstrating an inappropriate relaxation of the sphincter as a result of stimulation by fluid.[31]

Perineometry assesses the degree of perineal descent using a mechanical device.[40] It is a simple, rapid, and noninvasive method. At times it underestimates the degree of descent compared to radiologic studies in the erect position.

Defecography is a radiologic investigation of the anorectum and pelvic floor at rest and during straining at defecation.[41] It provides objective information about the rectal wall, perineal descent, anorectal angle, internal intussusception, and rectal prolapse. Its role in incontinence seems of limited value in the

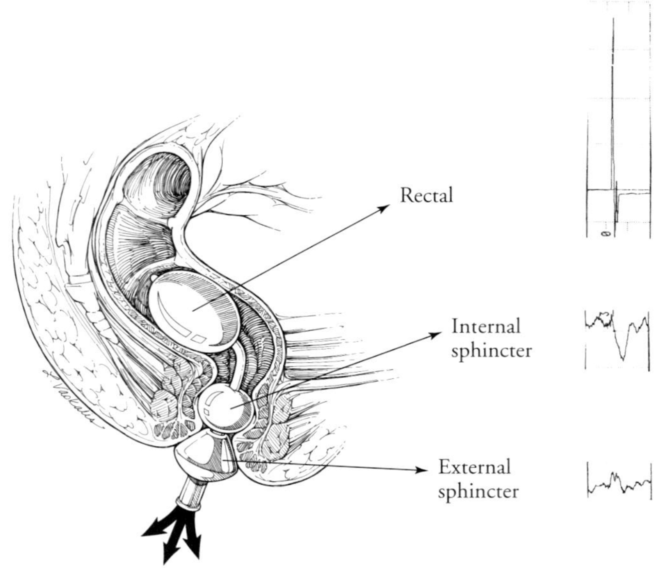

FIGURE 15.4 Schematic diagram of Schuster's balloon in place demonstrating internal sphincter relaxation and simultaneous external sphincter contraction with rectal balloon distention.

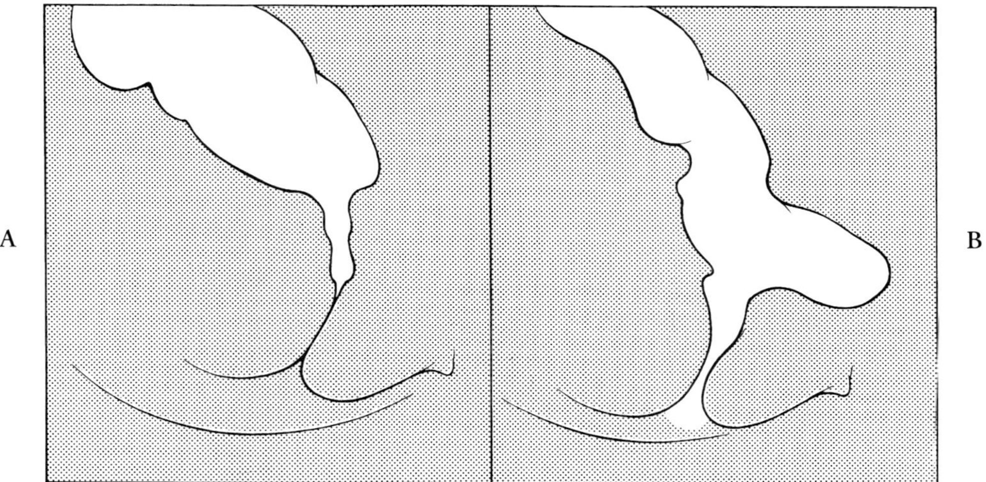

FIGURE 15.5 Schematic diagram of defecography showing persistent outpouching of an anterior rectocele. **A**, At rest. **B**, During defecation.

absence of obstructive symptoms.[31,42-44] This remains one of the best radiologic means of investigation of the anorectal function, demonstrating abnormalities in rectal wall configuration during evacuation, including the presence of rectocele, anteriorly or posteriorly, the relaxation of the puborectalis during straining, resulting in opening of the anorectal angle, and the coexistence of perineal descent (Figure 15.5). Bartolo and others have raised doubts concerning the validity of the flat valve theory regarding the mechanism of continence. Using defecography, they were unable to show the approximation of the anterior rectal wall to the upper anal canal during periods of raised intraabdominal pressure.[45] Its combination with visualization of the bladder and vagina provides a good dynamic imaging of the relation and support of the pelvic organs involved and can be helpful in preoperative evaluation of concomitant pathology.[20]

Endosonography provides information

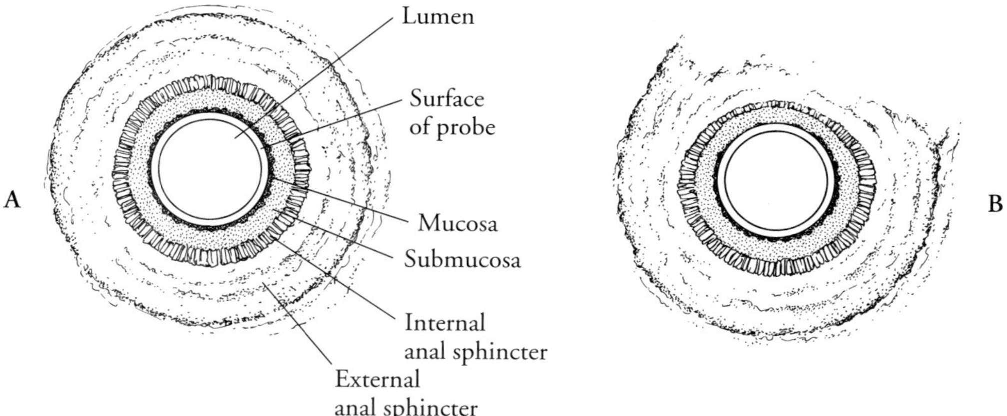

Figure 15.6 Schematic representation of sonographic anatomy of the anal sphincter. **A**, Normal. **B**, Abnormal.

useful in planning surgical intervention in patients with sphincter defects and in the evaluation of patients who have failed corrective surgeries.[13] Indeed, it allows a better definition of the sphincter muscles (Figure 15.6) and their integrity because the internal and external anal sphincters present distinct characteristics. The assessment of both sphincter anatomy and function are important in the evaluation of the continence mechanism. In some studies the thickness of the internal anal sphincter correlated with the resting anal pressure, as incontinent patients with a thin band of sphincter muscles also have a reduced anal sphincter pressure.[23] In other studies pathologic lesions of the anal canal and perianal region can be readily demonstrable using this technique, particularly abscesses and fistulas. Good correlation between acoustic and electrical defects of the external anal sphincter has been demonstrated. The combination of endosonography and pudendal nerve terminal motor latency provides the most significant information in selecting patients for surgery.[24]

Endoscopic examination is important to rule out an inflammatory or neoplastic lesion, a fistula, rectal prolapse, or other anorectal disorders.

Differential Diagnosis

The complete history and physical examination along with the pelvic and digital rectal examination should allow for the diagnosis of the most common cause of fecal incontinence in women, that is, sphincter defect. Anoscopy and proctoscopy rule out an intrinsic bowel disorder, whereas in those patients in whom a sphincter defect is not obvious, anal manometry may help assess the sphincteric function while ruling out a sensory deficit or altered rectal compliance. Presumably suitable examinations of patients with recurrent anal incontinence have excluded rectovaginal fistula, ulcerative colitis, and Crohn's disease of the colon.

Functional disorders of the anorectal area consist primarily of dysfunctions of the striated pelvic floor muscle through which the bowel passes. As demonstrated by Holmberg and others,[29] any reduction in rectal compliance is likely to be a secondary phenomenon.

Encopresis is the loss of stool from the anus at an inappropriate time. It represents incontinence without known physical causes as opposed to that which is secondary to neurologic injuries or congenital malformations. It is associated with or due to constipation in over 96% of the cases. It is important to rule out encopresis as the source of incontinence. The diagnosis usually is suggested by soiling in association with constipation when the diagnosis of Hirschsprung's disease, rectal prolapse, willful soiling, and incompetence due to mental retardation, dementia, and psychosis have been ruled out. On examination the anus is gaping and the sphincter tone is lax, while a large mass is present in the rectum. The treatment includes habit training and biofeedback.

Habit training is important at an early stage

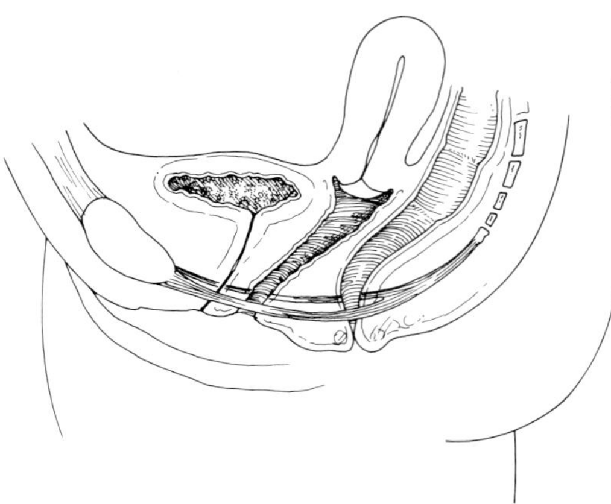

FIGURE 15.7 A sagittal section of the pelvis shows elongation and sagging of the levator plate. The usual angle between the anal canal and the rectum, as well as the horizontal axis of the rectum and the upper portion of the vagina, have been lost. (Redrawn from Nichols DH and Randall CL: Vaginal surgery, ed 4, Baltimore, 1996, Williams & Wilkins.)

as it is known that the pelvic diaphragm and its innervation by the pudendal nerve may be damaged to varying degrees by pathologic stretching, either as might result from bearing down during childbirth or, more commonly, chronic straining at stool. These mechanical stresses appear to stretch the pudendal nerve at its angulation around the ischial spine. The resulting progressive damage to the pudendal nerve over a period of time may compound the inability of the pelvic diaphragm and external anal sphincter to function at maximum efficiency. Pathologic funneling of the pelvic diaphragm is produced and is manifested by a visible descent of the perineum and anus (Figure 15.7). The patient then actually sits on her anus, which becomes the most dependent portion of the perineum. With straining, the perineum and anus may descend further as the pelvic diaphragm becomes more and more funneled.

Initially this excessive funneling reduces the width of the hiatus between the levatores ani. In some patients obstipation, an inability to empty the rectum no matter how the patient strains, may develop. Difficulty evacuating may become progressively worse, and the diameter of the stool noticeably decreases to an almost ribbonlike extrusion.

Descending perineum syndrome[46] is suggested by the finding that the anus is the most dependent portion of the patient's perineum, a situation made worse by voluntary straining, as the funneling of the muscles pathologically increases. During the development of this syndrome there may be at first no symptoms, but later there will be progressive obstipation and narrowing of stool. These symptoms are made worse the harder the patient strains. If the condition at this stage remains undiagnosed and untreated, further progression is a distinct possibility with the development of a progressive pudendal neuropathy. If the condition becomes permanent, the mechanism of anal continence will be severely disturbed.

The function of the levator ani can be measured by electromyography as noted above, but it also can be evaluated more simply by asking the patient to contract her pelvic diaphragm voluntarily during pelvic examination. Failure in the ability to voluntarily contract her pubococcygei suggests the presence of a pudendal neuropathy. Such damage may be permanent. For such a patient, the sole means for rectal continence may lie with the already described involuntary mechanism within her internal anal sphincter. Continence and evacuation will depend on her ability to program the necessary relaxation of her internal anal sphincter. If this last mechanism is lost, there may be total sphincter deficiency, and the patient may become rectally incontinent, an unwelcome event for which effective treatment is almost impossible. The patient may present anywhere along the spectrum of symptoms from evacuation difficulty to complete incontinence. Early diagnosis is essential to encourage reeducation about bowel habit to eliminate straining and prevent incremental pudendal nerve damage.

Coincident rectal prolapse suggests pathologic elongation of the large intestine and its mesentery, allowing an actual intussusception of the bowel. As mentioned before, the leading edge of the intussusception may constitute a dilating wedge of tissue pushing through the anorectal valve and external anal sphincter. Coincident progressive anal incontinence often results. Henry and Swash[47] suggested this relationship as follows:

> I think the primary pathology is one of neuropathy affecting the pelvic floor—in many patients a consequence of damage to the pudendal

nerve inflicted by traumatic childbirth. Incontinence may not develop initially if the internal anal sphincter is functioning normally. Pelvic floor denervation initiates rectal prolapse because of disruption of the anorectal flap valve. The prolapse starts with descent of the anterior rectal wall and at a later stage a circumferential complete prolapse intussuscepts through the anus. The dilatation of the internal anal sphincter caused by the prolapsing rectum then destroys the only mechanism protecting anorectal continence and a major functional problem results. Because the internal sphincter recovers, many patients recover a reasonable degree of control after successful repair of the prolapse. If continence is not recovered within 6 months, we will offer the patient a transperineal postanal repair [of the puborectalis and the pelvic diaphragm].

Conservative Management

The management of recurrent anal incontinence depends on the degree of disability resulting therefrom. The majority of cases will be helped by a conservative approach inasmuch as a fistula has been ruled out and/or corrected. The patient's disability and expectation of therapy remains the best indicator for the degree of aggressiveness of the therapy. Indeed, lack of control of flatus may be more significant to some patients whereas considerable soiling is to others. A careful evaluation of the patient's degree of disability and definition of bowel control is a critical part of the patient's management.

Conservative management represents the first and often the sole line of therapy for patients with recurrent anal incontinence. This is particularly so if a successful operative repair is not feasible or if the operative repair has been only partially successful and the patient remains with borderline incontinence that could be improved by these simple measures. Finally, for the patient in whom an operative procedure is not indicated, particularly when the likelihood of muscle retraining is promising, conservative measures in strengthening the residual sphincter might be adequate prior to consideration of any further aggressive therapy.

The patient may be placed on dietary fiber supplements, such as bran used daily at breakfast.

Redevelopment of good bowel habits should include heeding the morning gastrocolic reflex with adequate time for effective evacuation at the same time every day in habit retraining.

Estrogenic hormone stimulation for the postmenopausal woman may increase the pelvic blood supply and muscular nutrition. When the pubococcygei can be contracted, even though weakly and ineffectively at first, an intense program of Kegel perineal resistive exercises can be useful. A series of 15 voluntary firm contractions of this muscle for 3 seconds each 6 times daily should be employed. Increased muscular strength is often reflected in an improvement in rectal continence. The exercise should be continued indefinitely. In some resistive cases, some improvement may be obtained from courses of galvanic stimulation of the anal sphincter and pelvic diaphragm.

Finally, biofeedback using an intraanal electrode connected to an electromyometer may be effective. The success of biofeedback is dependent on the contraction of the adequate musculature, as often patients are unaware of which muscle to contract. Motivation and supervision, along with a maintenance program, are important.

In patients with partial incontinence, drug therapy to decrease intestinal motility, including anticholinergic drugs, may be helpful. In patients with leakage, a small tap water enema after a bowel movement may be of help. Finally, in neurogenic incontinence, rectal irritation by a gloved finger or suppository or rubbing the thigh or abdomen to initiate an emptying reflex may be useful.

Surgical Management

The surgical treatment of recurrent anal incontinence is dependent on the cause of the incontinence as defined by the history, physical examination, and laboratory evaluation. When mechanical disruption of the levator ani or external anal sphincter has been demonstrated, the treatment is surgical. Though unusually patulous, a sphincteroplasty, either anterior or posterior, may be performed with or without coincident perineorrhaphy (Figure 15.8). Correction of any defect of the supports

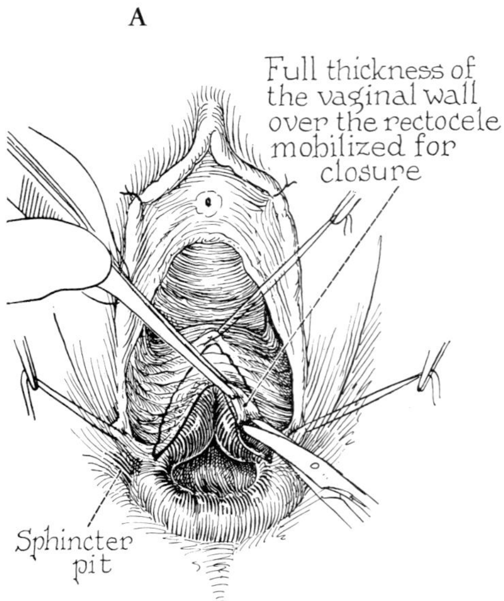
A
Full thickness of the vaginal wall over the rectocele mobilized for closure
Sphincter pit

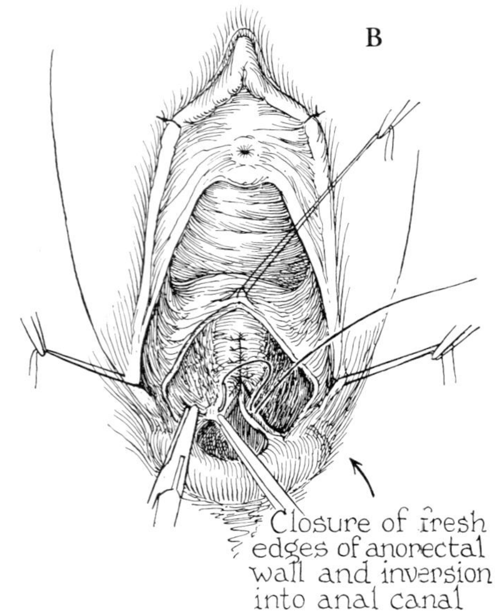
B
Closure of fresh edges of anorectal wall and inversion into anal canal

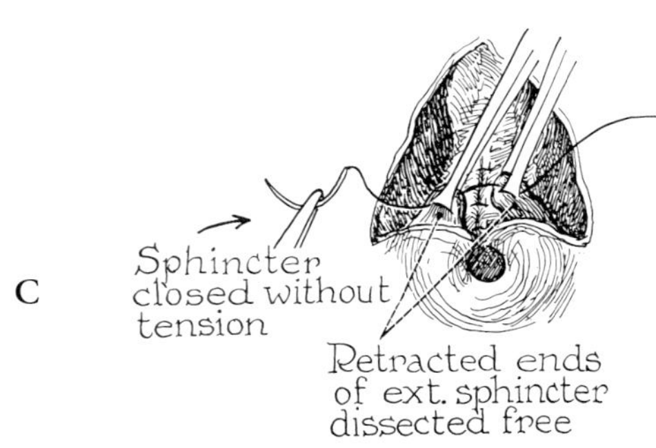
C
Sphincter closed without tension
Retracted ends of ext. sphincter dissected free

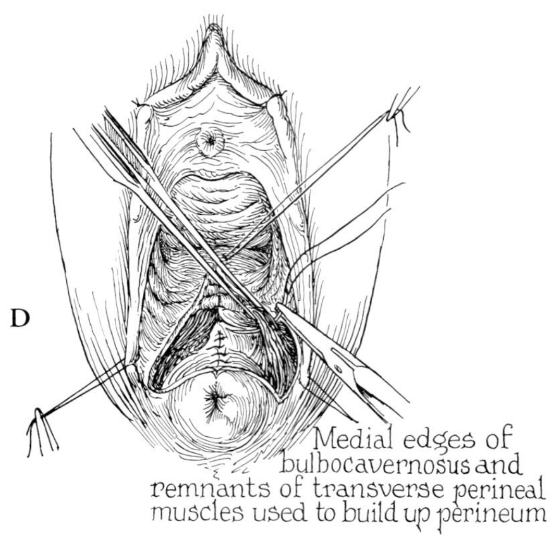
D
Medial edges of bulbocavernosus and remnants of transverse perineal muscles used to build up perineum

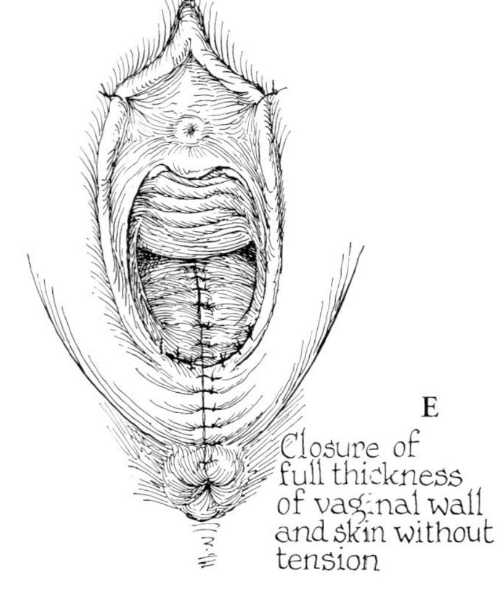
E
Closure of full thickness of vaginal wall and skin without tension

of the posterior vaginal wall, including treatment of such rectocele as may be present, may thus be done during the same procedure. Failures of prior sphincteric repair have been ascribed to a persistent sphincteric defect.[9,10,13] Careful evaluation and treatment of these patients is mandatory if the surgical procedure is to be corrective. The principles of sphincteric repair are important and should be adhered to in an attempt to optimize the possible results. This includes an adequate bowel preparation, and an aseptic and atraumatic technique of repair. Any excessive scarring should be removed, although the scar on the muscle is best left intact and used to suture the muscle. It is crucial to repair the entire sphincteric muscular complex. The importance of repairing the perineal body cannot be overemphasized in repairing the entire sphincteric complex. Such repair should be carried out without tension and with adequate hemostasis and drainage. It is important to keep in mind that in anterior sphincteric defects the anterior segment of the anal sphincter, the perineal body, and the rectovaginal septum should all be repaired in order to optimize the result. It can be carried out by the layer technique or the Warren flap method in the event of extensive tissue loss.[48] An apron of posterior vaginal mucosa is dissected off the rectovaginal fascia and used to cover the reconstructed perineal body and external anal sphincter.[49]

In direct anal sphincter injury, a direct anal sphincter repair is indicated as long as neurologic disease or destruction of the sphincter by inflammatory disease (Crohn's disease, abscess, or malignancy) has been ruled out. The presence of a functioning sphincter muscle is critical to the success of the operation. The purpose of the procedure is to eliminate the scarred segment and recreate an active sphincter muscle surrounding the anal canal. Identification of the muscle ends is the critical part of the procedure in addition to resection of the excessive scar and possibly overlapping the muscle without tension. It is helpful to start identifying normal muscle along with the proper plane of dissection and then advance to a scarred area. It is always better to leave the scar on the muscle as it will help in suture placement. In partial fecal incontinence, idiopathic or following internal sphincterotomy, perianal injection of bulking agents has proved successful in over 50% of patients.[50]

Strong consideration should be given to correcting the symptomatic perineal descent by a coincident retrorectal levatorplasty.[52,53] This operation, which includes the steps of the Parks postanal repair, may correct the descending perineal syndrome before a total neuropathy has developed.[51] In this operation an incision is made between the anus and the tip of the coccyx, the anococcygeal ligament is divided, and the dissection is carried directly into the retrorectal space (Figure 15.9). A series of plication stitches is placed in the posterior wall of the rectum and tied but not cut. When all of these have been placed, they are sewn to the periosteum of the undersurface of the sacrum with care taken to avoid the middle

FIGURE 15.8 Traction sutures are placed outlining a triangular area to be denuded. The apex of this triangle is above any scar tissue in the vagina, while the angles of the base are over the sphincter pits (**A**). The incision is carried high enough so the full thickness of the vaginal wall over a rectocele or lateral vaginal wall relaxation can be mobilized to aid in the closure. The dissection is continued until the full thickness of the vagina is mobilized and separated from the rectal wall and mucosa. The scar tissue in the vaginal and rectal walls is excised so that fresh edges are approximated, and the rectal and anorectal walls are inverted into the canal by interrupted sutures of 00 PGA on atraumatic needles (**B**). These sutures extend just to the submucosa and precisely approximate the tissues. The retracted ends of the external sphincter are located and mobilized sufficiently for approximation in the midline without tension (**C**). They are sutured together with interrupted sutures of 00 PGA on atraumatic needles. The medial edges of the bulbocavernosi and remnants of the transverse perineal muscles are used to build up the perineal body over and above the reunited external sphincter (**D**). The anterior edges of the levators are approximated in the midline to give additional support. The full thickness of the vaginal wall and the skin of the perineum are closed by interrupted sutures (**E**). They are approximated without tension and inspected again so that scar tissue is not incorporated into the wound. (From Ball TL: Gynecologic surgery and urology, ed 2, St Louis, 1963, Mosby.)

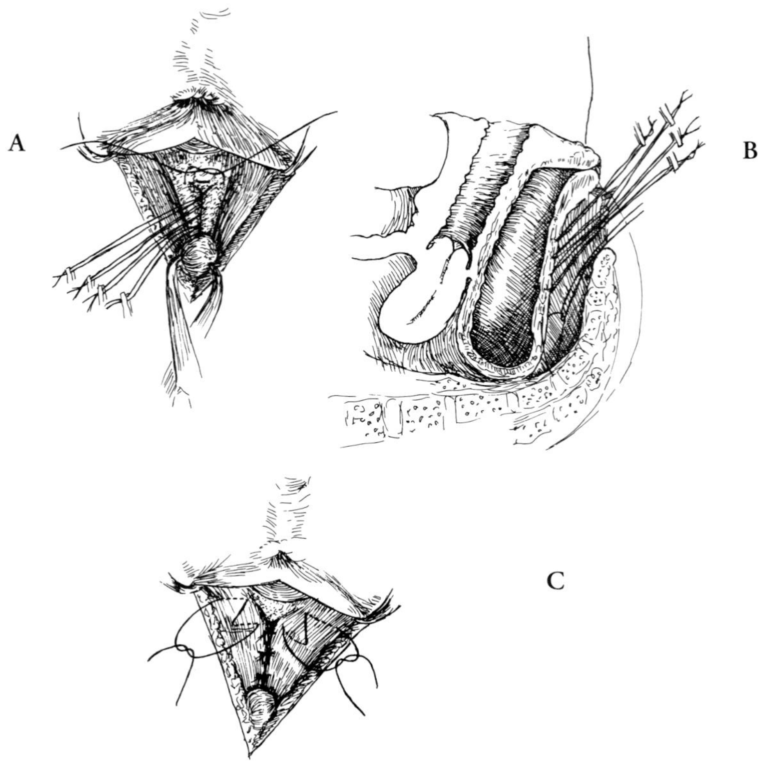

FIGURE 15.9 The essential steps of retrorectal levatorplasty include an incision through the skin beneath the anus and the coccyx, transection of any anococcygeal ligament that may be present, and establishing an opening into the retrorectal space. A series of plication stitches is placed in the posterior wall of the rectum and tied (**A**). These are then sewn to the periosteum of the hollow of the sacrum and tied (**B**). A number of interrupted stitches is placed reuniting the right to the left pubococcygeus (**C**) and reestablishing the levator plate and helping to form a new anorectal angle. These are tied loosely so as to avoid strangulation. A markedly elongated pubococcygeus may be further shortened by a Z stitch on each side, which, when tied, will shorten the pubococcygeus. (Redrawn from Nichols DH and Randall CL: Vaginal surgery, ed 4, Baltimore, 1996, Williams & Wilkins.)

sacral artery. When tied, the sutures will bring the rectum back into the hollow of the sacrum. The bellies of the pubococcygei are brought together behind the rectum with a series of interrupted stitches tied only tightly enough to hold them together but not to strangulate the tissue. This surgery reestablishes and lengthens the levator plate (which is the fusion of the pubococcygei posterior to the rectum).

Each elongated pubococcygeus may be shortened by a Z stitch or two as necessary to reestablish the horizontal orientation of the levator plate. An effective anorectal angle is thus reestablished but in a fashion by which it can be temporarily and voluntarily straightened out during the normal evacuation process, unlocking its protective valve–like function. Repair of coincident cystocele, rectocele, enterocele, and uterine prolapse follows immediately. If a reconstruction of this sort is not performed in a symptomatic patient, the perineal descent and pudendal nerve damage will progress. There should be a meticulous attempt to correct abnormal bowel habits to lessen the need for straining at stool. If such reeducation is neglected, increased damage to the pudendal nerve is likely to result.

Both perineal descent syndrome and genital prolapse may be associated with coincident rectal prolapse, an actual intussusception of the bowel on itself. When present, rectal prolapse should be treated by a separate surgical procedure, usually transabdominal, and the intussusception reduced either by large bowel resection or by suspension as in a Ripstein-like procedure.[54,55] Indeed, the treatment of rectal

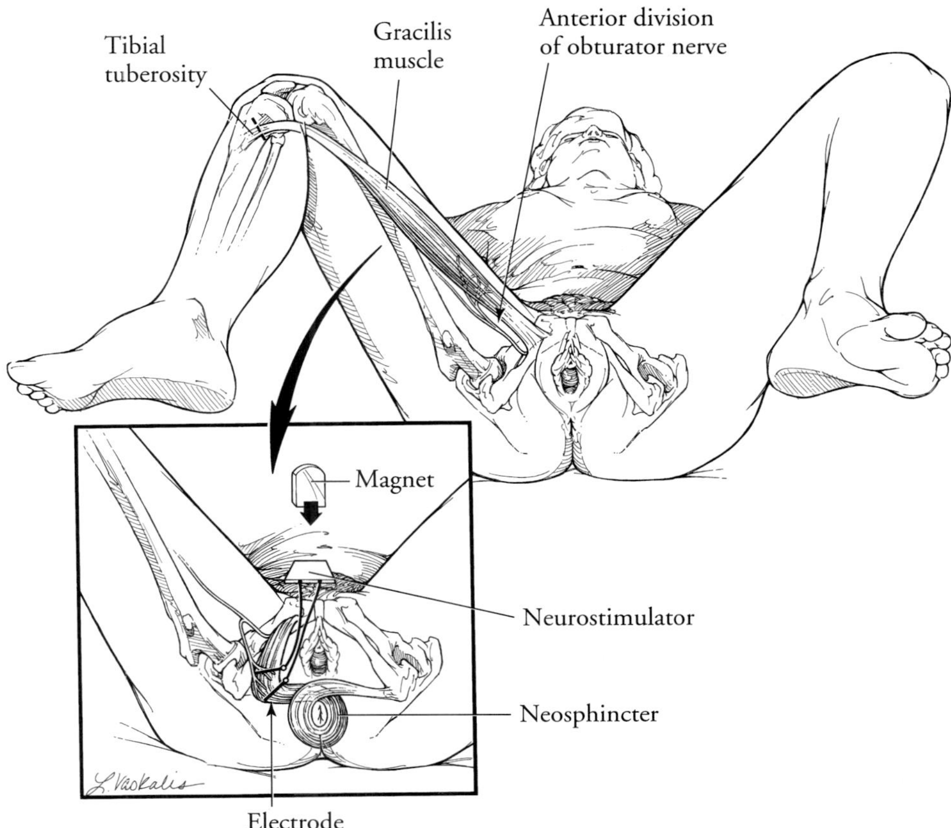

FIGURE 15.10 Schematic representation of anal dynamic graciloplasty.

prolapse is primarily surgical. It usually involves a transabdominal rectopexy using the Ripstein-type pinup operation. And when there is an unusually long segment of bowel, treatment is an appropriate transabdominal resection of this extra intestine with reanastomosis and sacral fixation of the colon. The transperineal bowel resection of Dunphy may be considered as a second choice, though it is technically more difficult to judge the amount of intestine to be removed, and proximal sacral fixation cannot be done.[56] A modification of Delome's procedure has been reported with the benefit of reduced recurrence rate, absent coloanal anastomosis, and better functional results.[57] For the elderly or infirm, the insertion of a Thiersch's wire or more elastic material[58,59] reinforcement of the external anal sphincter may be performed. The latter may be very delicately gauged, however, so as to not create a mechanical obstruction that would precipitate increased straining at stool. A postanal pelvic floor repair can also be used to alleviate incontinence remaining after correction of rectal prolapse.[56] In those situations, the external anal sphincter is patulous with little contraction, and although the puborectalis contracts, it is lengthened backward. The anorectal angle is thus abolished. The aim of the procedure is to restore the anorectal angle.

In neurogenic incontinence a gracilis muscle transplant is indicated where direct repair will not be successful and biofeedback is ineffective (Figure 15.10). This muscle takes its origin from the pubic tubercle, and the lateral pubic ramus courses down the medial aspect of the thigh to insert on the medial tibial condyle. As its neurovascular bundle containing the branches of the deep femoral artery and of the obturator nerve (L2,L3, and L4) enters the upper fourth of the muscle from its lateral side, as much as 75% of the muscle can be mobilized without compromise. The results of this procedure have been disappointing since the muscle is incapable of sustained contraction. The reported success

Table 15.4 Functional outcome of repair

Etiology	Repair	Results
Obstetric	Anterior sphincter repair	Excellent
Anorectal insult	Direct repair	Good
Neurogenic	Postanal repair	Fair
Neurovascular	Gracilis muscle transplant	Poor to fair
Fistulas	Warren flap	Good

of such conventional transposition has been explained by a tightening of the anal canal resulting in outlet obstruction. This is associated with moderate success. Long-term results have been less than optimal in patients with obstetric and/or gynecologic trauma.[60] More recently, added electrical stimulation has been shown to replace voluntary contraction by a sustained contraction leading to the transformation of Type II fatigue-prone muscle fibers into Type I fatigue-resistant fibers.[61] A recent series reporting on 52 patients showed a success rate of 73%.[62]

The reported functional outcome of repair varies with the cause and is listed in Table 15.4.

In intractable incontinence a colostomy can be effective as a last resort.

Some patients may require a combination of procedures. The surgeon should be mindful of the coincident or future development of SUI in such patients, as well as the possibility of progression of bowel symptoms. Patients should be encouraged to participate in long-term follow-up programs that include attention to improving bowel habits and elimination of straining at stool so that the natural progression of this most troublesome disorder can be arrested.

References

1. Nelson R, Norton N, and Cantley E: Prevalence of fecal incontinence in Wisconsin households, Dis Colon Rectum 37(S):89, 1994 (abstract).
2. Snooks S and others: Risk factors in childbirth causing damage to the pelvic floor innervation, Br J Surg (suppl)72:S15, 1985.
3. Sultan A and others: Anal sphincter disruption during vaginal delivery, N Engl J Med 329:1905, 1993.
4. Goldaber K and others: Postpartum perineal morbidity after fourth-degree perineal tear, Am J Obstet Gynecol 168:489, 1993.
5. Kamm M: Obstetric damage and faecal incontinence, Lancet 344:730, 1994.
6. Cornes H, Bartolo D, and Sirrat G: Changes in anal canal sensation after childbirth, Br J Surg 78:74, 1991.
7. Bek K and Laurberg S: Risks of anal incontinence from subsequent vaginal delivery after a complete obstetric anal sphincter tear, Br J Obstet Gynaecol 99:724, 1992.
8. Sultan A and others: Anal sphincter trauma during instrumental delivery, Int J Gynaecol Obstet 43:263, 1993.
9. Nielsen M, Dammegaard L, and Pedersen J: Endosonographic assessment of the anal sphincter after surgical reconstruction, Dis Colon Rectum 37:434, 1994.
10. Engel A and others: Anterior anal sphincter repair in patients with obstetric trauma, Br J Surg 81:1231, 1994.
11. Penninckx F: Fecal incontinence: indications for repairing the anal sphincter, World J Surg 16:820, 1992.
12. Hamalainen K-P and others: Biofeedback therapy in rectal prolapse patients, Dis Colon Rectum 39:262, 1996.
13. Felt-Bersma R and others: Unsuspected sphincter defects shown by anal endosonography after anorectal surgery, Dis Colon Rectum 38:249, 1995.
14. Infantino A and others: Striated anal sphincter electromyography in idiopathic fecal incontinence, Dis Colon Rectum 38:27, 1995.
15. Thorpe A and others: Pelvic floor physiology in women with faecal incontinence and urinary symptoms, Br J Surg 82:173, 1995.
16. Jorge JM and others: Does perineal descent correlate with pudendal neuropathy? Dis Colon Rectum 36:475, 1993.
17. Orr W and Schuster M: Clinical applications of anorectal manometry. In Barkin J and O'Phelan CA, editors: Advanced therapeutic endoscopy, New York, 1990, Raven Press.
18. Whitehead W and Schuster M: Anorectal physiology and pathophysiology, Am J Gastroentrol 82:487, 1987.
19. Gantke B and others: Sonographic, mano-

metric, and myographic evaluation of the anal sphincters morphology and function, Dis Colon Rectum 36:1037, 1993.

20. Hock D and others: Colpocystodefecography, Dis Colon Rectum 36:1015, 1993.
21. Hallan R and Marzouk D: Comparison of digital and manometric assessment of anal sphincter function, Br J Surg 76:973, 1986.
22. Smith LE, editor: Practical guide to anorectal testing, ed 2, New York, 1995, Igaku-Shoin Medical Publishers, Inc.
23. Felt-Bersma R and others: Anal endosonography: relationship with anal manometry and neurophysiologic tests, Dis Colon Rectum 35:944, 1992.
24. Falk P and others: Transanal ultrasound and manometry in the evaluation of fecal incontinence, Dis Colon Rectum 37:468, 1994.
25. Hashimoto B and Botoman V: New challenge for endorectal sonography: diagnosis of fecal incontinence, J Ultrasound Med 12:375, 1993.
26. Goes RN, Simons AJ, and Beart RW Jr: Level of highest mean resting pressure segment in the anal canal: a quantitative assessment of anal function, Dis Colon Rectum 39:289, 1996.
27. Lawson J and Nixon H: Anal canal pressures in diagnosis of Hirschprung's disease, Paediatr Surg 2:544, 1967.
28. Ger G-C and others: Anorectal manometry in the diagnosis of paradoxical puborectalis syndrome, Dis Colon Rectum 36:816, 1993.
29. Holmberg A and others: Anorectal manovolumetry in the diagnosis of fecal incontinence, Dis Colon Rectum 38:502, 1995.
30. Browning G and Parks A: Postanal repair for neuropathic faecal incontinence: correlation of clinical result and anal canal pressures, Br J Surg 70:101, 1983.
31. Parks T: The usefulness of tests in anorectal disease, World J Surg 16:804, 1992.
32. Scheuer M and others: Postanal repair restores anatomy rather than function, Dis Colon Rectum 32:960, 1989.
33. Kumar D and others: Prolonged manometric recording of the anorectal motor activity in ambulatory human subjects: evidence of periodic activity, Gut 30:1007, 1989.
34. Pinho M and others: Assessment of noninvasive intra-anal electromyography to evaluate sphincter function, Dis Colon Rectum 34:69, 1991.
35. Burnett S and others: Confirmation of endosonographic detection of external anal sphincter defects by simultaneous electromyographic mapping, Br J Surg 78:448, 1991.
36. Niell M and Swash M: Increased motor unit fiber density in the external anal sphincter muscle in anorectal incontinence: a single fiber EMG study, J Neurol Neurosurg Psychiatry 43:343, 1980.
37. Swash M: Anorectal incontinence: electrophysiological tests, Br J Surg (suppl Sept)72: S14, 1985.
38. Roe A and others: New method for assessing of anal sensation in various anorectal disorders, Br J Surg 25:1279, 1986.
39. Miller R and others: Anorectal temperature sensation: a comparison of normal and incontinent patients, Br J Surg 74:511, 1987.
40. Henry M and others: The pelvic musculature in the descending perineum syndrome, Br J Surg 69:470, 1982.
41. Mahieu P and others: Defecography: contribution to the diagnosis of defecation disorders, Radiology 9:253, 1984.
42. Rex D and Lappas J: Combined anorectal manometry and defecography in 50 consecutive adults with fecal incontinence, Dis Colon Rectum 35:1040, 1992.
43. Kelvin F, Maglinte D, and Benson T: Evacuation proctography (defecography): an aid to the investigation of pelvic floor disorders, Obstet Gynecol 83:307, 1994.
44. Hiltunen K-M, Kolehmainen H, and Matikainen M: Does defecography help in diagnosis and clinical decision-making in defecation disorders? Abdom Imaging 19:355, 1994.
45. Bartolo C and others: Flap valve theory of anorectal continence, Br J Surg 73:1012, 1986.
46. Parks A and others: The syndrome of the descending perineum, Proc R Soc Med 58:477, 1966.
47. Henry M and Swash M: Coloproctology and the pelvic floor, London, 1985, Butterworth.
48. Rosenshein N and others: An anatomic classification of rectovaginal septal defects, Am J Obstet Gynecol 137:439, 1980.

49. Warren J: A new method of operation for the relief of rupture of the perineum through the sphincter and rectum, Trans Am Gynecol Soc 72:322, 1882.

50. Shafik A: Polytetrafluoroethylene injection for the treatment of partial fecal incontinence, Int Surg 78:159, 1993.

51. Parks A: Anorectal incontinence, Proc R Soc Med 68:681, 1975.

52. Nichols DH: Retrorectal levatorplasty for anal and perineal prolapse, Surg Gynecol Obstet 154:251, 1982.

53. Nichols DH: Retrorectal levatorplasty with colporrhaphy, Clin Obstet Gynecol 25:939, 1982.

54. Ripstein CB: Procidentia: definitive corrective surgery, Dis Colon Rectum 15:334, 1972.

55. Schultz I and others: Continence is improved after Ripstein rectopexy: different mechanisms in rectal prolapse and rectal intussusception? Dis Colon Rectum 39:300, 1996.

56. Williams J and others: Treatment of rectal prolapse in the elderly by perineal rectosigmoidectomy, Dis Colon Rectum 35:830, 1992.

57. Lechaux JP and others: Results of Delorme's procedure for rectal prolapse: advantages of a modified technique, Dis Colon Rectum 38:301, 1995.

58. Larach S and Vazquez B: Modified Thiersch procedure with silastic mesh implant: a simple solution for fecal incontinence and severe prolapse, South Med J 79:307, 1986.

59. Labow S and others: Perineal repair of rectal procidentia with an elastic fabric sling, Dis Colon Rectum 7:467, 1980.

60. Corman ML: Gracilis muscle transposition for anal incontinence: late results, Br J Surg (suppl Sept)72:S21, 1985.

61. Konsten J and others: Morphology of dynamic graciloplasty compared with the anal sphincter, Dis Colon Rectum 36:559, 1993.

62. Baeten C and others: Anal dynamic graciloplasty in the treatment of intractable fecal incontinence, N Engl J Med 332:1600, 1995.

16

Recurrent Breast Disease

Douglas J. Marchant

In describing the management of reoperative breast disease, we assume that the patient has been referred following a surgical procedure, such as an open biopsy, aspiration of a cyst, or fine needle aspiration (FNA). The initial discussion will describe recurrent surgical procedures for the following benign conditions: (1) recurrent fibroadenomas, (2) recurrent squamous metaplasia, and (3) recurrent macrocyst.

The evaluation of the occult lesion and the management of the patient referred following an inadequate biopsy or incomplete surgery for breast cancer constitute an increasing number of referrals.

Recurrent Fibroadenomas

The fibroadenoma is a benign neoplasm of the breast, frequently discovered by accident in the postpubertal female. Surgery is recommended, because once a patient has discovered such a mass, sooner or later she will demand removal. These lesions, though small when discovered, continue to grow and often can be removed with a smaller incision at the time of the initial diagnosis. In addition, we live in a mobile society; patients may move, become pregnant, and be examined by their obstetrician/gynecologist, who then "discovers" the mass. The patient indicates that it has been present for many years. What is the responsibility of the primary care physician?

A single fibroadenoma is easily removed on a day surgery basis under local anesthesia. A cosmetic incision is chosen with the patient in the sitting or standing position. The problem occurs when more than one fibroadenoma is discovered, often some months or years following the first operation. It has been my practice in young patients to order an automated ultrasound of both breasts to determine how many additional fibroadenomas are present before recommending surgical removal of the "new" lesion. This diagnostic study presents a detailed "road map" for future biopsies, and often a period of watchful waiting is in order to determine whether additional lesions occur. When the lesions are stable, a decision concerning the removal of all or some of these masses, depending on their location and size, can be made.

One final point should be made. I have reoperated on a number of patients who have had a fibroadenoma removed but who have a "new" mass at the biopsy site. Fibroadenomas often feel quite superficial; however, they are located deep in the breast tissue, and unless one is careful during the dissection, only a small part of the lesion may be removed. The surgeon should be certain before the wound is closed that the entire lesion has been removed and submitted to the pathology department. The pathologist should be notified if the patient is pregnant since considerable hypertrophy occurs, erroneously suggesting the diagnosis of cystosarcoma phyllodes.

Recurrent Squamous Metaplasia

Squamous metaplasia, or nonpuerperal mastitis, is more common than the literature suggests. In older textbooks the lesion is referred to as plasma cell mastitis. The characteristic history is one of recurrent drainage adjacent to the nipple or the periphery of the nipple. Drainage has been performed one or more times, usually in an emergency room or office setting. The patient is asymptomatic for several weeks or months, and the condition recurs. Antibiotics or another drainage is attempted, and again the lesion recurs.

As the name implies, the histology is related to squamous metaplasia of the ducts. Whether this occurs as a result of infection or infection occurs following squamous metaplasia is unknown. Cultures taken at the time of surgery usually are negative. The symptom complex is not associated with pregnancy or lactation, nor does it seem to be related to trauma. There is no known relationship between this condition and the later development of breast cancer. The principal problem is recurrent pain and drainage requiring repetitive medical visits.

When a patient is referred for recurrent drainage, I take a culture. If the patient is more than 30 years of age, I obtain a mammogram and, on some occasions, an automated ultrasound to more clearly delineate the involved area. The patient is scheduled for removal of the duct system under general anesthesia on a day surgery basis. General anesthesia is preferred because of the extensive dissection required. The operation can be done under local anesthesia, but with recurrent infection it is difficult to penetrate all of the involved areas with adequate amounts of local anesthesia.

A circumareolar incision is made in the general area of the drainage, and any sinus tract is identified and removed. The nipple areolar complex is elevated with skin hooks, and by use of sharp dissection the duct system is removed until normal breast tissue is encountered. This may require extensive dissection toward the chest wall and beyond the nipple areolar complex. Bleeding is controlled with fine ligatures. A culture is taken, and the tissue is always submitted for rapid section diagnosis to rule out carcinoma. If the wound is dry, I do not routinely employ a drain unless the remaining cavity is quite large, in which case a ¼-inch Penrose drain is inserted and let out through the wound with a skin suture left long, to be tied 24 hours later. I close the skin with no. 5-0 nonabsorbable sutures. The suture adjacent to the drain is tied when the drain is removed 24 hours after the surgery, and all skin sutures are removed in 5 to 7 days. A pressure dressing is placed over the incision for the first 24 to 48 hours.

Even with extensive surgery, success cannot be guaranteed. I have had a few instances in which the initial cultures were negative, the pathology report confirmed the diagnosis, and wide local excision was performed, yet months or years later, recurrent drainage occurred. In this situation, permanent cure can be assured only with a wide local excision of the nipple areolar complex. The procedure is best performed under general anesthesia and with the use of appropriate prophylactic antibiotics.

The recurrent fistulous tract is identified (Figure 16.1, *A*). The line of excision is established, including the nipple areolar complex (Figure 16.1, *B*). The entire nipple areolar complex is removed, and the wound closed (Figure 16.1, *C*). If the remaining cavity is large, a small Penrose drain may be inserted before closure and removed in 48 hours. Usually this is not necessary, and it should be avoided whenever possible. The exit point of the drain may result in yet another sinus tract.

RECURRENT MACROCYST

The etiology of macrocysts is unknown. They are not associated with the later development of breast cancer. A number of studies have attempted to address the composition of the cyst fluid, but to date they have resulted in very little additional information concerning the etiology or the treatment of this condition. A palpable cyst probably does not increase beyond the initial size because of the atrophy of the epithelial lining produced by the pressure of the cyst fluid, and if the cyst is completely aspirated, no additional fluid will occur. In our Breast Health Center, we recommend that patients return 1 month after aspiration. If a mass is discovered at the site of aspiration, open biopsy is recommended. Evaluation of the cyst fluid seldom is helpful, although for medicolegal purposes, it may be wise to send the fluid for analysis.

Asymptomatic macrocysts should not be aspirated. We have seen a number of patients who have developed infection following repeated aspirations, and, in at least one instance, mastectomy was required. It is our practice to document the presence of a recurrent cyst, and if it is symptomatic, large, or painful, to aspirate it for symptomatic relief.

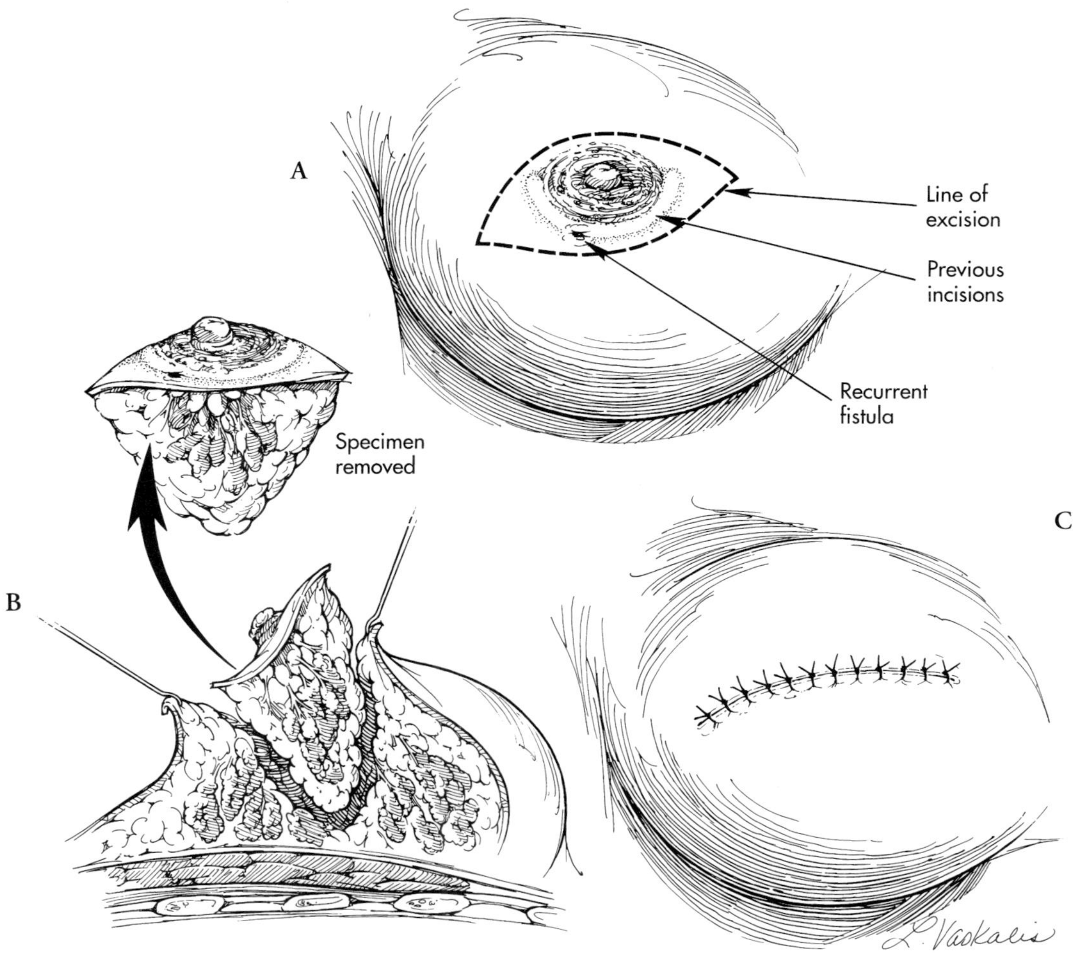

Figure 16.1 Recurrent squamous metaplasia. **A**, Fistula tract. **B**, Extent of reexcision. **C**, Completed surgical closure.

Reoperative Techniques for Breast Cancer

Occult Lesion

With increasing utilization of screening mammography, diagnosis of an occult lesion is not uncommon. Management depends on the expertise of the mammographer and the experience of the surgeon. Proper handling of an occult lesion, whether it represents an asymmetric density or a geographic cluster of microcalcifications, requires careful interpretation by an experienced mammographer followed by consultation with the responsible surgeon. We perform all of our localizations and biopsies under local anesthesia on a day surgery basis. The patient is taken to the radiology suite where a needle localization is performed using a Homer mammalock system (Figures 16.2 and 16.3).

The patient is then taken to the day surgery area for the operative procedure. The x-ray films are reviewed, and measurements are taken to locate the needle relative to the skin surface. This is helpful in deciding where to make the incision (Figure 16.4, *A* to *C*). Local anesthesia is used—2% lidocaine without epinephrine. The previously marked incision is injected, and the dissection is begun (Figure

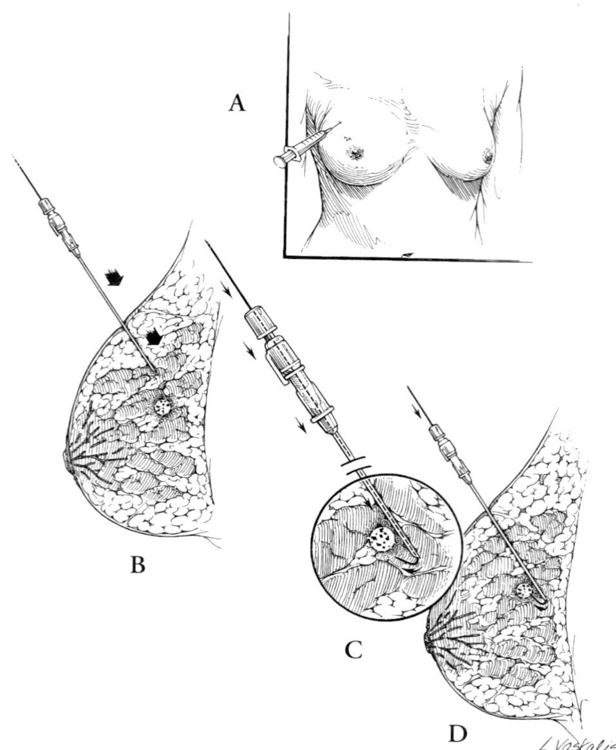

FIGURE 16.2 Localization and biopsy. **A,** Local anesthesia injected. **B** through **D,** Homer mammalock needle inserted and positioned. (From Marchant DJ: Breast biopsy. In Nichols DH, editor: Gynecologic and obstetric surgery, St Louis, 1993, Mosby.)

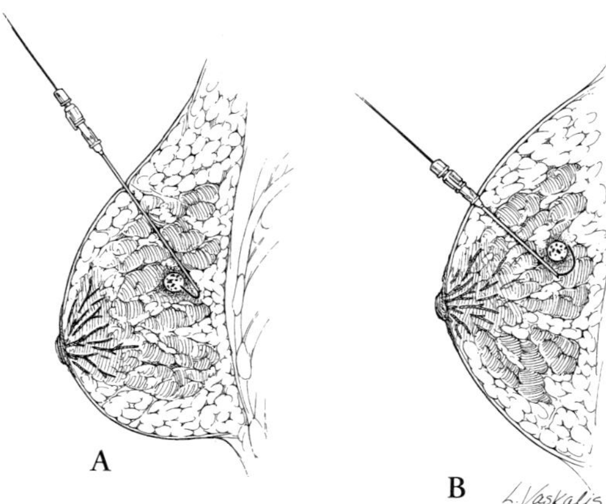

FIGURE 16.3 Needle in mediolateral and craniocaudal positions. **A,** Mediolateral view. **B,** Craniocaudad view. (From Marchant DJ: Breast biopsy. In Nichols DH, editor: Gynecologic and obstetric surgery, St Louis, 1993, Mosby.)

16.4, *D* and *E*). During the dissection care must be taken not to disturb the needle. When the proper distance has been reached, the needle is freed from the dermis and the tissue stabilized with a single Allis' clamp. Using the films as a guide, the area in question is removed by sharp dissection. Once the lesion has been removed, preferably with the needle, it is placed on an appropriate tray with wet sponges and delivered with the films to the radiologist for specimen radiography (Figure 16.5).

If an invasive cancer has been diagnosed by biopsy and involves one or more margins, we recommend reexcision. Alternative treatments are discussed with the patient, and if she is a candidate for wide local excision and axillary dissection, these procedures are scheduled under general anesthesia.

An important consideration is the condition of the biopsy site. This point often is overlooked since the majority of patients in the past had a modified mastectomy, and the location or condition of the biopsy site had little or no bearing on the outcome of the proposed surgery or the prognosis of the patient. Because of the possibility of conservative treatment, the location of the incision and the condition of the biopsy site are important. If there is a large hematoma at the biopsy site

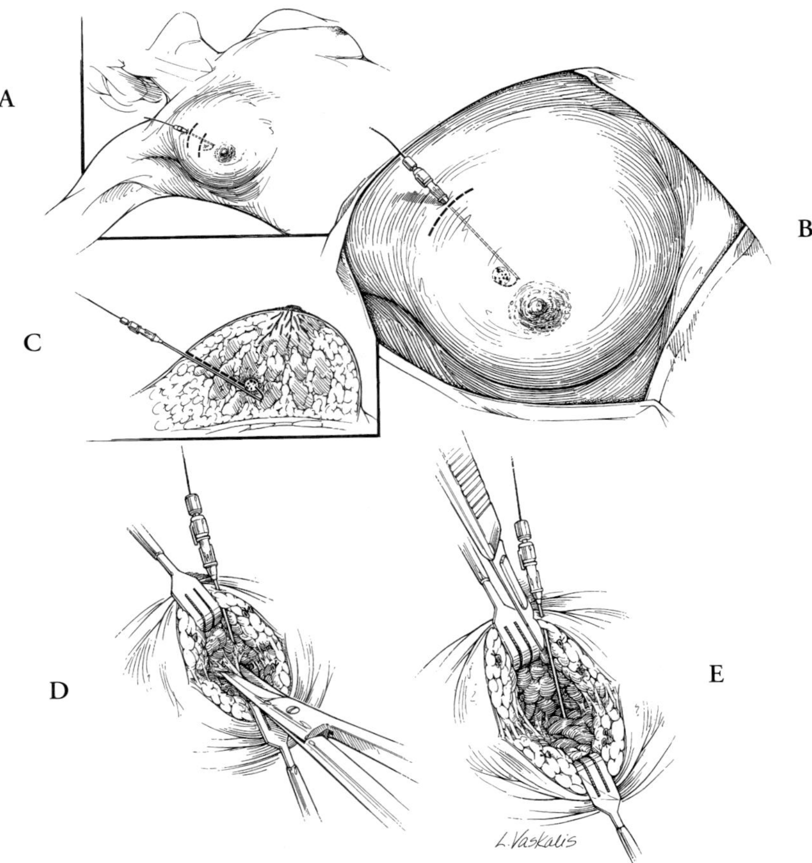

Figure 16.4 Localization and biopsy, operative procedure. **A** and **B**, Incision site chosen and incision made. **C** and **D**, Sharp dissection continues along needle toward lesion. **E**, Needle freed from dermis. (From Marchant DJ: Breast biopsy. In Nichols DH, editor: Gynecologic and obstetric surgery, St Louis, 1993, Mosby.)

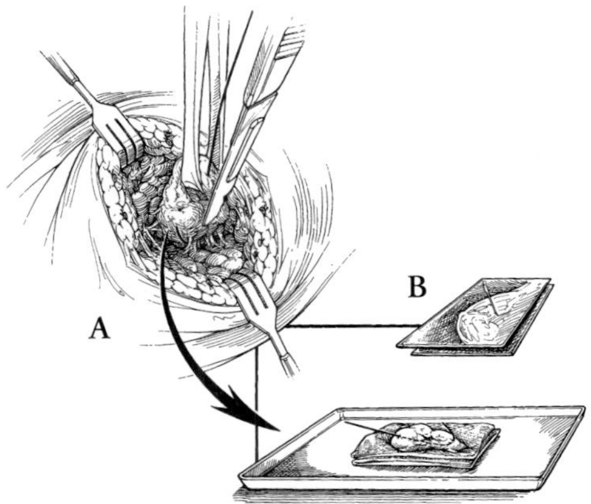

Figure 16.5 **A** and **B**, Lesion removed and sent with film to the radiology department. (From Marchant DJ: Breast biopsy. In Nichols DH, editor: Gynecologic and obstetric surgery, St Louis, 1993, Mosby.)

or if there is considerable induration and erythema, it is difficult for the surgeon to determine accurately the extent of the tumor. Occasionally more tumor is removed than is absolutely necessary, compromising what might otherwise be a cosmetic closure. It is therefore essential that the open biopsy be performed by an experienced surgeon who understands the implications of the biopsy and the necessity for complete healing without undue induration and ecchymosis.

For most patients, in addition to the reexcision of the biopsy site, an axillary dissection is performed. I prefer to mark my incision with the patient sitting or standing (Figure 16.6, *A*). The axillary dissection is performed first with a separate set of instruments. Exposure is facilitated by placing the arm on a crossbar to relax the pectoralis major (Figure 16.6, *B*). The pectoralis major and the costocoracoid fascia are identified. Sharp dissection is performed, removing the axillary contents distal to the axillary vein and its tributaries. Level 1 and 2 nodes are removed with this operation,

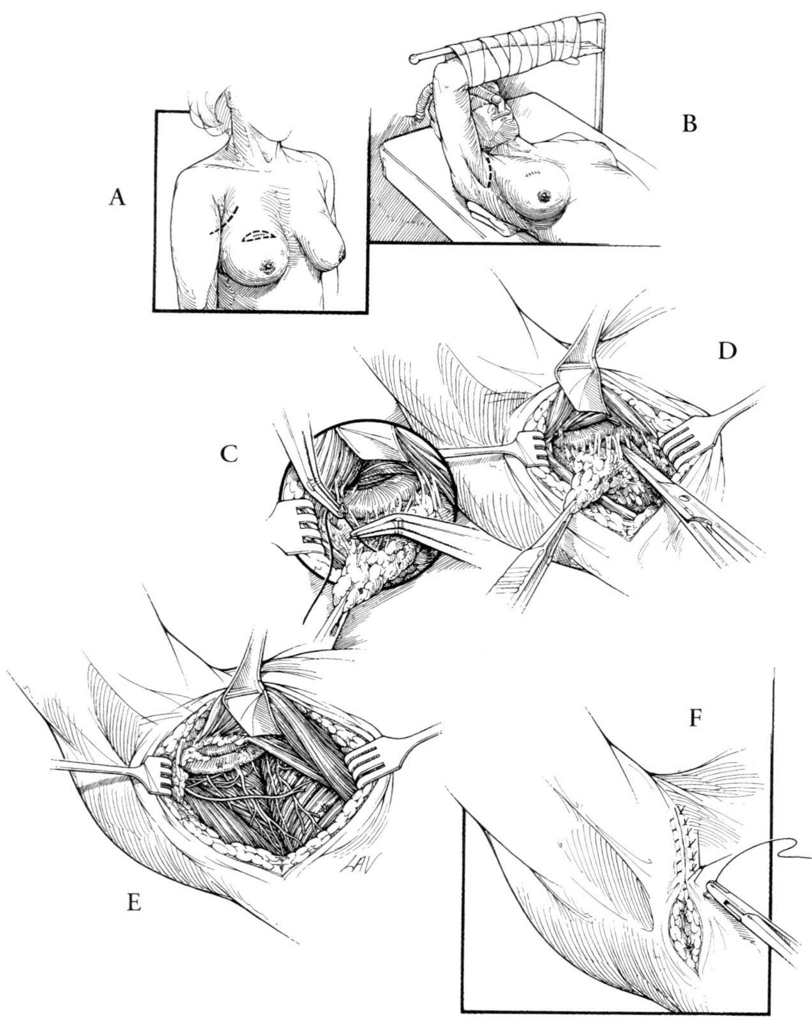

Figure 16.6 Axillary dissection. **A,** Cosmetic incisions marked with patient in sitting position. Note that axillary incision can be placed in "skin fold." **B,** Position of patient before draping. Note that arm is elevated on a crossbar to relax major pectoral muscle. **C,** Costocoracoid fascia is entered, and dissection is begun. **D,** Axillary vein and tributaries exposed. Vessels are ligated with 3-0 silk (hemoclips optional). **E,** Axillary dissection is completed. Note similarity to modified radical mastectomy dissection. **F,** Skin closure with 4-0 or 5-0 nylon. No drain is employed. (From Marchant DJ: Treatment options for breast cancer. In Nichols DH, editor: Gynecologic and obstetric surgery, St Louis, 1993, Mosby.)

and this usually is satisfactory for diagnostic purposes. With careful evaluation by a competent pathologist, 12 or more nodes are removed with this technique. If the wound is dry, I usually do not insert a drain (Figure 16.6, *C* to *F*).

The wide reexcision is then performed with a separate set of instruments. The arm is brought to the patient's side or placed on an arm board, and a temporary dressing is placed over the axillary incision (Figure 16.7, *A*). The previous incision is removed, and flaps are developed very similar to a modified mastectomy (Figure 16.7, *B* and *C*). The dissection is carried to the chest wall, and all indurated tissue is removed (Figure 16.7, *D* and *E*). Bleeding is controlled with ligatures of fine absorbable catgut or the actual cautery. It is best to proceed quickly with the removal of the specimen to prevent distortion of the anatomy by repeated attempts to ligate vessels and by repositioning of the retractors. Once the specimen has been removed, hemostasis can be achieved either with the actual cautery or ligatures of absorbable catgut.

The specimen is carefully marked, usually with a variety of sutures. Some pathology departments then use different colored ink to identify the appropriate margin for histologic evaluation.

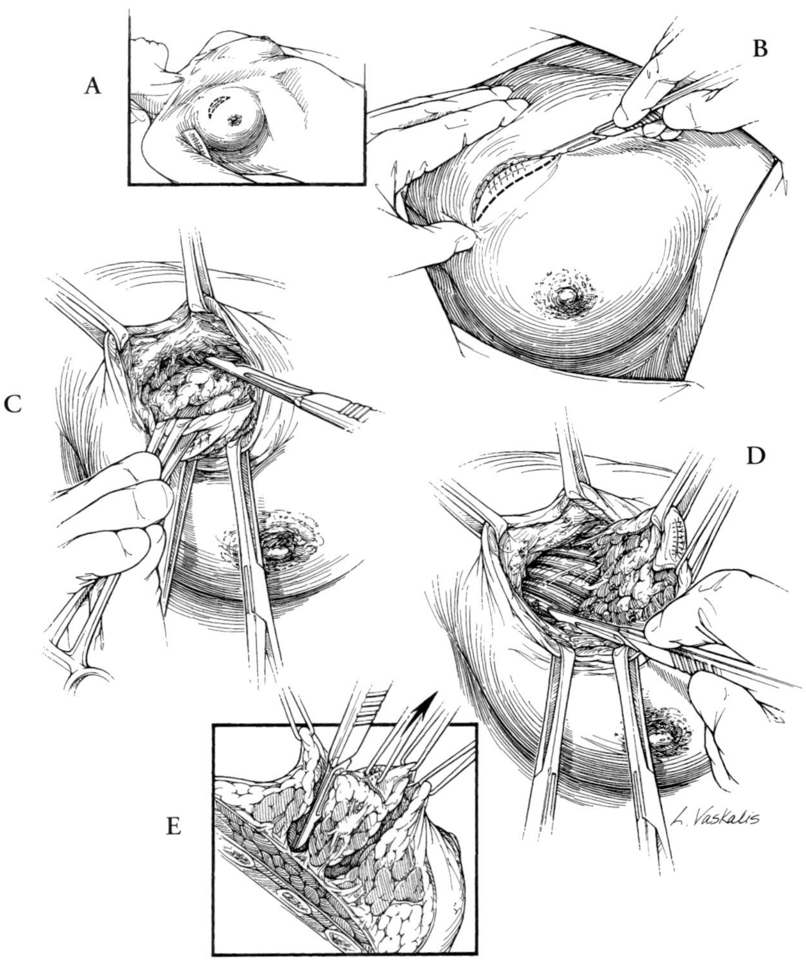

FIGURE 16.7 Wide local excision. **A,** Arm is brought to patient's side and covered with temporary pressure dressing. **B,** Incision is made, removing small amount of skin, including previous incision. **C,** Skin flaps are developed by sharp dissection. **D,** Dissection continues to anterior chest wall. **E,** Sagittal view showing extent of dissection. (From Marchant DJ: Treatment options for breast cancer. In Nichols DH, editor: Gynecologic and obstetric surgery, St Louis, 1993, Mosby.)

Once hemostasis has been achieved, no attempt should be made to obliterate completely the dead space in the central portion of the excision. It may be useful to "mark" the area of excision with a silver clip. A few milliliters of 0.25% bupivicaine without epinephrine are injected into the incision. The subcutaneous tissues are closed with fine absorbable catgut and the skin closed with vertical mattress sutures of 4-0 or 5-0 nylon. Before tying the last suture, I usually insert the suction to remove any fresh bleeding, and then an immediate pressure dressing is applied. The specimen is handed off appropriately marked for histologic evaluation (Figure 16.8).

I do not employ suction drainage, which inevitably results in retraction of the skin and a less-than-perfect cosmetic result. With the use of a pressure dressing, the breast is "molded" into its normal configuration. Most of these patients can be discharged within 24 to 48 hours, and the pressure dressing is left in place for 48 hours. Before discharge, the patient should be instructed in arm and chest exercises. This is important because of the fibrosis that may be associated with the subsequent radiation therapy.

There is some debate as to whether an axillary dissection is necessary for all patients, particularly older patients with normal axillas. If the receptors are positive, most of these patients will be given tamoxifen, and the axillary dissection is superfluous. Recent evidence suggests that patients with negative nodes should be offered adjuvant chemotherapy or hormonal therapy. In our Breast Health Center, we individualize the treatment of our patients. We recommend adjuvant chemotherapy in younger patients and patients who have negative receptors and those with a high mitotic

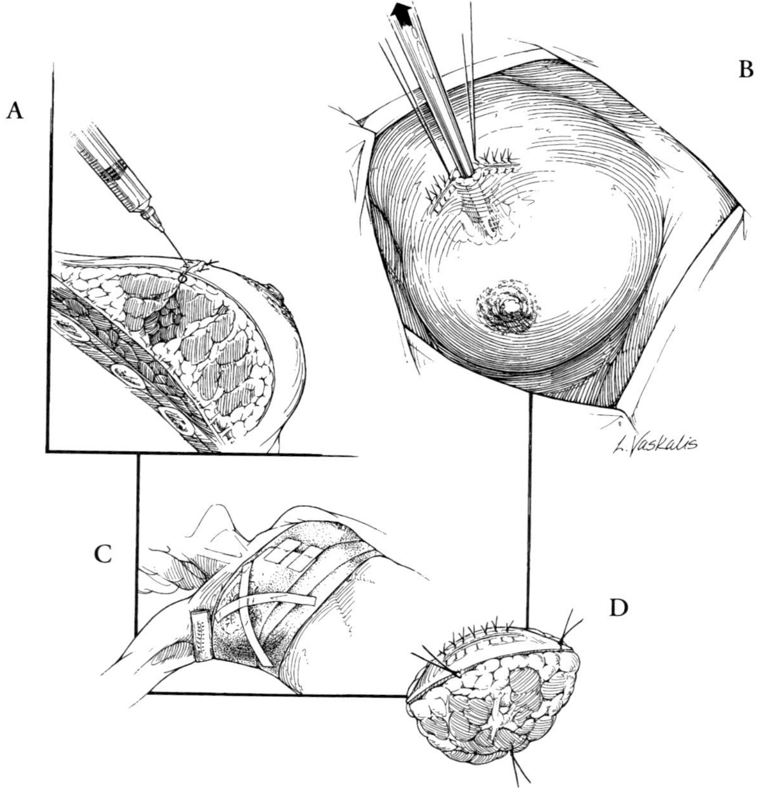

FIGURE 16.8 **A,** Solution of 0.25% bupivicaine is injected into the incision. No attempt is made to obliterate the cavity. Only subcutaneous fat is approximated. **B,** Wound is partially closed with vertical mattress sutures of fine nylon. One suture is left "long" to permit suction before closure is completed. **C,** Pressure dressing with "fluffs" and a 6-inch Ace bandage is applied. Depending on location of axillary incision, this may or may not be included in the dressing. **D,** Final specimen is appropriately marked for orientation by pathologist. (From Marchant DJ: Treatment options for breast cancer. In Nichols DH, editor: Gynecologic and obstetric surgery, St Louis, 1993, Mosby.)

index or aneuploidy demonstrated by flow cytometry. Since tamoxifen has fewer side effects, it is recommended for node-negative postmenopausal patients, and for the present, we continue to treat them indefinitely.

In Situ Carcinoma

By definition, in situ carcinoma should be 100% curable. Unfortunately, there often is a difference of opinion concerning the cell type and the possibility of "early invasion." There is always the possibility of extensive disease noted on the mammogram, and the significance of a palpable mass associated with the lesion must be considered. We have adopted our own protocol for handling these lesions (Table 16.1).

Recently there has been considerable interest in the treatment of in situ cancer, particularly with the release of the findings from the National Surgical Adjuvant Breast Project (NSABP) protocol B-17. Based upon the recommendations from this protocol, for most patients successful treatment of duct cancer in situ consists of wide local excision or reexcision followed by radiation therapy. This is in an effort to reduce a second ipsilateral breast tumor, which in some instances may in fact be an invasive tumor. There is considerable discussion concerning these recommendations as evidenced by an increasing number of critical reviews of this position.

For patients with discontinuous areas of disease or multifocal in situ disease, we recommend simple mastectomy. This is particularly true in those patients with comedo carcinoma. If there is any question of early invasion, axillary dissection is performed.

For patients with lobular cancer in situ (lobular neoplasia), usually found as an incidental lesion, we do not recommend reexcision nor do we recommend mirror image biopsies. There is some debate as to whether lobular neoplasia represents a true neoplasm or simply a marker or risk factor for the later development of breast carcinoma.

Role of Mastectomy

With the increasing utilization of second opinion, we are seeing more and more patients in our Breast Health Center requesting a discussion of alternative treatments. This has brought into focus the role of wide local excision versus the modified mastectomy. We provide second opinions only after a careful review of the mammograms and the microscopic slides. Often conservative treatment has been recommended, but we have noted extensive disease on the mammogram; because of this, we have chosen either total (simple) mastectomy or mastectomy with axillary dissection. The axillary dissection is recommended because, with a large area of involvement, it is possible that one or more areas in the breast will contain early invasive tumor. We do not routinely recommend axillary dissection

TABLE 16.1 Duct cancer in situ treatment guidelines

Lumpectomy
Lesion size 2 cm in diameter (specify whether nonpalpable or palpable)
Associated microcalcifications determined mammographically
Microscopically normal tissue margin 0.5 cm
If lesion is subareolar, removal of entire nipple-areolar complex

Lumpectomy plus radiotherapy or simple mastectomy
Lesion size no more than 2 cm in diameter (specify whether nonpalpable or palpable)
No associated microcalcifications
In patients treated with lumpectomy plus radiotherapy:
Radiotherapy to breast only
Excision margins to be appropriately evaluated and therapy appropriately tailored as per current Breast Health Center guidelines for invasive carcinoma

Mastectomy with level I/II lymph node dissection
Histologically confirmed multicentric disease that is detected grossly or mammographically
Margin positive (more than one focus or diffusely continuous) after reexcision, implying extensive disease

for in situ disease that has been completely removed with adequate margins and for which there is no question of early invasion.

Another consideration concerns the location of the lesion. Often even small lesions in the upper inner quadrant require mastectomy because of the inability to perform a cosmetic wide local excision. In some instances, with a large lesion immediately beneath the nipple areolar complex, we have recommended mastectomy, particularly for those patients with very small breasts for whom a wide local excision would leave very little tissue. In these cases, modified mastectomy with immediate or delayed reconstruction is preferable.

CONCLUSION

It is important that the surgeon understand the natural history of benign breast disease and avoid unnecessary surgery, particularly in the young patient. On the other hand, aggressive surgery is required for squamous metaplasia. For those patients suspected of having cancer, it is immediately obvious that the surgeon must understand the implications of the biopsy and participate in a multidisciplinary team that includes not only input from the medical oncologist and radiotherapist but the pathologist and radiologist as well. With this approach we can minimize the trauma to a patient already devastated by the knowledge that she has cancer and for whom the initial decision regarding treatment is most important.

BIBLIOGRAPHY

Fisher ER and others: Pathologic findings from the National Surgical Adjuvant Breast Project (NSABP) protocol B-17, Cancer 75:1310, 1995.

Fisher ER and others: Response: blunting the counterpoint, Cancer 75:1223, 1995.

Harris JR, Hellman S, and Kinne DW: Special report: limited surgery and radiotherapy for early breast cancer, N Engl J Med 313:1365, 1985.

Homer MJ: Non-palpable breast lesion localization using a curved end retractible wire, Radiology 157:259, 1985.

Homer MJ, Marchant DJ, and Smith TJ: The geographic cluster of breast microcalcifications—is it really intramammary? Surg Gynecol Obstet 161:532, 1985.

Homer MJ and Pile-Spellman ER: Needle localization of non-palpable breast lesions: the importance of communication. Special report: breast imaging, Applied Radiology, November 1987.

Homer MJ and others: Residual breast carcinoma after biopsy: role of mammography in evaluation, Radiology 170:75, 1989.

Johnson JE and Page DL: Response to the counterpoint, 75:1566, Cancer 1995.

Johnson JE and others: Recurrent mammary carcinoma after local excision: a segmental problem, Cancer 75:1612, 1995.

Kearney TJ and Morrow M: Effect of re-excision on the success of breast conserving surgery, Ann Surg Oncol 2(4):303, 1995.

Lagios MD and others: Duct carcinoma in situ: relationship of extent of non-invasive disease to the frequency of occult invasion, multicentricity, lymph node metastases and short-term treatment failure, Cancer 50:1309, 1982.

Lagios MD and others: Mammographically detected duct carcinoma in situ: frequency of local recurrence following tylectomy and prognostic effects of nuclear grade on local recurrence, CA 63:618, 1989.

Osteen RT: Strategies for breast-conserving surgery: an unresolved dilemma, Cancer 75:1563, 1995.

Page DL and Lagios M: Pathologic analysis of the National Surgical Adjuvant Breast Project (NSABP) B-17 trial: unanswered questions remaining unanswered considering current concepts of ductal carcinoma in situ, Cancer 75:1219, 1995.

Peters F: Failure of danazol to prevent recurrent periareolar abscesses, Breast Dis 1:283, 1989 (letter to the editor).

Rose MA and others: Conservative surgery and radiation therapy for early breast cancer, Arch Surg 124:153, 1989.

Rosenberg AL and others: Clinically occult breast lesions: localization and significance, Radiology 162:167, 1987.

Schuh ME and others: Intraductal carcinoma, analysis of presentation, pathologic findings and outcome of disease, Arch Surg 121:1303, 1986.

17

Gynecologic Malignancies

BRADLEY J. MONK
PHILIP J. DISAIA

In spite of current diagnostic techniques and excellent clinical acumen, a gynecologist will occasionally make a diagnosis of invasive cancer after an operative procedure that is inadequate as complete treatment for that particular malignancy. For example, a gynecologic surgeon may perform a vaginal hysterectomy on a postmenopausal woman with uterine descensus and no history of abnormal bleeding only to discover an occult endometrial cancer after histopathologic review of the specimen. Such a situation makes surgical evaluation of the pelvic and paraaortic lymph nodes and oophorectomy a consideration. Not only is the indication for further surgery controversial but so is the appropriate surgical approach, laparotomy versus laparoscopy.[1]

A more common situation is that of a patient with a gynecologic malignancy that has been appropriately treated and a recurrence is diagnosed. Reoperation can be an important part of the curative or palliative treatment for the recurring cancer. For instance, early diagnosis of locally recurrent squamous cancer of the vulva results in a 75% cure rate with immediate local reexcision.[2,3]

Finally, gynecologic surgeons are often faced with the need to carry out operative procedures for palliation. The best example is when a patient with recurrent cervical cancer suffers from a complete obstruction of the rectosigmoid and can be successfully palliated with fecal diversion. Not only can intestinal symptoms be relieved with such a procedure but survival also may be prolonged.

In this chapter the major sites relating to gynecologic oncology will be discussed. In addition, reoperative procedures with the intent of primary curative surgery, as well as curative and palliative operations for those with recurrent cancers, are reviewed.

VULVA

The vulva includes the labia majora, labia minora, the vestibule, and the clitoris. Squamous cell carcinoma is the most common malignancy in this area. Other neoplasms include melanoma, adenocarcinoma, Paget's disease, and metastatic cancer. The majority of patients with carcinoma of the vulva are postmenopausal and have presenting symptoms of itching, burning, mass effect, or bleeding. Aggressive biopsies of vulvar lesions should always be performed to ensure accurate diagnosis and appropriate therapy. Blue-black lesions on the vulva should be removed. Most investigators believe that typical small vulvar warts can be treated conservatively with local ablation. However, if condyloma persists or if the patient has massive or atypical warts, it is critically important that multiple biopsies be performed prior to any therapy not otherwise yielding a histologic specimen. For this reason, most gynecologic oncologists recommend surgical excision over laser therapy since surgery allows pathologic confirmation. This is especially important in patients with recurrent or persistent lesions, since recent data indicate that up to 17% of patients with what is thought to be vulvar intraepithelial neoplasia (VIN) will have an invasive component upon histologic review of the excised lesion. This emphasizes the importance of careful patient selection when considering the use of a laser to treat condyloma or other human papillomavirus (HPV)–associated lesions such as VIN.[4]

The surgical approach to vulvar carcinoma is dependent on lesion size and location as well as the risk of lymph node metastasis.[5] Cancers without lymphovascular invasion and with less than 1 mm of invasion rarely demonstrate lymphatic spread and are generally curable with a radical local excision (2 to 3 cm margin).[6,7] Lesions with more extensive invasion, either by direct extension or by metastases to the inguinal lymph nodes, ultimately may progress to the deep pelvic lymph nodes.[8] Direct spread to the deep pelvic nodes without inguinal involvement is exceedingly rare.

Until recently the standard operative procedure for any invasive cancer of the vulva or Bartholin's gland was a radical vulvectomy with bilateral inguinal and pelvic lymphadenectomy. Recent data indicate that if the inguinal lymph nodes are free of disease, the incidence of pelvic lymph node metastasis is extremely low, making routine pelvic lymphadenectomy unwarranted. In addition, the Gynecologic Oncology Group (GOG) has demonstrated that adjuvant pelvic radiotherapy is preferable to pelvic node dissection when inguinal metastases are documented.[9] Thus the appropriate treatment of frankly invasive vulvar cancers with invasion greater than 1 mm or with microscopic evidence of lymphovascular invasion is some sort of radical vulvectomy and bilateral inguinal lymphadenectomy with or without radiation therapy, depending on node status.

Finally, for unilateral T_1 (less than 2 cm) and perhaps even unilateral T_2 (2 cm or greater) lesions confined to the vulva, with less than 5 mm depth of invasion, radical local excision with unilateral superficial groin dissection has been recommended.[10] This is also true for early melanomas. Radical local excision commonly approximates a modified radical hemivulvectomy to ensure local control and should include a 2-cm margin circumferentially and at least 2 cm of fat and muscle deep to the tumor.[10,11] When surgical therapy less than that outlined above has been performed, additional surgery may be necessary to avoid the risk of recurrence and compromising survival.

Primary Cancer

For patients with invasive squamous carcinoma of the vulva, three situations suggest the need for an immediate more radical procedure. First, the patient who undergoes wide local excision of VIN or condyloma whose final pathology report indicates an invasive squamous carcinoma should immediately undergo either a radical local excision with superficial groin dissection or radical vulvectomy with bilateral inguinal lymphadenectomy. The type of surgery recommended will depend on the size, location, and depth of invasion. Second, patients with a persistent Bartholin's abscess will occasionally undergo excision of the Bartholin's gland. The final pathology report may reveal an invasive carcinoma of the Bartholin's gland, and in this situation the patient should immediately undergo radical vulvectomy and bilateral inguinal lymphadenectomy.[12] Whenever persistent Bartholin's gland infection occurs, especially in patients more than 40 years of age, multiple biopsies should be taken before performing a marsupialization or simple excision of the gland. Finally, although the majority of patients with Paget's disease of the vulva have an intraepithelial lesion that can be excised by simple vulvectomy, occasionally an underlying invasive adenocarcinoma will be discovered.[13,14] This patient should be returned to the OR for radical vulvectomy and bilateral inguinal lymphadenectomy. It is critically important to understand that although the pink velvety areas are definitely Paget's disease, normal skin also can contain pagetoid cells; thus wide margins are mandatory to decrease local recurrence. Moreover, rapid frozen section may be useful to assess the adequacy of the skinning vulvectomy at the time of primary operation in an attempt to decrease the need for reoperation.[15] Nevertheless, an occasional patient must be returned to the OR for more extensive excision because of positive margins.

Recurrent Cancer

Most vulvar cancer recurrences occur within 2 years of primary therapy, making careful postoperative surveillance at close intervals critically important. If nodal metastasis is absent at the time of primary therapy, the majority of recurrences will be along the surgical margins on the vulva. Several authors have reported as high as a 75% long-term survival following wide local reexcision of early recurrences on the vulva.[2,3] Aggressive biopsy of any abnormality seen along the healing scar will allow for early intervention. The reexcision should be deep and wide; thus skin flaps or grafts are frequently necessary since much of the skin may have been removed at the time of initial surgery, making reexcision quite extensive and normal anatomy distorted. One should again attempt to obtain at least 2-cm margins laterally and deep. If the recurrence is in the groin or is distal, surgical extirpation will be extremely difficult and rarely beneficial. Radical excision of recurrent groin disease or isolated systemic metastasis has been reported but with limited success since other subclinical metastasis are frequently present.[16,17]

Palliative Surgery

In vulvar cancer patients with widely metastatic disease, it is frequently appropriate to carry out wide local removal of symptomatic disease on the vulva as a comfort procedure, especially where operative risk is not excessive and the performance status and life expectancy of the patient are reasonable. If left untreated for just a few months, cancer on the vulva will almost undoubtedly progress to involve significant necrosis with foul-smelling discharge along with infection, severe pain, and difficulty with elimination. Thus the partial vulvectomy or excision can significantly palliate local symptoms and generally improve quality of life. The surgeon should remove the lesion with a narrower margin than that associated with an operation for curative intent and perform the procedure as rapidly as possible with the least traumatic anesthesia. Older patients will usually maintain rectal continence in spite of removal of the anterior portion of the rectal sphincter and urinary continence in spite of removal of the distal third of the urethra.

Cervix

Squamous cancer accounts for 70% of all invasive cancers of the cervix. Adenocarcinomas account for the majority of the remaining cases, although one occasionally sees a lymphoma, sarcoma, or primary melanoma.[18] Patients with primary cervical carcinomas generally range in age from 18 to 80 years, with the majority being in the 30- to 50-year-old age group. In developed countries, most invasive cervical lesions are diagnosed in their early asymptomatic stages since widespread Papanicolaou cytologic screening has become common; however, among patients with more advanced cancers, vaginal bleeding is a common symptom. All patients with Papanicolaou smears suggesting a squamous intraepithelial lesion should undergo colposcopy with biopsy and endocervical curettage before any conservative therapy is considered. Patients with persistent cervical discharge, vaginal bleeding, or presumed cervicitis should also undergo colposcopy and endocervical curettage before cryotherapy or laser treatment. This is important since cytologic screening has an inherent false negative rate, making the thorough evaluation of the symptomatic patient a critical part of early cervical cancer diagnosis. Endocervical curettage is part of a complete evaluation of the abnormal Papanicolaou smear, since adenocarcinoma of the endocervix is less often colposcopically visible and more difficult to pick up through cytologic screening.

Cancer of the cervix spreads in a stepwise fashion with local extension into paracervical tissues, followed by lymphatic metastasis. Early disease is successfully treated with either radical hysterectomy and bilateral pelvic lymphadenectomy or radical radiation therapy, which includes external irradiation therapy and brachytherapy.

Primary Cancer

In spite of a careful preoperative work-up, it is not uncommon for a gynecologic oncologist or radiation therapist to be referred a patient with invasive cancer of the cervix who has recently undergone a simple abdominal or vaginal hysterectomy. As with primary early invasive cancer of the cervix, radical reoperation, consisting of radical upper vaginectomy/parametrectomy with bilateral pelvic lymphadenectomy, and radiation therapy seem to have equal cure rates.[19-22] Since many of these patients are good surgical candidates, a surgical approach is usually reasonable, thus allowing preservation of ovarian activity and improved sexual function. The operative approach is very similar to a radical hysterectomy once the bladder and rectum have been dissected from the vaginal cuff. This initial dissection can be facilitated if a povidone-iodine (Betadine)–soaked pack is placed in the vagina at the time of surgery to expand the cuff of the vagina and facilitate its identification and isolation from the surrounding organs by the surgeon via the abdomen. By delaying the surgery at least 6 weeks after the hysterectomy, inflammation and tissue reaction will be greatly reduced, facilitating the dissection. However, any delay must be weighed against the possibility of tumor progression during the intertreatment interval. The literature would indicate that a delay in appropriate therapy of more than 6 months may portend a significant decrease in survival. The specimen should always include an adequate vaginal and parametrial margin. The lymph node dissection should be a complete lymphadenectomy, which includes all fat-bearing tissue surrounding the common iliac vessels, the external iliac and hypogastric vessels, and the obturator fossa, with the dorsal margin being at least the obturator nerve.

Recurrent Cancer

Patients with documented centrally recurrent cervical cancer can have long-term survival after an exenterative procedure. Recent reviews indicate that operative mortality is less than 2%, and 5-year cure rates range from 40% to 60% among selected patients.[23-26] Most gynecologic oncologists would recommend that a pelvic exenteration be performed only when a patient experiences a histologically confirmed recurrence in the central pelvis after radiotherapy for cervical carcinoma. Many of these patients also will have been previously treated with surgery consisting either of a radical hysterectomy or perhaps a surgical staging procedure to assess nodal spread.[27] Obviously, patients with long intertreatment intervals and those with smaller central recurrent tumors have a more favorable prognosis than those with a shorter interval following primary radiation, those with persistent disease after radiotherapy, and/or those with large lesions.[23-26] In addition, hydronephrosis and symptoms such as leg or back pain portend an increased risk of cancer outside the surgical field and thus are also poor prognostic factors. Spread to the pelvic sidewall and/or multiple lymph node metastasis is generally considered to be a contraindication for this radical surgical procedure. In selected patients with an anterior recurrence, the rectum can be spared by doing an anterior exenteration.[24] Before an exenterative procedure, the patient should undergo an extensive work-up to determine the feasibility of a successful operation. This should include a metastatic survey (CT of the abdomen and pelvis, chest radiograph) and an extensive medical and psychologic assessment to ensure her ability to withstand the operative procedure along with the prolonged morbidity and body changes that result from this operation.

On entering the abdomen, the surgeon must carefully evaluate the entire peritoneal cavity to ensure that the recurrence is localized to the planned area of surgical extirpation. Next, the area over the aorta and vena cava should be identified and the retroperitoneal space opened. Laterally, the surgeon should identify the ureters and ensure that they are not injured. A careful dissection of all fatty tissue containing lymph nodes from the bifurcation of the aorta and vena cava to the renal vessels is done, and this tissue is sent for frozen section. If these nodes are normal, the surgeon proceeds to the pelvis, where the retroperitoneal spaces are entered and all lymph-bearing tissue is removed from the external iliac artery and vein, the hypogastric artery and vein, and the obturator fossa. Finally, the perirectal and perivesical spaces are opened, and the surgeon ensures a tumor-free margin between the biopsy-proven disease and the pelvic sidewall (Figure 17.1). Only at this point does the surgeon proceed with removal of the bladder, uterus, cervix, vagina, and rectum if a total exenteration is to be carried out (Figure 17.2). A majority of patients can undergo immediate reconstruction of the vagina. Multiple flap procedures have been described for this purpose.[28,29]

Palliative Surgery

Occasionally, after a prolonged disease-free interval, a single pulmonary nodule or several clustered unilateral pulmonary nodules will be noted, and it may be appropriate to remove these for long-term palliation, although the exact role of thoracotomy in this situation is not known.[30] Furthermore, some authors

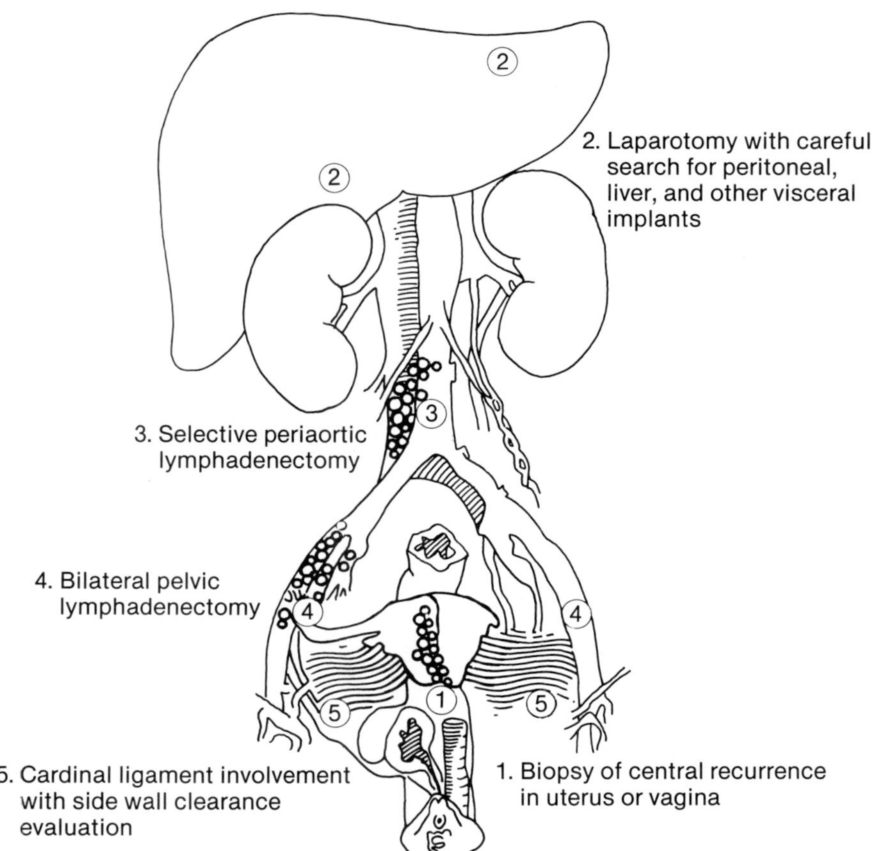

Figure 17.1 Steps in evaluation of patients for an exenterative procedure. (From DiSaia PJ and Creasman WT: Clinical gynecologic oncology, ed 4, St Louis, 1993, Mosby.)

have recommended performing an exenteration for a pelvic recurrence, even if disease outside of the operative field is documented, to palliate pain, bleeding, and/or infection.[31] However, most gynecologic oncologists would not carry out this extensive procedure without a curative intent given the inherent degree of morbidity associated with exenteration.

Great controversy exists as to the appropriateness of urinary diversion for palliation of recurrent or widespread cancer of the cervix.[32] These patients are significantly different from those untreated patients who present with ureteral obstruction since some of these can be salvaged with primary therapy. The patient with bilateral ureteral obstruction following a full dose of pelvic radiation is a more complicated problem since very few (less than 5%) will have obstruction caused by radiation fibrosis alone, and therefore it is uncommon for such patients to receive long-term benefit from urinary diversion.[33] Indeed, bilateral ureteral obstruction following radiation is usually a result of recurrent disease leading to death in essentially every patient. It is well known that death due to recurrent cervical cancer is often very painful, making uremia a preferable method of expiration. Unfortunately, there are no significant chemotherapeutic agents or regimens to date that produce long-term survival among patients with recurrent metastatic cervical cancer. Therefore urinary diversion prolongs life in most patients with recurrent cancer only with significant side effects, such as pain and infection. On the other hand, uremia usually results in a significant decrease in the sensation of pain and even euphoria among some patients. This may allow for a more pleasant terminal period. Colostomy or ileostomy may be appropriate in carefully selected patients to palliate severe side effects such as bowel obstruction or significant enteral vaginal fistula. Each of these patients should be thoroughly counseled and each decision should be individualized.

ENDOMETRIUM

Adenocarcinoma of the endometrium is the most common gynecologic malignancy, and the cure rate is high. For this reason there is a tendency to be initially conservative in the treatment of this disease. These patients are often between the ages of 40 and 80, obese, and frequently nulliparous. They most often present with abnormal or postmenopausal vaginal bleeding. The standard therapy for carcinoma of the uterine corpus is TAH, BSO with pelvic and paraaortic lymph node sampling among selected patients with tumors that are deeply invasive or poorly differentiated.[34] Radiation therapy is reserved for those with nodal metastasis. The GOG is currently prospectively investigating the role of adjuvant pelvic radiation among those with intermediate risk cancers such as those involving the cervical stroma and those that are either deeply invasive or poorly differentiated but without nodal spread. Recent large studies have indicated that prognostic factors include differentiation of the tumor, depth of myometrial invasion, and pelvic and paraaortic lymph node status.[35,36]

Currently the most common procedure for the diagnosis of corpus cancer is an office endometrial biopsy following an endocervical curettage. If the diagnosis of endometrial cancer is made and tissue is sufficient for grading, formal fractional dilatation and curettage (D & C) is unnecessary. However, when the curettage specimen from the office biopsy is equivocal, a formal fractional D & C is indicated.

Two pathologic variants, papillary serous adenocarcinoma and clear cell carcinoma, behave more like ovarian cancer.[37,38] It is important to evaluate the omentum and

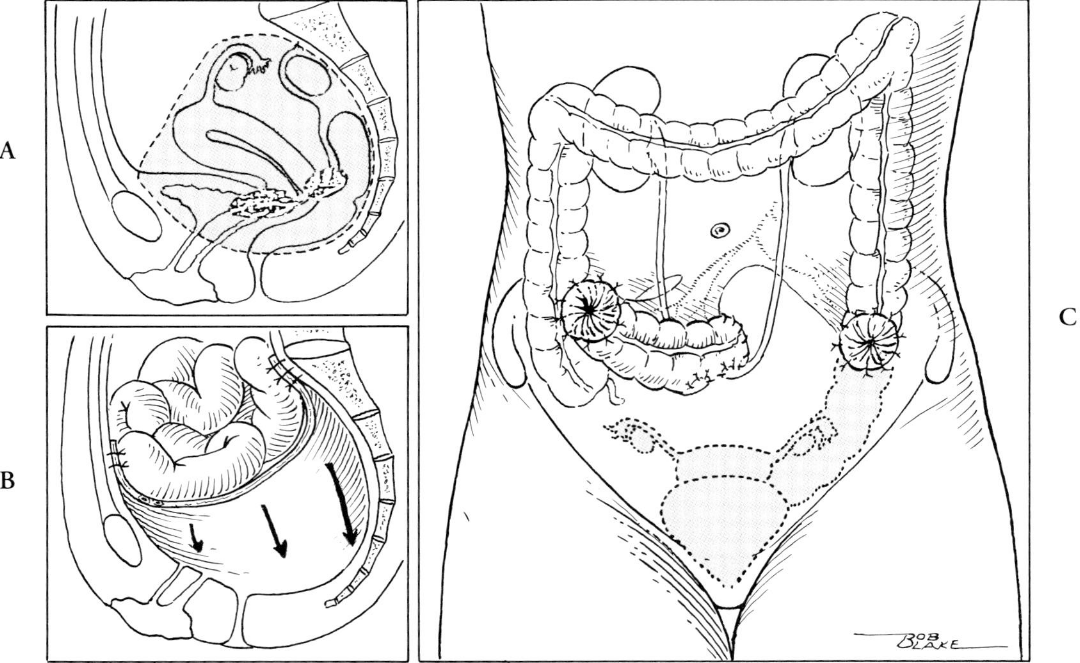

FIGURE 17.2 A, Lateral view of recurrent cancer involving cervix and upper vagina with extension into the bladder and rectum. Stippled area is tissue to be removed by exenteration. B, Lateral view after pelvic viscera have been removed. Omental "carpet" is used to keep intestines out of the pelvis during immediate postoperative period. With time, omental "carpet" will descend into pelvis, and "carpet" will adhere to pelvic floor. C, Urinary conduit and colostomy diversion after exenteration. Dotted areas of sigmoid, bladder, and internal genitalia have been removed. (From DiSaia PJ and Creasman WT: Clinical gynecologic oncology, ed 4, St Louis, 1993, Mosby.)

peritoneal surfaces in these situations. The optimal adjuvant postoperative treatment regimen for these unique histologic subtypes has not been identified.

Unsuspected Primary Cancer Diagnosed after Hysterectomy

Occasionally patients will undergo a total abdominal or vaginal hysterectomy and subsequent histologic review will reveal adenocarcinoma of the endometrium. At this point, the gynecologic surgeon is confronted with the need either to reoperate and surgically stage the patient, thereby evaluating metastatic spread, or simply to administer empiric postoperative therapy, usually consisting of pelvic irradiation. With the extensive prognostic data collected over the last 20 years, this question has become less difficult in that the risk of adnexal or lymphatic spread is exceedingly low for the patient with well-differentiated endometrial cancer (Table 17.1) and no or minimal myometrial invasion (Table 17.2). Therefore most clinicians would recommend careful follow-up with neither further surgery nor postoperative irradiation therapy among these low-risk patients. On the other hand, if negative prognostic factors such as poor differentiation, deep myometrial invasion, or extension to the lower uterine segment or cervix are present, many clinicians would recommend reoperation and/or postoperative radiation therapy. Retrospective data suggest that adjuvant therapy in this setting may decrease the risk of local recurrence.[39] When radiation therapy is being seriously considered, reoperation may be prudent to collect additional data on the extent of the disease and to better plan adjuvant therapy. The impact of postoperative radiation on overall survival is less clear. Since a survival benefit for postoperative radiation is unproven, the clinician may prefer to observe a patient with deeply invasive or poorly differentiated uterine cancer after hysterectomy and surgical staging. Surgical assessment may be helpful to identify a category of low-risk patients where such a posture is reasonable.[40,41] Premenopausal patients with intact ovarian function should be considered for reexploration to remove the ovaries and carry out lymph node sampling, especially if postoperative radiation therapy is not planned. A recent retrospective institutional review has complicated this controversy by demonstrating a survival benefit among those patients with endometrial cancer who undergo extensive surgical staging with lymphadenectomy whether or not nodal disease is found histologically. The authors suggest that lymphadenectomy may have both a prognostic and therapeutic role by removing occult lymphatic cancer.[42] If this finding is confirmed, all patients with an intermediate risk of lymphatic spread, such as those with moderately or poorly differentiated cancers and those with involvement of the outer half of the myometrium or cervical extension, may benefit from comprehensive surgical staging. We are inclined to recommend reoperation and full staging in this group of patients (when surgery is reasonably safe) because it permits a more rational prescription of adjuvant therapy versus observation.

Table 17.1 Endometrial cancer grade versus positive pelvic and aortic nodes

Grade	Pelvic	Aortic
G1 (N = 180)	5 (3%)	3 (2%)
G2 (N = 288)	25 (9%)	14 (5%)
G3 (N = 153)	28(18%)	17(11%)

Modified from Creasman WT and others: Cancer 60:2035, 1987.

Table 17.2 Maximal depth of invasion for endometrial cancer and its relationship to node metastasis

Maximal invasion	Pelvic	Aortic
Endometrium only (N = 87)	1 (1%)	1 (1%)
Superficial muscle (N = 279)	15 (5%)	8 (3%)
Intermediate muscle (N = 116)	7 (6%)	1 (1%)
Deep muscle (N = 139)	35(25%)	24(17%)

Modified from Creasman WT and others: Cancer 60:2035, 1987.

With the advent of modern laparoscopic technology, some surgeons have begun laparoscopic staging of patients with endometrial cancer. This is done either at the time of a laparoscopically assisted vaginal hysterectomy or following a previous hysterectomy for an unsuspected corpus cancer. Childers and others have demonstrated the feasibility of this approach,[1] and further study is currently underway within the GOG.

Recurrent Cancer

Numerous studies have looked at the use of total pelvic exenteration for recurrent endometrial cancer in the central pelvis. The majority of these studies have indicated a very poor prognosis because these patients routinely die from distant metastasis. Recent data indicate that radiation therapy alone is effective for very small central pelvic recurrences, but cytoreductive surgery plus radiation therapy may be more beneficial in patients with vaginal lesions greater than 1 to 2 cm.[43] In this situation an exploratory laparotomy with evaluation of the paraaortic and pelvic nodes with removal of the vaginal cuff mass (without radical pelvic dissection) is carried out, followed by postoperative radiation therapy. In addition, creation of an omental pedicle graft to the pelvis can be performed at the time of laparotomy in an attempt to improve dosimetry to residual disease and reduce intestinal complications.[44] Recurrent disease in areas other than the vaginal cuff is traditionally treated with radiation therapy, chemotherapy (cytotoxic and hormonal), or both.

Palliative Surgery

Palliative surgery is appropriate in endometrial cancer because many patients develop a slow-growing, prolonged illness. Colostomy, ileostomy, or urinary diversion is appropriate in selected individuals. Debulking of lymph node metastases, followed by radiation therapy or chemotherapy, is also appropriate in selected patients. Occasionally a patient with recurrent corpus cancer will present with bowel perforation because this cancer can invade the intestinal wall. This situation requires emergency bowel bypass, but the procedure should be as safe and conservative as possible.

OVARY

There are three general histologic categories of primary ovarian cancer. First, epithelial ovarian cancers arise from the surface epithelium and tend to present in middle-aged women as widespread intraperitoneal disease. Serous, endometrioid, and mucinous carcinomas are the three most common histologic patterns. Second, germ cell cancers present in the teenage years, often with pain and a rapidly expanding pelvic mass. These tumors are usually unilateral, and prognosis over the last several years has significantly improved with the use of aggressive postoperative combination chemotherapy. Finally, stromal tumors of the ovary tend to produce hormones and follow a more indolent course. The majority of these tumors are treated with surgery alone because recurrence is rare and chemotherapy is generally ineffective in these slow-growing cancers.

Over the last 20 years, a significant amount of basic science and clinical research has led to a better understanding of the epidemiology and treatment of ovarian cancer. Three significant areas require comment. First, the understanding of the routes of ovarian cancer spread and the areas where microscopic metastases may be found has led to a better operative staging procedure. Second, excellent postoperative chemotherapy in combination with aggressive tumor-reductive surgery has led to prolonged survival for some patients. Finally, tumor markers such as α-fetoprotein, human chorionic gonadotropin, and CA-125 assist the clinician in the management of these patients.

Primary Cancer

Patients referred with apparently localized well or moderately differentiated epithelial ovarian cancer who have had incomplete surgical evaluation are candidates for immediate reexploration. This approach is justified by the fact that a prospective study completed by the National Cancer Institute and the GOG[45] indicates that some patients who have been properly surgically staged do not require postoperative therapy. The 5-year survival for these low-risk patients is excellent (greater than 90%) even without adjuvant therapy. The initial operation or reoperation should always include four peritoneal washings for cytologic examination (diaphragm, right and left abdomen, pelvis), careful inspection of all peritoneal surfaces, biopsy or smears from the undersurface of the right diaphragm, biopsies of both paracolonic recesses (to the right of the ascending colon and to the left of the descending colon), biopsies of the peritoneum covering the bladder/cul-de-sac/right pelvis/left pelvis, biopsy of all suspicious lesions, including biopsy or resection of any adhesions, omentectomy, and pelvic and paraaortic lymph node sampling to the level of the renal vessels.[46,47]

In a patient who has not completed her family, the uterus and contralateral tube and ovary can be preserved in Stage I disease with some risk. This conservative surgery is very reasonable in patients with germ cell or stromal tumors. It is less prudent among patients with epithelial cancers. Patients with poorly differentiated epithelial lesions, as well as those with evidence of extraovarian spread, including rupture of the tumor before or at the time of surgery or excrescences on the surface of the ovary, are less likely candidates since they should receive postoperative chemotherapy or radiation therapy. Conservative surgery for epithelial cancer is therefore fruitless since in these situations adjuvant therapy usually causes sterilization. Finally, when ovarian-sparing surgery is performed in a patient with an ovarian malignancy, close follow-up is mandatory and the remaining ovarian tissue should be removed following completion of childbearing.

Patients with widespread ovarian cancer who have undergone surgical exploration without an aggressive attempt at maximal tumor reduction may be candidates for immediate reexploration and cytoreductive surgery. Another option is to administer aggressive chemotherapy (neoadjuvant) usually for two to three cycles, followed by tumor reduction at a later date. To date, there is no evidence that either of these approaches is more appropriate; however, the majority of patients usually undergo immediate reexploration. If bulky residual tumor remains even after an aggressive attempt at debulking, another attempt at cytoreduction may prolong survival after an induction phase of chemotherapy (usually two to four cycles).[48] This concept of interval debulking of patients with suboptimal ovarian cancer is currently under prospective study by the GOG. Whether at primary or reoperation, maximal surgical debulking of advanced untreated ovarian cancer should be attempted by an experienced pelvic surgeon familiar with the biology of ovarian malignancies. It is now generally accepted that the amount of residual tumor remaining after cytoreductive surgery is a major prognostic factor among those with advanced epithelial ovarian cancer.[49,50] If it is judged that all bulky disease can be removed, it is appropriate to resect areas of bowel with reanastamosis. If the last visible residual disease is on the right hemidiaphragm, some surgeons would aggressively remove the disease from this area as well.[51,52]

Recurrent Cancer

Secondary Tumor Debulking. Since primary cytoreduction has been firmly established as initial therapy by almost every clinical review of patients with advanced ovarian cancer, investigators have proposed that secondary tumor reduction for recurrent cancers may be equally effective. The survival benefit and morbidity of these secondary procedures has been difficult to analyze since all of the data have been retrospective. Studies investigating the role of secondary debulking have frequently included mixed populations such as (1) those that progress during primary chemotherapy[53]; (2) patients undergoing debulking procedures for clinically occult disease discovered at the time of second-look laparotomy[53,54]; (3) individuals with chemoresistant tumors that recur shortly after the completion of first-line chemotherapy (within 6 months); and (4) patients whose tumors recur after long intertreatment intervals, usually having tumors still sensitive to chemotherapeutic agents.[55] Clearly, the survival benefit of secondary cytoredutive surgery in ovarian cancer depends on which of these clinical situations applies and the effectiveness of second-line chemotherapy (Table 17.3).

TABLE 17.3 Factors to consider in deciding for or against secondary cytoreduction of ovarian cancer

Clinical situation	No. prior regimens	Response to last therapy	Likelihood of successful cytoreduction	Benefit to patient
Progression	1	Poor	~50%	Unlikely
Interval cytoreduction	≤1	Poor/Good	~70%	Probable
Second look	1	Good	~70%	Unknown
Recurrence	≥1	Good	~50%	Probable

Second-Look Operation. The second-look operation in ovarian cancer has been evaluated in a large number of studies. Presently it is reserved for patients who have completed a required course of chemotherapy and have no evidence of persistent disease either on physical examination, radiologic testing, or CA-125 testing.[56-59] Patients who are candidates for further therapy either via protocol or as further palliative therapy in the form of intraperitoneal radioactive substances or chemotherapy may undergo a second-look operation. Unfortunately, no individual therapeutic approach has been unequivocally demonstrated to affect survival when recurrent cancer is documented at second-look surgery. For this reason, surgical reassessment is generally reserved for protocol settings or limited to other unique scenarios. When indicated, this operation is performed through a generous incision and involves careful evaluation of the entire peritoneal cavity and the retroperitoneal spaces. Extensive biopsies are taken from the diaphragm, all peritoneal surfaces, all adhesions, and the retroperitoneal lymph nodes or retroperitoneal spaces not explored at the time of primary surgery. Multiple pelvic peritoneal biopsies are mandatory. Usually this operation will result in 30 to 50 separate histologic specimens for evaluation. Simply opening the peritoneal cavity, taking a look around, and removing a couple of adhesions is inappropriate and should not be considered a negative second-look operation.

Palliative Surgery

Although epithelial ovarian cancer is a surface-spreading disease that rarely invades vital organs, partial or complete bowel obstruction is often seen. This is secondary to extrinsic compression of the small bowel or hypoperistalsis due to mesenteric and bowel surface implants. In most cases, nausea and vomiting can be relieved by conservative measures. However, occasionally long-term palliation can be afforded by reexploration and bowel bypass.[60-66] Patients must be carefully selected, and surgery should be as conservative as possible. Preoperatively a long tube is passed, and intraoperatively the bulb of the tube is identified to find the small bowel above the obstruction. This small bowel is then anastomosed in a side-to-side fashion to the most appropriate area of colon. It is paramount to obtain a preoperative barium enema to ensure that there is no obstruction of the lower colon.

SUMMARY

Although an awareness of appropriate techniques for diagnosis and evaluation of gynecologic cancer has been stressed over the last 20 years, a small number of patients continue to require immediate reexploration for evaluation and/or treatment of their cancer. Every obstetrician and gynecologist should be fully aware of these situations and understand the need for further surgery. Unnecessary delay can result in decreased survival and potentially compromise cure. More important, careful follow-up at close intervals of the recently treated oncology patient may lead to the early diagnosis of recurrence at a point where reoperation may be curative. Finally, it is critically important that each patient be afforded the best possible palliative care, which may include operative procedures that will extend life or alleviate significant symptoms without creating severe complications.

References

1. Childers JM and others: Laparoscopic staging of the patient with incompletely staged early adenocarcinoma of the endometrium, Obstet Gynecol 83:597, 1994.
2. Buchler DA and others: Treatment of recurrent carcinoma of the vulva, Gynecol Oncol 8:180, 1979.
3. Hopkins MP, Reid GC, and Morley GW: The surgical management of recurrent squamous cell carcinoma of the vulva, Obstet Gynecol 75:1001, 1990.
4. Chafe W and others: Unrecognized invasive carcinoma in vulvar intraepithelial neoplasia (VIN), Gynecol Oncol 31:154, 1988.
5. Thomas GM and others: Changing concepts in the management of vulvar cancer, Gynecol Oncol 42:9, 1991.
6. DiSaia PJ, Creasman WT, and Rich WM: An alternate approach to early cancer of the vulva, Am J Obstet Gynecol 133:825, 1979.
7. Burke TW and others: Radical wide excision and selective inguinal node dissection for squamous cell carcinoma of the vulva, Gynecol Oncol 38:328, 1990.
8. Homesley HD and others: Assessment of current International Federation of Gynecology and Obstetrics staging of vulvar carcinoma relative to prognostic factors for survival (a Gynecologic Oncology Group study), Am J Obstet Gynecol 164:997, 1991.
9. Homesley HD and others: Radiation therapy versus pelvic node resection for carcinoma of the vulva with positive groin nodes, Obstet Gynecol 68:733, 1986.
10. Stehman FB and others: Early stage I carcinoma of the vulva treated with ipsilateral superficial inguinal lymphadenectomy and modified radical hemivulvectomy (a prospective study of the Gynecologic Oncology Group), Obstet Gynecol 79:490, 1992.
11. Heaps JM and others: Surgical-pathologic variables predictive of local recurrence in squamous cell carcinoma of the vulva, Gynecol Oncol 38:309, 1990.
12. Leuchter RS and others: Primary carcinoma of Bartholin gland (a report of 14 cases and review of the literature), Obstet Gynecol 60:361, 1982.
13. Bergen S and others: Conservation management of extramammary Paget's disease of the vulva, Gynecol Oncol 33:151, 1989.
14. Feuer GA, Shevchuck M, and Calanog A: Vulvar Paget's disease: the need to exclude an invasive lesion, Gynecol Oncol 38:81, 1990.
15. Stacy D, Burrell MO, and Franklin EW: Extrammammary Paget's disease of the vulva and anus: use of intraoperative frozen-section margins, Am J Obstet Gynecol 155:519, 1986.
16. Powell JL, Donavan JT, and Reed WP: Hip disarticulation for recurrent vulvar cancer, Gynecol Oncol 47:110, 1992.
17. Podratz KC, Symmonds RE, and Taylor WF: Carcinoma of the vulva: analysis of treatment failures, Am J Obstet Gynecol 143:340, 1982.
18. DiSaia PJ and Creasman WT: Invasive cervical cancer. In Clinical gynecologic oncology, ed 4, St Louis, 1993, Mosby.
19. Chapman JA and others: Surgical treatment of unexpected invasive cervical cancer found at total hysterectomy, Obstet Gynecol 80:931, 1992.
20. Andras EJ, Fletcher GH, and Rutledge F: Radiotherapy of carcinoma of the cervix following simple hysterectomy, Am J Obstet Gynecol 115:547, 1973.
21. Heller PB and others: Cervical carcinoma found incidentally in a uterus removed for benign indications, Obstet Gynecol 67:187, 1986.
22. Orr JW and others: Surgical treatment of women found to have invasive cervix cancer at the time of total hysterectomy, Obstet Gynecol 68:353, 1986.
23. Barber HR: Pelvic exenteration, Cancer Invest 5:331, 1987.
24. Hatch KD and others: Anterior pelvic exenteration, Gynecol Oncol 31:205, 1988.
25. Jones WB: Surgical approaches for advanced or recurrent cancer of the cervix, Cancer 60:2094, 1987.
26. Lawhead RA and others: Pelvic exenteration for recurrent or persistent gynecologic malignancies: a 10-year review of the Memorial Sloan-Kettering Cancer Center experience (1972-1981), Gynecol Oncol 33:279, 1989.
27. Lagasse LD and others: Results and complications of operative staging in cervical cancer: experience of the Gynecologic Oncology Group, Gynecol Oncol 9:90, 1980.
28. Morley GW, Lindenauer SM, and Young D: Vaginal reconstruction following pelvic exenteration, Am J Obstet Gynecol 116:996, 1973.

29. Wheeless CR Jr: Neovagina constructed from an omental J flap and a split thickness skin graft, Gynecol Oncol 35:224, 1989.
30. Gallousis S: Isolated lung metastases from pelvic malignancies, Gynecol Oncol 7:206, 1979.
31. Stanhope CR and Symmonds RE: Palliative extenteration: what, when, and why? Am J Obstet Gynecol 152:12, 1988.
32. Carter J and others: Percutaneous urinary diversion in gynecologic oncology, Gynecol Oncol 490:248, 1991.
33. Graham JB and Abab RS: Ureteral obstruction due to radiation, Am J Obstet Gynecol 99:409, 1967.
34. DiSaia PJ and Creasman WT: Adenocarcinoma of the uterus. In Clinical gynecologic oncology, ed 4, St Louis, 1993, Mosby.
35. Aalders JG, Abeler V, and Kilstad P: Recurrent adenocarcinoma of the endometrium: a clinical and histopathological study of 379 patients, Gynecol Oncol 17:85, 1984.
36. Creasman WT, Morrow CP, and Bundy L: Surgical pathological spread patterns of endometrial cancer, Cancer 60:2035, 1987.
37. Jeffrey JF, Krepart GV, and Lotocki FU: Papillary serous adenocarcinomas of the endometrium, Obstet Gynecol 67:670, 1986.
38. Photopulos GJ and others: Clear cell carcinoma of the endometrium, Cancer 43:1448, 1979.
39. Bond WH: Early uterine body carcinoma: is postoperative vaginal irradiation any value? Clin Radiol 36:619, 1985.
40. Chen SS: Operative treatment in stage I endometrial carcinoma with deep myometrial invasion and/or grade 3 tumor surgically limited to the corpus uteri: no recurrence with only primary surgery, Cancer 63:1843, 1989.
41. DiSaia PJ and others: Risk factors and recurrent patterns in stage I endometrial cancer, Am J Obstet Gynecol 151:1009, 1985.
42. Kilgore LC and others: Adenocarcinoma of the endometrium: survival comparisons of patients with and without pelvic node sampling, Gynecol Oncol 56:29, 1995.
43. Greven K and Olds W: Isolated vaginal recurrences of endometrial adenocarcinoma and their management, Cancer 60:419, 1987.
44. Monk BJ and others: Open interstitial brachytherapy for the treatment of local-regional recurrences of uterine corpus and cervix cancer after primary surgery, Gynecol Oncol 52:222, 1994.
45. Young RC and others: Adjuvant therapy in stage I and stage II epithelial ovarian cancer: results of two prospective randomized trials, N Engl J Med 322:1021, 1990.
46. Piver MS, Barlow JJ, and Lele SB: Incidence of subclinical metastasis in stage I and II ovarian carcinoma, Obstet Gynecol 52:100, 1978.
47. Young RC and others: Staging laparotomy in early ovarian cancer, JAMA 250:3072, 1984.
48. Favalli G and others: The effect of debulking surgery after induction chemotherapy on the prognosis in advanced epithelial ovarian cancer. Gynecological Cancer Cooperative Group of the European Organization for Research and Treatment of Cancer. N Engl J Med 332:629, 1995.
49. Hacker NF and others: Primary cytoreductive surgery for epithelial ovarian cancer, Obstet Gynecol 61:413, 1983.
50. Delgato G, Aram DH, and Petrilli ES: Stage III epithelial ovarian cancer: the role of maximal surgical reduction, Gynecol Oncol 18:293, 1984.
51. Montz FJ, Schlaerth JB, and Berek JS: Resection of diaphragmatic peritoneum and muscle: role in cytoreductive surgery for advanced ovarian cancer, Gynecol Oncol 35:338, 1989.
52. Deppe G, Malviya VK, and Malone JM: Dubulking surgery for ovarian cancer with the cavitron ultrasonic surgical aspirator (CUSA): a preliminary report, Gynecol Oncol 31:223, 1988.
53. Morris M, Gershenson DM, and Wharton JT: Secondary cytoreductive surgery in epithelial ovarian cancer: non-responders to first-line therapy, Gynecol Oncol 33:1, 1989.
54. Hoskins W, Rubin S, and Dulaney E: The influence of secondary cytoreduction at the time of second-look laparotomy on the survival of patients with epithelial ovarian carcinoma, Gynecol Oncol 34:365, 1989.
55. Morris M and others: Secondary cytoreductive surgery for recurrent epithelial ovarian cancer, Gynecol Oncol 34:334, 1989.
56. Berek JS and others: CA 125 serum levels correlated with second-look operations among ovarian cancer patients, Obstet Gynecol 67:685, 1986.

57. Chambers SK and others: Evaluation of the role of second-look surgery in ovarian cancer, Obstet Gynecol 72:404, 1988.

58. Podezaski ES and others: Use of second-look laparotomy in the management of patients with ovarian epithelial malignancies, Gynecol Oncol 28:205, 1987.

59. Podratz KC and others: Evaluation of treatment and survival after positive second-look laparotomy, Gynecol Oncol 31:9, 1988.

60. Castaldo TW and others: Intestinal operations in patients with ovarian carcinoma, Obstet Gynecol 139:80, 1981.

61. Krebs HB and Goplerud DR: Surgical management of bowel obstruction in advanced ovarian carcinoma, Obstet Gynecol 61:327, 1983.

62. Makela J, Kairaluoma MI, and Kauppila A: Palliative surgery for intestinal complications of advanced recurrent gynecologic malignancy, Acta Chir Scand 153:57, 1987.

63. Piver MS and others: Survival after ovarian cancer induced intestinal obstruction, Gynecol Oncol 13:44, 1982.

64. Rubin SC and others: Intestinal surgery in gynecologic oncology, Gynecol Oncol 34:30, 1989.

65. Rubin SC and others: Palliative surgery for intestinal obstruction in advanced ovarian cancer, Gynecol Oncol 34:16, 1989.

66. Tunca JC and others: The management of ovarian-cancer-caused bowel obstruction, Gynecol Oncol 12:186, 1981.

18

Minor Surgery

HAROLD MICHLEWITZ

This chapter will deal with some relatively minor procedures that are technically simple but require some element of precision. Knowledge about the purpose of the procedure will help to avoid the need to repeat the procedure.

VULVAR BIOPSY

The practitioner has frequently bypassed the vulva on the way to the Papanicolaou smear collection and in so doing has missed numerous diagnoses. Current practice requires a careful inspection of the vulva, frequently with a colposcope. After significant experience with a colposcope, examiners may be able to train their eyes sufficiently to dispense with using a colposcope on a routine basis.

Identifying what to excise is as important as knowing how to do it. If the lesion to be excised is an exophytic growth such as condyloma acuminatum, the instrument could be an appropriately sized circular punch biopsy or other instruments (forceps and scapel) to achieve a superficial and deep margin of normal tissue. A more extensive condition such as lichen sclerosus requires excision of the most abnormal-looking area, such as a site of erosion, as well as a margin of noneroded tissue for epithelial comparison. In the case of no epithelialized tissue, the biopsy should be deep enough to identify a possible underlying carcinoma. Some observers believe that carcinomas might be found in 4% to 7% of the patients with vulvar lichen sclerosus. When dealing with lesions such as lichen planus, the erosive version requires identification of the epithelium adjacent to the erosive margin. This epithelium might have the characteristic white linear or latticelike striae associated with lichen planus. Management of the pigmented lesion requires achieving good clear margins of the pigmented portion so that on pathologic evaluation the margins are free. If they are not, reexcision may be required. If delayed long enough for healing, the original site might not be recognizable, thus creating a significant dilemma.

Special consideration must be given to evaluating the clitoral region. The hood needs to be lifted back in order to expose any clitoral lesions. Biopsy of this area can be particularly sensitive and emotionally distressing. Appropriate sampling should take this into account. Lesions of the perineal body region often involve lesions of the perianal location, and full evaluation of this site should direct the practitioner to the best site for diagnosis. In very extensive conditions such as intraepithelial neoplasia or lichen sclerosus, more than one site should be sampled to fully evaluate the condition.

The punch biopsy site can be treated with Monsel's solution (ferric subsulfate in a mustardlike consistency) to achieve hemostasis. Larger excisions in fact require elliptical incisions to allow for suture closure. For the larger excisions interrupted Vicryl 4-0 sutures could be placed as a subcuticular running stitch. These biopsies can be done under 1% to 2% lidocaine injections (with or without epinephrine). They can also be done under Enteric Mixture of Local Anesthetics Lidocaine and Prilocaine (EMLA) cream application after adequate anesthesia is achieved.

In conclusion, the vulvar biopsy is the first line of defense against an error in diagnosis. Making the task of biopsy easy will avoid the potentially disastrous decision to treat without biopsy.

CYSTIC VULVAR DISEASE

There are two categories of cystic vulvar disease: the infection-related lesion and the noninfected variety. The most frequently encountered vulvar inflammation is related to an abscess. This can arise from a break in the integrity of the skin with secondary infection. The vulvar area is prone to moisture from sweating and heat and can easily become infected. As with any abscess formation, the area should be incised and drained. If the abscess cavity is large enough, iodoform packing should be left in for sufficient time to allow continual drainage. Antibiotic coverage may be required if the condition is extensive or in a diabetic patient. The diabetic status confers special risks in this setting because of the increased risk of necrotising fasciitis. Aggressive management is necessary.

Infections in this area might represent cutaneous drainage of an intestinal condition such as regional enteritis. Intestinal evaluation should be considered in order to explain cases of insufficient healing or recurring abscesses. In the area of the posterior fourchette/perineal body, an abscess might represent a cutaneous manifestation of a perirectal abscess. Drainage may best be accomplished by treating the perirectal abscess.

The most common vulvar abscess is the Bartholin's gland duct abscess. The Bartholin's gland lies deep to the vulvar vestibule at 4 and 8 o'clock. The circuitous duct opens in the vulvar vestibule to expel its mucousy effluent. If the duct opening is occluded through infection (whether a sexually transmitted disease [STD] or not), the mucus production from the deeper gland continues with subsequent distension of the duct. With infection the area becomes fluctuant and tender. There may be spontaneous drainage or intervention, which will require incision and drainage over the mucosal surface. The abscess opening can be maintained in a patent condition with a Word catheter or by marsupialization. During marsupialization the abscess cavity wall is sewn to the skin surface. If the opening is not sufficiently large, it may close prematurely. It is important that adhesions inside the abscess are lysed to prevent pocketing and recurrence. The abscess cavity may extend anteriorly as high as the mons pubis, giving rise to concerns about where the origin of the abscess is. Recurrent abscess formation is frequently encountered, or an abscess may occur on the opposite side at a future date. In the older patient, a sample of the wall should be sent to exclude a Bartholin's gland carcinoma.

The cystic lesion that is not infected in the posterior perineal region is frequently the Bartholin's gland duct cyst. Anteriorly this might represent a hydrocele, a hernia, or lymphangiectasia (especially if prior surgery in the area has occurred.) Whenever there is swelling of the labia majora—either unilateral or bilateral—the possibility of hernia exists. The round ligament passes through the inguinal canal and creates the potential for hernias. Examination in a standing position or with Valsalva can exaggerate the hernial defect. Intestinal contents can make this an emergency discovery and referral for repair to a general surgeon. At times the swelling may be free of association with the inguinal canal, but located high on the labia majora. In this case it may be a hydrocele representing an isolated persistence of the Canal of Nuck with a peritoneal sac. The area may be nontender and troublesome solely due to its presence. It can be left alone. If enlarging, it may need to be excised. Here complete excision is necessary to prevent recurrence. The cyst neck should be identified and closed. Absence of intestinal contents should be assured when first opening the hydrocele. If a recurrence does occur, the use of indigo carmine injection into the cyst to identify the whole structure is advisable. Similarly, if the cystic mass is a form of lymphangiectasia, it would be helpful to inject indigo carmine to identify the multiple cystic component.

The previously noted structures can be differentiated from a Bartholin's cyst, even if the cyst is large and extends up the labia majora. Since it is typically located in the posterior aspect of the fourchette, its predominant swelling will be noted toward the vulvar vestibule and just inside the hymenal ring. It is at this site that the incision, drainage, and placement of a Word catheter (a small Foley-type device designed to keep the incision site patent) is most helpful. It is preferable not to have further effluent from the duct to be toward the external cornified skin. The catheter should be left in place at least 2 weeks. The Bartholin's cyst may swell towards the ischiorectal fossa and superiorly under the labia majora. If the cystic distension is not tense, the full extent of the structure may not be appreciated. During the dissection the surgeon might more successfully accomplish this if the cyst is made tenser by injecting indigo carmine into it. When the cyst is not infected, the tract is not expected to extend superiorly. Word catheter placement or marsupialization will allow shrinkage of the distended duct within a few days. Recurrence is not uncommon when infected, otherwise it is unusual. A cystic wall sample should be examined histologically to determine its benign nature. Even when not dramatically swollen, that is, greater than 2 cm, its benign nature must be determined in the postmenopausal woman. If the structure feels rubbery or an attempted drainage of fluid is not released, it is important to perform a biopsy. This might represent an unusual pathologic entity such as a fibroid or sarcoma.

Vulvar Vestibulitis Syndrome

The vulvar vestibule is anatomically the area of minimally cornified inner aspect of the labia minora and the mucous membrane–covered area outside the hymenal ring. The anterior vestibule includes the area between the labia minora just below the clitoris and extending to the Skene's duct/crypts adjacent to the urethra. The posterior vestibule includes the posterior fourchette, where one finds the opening to the major vestibular gland (Bartholin's gland) bilaterally. Hart's line usually defines the junction between the cornified and noncornified region of the inner aspect of the labia minora when viewed after the application of 3% acetic acid. The cornified area appears white.

The syndrome of note is a category of the umbrella syndrome vulvodynia–vulvar pain syndrome (VVS). The symptom of vulvodynia is either pain or burning. When applying the term vulvar vestibulitis (VV), the constellation of symptoms is limited to introital contact pain either from sexual intercourse or on insertion of speculum/tampon. In addition, the exquisite areas of tenderness are limited to focal areas of the vulvar vestibule. These sites may appear erythematous but not exclusively so. Tenderness in the vulvar vestibule can be elicited by touch with a wet cotton swab.

The recognition of this syndrome in the mid 1980s belies the fact that the syndrome probably represents similar conditions reported in the 1890s and 1950s without a wide recognition of the disease. The preponderance of literature appeared after 1983. The pain and burning was thought to follow a particularly difficult period of vulvar infection with either yeast, *Trichomonas,* or other inciting agents. This was never a consistent finding and certainly did not explain the group of patients who had this condition prior to any sexual activity. Extensive study during the last 10 to 15 years has failed to identify an etiology. During the early 1990s, it was commonly felt that koilocytotic changes on histologic examination represented HPV. Subsequent DNA probes have essentially eliminated HPV as the responsible agent.

Patients typically report normal sexual function until the development, either gradually or acutely, of severe pain with sexual contact, resulting in a rapid diminution of sexual activity. Prior to the current awareness of this condition many patients were led to believe that it was a psychologically based condition. With local anesthesia the patients could function normally, which established the pathologic nature of the complaint. Careful interviews had not uncovered a latent sexual abuse history.

Curiously the demographics revealed an overwhelming preponderance of white women aged 18 to 45. A large percentage had never been pregnant, though the condition had been seen in parous women and on occasion first became manifest after a vaginal delivery (with episiotomy). Patients frequently have complaints of sexual discomfort but fail to raise the issue with practitioners, which accounts for underestimation of the prevalence of this condition.

A number of patients who were examined on a routine visit showed focal vestibular tenderness (20%) without complaining of dyspareunia. This group may join the patients with dyspareunia at some point in the future. Visual inspection noting focal erythema does not necessarily identify a patient with dyspareunia. A number of studies have shown that areas of tenderness in the vulvar vestibule when examined histologically reveal an infiltration with chronic inflammation—predominantly lymphocytes—but plasma cells have also been noted. A recent European study was conducted in which a biopsy of asymptomatic patients also revealed the presence of chronic inflammation. Thus the histologic finding is characteristic of but not specific for VV. Attempts at identifying etiologic agents by histologic examination have been unsuccessful. HPV-DNA evaluation has failed to reveal an etiologic agent. HPV was popularly thought to be the obvious culprit because the syndrome of VV exploded in the late 1980s as the HPV epidemic was being evaluated. Occasional cases of VV seemed to have followed the perineal ablation of what was thought to be micropapillation. These micropapillations do not need to be treated and do not reflect microscopic HPV. We are left with a syndrome that has qualities that are also present in asymptomatic patients. Thus it has become difficult to ascertain the exact treatment of this condition. I will therefore review what the various approaches have been and their current level of effectiveness.

The syndrome has varying levels of severity. Certainly the milder forms of the disease can spontaneously resolve, but this type of resolution fails to occur after a 6-month interval. Local injectible anesthesia provides only temporary relief and carries the reassurance that it is not a psychologic illness. Some patients can function with the use of Xylocaine topical products with either 2% or 5% active ingredients. The EMLA product is better suited for sexual function because of its longer anesthetic action, but it can on occasion cause significant skin-burning sensation prior to the anesthetic effect. It also has not been released for use on mucous membranes. Injections of steroids locally have been unsuccessful. Multiple oral antibiotics, antibiotic creams and jellies, and steroid applications have been ineffective. Despite the inability to identify HPV, there has been some limited success using acyclovir. (There is no evidence of herpes genitalis activity.) A very successful application of interferon injections has helped on a temporary basis. There is now less enthusiasm about this therapy, especially in light of the negative DNA probes for HPV. A number of advocates still feel considerable relief can be achieved with interferon injections. The use of tricyclic antidepressants (TADs) has found wider success in the vulvodynia patient who does not have the focal tenderness associated with VVS. For those patients who have diffuse complaints but also have focal tenderness, the use of TADs may limit the diffuse pain to only the focally tender sites. In that case the practitioner may proceed to the therapy felt to be most effective in VVS after TAD use.

The most successful therapy to date has been the elimination of the focally tender sites: en bloc surgical resection of the posterior vestibular tissue in an elliptical specimen followed by partial exteriorization of the vaginal mucosa. This has met with 65% to 90% success, especially if the anterior vestibular tender foci are also removed. The anterior surgical site, if located between the clitoris and the urethra, is allowed to heal by secondary intention. The posterior vestibule and periurethral sites are sutured with interrupted 4-0 Vicryl stitches. The complications of this procedure include local bleeding, hematoma formation and surgical site disruption. This does not impair the success of the procedure. Of concern in approximately 5% to 10% of patients is the risk of Bartholin's duct occlusion. If this subsequently results in duct swelling, unroofing of this duct swelling may return the area to more normal anatomy. For those patients who do not get relief or who experience recurrence at some point in the future, either reoperation or an alternative form of therapy would be needed. A more recent suggestion that the skin of the vulvar vestibule be undermined, thus denervating the area (vestibuloplasty) has failed to achieve the success of actually removing the epithelium.

There is a suggestion that a number of patients might finally get relief with vaginal delivery. A natural avulsion of the vestibule during delivery or a widening of the introitus might be the natural therapy for this condition. Patients who have undergone perineoplasty are naturally anxious about subsequent vaginal delivery, but to date this has not been a problem.

Since the etiology of the condition is unknown and success with surgery is not universal, alternative approaches have been suggested and are under wider review. First among these is the use of biofeedback. Patients undergo biofeedback using a portable electromyographic instrument to allow for pelvic floor muscle exercises. After 4 months the resting tension levels decrease 68%. Electrical stimulation is used to treat pelvic floor dysfunction that arises from spastic muscles, leading to ligamental strain.

Some investigators have been exploring the use of flash lamp–excited dye lasers, which emit energy selectively absorbed by the oxyhemoglobin absorption peak at 585 nm wavelength. This destroys the vascularity that may have been hyperemic near the involved neural elements. These neuronal elements are thought to excite sympathetic autonomic pain. There is not extensive experience with this therapy. The literature with respect to the efficacy of limiting calcium oxalate in the diet and replacing it with calcium citrate has been confusing and unexplainable in its limited application. The lack of obvious harm from this approach has gained public attention, demanding further evaluation of its scientific significance.

In conclusion, the various conditions discussed here require that the operator pay close attention to the unique aspect of each disease. Then the retrieval of information or application of surgical therapy will be maximized with little need to revisit the issue.

BIBLIOGRAPHY

Bornstein J, Zarfati D, and Abramovici H: Perineoplasty compared with vestibuloplasty for severe vulvar vestibulitis, Br J Obstet Gynaecol 102:652, 1995.

Crawford RAF and others: Outpatient vulval biopsy: a note of caution, Br J Obstet Gynaecol 102:487, 1995.

Friedrich EG Jr: Vulvar vestibulitis syndrome, J Reprod Med 32:110, 1987.

Frits L: Iatrogenic lymphangiectatic cysts. Paper presented at the Thirteenth Congress of the International Society for the Study of Vulvar Disease, Iguazw, Argentina, September, 1995.

Glazer HI and others: Treatment of vulvar vestibulitis syndrome with electromyographic biofeedback, J Repro Med 40:283, 1995.

Goetsche M: Vulvar vestibulitis prevalence and historic features in a general gynecologic practice population, Am J Obstet Gynecol 164:6, 1991.

Hart WR, Norris HJ, and Helwig EB: Relation of lichen sclerosus et atrophicus of the vulva to development of carcinoma, Obstet Gynecol 45:369, 1975.

Horowitz BJ: Interferon therapy for condylomatous vulvitis, Obstet Gynecol 73:446, 1989.

McKay M: Vulvodynia: a multifactorial clinical problem, Arch Dermatol 12S:256, 1989.

Monif GGRG and Belatti RG: Intercourse related vaginal pain syndrome: a variant of vulvar vestibulitis syndrome, Am J Obstet Gynecol 169:194, 1993.

Reid R and others: Flash lamp–excited dye laser therapy for idiopathic vulvodynia, Am J Obstet Gynecol 1722:1684, 1995.

Riva JM and others: Extended carbon dioxide laser vaporization in the treatment of subclinical papillomavirus of the lower genital tract, Obstet Gynecol 73:25, 1990.

Salvino C, Harford F, and Dobrin P: Necrotizing infections of the perineum, South Med J 86:908, 1993.

Skene AJ: Treatise on the diseases of women, New York, 1889, D Appleton and Co.

Solomons CC, Melmed MH, and Heitler SM: Calcium citrate for vulvar vestibulitis, J Reprod Med 36:879, 1991.

Woodruff JD and Parmley TH: Infection of the minor vestibular gland, Obstet Gynecol 62:609, 1983.

19

Postoperative Hemorrhage

James L. Breen
Jennifer Y. Choe

With the exception of evisceration and hemorrhage, few surgical complications necessitate reoperation as an emergent procedure. Reviewing the literature on postoperative hemorrhage, we are impressed by the volumes of blood that are required to stabilize patients before they are brought to a successful hemostatic outcome. This may reflect the natural tendency of surgeons to initially deny the need for reoperation in the immediate postoperative period or the difficulties encountered by the surgeon in controlling hemorrhage because of the extensive primary and collateral circulation surrounding the operative field.

Postoperative hemorrhage may occur in any patient despite the most careful surgical techniques. The stage for it, however, may be set by the following: an inappropriate abdominal incision, speed or impatience on the part of the surgeon, improper handling of tissues, poor surgical technique, and failure to closely inspect the operative field before closure.

Three specific surgical principles regarding the handling of tissue pedicles are essential to reduce the risk of intraoperative and postoperative bleeding. Recall that the purchase point of surgical clamps is limited to their distal third or half; therefore incorporating an entire pedicle or overloading the clamp to its crotch leads to slippage of the suture or rotation of vasculature within the pedicle. Second, regardless of the suture material or the methodology of suture ligature, the surgeon should place the needle as close to the clamp as possible. This is facilitated by rolling the clamp to expose the tissue-clamp interface and placing the needle through the pedicle riding the surface of the clamp. Finally, once pedicles have been ligated, and this is particularly true for vascular pedicles, they should not be tagged because traction may cause ligature slippage or tissue tearing. Careful suturing and handling of pedicles are paramount in the prevention of postoperative hemorrhage.

The gynecologic surgeon should be prepared to recognize hemorrhagic complications early to resolve them with appropriate techniques—techniques that obviate the need to refer to other chapters in this text. The surgeon may expect, when reoperation is necessary, that the presence of large dissecting hematomas, friable tissues, disseminated intravascular coagulation, and consumption coagulopathy will further complicate the surgical picture. It is reassuring that large documented series regarding the management of postoperative hemorrhage are rare. The recommendations made in this chapter are based on personal experiences and articles that consist of case reports and limited, uncontrolled studies. These recommendations will range from simple ligation of offending vessels to newer approaches, such as interventive radiology.

Anatomy and Physiology of Pelvic Bleeding

Familiarity with the vascular anatomy of the pelvis is imperative not only for performing pelvic surgery but also for understanding the approaches to control intraoperative or postoperative hemorrhage. There is an intricate primary and collateral circulation to pelvic structures (Figure 19.1). Branches of the anterior division of the internal iliac (hypogastric) artery provide the major blood supply to the organs of the female pelvis. The hypogastric artery arises at the bifurcation of the common iliac artery, at a point opposite the lumbosacral intervertebral disk and in front of the sacroiliac joint. It then descends to the upper part of the

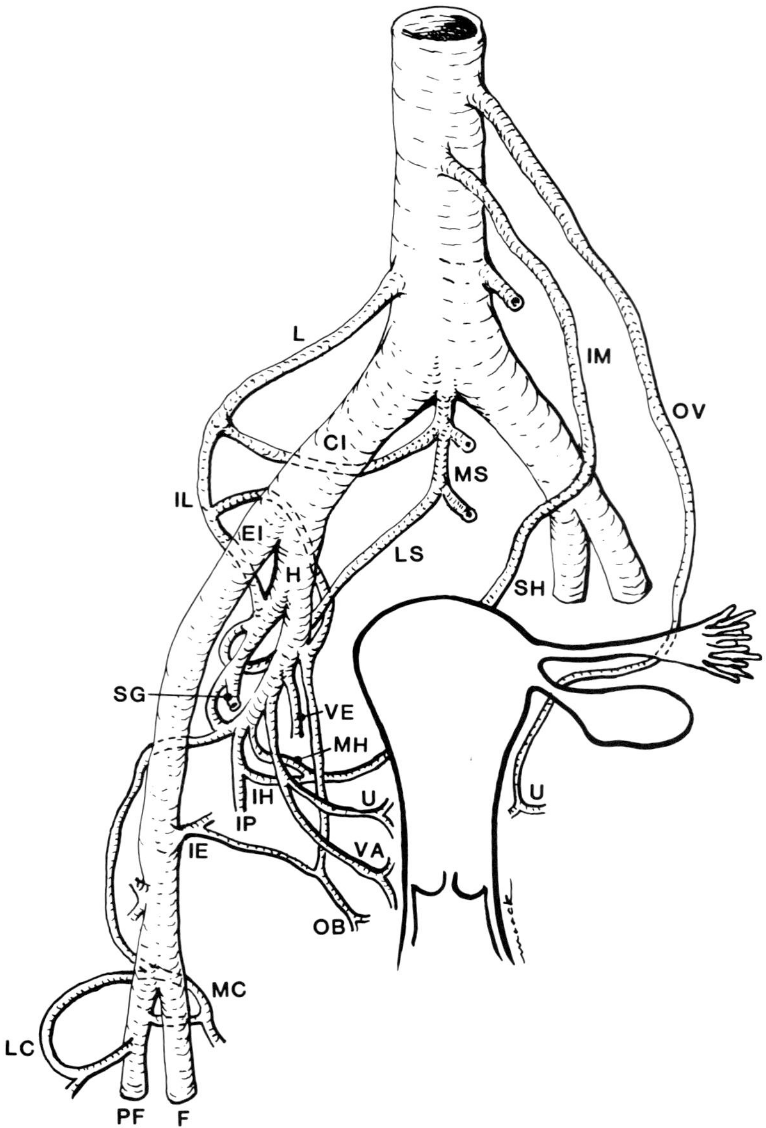

Figure 19.1 Primary pelvic arterial circulation and pertinent collateral vessels. *IM,* Inferior mesenteric; *L,* lumbar; *OV,* ovarian, *CI,* common iliac; *MS,* middle sacral; *IL,* iliolumbar; *EI,* external iliac; *LS,* lateral sacral; *H,* hypogastric (internal iliac); *SH,* superior hemorrhoidal; *SG,* superior gluteal; *VE,* vesical; *MH,* middle hemorrhoidal; *U,* uterine; *IH,* inferior hemorrhoidal; *IP,* internal pudendal; *VA,* vaginal; *IE,* inferior epigastric; *OB,* obturator; *MC,* middle femoral circumflex; *LC,* lateral circumflex; *F,* femoral; *PF,* deep femoral.

greater sciatic foramen, where it divides into the anterior and posterior trunks. The latter gives off the iliolumbar and lateral sacral arteries before leaving the pelvis through the greater sciatic foramen as the superior gluteal artery. The anterior division leaves the pelvis through the lesser sciatic foramen as the inferior gluteal artery. In the process it gives off the obturator, superior vesical, inferior vesical, uterine, vaginal, middle hemorrhoidal, inferior hemorrhoidal, and pudendal arteries.

The initial approach to any patient with significant postoperative bleeding is to maintain or restore hemodynamic stability, followed immediately by a search for the offending vessel. The rate of blood loss from injured or unligated blood vessels can be quantitated by a simple equation:

$$Q = S\sqrt{\frac{P_I - P_E}{e} + V^2}$$

Q is the rate of blood loss, S is the surface area of the laceration, P_E is the extravascular pressure, P_I is the intravascular pressure, e is the density of the blood, and V is the velocity of blood flow in the vessel. Clearly a suture that reduces S to zero will cease all flow. For example, hypogastric artery ligation reduces flow by decreasing both V and P_I. P_E can be increased to equal P_I by pressure packs or military or medical antishock trousers (MAST) suits. Arterial embolization reduces S to zero in terminal vessels and is similar to a hypogastric artery ligation. Patients in shock have low P_I and V values and therefore may present a problem to the surgeon trying to identify the offending vessel during extreme hypotensive periods. This situation may explain the occasional need for a second reoperation. This formula does not take into consideration the status of the patient's coagulation system.

Posthysterectomy Bleeding

Postoperative hemorrhage may complicate any operation whether it be a simple or extensive procedure. Postoperative hemorrhage requiring reoperation complicates approximately 0.8% of hysterectomies.[1]

Inapparent postoperative intraabdominal bleeding may be difficult to diagnose. Suspicion should be aroused if any of the following occurs: excessive postoperative pain; persistent oliguria; abdominal rigidity or distention; shoulder, vaginal, or scapular pain; tachycardia; or hypotension. In these situations, serial evaluations of the hemoglobin and hematocrit values are helpful. Ultrasound studies, culdocentesis, or an abdominal tap may aid in the diagnosis. Once the diagnosis is made or the index of suspicion is high without supporting evidence, celiotomy with complete exploration of the abdomen is mandatory.

Hysterectomy techniques that extraperitonealize vascular pedicles and leave the vaginal cuff open increase the likelihood that postoperative bleeding will be recognized early. Bleeding that is retroperitoneal or intraabdominal, without access to the vagina, is usually diagnosed after the patient has lost a significant volume of blood. In 1219 vaginal hysterectomies reported by Smith and Pratt, 7 patients who required reoperation for hemorrhage developed symptoms 5 to 11 hours postoperatively.[2] Physical examination may reveal a distended abdomen with decreased bowel sounds or differential dullness on percussion, which may or may not shift (the latter is true of retroperitoneal bleeding). Ultrasound scanning may be useful in locating the site of hematoma, but the ultimate discovery is at reoperation.

Patients who manifest postoperative bleeding early (i.e., within the first 24 hours) generally bleed from a pedicle that was inadequately sutured or from a pedicle in which suture breakage or slippage occurred. Bleeding after the first 24 hours is usually due to tissue or suture sloughing, but this has decreased with the advent of synthetic absorbable sutures that retain their tensile strength for up to 30 days.

Although the most common site of significant postoperative bleeding following hysterectomies is the vaginal vault, any vascular pedicle may be implicated.

Bleeding that occurs within the first 24 hours is best managed by appropriate reexploration and resuturing of the offending vessels. Those cases where postoperative bleeding is more indolent (i.e., presenting as a hematoma, both confined and self-tamponading) may require reoperation or merely observation. The reoperative procedure—hematoma evacuation and placement of hemostatic sutures—diminishes the risk of secondary infection and abscess formation. Conversely, many hematomas may self-tamponade and stabilize without additional bleeding or subsequent infection. The decision to operate on stable hematomas is highly individualized and is based primarily on how stable the patient is and what the risks of infection are. The risk of infection relates to the indication for the original surgery, the use of antibiotics, and the general metabolic status of the patient.

Postoperative hemorrhage of significance is almost always arterial in origin and must be controlled. The first step in management includes the restoration of blood volume with fluid, blood, and specific blood products. An initial examination should be attempted especially if bleeding from the vagina is noted. With the patient in a lithotomy position, clots are removed and the vaginal cuff is examined closely. If a bleeding vessel is identified at or near the cuff, one or more superficial sutures may suffice. If a vaginal examination fails to reveal the bleeding site, then a nonsurgical option of angiographic arterial embolization should be attempted.

ANGIOGRAPHIC ARTERIAL EMBOLIZATION

Selective angiographic arterial embolization is a useful alternative to bilateral hypogastric artery ligation in the control of pelvic hemorrhage that has failed other modes of therapy.[3-6] Historically angiography was attempted as a last resort in patients who were considered poor surgical risk, but now with increasing experience and success, some authors recommend that the technique be considered prior to surgical intervention.[6] It should be remembered, however, that embolization requires 1 to 2 hours, so in severe hypotensive shock it is not an appropriate option.

The advantages of angiographic embolization are that bleeding points that are impossible to find at surgery may be easily identified by angiography and working with friable tissues can lead to complications such as ureter and bladder injury, which may be avoided with embolization.[6] Previous hypogastric artery ligation makes embolization more difficult. Conversely, the surgical option is still open for failures of embolization without having compromised the patient. Thus angiographic embolization should be considered before hypogastric artery ligation.[7]

The branches of the anterior division of the internal iliac arteries usually are the cause of posthysterectomy bleeding. These vessels can be evaluated by angiography, and when contrast extravasation is present, embolization can be expected to control the hemorrhage.[8]

The procedure involves the following steps:

1. Taking a baseline aortogram to outline the hypogastric arteries bilaterally, and identifying the bleeding branch
2. Advancing the catheter tip distally to the bleeding site to maximize hemostasis and minimize ischemia to other surrounding tissues
3. Embolizing with the material
4. Taking a postembolization film to make certain there is obstruction of the vessel
5. Withdrawing the catheter and inserting it into the contralateral hypogastric artery to ensure that one of the branches is not bleeding or supplying a bleeding collateral vessel
6. Taking a postembolization aortogram to demonstrate no further extravasation[5] (Figures 19.2 and 19.3)

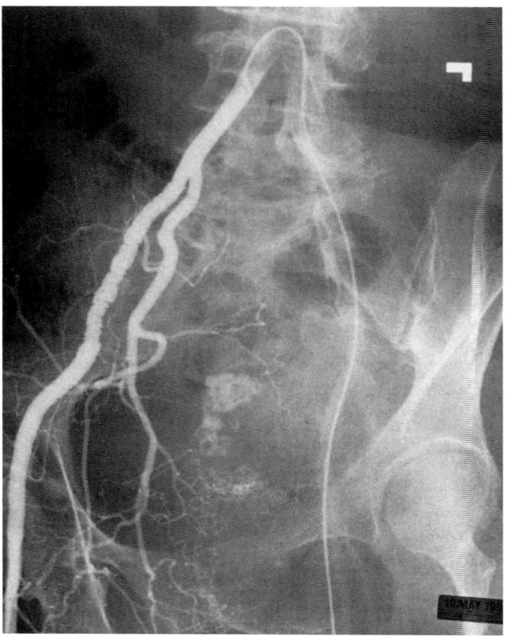

FIGURE 19.2 Angiography revealing the outline of the hypogastric artery.

Many agents are available for arterial embolization. The agent used is determined by the size of the vessel to be embolized, the desired duration of occlusion, the rate of blood flow through the vessel, and whether or not the vessel tapers or branches.[8] The four most common particles used clinically include autologous clot, Gelfoam, polyvinyl alcohol, and Avitene.[9] Gelfoam, an absorbable gelatin sponge, is the most widely used and acts as a matrix for the formation of thrombus. It is used to occlude small tapering vessels for short-term occlusion (10 to 30 days). Larger nontapering vessels are occluded with a de-

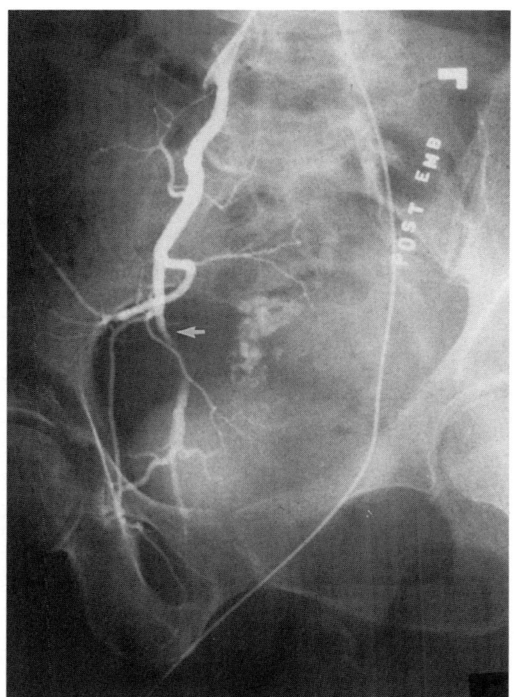

Figure 19.3 Angiography. Postembolization film to demonstrate no further extravasation.

tachable balloon or Gianturco coil. A large number of Dacron fibers are attached to the metal coil to promote thrombosis.

Some uncommon complications of the procedure are related to the puncture site and include arterial thrombosis, arterial venous fistulas, local infection, and pseudoaneurysm formation. Ischemic complications such as fever, pain, and tissue necrosis should be considered in patients who are compromised within their vascular system such as those with atherosclerosis, extensive radical surgery, or previous radiation therapy.[10] Necrosis of the bladder and rectum as well as sciatic nerve injury have been reported.[20]

Selective angiographic arterial embolization provides a safe and effective means of controlling hemorrhage. If, however, the patient is not stable hemodynamically or if the procedure is not immediately available to the patient, reoperation is the next obvious step. Once the decision to explore the patient is made, a midline incision of sufficient size should be made to facilitate adequate exploration of all pelvic and abdominal structures. After all clots are evacuated, exploration of the abdomen along with careful localization of all previous pedicle sites will usually suffice and allow for religature. The cyclic spurting of blood from arteries facilitates their location and allows for precise clamping compared with a diffuse venous ooze, which does not allow for clamping. Regardless of the severity of bleeding, blind haphazard clamping and suturing of tissues is to be condemned. Direct compression with a finger or pack and releasing the compression slowly will aid in accurate clamp and suture placement. These conventional steps will resolve most cases of postoperative bleeding. If the bleeding, however, is diffuse or the bleeding vessels are located deep in the pelvis where they either cannot be located or, if located, are not amenable to suturing, direct pressure with a pack and a hypogastric artery ligation should be performed.

Hypogastric Artery Ligation

Once the surgeon exhausts the conventional means of controlling postoperative hemorrhage without success, the ultimate resolution of bleeding may be accomplished by ligating the internal iliac (hypogastric) artery.[11] Bilateral ligation of these arteries is an integral part of the management of massive obstetric and gynecologic hemorrhage, and all surgeons should be familiar with its technique. The procedure, while decreasing the mean uterine artery pressure and blood flow by only 24% and 48%, respectively, produces its most significant physiologic effect by reducing the arterial pulse pressure by 85%.[12] Hypogastric artery ligation does not control hemorrhage from branches of the ovarian artery, which if bleeding must be ligated separately, or from generalized venous oozing.

Hypogastric arteries may be exposed either extraperitoneally or intraperitoneally, the latter being the preferred approach if there is extensive intraperitoneal bleeding. The common iliac artery and its two main branches are easily palpable and visualized along the pelvic sidewall. Care should be taken to retract the ureter and its peritoneum medially during the procedure. An attempt should be made to ligate the hypogastric artery distal to its posterior division, but many times it is easier to tie the hypogastric near its origin from the common iliac artery. The origin of the division is not always obvious but generally occurs within the first 2 to 3 cm from the iliac bifurcation. Once the site for ligation is determined, the loose areolar tissue and adventitia are dissected from the artery. In an effort to avoid injury to the hypogastric vein, a Babcock's clamp is used to elevate the artery. A right angle or Mixter's clamp is passed beneath the artery, hugging its surface (lateral to medial clamp may add additional protection to the underlying vein) A no. 2 synthetic polyglycolic suture is passed to the tip of the right angle clamp and drawn up for tying (Figure 19.4). The vessel should be doubly ligated, but transection is never recommended (Figures 19.5 and 19.6). Technical problems associated with hypogastric artery ligation include ligating the external iliac ar-

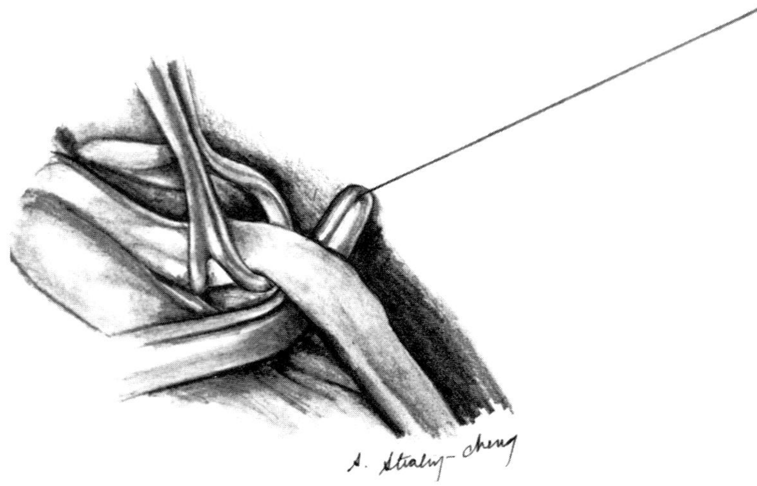

FIGURE 19.4 Right hypogastric artery ligation. Hypogastric artery held by a Babcock's clamp and a suture placed on tip of Mixter's clamp, ready to be passed under the artery.

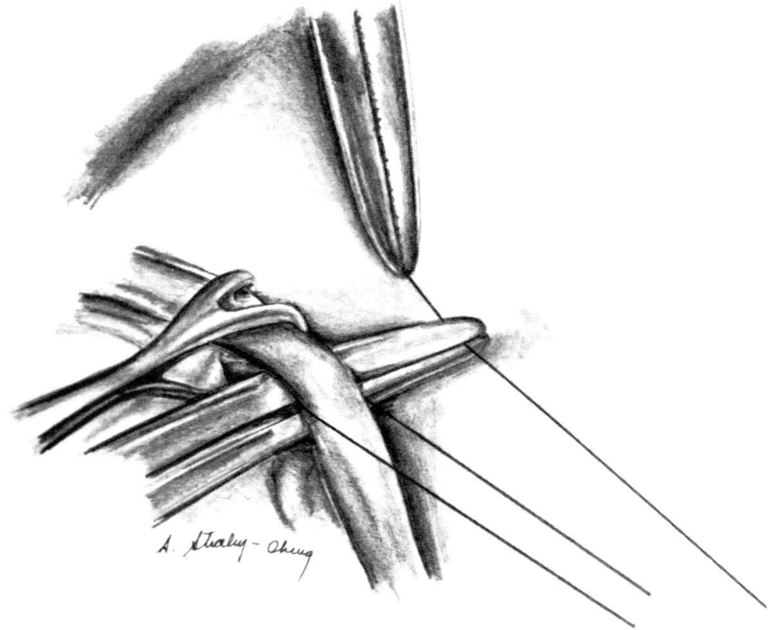

FIGURE 19.5 Hypogastric artery ligation. Mixter's clamp is repositioned below hypogastric artery and suture on tonsil clamp is brought down and grasped by Mixter's clamp for second pass below hypogastric artery.

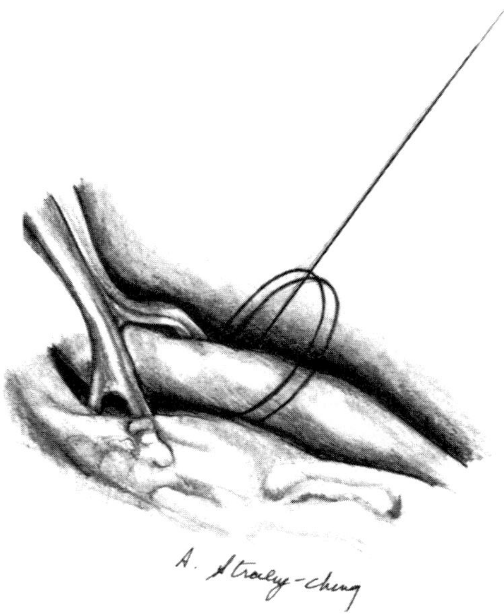

Figure 19.6 Hypogastric artery ligation. The doubly passed suture is ready to be tied.

Table 19.1 Hypogastric artery ligation indications

Procedure	No. of patients
Radical gynecologic surgery	
Therapeutic	5
Prophylactic	35
Teaching	358
Total abdominal hysterectomy	7
Uterine rupture	6
Vaginal hysterectomy	4
Hot knife conization of the cervix	4
Cold knife conization of the cervix	3
Cryosurgery of the cervix	3
Placenta accreta	3
Uterine atony	3
Anterior colporrhaphy	1
Total	432

Data from Saint Barnabas Medical Center, Livingston, NJ, 1969-1989.

tery or the ureter and lacerating the hypogastric vein. The operator should palpate the femoral pulses, identify the ureter both before and after the ligation, and use extreme care around the hypogastric vein. The most common error associated with this procedure, however, is waiting too long to perform it.

The success rate of hypogastric artery ligation in postoperative hemorrhage is difficult to assess. Approximately one half of the patients with hemorrhage will respond successfully.[13] Table 19.1 lists the indications for hypogastric ligation at the Saint Barnabas Medical Center over a 20-year period. Note that the leading indication was for teaching. It is better to learn under a controlled situation rather than when truly indicated. Should this procedure fail, the following techniques may prove useful.

Pelvic Packs

The surgeon is occasionally faced with controlling hemorrhage from large raw surfaces, venous plexuses, or inaccessible areas within the pelvis, often with the added problem of a coagulopathy. In these situations, the surgeon may employ a pack to produce a pelvic tamponade. The variably known umbrella or mushroom pack was described by Logothetopulos in 1926 to control bleeding, primarily after radical surgical procedures.[14-16] He demonstrated its effectiveness by placing the pelvic pack to control bleeding in a patient who had a hysterectomy without vessel ligation! The pack consists of a square, fine-mesh gauze laparotomy pad of cotton or nylon 24 inches to a side. Fifteen to 20 yards of 2-inch gauze tape or 6 yards of 4-inch head-roll gauze are layered into the center of the pack, taking care to prevent tangling, which may prevent removal. A funnel-shaped sling is then formed when the four corners of the pad are brought together, with a short tail of the gauze left free and tagged with a suture. The diagonal corners of the pack are brought over the pack and tied (Figure 19.7). This bolus of gauze is then placed in the true pelvis with the tail exiting the vagina (Figure 19.8). If bleeding points are observed near the pelvic brim, additional gauze may be necessary. This pack also may be applied through the vagina and formed inside the pelvis. Here the pad is held in front of the vulva by the corners, and the center is pushed through the vagina into the pelvis by inserting gauze with a ring forceps. The four corners are brought together and pulled down to seat the pack.[14] Approximately 2 to 5 kg of traction weight are applied to the tails of the pack for 48 to 72 hours, with the tension released every 8 hours to prevent pressure necrosis of pelvic tissues. Passing the tails through a no. 80 doughnut pessary and cross-clamping the tails with a Kelly's clamp after applying sufficient

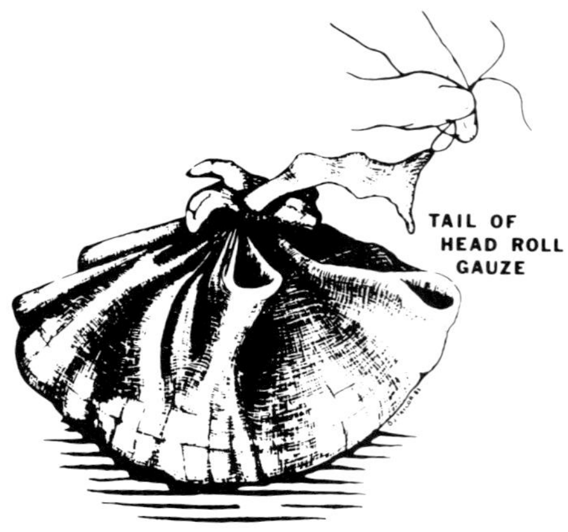

FIGURE 19.7 Umbrella pack ready for pelvic tamponade. Diagonal corners of the laparotomy pad are brought together and secured after carefully filling with layered gauze. The tagging suture should be placed through the cuff into the vagina. (From Cassels JW, Greenberg H, and Otterson WN: J Reprod Med 30:689, 1985.)

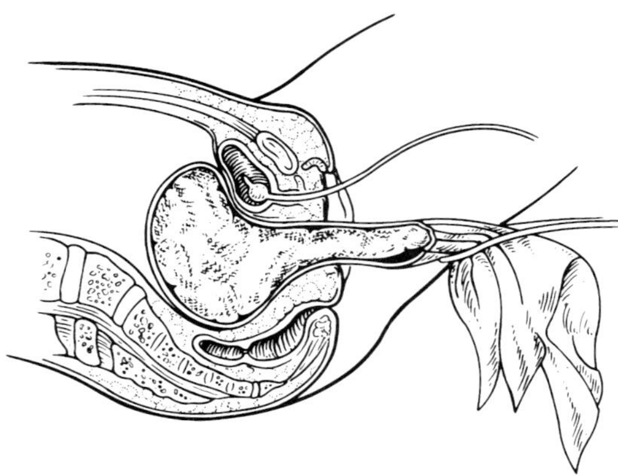

FIGURE 19.8 Umbrella pack used to tamponade the pelvis with the tail exiting the vagina.

traction to seat the pack are satisfactory. A Foley catheter is placed in the bladder so that the bulb is above the pack (Figure 19.9). Decreased urine output after restoring circulating volume may indicate excessive traction. Broad-spectrum antibiotics are advisable during its use. Regardless of the technique of insertion, the pack is removed vaginally. Before its removal, the ends are soaked in saline and hydrogen peroxide. The pack may be removed under analgesia on the following day.

More conventional packing, however, may be appropriate. In a patient with broad surface bleeding or bleeding in areas inaccessible to conventional suturing or clamping, transabdominal placement of 2-inch packs in the pelvis is highly effective.[11] The technique is to take a 2-inch pack, and moving it from right to left to center, place it over the entire pelvis, bringing it out through a stab wound in the groin. The inferior pack should be placed at the most dependent portion of the pelvis. When bleeding is extensive, it is usually necessary to use five or six 2-inch packs. The second pack is placed over the first and brought out through a separate stab wound. Never tie two packs together because they have to be removed through the incisions in the groin. If six packs are used, there will be six exit sites within the groin.[13] It is important to tag each pack with either a safety pin or a suture, so that the surgeon knows which pack is on the bottom and which is on the top. This is important because it is embarrassing for the surgeon to start removing what is thought to be the top pack the day after surgery and find that the bottom packs are being pulled on instead. The topmost packs should be removed within the first 24 hours and the bottom packs removed 72 hours after surgery. It is important to cover the patient with broad-spectrum antibiotics during this period.

MILITARY ANTISHOCK TROUSERS

Military antishock trousers (MAST) can be a life-saving measure in the management of hemorrhage when traditional therapies have failed or when the patient must be stabilized before surgery. Situations in which the MAST have been utilized successfully include rupture of the liver in pregnancy, ruptured ectopic pregnancy, postcesarean hysterectomy, disseminated intravascular coagulation, intractable intraoperative bleeding, and bleeding following radical pelvic surgery.[17]

The MAST suit consists of a pair of trousers with three inflatable balloons resembling a large blood pressure cuff created into a pair of pants. It consists of three components—two legs and an abdominal part—each of which can be inflated separately. The suit is inflated through a foot pump and has pressure gauges set at 104 mm Hg (Figure 19.10).[18]

Patients placed in MAST suits respond with

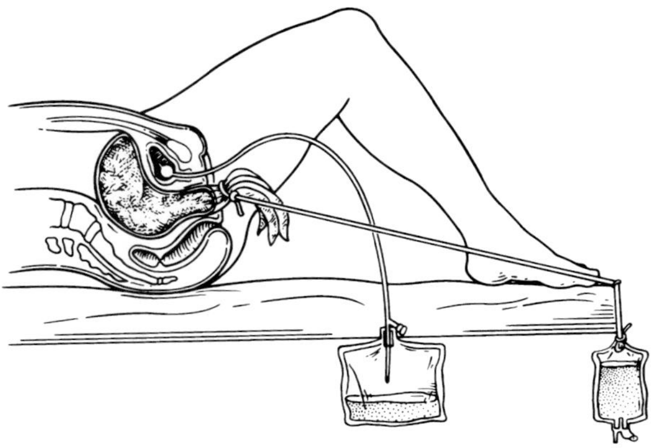

Figure 19.9 Umbrella pack in pelvis with the traction weight applied to the tails of the pack and the Foley catheter inserted in the bladder.

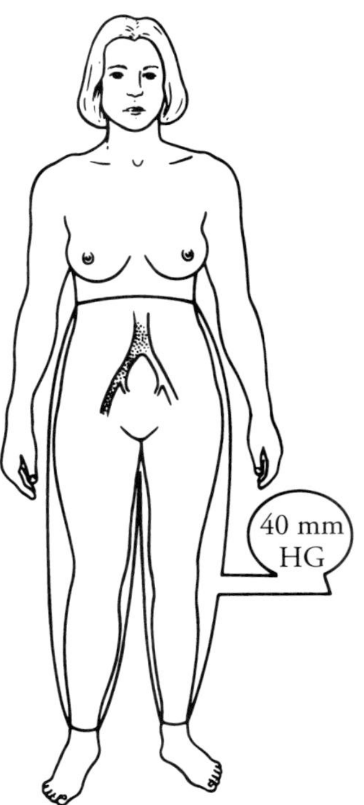

Figure 19.10 MAST suit.

an elevation in blood pressure by increasing total peripheral resistance rather than by augmenting cardiac output via autotransfusion. So the MAST inflation, which sacrifices perfusion in the lower half of the body, will increase flow to vital organs such as the heart, lungs, brain, and kidneys in the upper part of the body. In addition, it decreases the blood loss by increasing the intraabdominal pressure and thus decreasing the diameter of the venous and arterial vessels.[15] Patients with secondary coagulopathies in which surgical intervention has failed to control bleeding are prime candidates for the use of MAST because this provides time to correct coagulation-related bleeding disorders.

Once the decision to apply the MAST suit has been made, it is applied so that it extends from the ankles to the lower border of the lateral rib cage. It then is inflated from the legs to the abdominal compartment with an initial pressure of 30 to 40 mm Hg while blood pressure is monitored.[18] Twelve to 24 hours after the bleeding has stopped, the suit is removed by deflating the abdominal compartment first, followed by the legs, in 5 mm Hg increments. As pressure is released from the garment, the rate of IV fluid administration should be increased to maintain the systolic blood pressure at 100 mm Hg. If a drop of greater than 10 mm Hg of systolic blood pressure occurs, deflation should be suspended. The MAST should be reinflated if the blood pressure cannot be restored with IV fluids[19] (Table 19.2).

Presacral Bleeding

In performing procedures such as the presacral neurectomy and abdominal sacral colpopexy, the gynecologic surgeon should be aware of the life-threatening problem of hemorrhage from the presacral vessels. Hemostasis is usually difficult to obtain in this anatomic area because of the venous network not only on the

Table 19.2 Current recommendations for use of the medical g-suit in controlling intra-abdominal hemorrhage

Close wound snugly
Insert indwelling urinary catheter
Apply garment
Inflate to 20 to 25 mm Hg, legs first, then abdomen
Maintain pressure for 12 to 36 hours
During this interval:
- Correct hypovolemia (if replacement of large volumes is necessary, insert central venous pressure line or Swan-Ganz catheter)
- Replenish coagulation factors
- Maintain normal respiratory exchange and acid-base balance (if mechanical ventilation is necessary, insert endotracheal tube and arterial catheter)
- DO NOT DEFLATE GARMENT, EVEN MOMENTARILY

After this interval:
- Deflate garment slowly over 15 to 30 minutes, legs first (if systolic pressure falls more than 10 mm Hg, reinflate and correct hypovolemia before repeating)

From Sandberg EC and Pelligra R: Am J Obstet Gynecol 146:519, 1983.

surface but also below the sacral periosteum. When there has been injury to the veins, they retract beneath the surface, making hemostasis with sutures, metallic clips, cautery, bone wax, Gelfoam, or hypogastric vessel ligation difficult.[20] Packing is useful when it is in place, but once the pack is removed, there is oftentimes rapid accumulation of blood.

Reports that have been published in the general surgical literature on the use of thumbtacks for presacral bleeding have led to their use in gynecologic surgery (Figure 19.11).[21] It is important that stainless steel thumbtacks be used because they will not corrode. Pressure should be placed on the bleeding points, and beginning at the superior aspect, each vessel should be occluded with a thumbtack. No known complications have been reported, but there have not been large series. One important aspect is that the patient should be informed so that there will be no future confusion with abdominal films.

Another reported method of controlling presacral hemorrhage describes using electrocautery through a muscle fragment pressed on the bleeding vein.[22] The authors utilize a piece of muscle about 1.5 to 2.0 cm in length from the rectus abdominis. While holding the muscle in a long forceps, they guide it into the presacral space and apply it to the bleeding location. Then high-frequency electrical current is delivered to the muscle fragment by touching the hemostatic forcep. After hemostasis is obtained, the forceps is withdrawn.

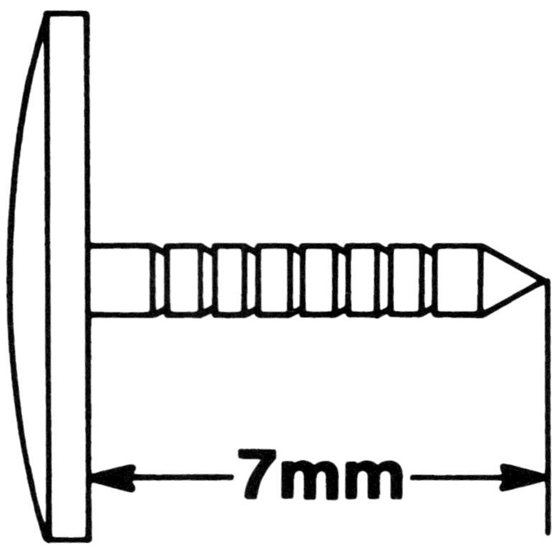

Figure 19.11 Stainless steel thumbtacks used in presacral bleeding.

Summary

Every gynecologic surgical procedure, regardless of how well planned and skillfully executed, is characterized by a certain irreducible loss of blood that is commensurate with the magnitude of the operation, the vascularity of the surgical field, and the capabilities of the surgeon. In most operations, blood loss may be kept to an acceptable minimum by applying the basic principles of hemostasis. Even a moderate amount of uncontrolled bleeding, involving in some situations up to 30% of the circulating blood volume, may not seriously alter circulatory dynamics. However, uncontrolled unanticipated excessive blood loss may be catastrophic.

Hemorrhage during or after surgery is usually not anticipated, but few gynecologists have not had a routine procedure abruptly transformed into a life-threatening drama. Under these circumstances, the attitude of the surgeon may be the deciding factor in the outcome of the situation. Though a degree of alarm is a normal reaction, the surgeon must keep a clear head, even in the presence of massive hemorrhage. One important factor is the surgeon's realistic appraisal of his or her personal limitations; it is a wise individual who accepts these limitations and seeks assistance.

References

1. Fehrman H: Surgical management of life-threatening obstetric and gynecologic hemorrhage, Acta Obstet Gynecol Scand 67:125, 1988.
2. Smith RD and Pratt JH: Serious bleeding following vaginal or abdominal hysterectomy, Obstet Gynecol 26:592, 1965.
3. Yamashita Y and others: Transcatheter arterial embolization in the management of postpartum hemorrhage due to genital tract injury, Obstet Gynecol 77:160, 1991.
4. Kivikoski AI and others: Angiographic arterial embolization to control hemorrhage in abdominal pregnancy: a case report, Obstet Gynecol 71:456, 1988.
5. Rosenthal DM and Colapinto R: Angiographic arterial embolization in the management of postoperative vaginal hemorrhage, Am J Obstet Gynecol 151:227, 1985.
6. Brown BJ and others: Uncontrollable postpartum bleeding: a new approach to hemostasis through angiographic arterial embolization, Obstet Gynecol 54:361, 1979.
7. Gilbert WM and others: Angiographic embolization in the management of hemorrhagic complications of pregnancy, Am J Obstet Gynecol 166:493, 1992.
8. Marx MV, Picus D, and Weyman PJ: Percutaneous embolization of the ovarian artery in the treatment of pelvic hemorrhage, Am J Radiol 150:1337, 1988.
9. Harrington DP: Particulate embolization materials. In Abrams: Angiography: vascular and interventional radiology, ed 3, Boston, 1983, Little, Brown & Co, Inc.
10. Behnam K and Jarmolowski CR: Vesicovaginal fistulas following hypogastric embolization for control of intractable pelvic hemorrhage, J Repro Med 27:304, 1983.
11. Breen JL, Kindzierski J, and Gregori C: Surgical hemorrhage and infection. In Current therapy in surgical gynecology, Philadelphia, 1987, BC Decker.
12. Burchell RC: Physiology of the internal iliac artery ligation, J Obstet Gynaecol Br Commonw 75:642, 1968.
13. Clark SL and others: Hypogastric artery ligation for obstetrical hemorrhage, Obstet Gynecol 66:353, 1985.
14. Cassels JW, Greenberg H, and Otterson WN: Pelvic tamponade in puerperal hemorrhage, J Reprod Med 30:689, 1985.
15. Guerre EF and others: Uncontrollable intra-abdominal hemorrhage treated with packing and use of a MAST suit, J Reprod Med 32:230, 1987.
16. Logothetopulos K: Eine absolut sichere Blutstillungs Methode bie vaginalen und abdominalen gynakologischen Operationen, Zentralbl Gynakol 50:3202, 1926.
17. Hall M and Marshall JR: The gravity suit: a major advance in management of gynecologic blood loss, Obstet Gynecol 53:247, 1979.
18. Kaback KR, Sanders AB, and Meislin HW: MAST suit update, JAMA 252:2598, 1984.
19. Slye DA: The physiologic response to the use of a pneumatic antishock garment (PASG) in the care of the patient experiencing shock, Orthopedic Nursing 9:43, 1990.
20. Qinyao W and Weijin Shu: New concepts in severe presacral hemorrhage during proctectomy, Arch Surg 120:1013, 1985.
21. Patsner B and Orr JW: Intractable venous sacral hemorrhage: use of stainless steel thumbtacks to obtain hemostasis, Am J Obstet Gynecol 162:452, 1990.
22. Xu J and Lin J: Control of presacral hemorrhage with electrocautery through a muscle fragment pressed on the bleeding vein, J Am Coll Surgeons 179:351, 1994.

20

Postoperative Infection

DAVID L. HEMSELL

CLASSIFICATION OF SURGICAL PROCEDURES

Surgical procedures and the likelihood of postoperative infection have been classified with regard to contamination by operative site flora and preservation of appropriate operative technique. There are four separate categories of surgical procedures, each associated with a range of postoperative infection.

Clean

Clean operative procedures are those performed for nontraumatic indications, and inflammation is not encountered. Surgical technique is maintained, and the respiratory, alimentary, and genitourinary tracts are not entered. Infection without antimicrobial prophylaxis ranges from 1% to 5%, and perioperative antimicrobial administration does not decrease the incidence of infection. Many laparoscopic and adnexal surgical procedures qualify for this category.

Clean Contaminated

The majority of gynecologic surgical procedures are classified as clean-contaminated cases since the vagina is entered or operated through in the absence of obvious clinical infection. Minor break in surgical technique is allowed without changing the category. The observed infection rate is between 5% and 15% for patients whose procedures are in this category. Antimicrobial prophylaxis is indicated for high-risk procedures and/or populations only; not all require prophylaxis, and risk identification is mandatory. For example, D & C and cervical conization are rarely followed by infection; antimicrobial prophylaxis is usually contraindicated. The opposite is true for vaginal hysterectomy. Abdominal hysterectomy, however, may fall into either a high-risk or a low-risk category in different hospitals, or in different patient populations in the same hospital, so individual determination is mandatory.

Risk factors potentially increasing the pelvic infection rate following hysterectomy are presented in Table 20.1. Immune system deficiencies are uniformly associated with an increased incidence of postoperative infection, irrespective of surgical classification. This deficiency may be the result of chemotherapy for malignancy, glucocorticosteroid therapy, or immunotherapy for transplant patients and may be a significant underlying factor contributing to a higher infection rate in socioeconomically deprived indigent populations.

Contaminated

Contaminated procedures are those in which there is a major break in surgical technique or gross spillage from the GI tract. Genitourinary or biliary tract entry in the presence of infected urine or bile results in placement in this category, but no mention was made in the original classification description regarding surgery in the acutely infected upper reproductive tract.[1] For example, laparoscopy or laparotomy for acute salpingitis should be included in this category. Infection rates in this category range between 10% and 25%, at least perioperative antibiotic administration is required, and delayed wound closure may be appropriate.

Dirty

Delayed wound closure also may be appropriate when procedures qualify for the classification of dirty or infected procedures. Such procedures are followed by infection 30% to

Table 20.1 Potential risk factors increasing pelvic infection after hysterectomy

Lower socioeconomic status
Patient age
Older age—abdominal hysterectomy
Younger age—vaginal hysterectomy
Patient weight
Obesity—abdominal hysterectomy
Emaciated—vaginal or abdominal hysterectomy
Diabetes
Excessive blood loss
Prolonged surgical procedure
Menstrual cycle phase—variable
Operator experience—rarely
Recent pelvic surgery
Catheter placement
Concomitant surgical procedure(s)
Preoperative anemia
Postoperative anemia

100% of the time; antimicrobial administration is therapeutic and not prophylactic, as is the case with contaminated procedures.

Classification of Postoperative Infections

Deep Incisional Surgical Site Infections

According to recent Centers for Disease Control and Prevention (CDC) wound infection definitions,[2] pelvic infections fall into the categories of deep incisional or organ/space surgical site infections (SSIs). Deep SSIs, by definition, occur within 30 days after an operative procedure when no foreign body (prosthetic heart valve, prosthetic joint, etc.) is permanently implanted. There must be at least one of the following: (1) purulent drainage from deep incision not from the organ or space component of the surgical site; or (2) a deep incision that spontaneously dehisces or is opened deliberately by a surgeon when a patient has at least one of the following signs or symptoms: temperature 38° C, localized pain or tenderness unless the incision is culture-negative, an abscess or other evidence of infection found at reoperation or by a histopathologic or radiologic examination, or a diagnosis of deep SSI by the surgeon or attending physician.

Organ/Space Surgical Site Infections

Organ/space SSIs develop in spaces or organs other than that opened by the original incision or manipulated during the operative procedure. Specific sites, which must be used to differentiate spaces, are listed in the original publication.[2] An example might be hysterectomy with subsequent pelvic infection and intraabdominal abscess. Specific pelvic sites of organ/space SSI listed include the following: vaginal cuff; endometrium; urinary tract; other (male or) female reproductive tract; and intraabdominal, not specified elsewhere. These infections also must occur with 30 days of the operative procedure if there are no implants, and at least one of the following must be present: purulent drainage from a drain placed through a stab wound into the organ/space; isolated organisms from an aseptically obtained culture of fluid or tissue in that organ/space; an abscess or other evidence of infection involving the organ/space found on direct examination during reoperation or by histopathologic or radiologic examination; or a diagnosis of an organ/space SSI by a surgeon or attending physician.

SSIs are classified by the CDC[2] as superficial or deep. The superficial infection must be diagnosed within 30 days of the operative procedure and must involve only the superficial tissues. Requirements for the diagnosis include the following: purulent drainage or organisms isolated from an aseptically obtained culture of tissue or fluid with at least one of the following signs or symptoms: tenderness or pain; heat or redness; localized swelling; requirement for deliberate opening of the superficial incision by a surgeon, unless the incision is culture-negative; or diagnosis of superficial infection by the surgeon or attending physician. Several infections not to be included in this category include stitch abscess, episiotomy infection, infected burns, or extension to deep layers. Deep infection has been defined previously.

Risk Factors

Operative site infections continue to account for about 40% of hospital-acquired infections, and they account for almost one fourth of adverse events leading to litigation in California.

Morbidity and monetary impact are significant. In our indigent patient population undergoing hysterectomy, pelvic operative site infection at least doubles the hospital stay and hospital bill; infection (and superficial dehiscence without infection) in the abdominal wall may triple those variables. Infection rates have been decreasing during the last several decades.

Emphasis on preoperative normalization of vaginal flora, decreased preoperative stay, improving surgical techniques, appropriate utilization of perioperative antimicrobial therapy, improved suture material, enhanced anesthesia techniques, early ambulation, and early return to the home environment, all contribute to the reduction in postoperative infection. The importance of surgical technique and its contribution to infection prevention were stressed by Richardson and others,[3] who reported a decrease in operative site infection after abdominal hysterectomy from 22% to 2.4% by technique alteration only. Gentle handling of tissue, small pedicles, and accurate hemostasis are imperative. Active rather than passive drainage is associated with a lower infection rate in those situations when drainage is indicated. Improved patient nutrition has undoubtedly contributed to diminished infection in indigent populations.

FEBRILE MORBIDITY

The incidence of asymptomatic temperature elevation, or febrile morbidity, after hysterectomy differs by surgical approach in our patients. It has been observed in up to 40% of women after abdominal hysterectomy and in as high as 27% of women after vaginal hysterectomy. This recurrent oral temperature elevation to 38° C or above occurs a mean of about 50 hours after either surgical approach. A retrospective review of the charts of women undergoing abdominal and vaginal hysterectomy revealed that in the early and mid-1970s, most women with this phenomenon were treated with parenteral antimicrobials, frequently without a diagnosis. Febrile morbidity is rarely observed after most other gynecologic procedures. Recurrent temperature elevation may certainly be one sign of infection, but it should not be the only one present prior to therapy for pelvic or abdominal incision infection. Operative site examination and an infection diagnosis are mandatory prior to antimicrobial therapy.

Origin

The exact origin of this early and asymptomatic temperature elevation is infrequently identified. Extremity phlebitis occurs rarely following elective gynecologic surgical procedures because IV lines are removed early. IV sites always should be investigated when the source of postoperative temperature elevation is sought. Microatelectasis is certainly a contributor; an x-ray film of the chest is usually normal even in the presence of decreased basilar breath sounds and crackles at auscultation, however. In the absence of pyelonephritis, the urinary tract is not a contributor to temperature elevation in our patients, including those with an indwelling transurethral catheter after surgical repair for SUI.

Evaluation

Thus a chest x-ray examination, urinalysis, and urine culture are not cost-effective or beneficial in the identification of the source of asymptomatic postoperative pyrexia in our patients. Leukocytosis is the rule after surgery, so a complete blood count (CBC) with differential does not usually guide us to the source. A thorough history and a careful physical examination are the appropriate evaluators for asymptomatic and symptomatic temperature elevation that occurs during the immediate or late postoperative period. The upper respiratory tract and middle ears also must be evaluated but are rarely the cause with the possible exception of viral upper respiratory tract infection (URI). A pelvic examination is infrequently necessary if gentle, deep palpation of the lower abdomen over the surgical site is "normal," with "expected tenderness." Administration of perioperative antimicrobial to prevent operative site infection after vaginal and abdominal hysterectomy did not alter the incidence of asymptomatic temperature elevation when compared to placebo in our patients.

Infection

Vaginal Cuff Cellulitis

The most common postoperative infection is a cellulitis in pelvic soft tissues. It is observed almost exclusively after hysterectomy. It is my belief that all women develop cellulitis at the vaginal surgical margin after hysterectomy. It is characterized by small vessel engorgement resulting in erythema and heat, stasis, and endothelial leakage with interstitial edema, which cause induration, and an inflammatory polymorphonuclear infiltrate. It is truly a vaginal cuff cellulitis, and it is more of a histologic diagnosis than a clinically important diagnosis, at least in our indigent patient population. Antimicrobial therapy is infrequently required for this diagnosis during the immediate postoperative period.

Women who require therapy for this diagnosis come to the clinic before their appointed follow-up visit complaining of central lower abdominal, pelvic, and/or lower back pain and foul-smelling vaginal discharge following discharge from the hospital after an uneventful postoperative course. There are purulent secretions in the vagina. At bimanual examination an indurated, erythematous, vaginal margin is identified, and it is more tender than anticipated. A temperature elevation also may be present. These findings are "the rule" during the immediate postoperative period, but at that time patients are not symptomatic. After discharge from the hospital, these are abnormal findings and will not disappear without antimicrobial therapy. Readmission to the hospital is unnecessary in most instances, and oral antimicrobial therapy as an outpatient is effective. The broadest spectrum of bactericidal coverage is afforded by amoxicillin and clavulanic acid (Augmentin). If the only complaint is vaginal discharge, and the only finding is purulent vaginal secretions, local therapy such as a povidone-iodine or vinegar douche usually results in resolution without requiring antimicrobial administration.

Pelvic Cellulitis

If host cellular and humoral-mediated defense mechanisms are unable to control the normal inflammatory process at the vaginal surgical margin, the process extends into the parametrial regions. This infection usually develops during the immediate postoperative period and prior to discharge from the hospital. It does not usually affect both parametria equally, but rather it is predominantly a unilateral phenomenon. Symptoms of increasing unilateral lower abdominal and/or pelvic pain with or without back pain precede or accompany recurrent temperature elevations and appear a mean of about 80 hours after hysterectomy in our patients, irrespective of surgical approach. There is lower abdominal tenderness over the affected area, and at bimanual examination the affected parametrial area is thickened and tender, but no mass is usually present. Peritonitis or ileus are usually absent, but anorexia is common.

Adnexitis

If adnexa are retained at hysterectomy, adnexitis may also develop; presentation is very similar to that of pelvic cellulitis. There is a difference in findings at pelvic examination: tenderness is absent in the lateral parametrial areas but rather is cephalad thereto, or central and above the vaginal cuff. This infection also is predominantly unilateral and may be associated with a palpable mass. Suturing adnexa to the areas adjacent to the vaginal cuff may increase the potential for subsequent infection. Postoperative pain secondary to adnexal attachment to the vaginal cuff area can be avoided by not extraperitonealizing the round ligament and utero-ovarian ligament.

The principal reason given for extraperitonealizing those pedicles is for identification and accessibility should bleeding occur postoperatively. In my experience, bleeding has been intraperitoneal even when these pedicles were extraperitonealized. For those two reasons, I do not extraperitonealize the round or utero-ovarian ligament. Some gynecologic surgeons extraperitonealize those ligaments at vaginal hysterectomy, but not at abdominal hysterectomy; if such were advantageous, the procedure should be performed irrespective of surgical approach. Adnexal infection may uncommonly develop after tubal ligation, surgical therapy for an ectopic pregnancy, or other adnexal surgery.

There is a collection of from 40 to 200 cc of serum, lymph, and/or blood between the vaginal margins and the pelvic peritoneum following hysterectomy. This is an excellent medium for the growth of bacteria inoculated during surgery. Before we began to evaluate antimicrobial prophylaxis in our patient population, the open cuff technique was associated with a significantly lower pelvic infection rate than was observed if the vagina was sutured closed. Evaluation of cuff management after the initiation of antimicrobial prophylaxis at hysterectomy revealed no difference in infection rates. Active drainage of that space to reduce the postoperative infection rate has been evaluated by several investigators. For some investigators, drainage was as effective at preventing postoperative infection as was perioperative antimicrobial therapy. For others, it was either ineffective in preventing postoperative pelvic infection or associated with an increased infection rate. These conflicting results underscore the importance of individual determination of factors contributing to postoperative pelvic infection, and the most efficient means of preventing that infection.

Obviously if we could avoid the perioperative administration of antibiotic and have low infection rates by utilization of mechanical measures, then potential complications of prophylaxis such as an allergic reaction (including anaphylaxis), superinfection, induction of antimicrobial resistance, and flora alteration at the operative site and other sites would be avoided. Compared with no prophylaxis, administration of a single dose of antimicrobial at hysterectomy does not adversely affect the postoperative lower reproductive tract flora or resistance patterns in those bacteria when prospectively evaluated. Multiple doses over even as short a period as 8 hours does alter the flora qualitatively and is associated with an increase in species that are resistant to the prophylactic regimen.

A single dose of cefazolin was the recommended prophylactic regimen for hysterectomy in a recent review.[4] We prospectively evaluated a 1 g parenteral dose of cefazolin in 539 women undergoing vaginal and abdominal hysterectomy. The overall postoperative infection rate was 7.6%. By historical comparison, that is significantly less than the rate of 45.1% observed with placebo, but greater than that observed (4.8%) in combined data from earlier prospective studies evaluating a single dose of an expanded-spectrum cephalosporin or penicillin. In a recent prospective, randomized blinded clinical trial involving 511 women, 1 g of cefotetan was followed by a significantly lower (relative risk 1.84; 95% confidence interval 1.03-3.29; $P < .05$) operative site infection rate after abdominal hysterectomy when compared with 1 g of cefazolin.[5] There were fewer abscesses ($P = .04$), and 234 fewer hospital days for women given cefotetan prophylaxis. A list of frequently used antibiotics approved by the FDA for single preoperative dosing at vaginal or abdominal hysterectomy is presented alphabetically in Table 20.2.

Pelvic Abscess

With antimicrobial prophylaxis, the development of pelvic abscess after gynecologic surgery is currently a rare infection. Before antimicrobial prophylaxis, the most common location for a pelvic abscess was in the space between the pelvic peritoneum and the vaginal

TABLE 20.2 FDA-approved single-dose antimicrobial regimens for prophylaxis at hysterectomy

GENERIC NAME	PRODUCT NAME	MANUFACTURER
Cefonicid	Monocid	SmithKline Beecham Pharmaceuticals
Ceforanide	Precef	ICN Pharmaceuticals
Cefotaxime	Claforan	Hoechst-Roussel Pharmaceuticals
Cefotetan	Cefotan	Zeneca Pharmaceuticals
Cefoxitin	Mefoxin	Merck & Co
Ceftriaxone	Rocephin	Roche Laboratories
Cefuroxime	Zinacef	Glaxo Pharmaceuticals

margin. The overall incidence of postoperative pelvic infection in retrospective studies was as high as 60%, and between 5% to 10% of women developed a cuff abscess. Mechanical drainage was established by opening the central portion of vaginal margins in the examination and/or treatment room. Abscess formation causes temperature elevation, and lower abdominal and pelvic pain, and it may cause back pain. It usually causes central rather than lateral pain, and a tender mass can be palpated above the vaginal apex at bimanual examination. These women may not appear more ill clinically than women with pelvic cellulitis. In fact, they may have less symptomatology early in the course.

An abscess can also develop in an adnexus following surgery. Classically, adnexal abscesses do not develop during the initial hospitalization but rather occur 1 to 2 weeks after discharge from the hospital. The immediate postoperative course in women who develop this life-threatening infection is usually uncomplicated, as is the postoperative period at home until the abscess, which is almost always ovarian, ruptures about 18 days after the surgical procedure. Patients deteriorate quickly and require immediate stabilization and surgery. It is assumed that the genesis of this infection following hysterectomy is ovulation adjacent to the normal inflammatory response in the pelvis. The corpus luteum becomes a perfect culture medium for the inoculated bacteria. To avoid the potential for an abscess, surgery should not be scheduled just prior to anticipated ovulation in the ovulatory female, and the adnexa should be as far away from the area of normal inflammatory response as possible. It is not just a break in ovarian integrity, because ovarian cystectomy at vaginal or abdominal hysterectomy is not a risk factor for infection.

Hematoma

An infected hematoma developing extraperitoneally above the vaginal cuff or in the lateral pelvis is an infection that has a relatively late onset during the hospital course or soon after discharge from the hospital. Initially it is not associated with symptoms or abnormal physical findings in the majority of patients. Temperature elevation in a patient who has no symptoms, who has a normal abdominal examination, and who wants to go home is the common presentation when manifestation occurs before discharge from the hospital. There is usually disparity between the patient's current hemoglobin concentration and what it should be, based on the preoperative hemoglobin concentration and the estimated blood loss during the surgical procedure.

Pelvic examination should be performed, but it may not result in detection of a hematoma because of its soft consistency. Ultrasonography will identify these structures, and it is more cost-effective than CT or MRI. Broad-spectrum antimicrobial therapy should be instituted, and drainage through the vagina should be performed if it can be done in a treatment room. If therapy is withheld, patients will eventually become symptomatic and physical evidence of infection will become clinically apparent. When the infection develops after discharge from the hospital, a tender mass is usually palpable in patients who have pain and are febrile.

Abdominal Incision

The diagnosis of abdominal incision infection is easier to make because of observational capability and the ability to more thoroughly evaluate the area. Erythema and tenderness at skin edges are usually associated with purulence in the incision, increasing pain, and temperature elevations that develop late on the third or fourth postoperative day, although the infection may not develop until after discharge from the hospital. Abdominal incision infection may develop in conjunction with pelvic infection, or it may be the only infection that develops. The incidence of abdominal incision infection is significantly lower than pelvic infection after hysterectomy, and it is rarely observed after other gynecologic procedures. Perioperative antimicrobial therapy does not appear to alter the already low incidence of abdominal incision infection. Rather, mechanical factors seem to be more important in preventing wound infection. Shaving the skin other than just prior to the procedure, occlusive drapes, excessive use of cautery, passive drains, and drains exiting through the incision have all been shown to be associated with an increased incidence of infection. Incision placement is also important; a transverse incision in the abdominal wall crease of a woman with a large panniculus will develop infection.

Drainage is the foundation of therapy for abdominal wall infections. Mechanical care with wet to dry dressing changes three times daily is usually sufficient, although parenteral antimicrobial therapy may be necessary. Fine-mesh gauze stimulates fibroblastic proliferation and granulation tissue development and should be carefully applied to wound margins. It can be held against the margins with gauze, which should be moistened with sterile saline after dressing change. Its use before the next debridement with hydrogen peroxide or povidone-iodine will make removing the fine-mesh gauze much less uncomfortable for the patient.

Hematoma or seroma formation in an abdominal incision may have the same impact on hospital stay because the incision separates. The tissue should be cultured as should the purulent material in an infected incision. One must be certain that infection is not present prior to reclosure of such wounds. Many times the entire incision is not involved by a seroma or hematoma as is the case when clinical infection occurs.

INFECTION SITE MICROBIOLOGY

The pelvic and abdominal incision infections that develop after hysterectomy are usually polymicrobial, as are the other occasional postoperative infections. Inoculation of the operative site occurs at vaginal transection. The fact that bacterial contamination occurs at the beginning of and throughout vaginal hysterectomy may explain why infection rates without prophylaxis are higher after that procedure. The contamination at abdominal hysterectomy occurs close to the end of the procedure, and the vaginal preparation agent has been in place until the vagina is entered. Contaminating bacteria are the normal flora of the lower reproductive tract; isolates recovered from pelvic and abdominal incision infection sites after hysterectomy in Parkland Memorial Hospital are presented in Table 20.3. Bacterial vaginosis flora has been identified as a risk factor for infection after hysterectomy. This condition should be treated preoperatively.

TABLE 20.3 Bacteria recovered from infection sites after gynecologic surgical procedures

Staphylococcus aureus
Staphylococcus epidermidis
Enterococcus faecalis
Group B streptococci
Escherichia coli
Enterobacter species
Klebsiella species
Proteus species
Pseudomonas species
Peptostreptococcus species
Prevotella bivius
Prevotella species
Bacteroides fragilis group
Fusobacterium species
Clostridium species

A mean of four bacterial species is recovered from a pelvic or abdominal postoperative infection site in our hospital, and 60% of the isolates are aerobic. Sixty-five percent of those bacteria are gram-positive, and *E. faecalis* accounts for almost one half of the species. *E. coli* is the predominant gram-negative aerobe (61%). *Proteus* and *Enterobacter* species account for about 17% each. *Peptostreptococcus* species comprise about one half of the anaerobic isolates, and *Prevotella* (previously *Bacteroides*) *bivius* is the predominant gram-negative anaerobe that is recovered. *B. fragilis* group isolates are recovered from less than 5% of patients with postoperative pelvic/abdominal incision infection. A mixture of aerobic and anaerobic bacteria is isolated from most infection sites; aerobes only or anaerobes only may be recovered, however.

INFECTION SITE THERAPY

A broad-spectrum therapeutic regimen is necessary to eradicate the majority of the important potential pathogens from operative site infections following gynecologic surgical procedures. Combination regimens are infrequently required for successful therapy of most postoperative infections that are not associated with abscess formation. Combination therapy has a greater likelihood of success when an

Table 20.4 Commonly used therapeutic regimens for operative site infections after gynecologic surgical procedures

Single-agent cephamycin/cephalosporin
Cefotetan
Cefoxitin
Cefotaxime
Ceftizoxime
Single-agent penicillin
Mezlocillin
Piperacillin
Ticarcillin
Penicillin/β-lactamase inhibitor
Ampicillin/sulbactam
Ticarcillin/clavulanate potassium
Piperacillin tazobactam
Combination regimens
Clindamycin plus aminoglycoside plus penicillin/ampicillin
Metronidazole plus aminoglycoside plus penicillin/ampicillin

abscess or infected hematoma is present. Frequently utilized empiric regimens are presented alphabetically in Table 20.4. Accumulating data from animal experiments and human clinical trials indicate that once-daily dosing of an aminoglycoside is as effective as, and possibly less toxic than, more frequent dosing.[6] Duration of antibiotic regimen administration is not well established. Ten to 14 days of therapy were recommended at one time without justifying data; prolonged therapy has been clinically proven to be unnecessary.

Our practice, based on experience and data in the literature, is to administer parenteral antimicrobial until the patient is afebrile at least 24 hours. The parenteral antimicrobial is discontinued, and the patient is discharged on no oral antimicrobial. If an abscess or infected hematoma is present, the parenteral regimen is administered until the patient has been afebrile for at least 48 hours. Prolonged administration invites superinfection, induced resistance, toxic side effects, and allergic reaction. Stopping therapy too early, however, invites recurrence, so clinical evaluation is mandatory.

There have been more reported clinical failures with clindamycin combination regimens in recent years. Substituting metronidazole as the antianaerobic agent is becoming more popular. The addition of a β-lactamase enzyme inhibitor to a β-lactam antibiotic was established to combat the most common defense mechanism of pelvic infection pathogens. Extended-spectrum penicillin plus β-lactamase enzyme inhibitor (ticarcillin/clavulanate potassium or piperacillin/tazobactam) is usually reserved for combination therapy with an aminoglycoside in the treatment of febrile neutropenic patients or patients who fail empiric therapy. The same is appropriate use for carbapenems. *B. fragilis* group species were among bacteria to be included in an antibiotic resistance surveillance program recommended by the American Society of Microbiology Task Force.[7] Other potential postoperative pelvic infection pathogens included enterococci, streptococci, staphylococci, and Enterobacteriaceae.

Controversy exists regarding the necessity to culture prior to therapy for postoperative pelvic infection, primarily because of the contamination potential and inaccessibility to sites of pelvic infection. Care must be taken to disinfect the area through which the sample is obtained. A protected sample obtained from cephalad to the vaginal margin would identify the most likely pathogens of extraperitoneal cellulitis. Any intraperitoneal infection site cannot be cultured without risk for potentially significant morbidity. Culture of purulent material that is drained from a space will accurately identify pathogens present. A sterile needle and a glass syringe should be utilized whenever possible. The needle should be plugged with a rubber stopper after the air is expelled from the syringe. Air can diffuse through a thin film of pus on a swab, killing most anaerobes; certain plastics may oxidize aspirated material. To culture the vaginal cuff will not result in clinically useful information.

Microbiologic information that is currently available is certainly more useful than what existed even 5 years ago. Anaerobic isolates were not reported by many laboratories. Later, species were identified, but sensitivity data were not provided. Now with automation, more and more laboratories are able to provide such data, but not for about 72 hours. If laboratories cannot provide suitable answers, there is certainly no need to perform cultures. When positive, blood cultures do yield invaluable information. The incidence of positive blood cultures accompanying postoperative infections in women undergoing gynecologic surgical procedures may be as high as 1%, certainly not high enough to justify routine blood culturing prior to parenteral antimicrobial therapy for all patients.

Other Infections

Endocarditis

Types of heart abnormalities requiring antimicrobial protection include valvular heart disease, prosthetic valves, congenital heart disease (excluding uncomplicated secundum atrial septal defect), idiopathic hypertrophic subaortic stenosis, and mitral valve prolapse with regurgitation. Regimens recommended to prevent valvular damage or endocarditis appear in Table 20.5. A one-time administration is proposed by some; others recommend an identical second dose 8 hours later or an oral dose of 1.5 g amoxicillin 6 hours after the initial dose.

Necrotizing Soft Tissue Infection

Several rare but devastating and potentially life-threatening infections can develop following elective gynecologic operative procedures. One such infection is necrotizing soft tissue infection. This infection can be divided into clostridial and nonclostridial, or synergistic gangrene, and its location can be superficial or deep. The superficial infection of the skin and subcutaneous tissues does not involve the fascia. The clinical presentation of nonclostridial infection is markedly different from clostridial infection, which is associated with gas production, muscle involvement, and marked symptomatology. Clostridial infection requires immediate drainage and surgical removal of damaged tissue. Myonecrosis may develop in pelvic or abdominal wall muscles. Large doses of parenteral penicillin G are required to eradicate the organisms not surgically removed. The infection not associated with *Clostridium* species is a very slowly progressive infection caused by microaerophilic streptococci, Enterobacteriaceae, hemolytic streptococci, *S. aureus,* and other mixed bacteria. Early care is not sought by the patient because of the indolent nature of the infection.[8] Parenteral antimicrobial and resection are necessary for cure, however.

Table 20.5 Endocarditis prophylaxis at gynecologic surgical procedures

Antimicrobial	Dose
Ampicillin plus	2 g IM or IV 30 minutes before procedure
gentamicin	1.5 mg/kg IM or IV 30 minutes before procedure
Vancomycin (penicillin allergy)	1 g IV infused slowly over 1 hour beginning 1 hour before procedure

Necrotizing Fasciitis

Necrotizing fasciitis was named by a University of Texas Southwestern Medical Center/Parkland Memorial Hospital surgeon.[9] This rapidly progressive infection has been also referred to as β-hemolytic streptococcal gangrene, synergistic necrotizing cellulitis, gangrenous erysipelas, hospital gangrene, Meleney's gangrene, gram-negative anaerobic cutaneous gangrene, or nonclostridial gas gangrene. It has acute onset, and systemic involvement is apparent early. Predisposing factors include diabetes, arteriosclerotic heart disease, age over 50 years, and debilitating disease of any type. Clinical clues as to its existence are the development of dermal blisters and/or ecchymotic areas in an area of cellulitis or gas in the tissues (crepitus). Excessive edema exists beyond the area of apparent mild cellulitis. A thin gray fluid may seep through the skin, which slips over underlying tissue and does not bleed when cut. Superficial vessels become occluded, thereby inducing local surface anesthesia and depriving the area of oxygen and making it impossible to deliver antibiotic to the affected area.

S. aureus, Enterobacteriaceae, *S. faecalis,* hemolytic streptococci, *Prevotella* and *Bacteroides* species, *Peptostreptococcus* species, and *Fusobacterium* species have been recovered from tissues involved with this infection. They produce large quantities of proteolytic enzymes, which allow rapid spread to contiguous tissues along fascial planes. Even massive doses of multiple antibiotics are ineffective; only frequently disfiguring but life-saving surgical debridement of affected areas and tissues exhibiting vigorous bleeding will halt the progress of and will result in the cure of this infection. Whirlpool baths may be useful and, for severe infections, a hyperbaric oxygen chamber. Broad-spectrum antimicrobial therapy should be administered preoperatively and continued until the area is covered with a good base of granulation tissue. This infection has been observed after tubal sterilization,[10] around a suprapubic catheter,[11] and after abdominal hysterectomy.[12]

Septic Pelvic Thrombophlebitis

Septic pelvic thrombophlebitis infrequently complicates a postoperative infection. The presentation that we observe is almost identical to that of a woman with an infected hematoma on the fourth postoperative day; she is asymptomatic and has a normal abdominal and pelvic examination but has a mild tachycardia and recurrent temperature elevations. The woman with phlebitis, however, has responded to and is still receiving parenteral antimicrobial therapy administered for a postoperative pelvic infection. Sonography does not detect a mass, and in most instances CT scan will detect thrombi. Perhaps this entity is just inflammatory phlebitis. Septic embolization is not observed. Altering the antibiotic regimen is not beneficial, but heparin administration frequently results in normocardia and disappearance of temperature elevations. As little as 5,000 units every 8 hours may be effective. Drug fever is in the differential diagnosis; eosinophilia and a positive direct Coombs' test are commonly present with this rare complication of antimicrobial therapy in the asymptomatic, febrile patient who is clinically cured by antimicrobial therapy.

This presentation is quite dissimilar to presentations observed when this entity was initially described in the early 1950s, before the introduction of the excellent antibiotics that are now available. Hectic alterations in temperature were observed in women who were clinically septic with headache, malaise, and chills. As septic embolization occurred, tachypnea, cough, and hemoptysis developed, and patients became anxious and restless. Chest x-ray films were positive in up to almost 50% of cases in some earlier reports. When surgery was the only means of diagnosing this potentially fatal complication, the mortality rate was about 50%. Diagnosis and therapy have changed from invasive surgery to noninvasive methods. The pelvic event is most accurately diagnosed by CT or MRI; embolization is confirmed by arterial blood gas determination and isotopic lung scan. Surgical ligation of the inferior vena cava and possibly the ovarian veins has been replaced by heparin therapy unless embolization occurs or persists after heparinization. Umbrella placement has replaced vena cava ligation in most instances.

Heparin therapy is not without potential sequelae. Careful attention must be given to dose and response as measured by the PT. If more heparin is required to achieve the same degree of anticoagulation, or if the platelet count falls, the white clot syndrome[13] should be suspected. Although it occurs in less than 1% of those given bovine or porcine heparin by any route, a 20% major-limb amputation rate can result, and the mortality rate may be as high as 50%. Broad-spectrum antimicrobial therapy should be continued until the patient has been afebrile for at least 48 hours.

Nonmenstrual Toxic Shock Syndrome

One last potentially devastating syndrome should be discussed since it relates to postoperative infections, although it is not an infection in the strictest definition but rather a response to a toxin produced by *S. aureus*. That is the toxic shock syndrome. Clinical symptomatology, physical findings, and laboratory results of non–menstrual related toxic shock are identical to those observed in women with menstrual-related syndrome; the median interval between surgical procedure and onset of symptoms is about 2 days. Signs of wound infection are usually minimal, but wound cultures are positive for *S. aureus*. Patients with chronic nonhealing surgical incisions are at risk for late development of the syndrome; such has been reported up to 65 days after a surgical procedure. Gynecologic surgical procedures that have been followed by toxic shock are presented in Table 20.6.[14]

Patients complain primarily of fever and malaise and have experienced diarrhea. Con-

TABLE 20.6 Gynecologic surgical procedures followed by toxic shock syndrome

Tubal ligation
Ovarian cystectomy
Marshall-Marchetti-Krantz
Urethral suspension
Laparotomy
D & C
Hysterectomy
Laser vaporization of condyloma
Laparoscopy

junctival and pharyngeal hyperemia without purulent exudate are present, and the tongue is "strawberry" or "raspberry." There is a nonpainful and nonpruritic erythema of the skin that is more prominent over the trunk. Orthostatic hypotension or overt shock may be present, and the temperature reading is equal to or greater than 38.8° C. There are laboratory signs of poor organ system perfusion and leukocytosis with a left shift. A collaborative definition for severe toxic shock syndrome is presented in Table 20.7. The patient must have all major criteria and at least three minor criteria to meet criteria for the strict definition. There are those who receive therapy early who may not manifest the fully developed syndrome. Bacterial sepsis, scarlet fever, enterovirus infection, meningococcemia, measles, Rocky Mountain spotted fever, leptospirosis, and Stevens-Johnson syndrome must be ruled out.

Therapy for this response to staphylococcal toxin is supportive and must be initiated before other diagnoses have been excluded. The cornerstone of therapy is large volumes of IV fluid and electrolytes to replace losses through diarrhea, insensible loss, and capillary leakage to the interstitial space. Severe edema may result, representing capillary leakage rather than vascular volume overload.

To differentiate and guide management, CVP and urinary output must be monitored. Dopamine administration may be necessary. A careful search must be made in incisions for the staphylococcal focus so that mechanical drainage can be accomplished and the toxin source eliminated. Antistaphylococcal antibiotic also must be administered and continued for perhaps up to 10 days to decrease recurrences.

TABLE 20.7 Toxic shock syndrome—definition criteria*

Major criteria
Temperature ≥ 38.8° C
Diffuse macular erythroderma
Late skin desquamation, particularly palms of hands and soles of feet (1-2 weeks)
Hypotension
Orthostatic syncope
Systolic blood pressure < 90 mm Hg for adults
Minor criteria—organ system involvement
GI (vomiting or diarrhea)
Muscular (myalgia or CPK > twice normal)
Mucous membrane involvement (conjunctival, oropharyngeal, vaginal)
Renal (BUN and creatinine > twice normal or > 5 WBCs/HPF without infection)
Hepatic (bilirubin, SGOT, SGPT > twice normal)
Hematologic (platelets < 100,000/mm^3)
Central nervous system (disorientation or consciousness alteration without focal localizing signs)
Negative results (if obtained)
Blood, CSF, and throat cultures
Serologic tests for measles, leptospirosis, Rocky Mountain spotted fever

**CPK*, creatinine phosphokinase; *BUN*, blood urea nitrogen; *WBCs*, white blood cells; *HPF*, high-power field; *SGOT*, serum glutamic oxaloacetic transaminase; *SGPT*, serum glutamic pyruvic transaminase; *CSF*, cerebrospinal fluid.

When administered early, there is evidence, albeit retrospective, that administration of corticosteroid significantly decreases the severity of and shortens the duration of the toxin-induced syndrome. In spite of appropriate resuscitation and management of the infected site, up to 5% of those with this syndrome are at risk for death, usually because of adult respiratory distress syndrome, disseminated intravascular coagulopathy, or unresponsive hypotension with myocardial failure.

SUMMARY

Fortunately, postoperative infections that develop after gynecologic surgery are infrequent and not serious and most respond promptly to the broad-spectrum antimicrobials that are available. Gynecologists must be aware of risk factors in their patient populations, and they must utilize antimicrobial prophylaxis as indicated. Antimicrobial therapy should not be initiated without operative site examination and a diagnosis that will be placed on the cover sheet of the patient's chart. Careful surveillance of response to therapy and awareness of devastating conditions will allow early diagnosis, appropriate therapy, and potential prevention of these rare postoperative infections and syndromes.

References

1. Ad Hoc Committee of the Committee on Trauma, Division of Medical Sciences, National Academy of Sciences, National Research Council: Postoperative wound infections: the influence of ultraviolet irradiation of the operating room and of various other factors, Ann Surg Suppl 160:1, 1964.
2. Horan TC and others: CDC definitions of nosocomial surgical site infections, 1992: a modification of CDC definitions of surgical wound infections, Infect Control Hosp Epidemiol 13:606, 1992.
3. Richardson AC, Lyon JB, and Graham EE: Abdominal hysterectomy: relationship between morbidity and surgical technique, Am J Obstet Gynecol 115:953, 1973.
4. Van Scoy RE and Wilkowske CJ: Prophylactic use of antimicrobial agents in adult patients, Mayo Clin Proc 67:288, 1992.
5. Hemsell DL and others: Cefazolin is inferior to cefotetan as single-dose prophylaxis for women undergoing elective total abdominal hysterectomy, *Clin Infect Dis* 20:677, 1995.
6. Prins JM and others: Once daily gentamicin in patients with serious infections, Lancet 341:335, 1993.
7. American Society for Microbiology Public and Scientific Affairs Board Task Force: Report of the ASM Task Force on Antibiotic Resistance, Antimicrob Agents Chemother 39 (Suppl):1, 1995.
8. Borkowf HI: Bacterial gangrene associated with pelvic surgery, Clin Obstet Gynecol 16:40, 1973.
9. Wilson B: Necrotizing fasciitis, Am Surg 18:416, 1952.
10. Badenoch DF: Meleney's gangrene following sterilisation by salpingectomy: case report, Br J Obstet Gynaecol 88:1061, 1981.
11. Bearman DM, Livengood CH III, and Addison WA: Necrotizing fasciitis arising from a suprapubic catheter site: a case report, J Reprod Med 33:411, 1988.
12. Henderson WH: Synergistic bacterial gangrene following abdominal hysterectomy, Obstet Gynecol Suppl 49:24, 1977.
13. Stanton PE Jr and others: White clot syndrome, South Med J 81:616, 1988.
14. Petitti O, D'Agostino RB, and Oldman MJ: Nonmenstrual toxic shock syndrome, J Reprod Med 32:10, 1987.

21

Foreign Bodies Left Behind

BRUCE H. DRUKKER

Surgeons often have a feeling of security in the OR that is based on long years of training. The surgeon must learn to use the OR to maximum advantage. Planning and attention to detail must always override even a modicum of complacency. The environment must be quiet, and all participants in the operative procedure must demonstrate a high level of professionalism. Everyone present has a unique, predetermined assignment focused toward an excellent outcome for the patient. Preoperative planning regarding positioning, lighting, and instruments will prevent unnecessary intraoperative delays with accompanying reduction in efficiency and excellence of surgical outcome. The craft of surgery cannot be permitted to undergo any deviations from the highest levels of excellence as a result of breaks in professionalism, pressures, shortcuts, or lack of appropriate or compromised equipment when economic incentives reduce OR budgets.

Sponge and laparotomy pad counts have been a ubiquitous part of surgery for years. Needle and instrument counts are new measures to ensure quality in the surgical theater. The institution of these counts is mandated by the occasional foreign body inadvertently left behind at surgery and discovered surreptitiously at a later date. These accounts, although infrequent, continue to permeate the substance of our specialty and can lead to disturbing interventions on behalf of the patient, as well as obvious concerns for the provider of care (i.e., physicians, nursing personnel, and hospitals). The purpose of this chapter is to review the implications of both purposeful and nonpurposeful foreign bodies that are left behind.

Purposeful Placement of Foreign Bodies

In gynecologic surgery, a number of foreign bodies can deliberately be incorporated into a surgical field and left for a brief or extended period. In some situations, permanency of the foreign body is the goal.

Catheters and Drains

Short-term foreign bodies, that is, those left in place a few days to 2 to 3 weeks, include latex rubber or silicone catheters and latex rubber or silicone drains, generally with suction. These structures are left in situ with an external point of egress or access. The traditional rubber urinary drainage catheter (Foley, Malecot), although a foreign body, is rarely left behind for extended periods in gynecologic surgery. However, as foreign bodies, catheters provide superb points of entrance for microorganisms to the urinary tract. UTI is directly related to the duration of indwelling catheter use, the location of the catheter, and its manipulation. Rubber catheters have been found as foreign bodies in the peritoneal cavity in gynecologic patients, usually as a complication of an illegal pregnancy termination. Silicone catheters are surmised to be less reactive but generally are fraught with the same types of problems that are associated with rubber catheters. Rubber and silicone catheters handled correctly do not break away or separate with a portion of the catheter left in the bladder. Thus retained portions of these surgical appliances are uncommon. If they do break and a portion is left behind, they can easily be retrieved at cystoscopy. If a catheter breaks and a portion of a silicone or rubber catheter is left in the peritoneal cavity, retroperitoneal space, or space of Retzius, the surgical incision must be opened sufficiently to permit exploration and removal of the catheter.

The ureteral stent, another form of catheter, is left behind purposefully for 6 to 8 weeks. Stents can be placed by the more common percutaneous route or by retrograde insertion. Stents are generally used for situations related to ureteral injury, which may be due to vascular problems, trauma, or iatrogenic interference. Urinary extravasation and urinoma formation are not acceptable and must be drained. The stent will preserve renal function, prevent urinoma formation, and encourage healing.

If severe infection occurs and antibiotic therapy is not helpful, the stent must be removed to permit clearing of the problem. Replacement can then be considered.

T-shaped or straight latex drains have been used in gynecologic surgery for decades, initially with trepidation, then with selective uniformity, and presently with discretion. They have been irrigated or left to drain independently for a few days. They are then advanced for arbitrary distances and at arbitrary times until they have been removed. These open drainage systems should be considered short-term foreign bodies and are not used frequently. Currently the majority of drains are tubes or perforated flat closed-system devices attached to negative suction reservoirs. They are usually sewed in place until removal. Plain latex drains may initially be sewed in place with the classic safety pin on the outer end. As the drain is removed, the safety pin prevents the drain from moving back into its drainage track, truly a rather unusual occurrence. Drains can cause problems from a retention standpoint if they are trapped inadvertently by a suture, particularly a permanent suture. If suture entrapment occurs, the surgeon can wait a few days if absorbable suture is used and again attempt removal. Eventually the drain will move, and the problem will be resolved. On the other hand, if the operator knows a permanent suture was used, there is no alternative other than reoperation and removal if a sharp tug does not remove the drain and it is visualized to be intact after removal. In general, the scrupulous gynecologic surgeon rarely has any difficulty with drains. Gore-Tex drainage systems thought to be quite inert should be handled in a similar fashion.

Meshes

Various forms of mesh are also purposefully left behind. Meshes can be nonpermanent, such as those made from polyglactin or polyglycolic acid. Permanent mesh used most commonly is knitted polypropylene. Polyglactin absorbable mesh was considered a useful item to install at the pelvic brim for patients who might require radiation therapy to the pelvis, particularly following TAH and BSO for adenocarcinoma of the endometrium. It is not used frequently at this time. Polypropylene mesh, on the other hand, usually has been used to repair extensive fascial defects or occasionally to support the urethrovesical junction in patients with recurrent and debilitating SUI. If the mesh erodes into the vagina, it can become infected, and removal is necessary. Polypropylene mesh or Gore-Tex has also been used for retroperitoneal placement in sacrovaginal suspensions for extensive vaginal prolapse. In these instances, it is appropriate to be sure there is no continuity between the polypropylene, Gore-Tex, or sutures used to place the mesh at the apex of the vagina and the vaginal epithelial mucous membrane. Should such a point of access for vaginal microorganisms exist, a serious potential for infection and retroperitoneal abscess does exist.

Lyophilized dura mater has also been used for these suspensions. Tissue reactivity is minimal, and there have been few complications.

Gauze Packing

The use of gauze packing in abdominal gynecologic surgery purposefully placed and left behind with intent is extremely uncommon. It is usually associated with emergent situations related to hemostasis where all other means of control have failed. It is by far the least desirable means of obtaining vascular control. Not only does it require secondary intervention for removal, but it has a notoriously poor track record with respect to maintenance of a sterile environment. It is a perfect culture site, superbly bathed in tissue fluid, where microorganisms can flourish. This technique should truly be identified as a last resort. It is in the realm of surgical heroics when all else fails.

On the other hand, long 3- or 4-inch gauze packing strips are used with some frequency following both minor and major vaginal surgery. Again, the theory relates to pressure with concomitant hemostasis of small vessels not visualized at surgery or those on the edge of transected tissue planes that are anticipated to spontaneously coagulate and not be troublesome. Occasionally the patient's vascular physiologic verve exceeds these coagulation expectations. Hemostasis achieved by suture or electrocoagulation is superior to packing. Generally, vaginal packing, regardless of the configuration of the gauze, is removed within 24 hours. After this brief "locum tenens in vaginum" even the less discriminating physician can appreciate the unique culture resource for vaginal organisms provided by the foreign body. Olfactory sensations critically reinforce this observation. Vaginal packing should be avoided and not made a standard part of a particular vaginal surgical procedure. On the other hand, it can occasionally be used to solve a hemostasis problem. In these situations it should be used carefully, slightly moistened by a solution of normal saline and dilute povidone-iodine. Prophylactic antibiotics used appropriately and with increasing frequency with some major vaginal procedures may reduce egress of deleterious organisms into open tissue planes. However, the best resolve for vaginal packing is timely removal.

In my estimation if the sun rises or sets twice on a pack, the problems of potential pelvic cellulitis or vaginal infection, regardless of antibiotics, are substantial. An exception relates to the necessity of vaginal packing associated with intravaginal and uterine intracavitary irradiation. Often this must be left in place for 48 to 72 hours. Since there are no open tissue planes during this procedure, serious infection is usually not a problem despite occasional vaginal mucosal abrasions that can occur during placement of the afterloading devices. Here again, moistening of the pack in a solution of normal saline and dilute povidone-iodine reduces to a degree bacterial growth. Symptoms developing are often subtle, with pelvic discomfort, pressure, and eventually pain and a febrile response. If any of these symptoms occur and do not respond to conservative treatment, removal is required.

Surgical Clips

Originally introduced by Harvey Cushing[1] and for years confined to intracranial procedures, surgical clips have been used with much more frequency following Samuels's introduction of metallic hemostatic clips in 1966.[2] In gynecologic surgery metallic clips, both small and large, are frequently used for hemostasis in the abdomen, pelvis, omentum, and retroperitoneal, periaortic, and pelvic areas.[3] These clips are also used for bowel anastomosis and maintenance of hemostatic control for some vessels, as well as in general surgical procedures on the stomach, pancreas, and biliary tract. The inert characteristics of the metal have led to no serious problems with infection. On the other hand, the clips have been known on occasion to migrate. Reports of deleterious effects of such migration in gynecologic patients are not available.

FOREIGN BODIES ACCIDENTALLY LEFT BEHIND

Fiber Products

Retained foreign bodies inadvertently left behind following gynecologic surgery are most frequently surgical sponges, laparotomy pads, and occasionally towels. This does not occur with great frequency, and retention of towels is very infrequent. If the retained foreign body is small, often an aseptic granuloma will form, and the patient has little or no discomfort.[4] In other situations, particularly when the foreign substance is larger, adhesions may form, with subtle symptoms of partial intestinal obstruction. The patient may experience minimal to moderate abdominal cramping, change in stool pattern, and generalized lower abdominal discomfort.

Some patients may develop symptoms of mild to moderate pelvic or abdominal inflammation. Fever, leukocytosis, point tenderness, and rebound, all may be present. The patient may be able to localize pain or perceive an area of fullness. These symptoms herald the presence of a pelvic or abdominal intraperitoneal or retroperitoneal abscess secondary to infection of a foreign body.

The diagnosis of a retained fiber-containing foreign body can be difficult, often requiring abdominal or pelvic imaging assessment. Diagnosis is particularly difficult if the foreign body has no radioopaque stripe or marker.

When plain radiographs are used, a whorl-like image may be produced for gauze both with and without markers. This appearance is attributed to "gas" trapped in the fibers of the gauze. Unfortunately the whorl-like appearance of the foreign body is not uniformly encountered. In fact, it is quite infrequent. Thus traditional radiographic imaging has not consistently aided in diagnosis.[5]

Ultrasonography also has been used to demonstrate the presence of fiber-containing foreign bodies.[6] Sonographic imaging of sponges is intense, with sharply described acoustic imaging. This acoustic shadowing may be inappropriately large in the presence of air or calcifications within the foreign body. On occasion some masses may have an alternative sonographic characteristic, with markedly diffuse and irregular internal echoes. Unfortunately, this is a rather nondescript and nonspecific appearance. Ultrasonography appears to assist definitely with diagnosis of a foreign body in less than 50% of patients with a retained fiber-containing foreign body.

CT appears to be the most useful tool for diagnosis of the fiber-containing foreign body. In most studies, CT scans image well-demarcated round or oval masses. Imaging characteristics most commonly encountered were low densities (approximating water or between water and blood). Low and medium complex masses (blood attenuation) have also been identified. High-density masses (greater than liver attenuation) have also been noted, but infrequently. Occasionally focal peripheral or central calcifications are noted, or gas bubbles can be seen. The use of IV contrast material at time of CT is particularly helpful since it can create an image enhancement at the periphery of the fiber foreign body. On occasion, but with considerably less frequency, the inner component of the mass will image as enhanced. Apparently the longer a fiber-containing foreign body remains in place, the greater the frequency of calcification. This has been documented in unusual situations, as when a diagnosis was made on CT but the patient refused operative intervention and remained asymptomatic. A repeat CT approximately 6 to 12 months later demonstrated new calcifications in the identified mass.

If a fiber-containing foreign body (sponge, laparotomy pad, or towel) is identified, it should be removed even if there is absence of symptoms. At the time of surgery, adhesions should be anticipated. Bowel preparation also is important to permit complete surgical extirpation of the foreign body with completion of any indicated bowel surgery at that time. Following removal of the foreign body, the area should be copiously irrigated before closure of retroperitoneal and peritoneal spaces. There are no strict guidelines for drainage, but if the area of removal is clean and there is no abscess formation, routine drainage does not appear to be indicated.

Metal Products

Inadvertent retention of metallic surgical instruments such as clamps, forceps, or scissors is infrequent (Figure 21.1). The current concept of operative instrument counts will virtually eliminate this problem. If any instrument is left behind, symptoms are not usually those of infection or abscess formation. In fact, patients may be asymptomatic or may have minimal vague abdominal pains.[7] Interestingly, however, these pains may be accentuated by certain postural changes, such as bending forward or backward. The surgeon has to have a very high degree of suspicion to make this diagnosis, which is verified by an abdominal or pelvic radiograph. In all situations, surgical removal is mandated.

Surgical needles are an additional problem. They can break, be misplaced, or fly off the needle holder. This occurs particularly when the needle is being returned to the person passing instruments. A broken needle with a small portion missing may be very difficult to locate with or without radiographs or magnets. If it is a small piece (< 1 cm) and cannot be located, it is better to leave it in place than to create a large amount of surgical morbidity with blind dissection. The metal can be treated like a retained clip with minimal anticipated

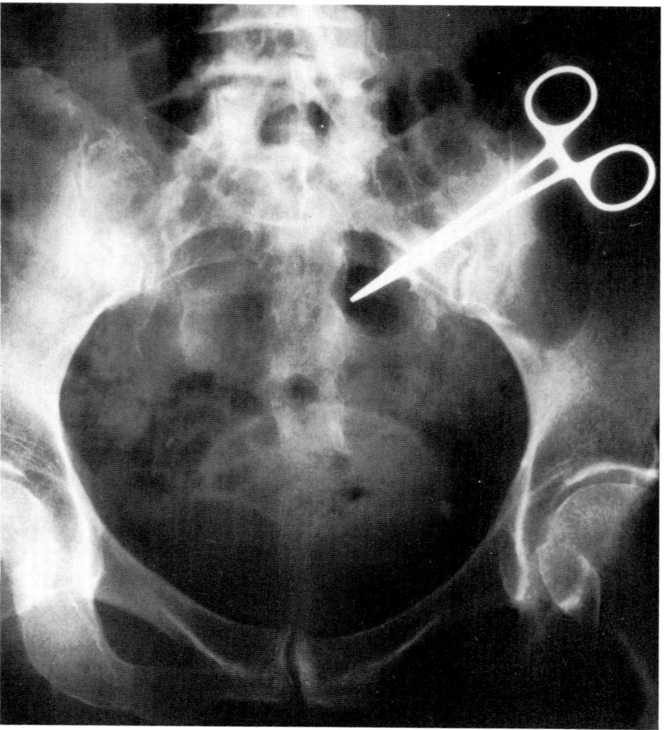

FIGURE 21.1 Hemostat inadvertently left in place during major gynecologic surgery. Removal required a second surgical procedure.

difficulty. The patient should be informed of the situation and advised of the rationale for the decision not to pursue a small fragment. On the other hand, a complete needle should be sought using all routine means and only as a last resort allowed to remain in the pelvic or abdominal cavity, as might occur rarely when a tiny microsurgical needle has been lost and cannot be retrieved even though it can be visualized on radiograph.

Despite counts of sponges, laparotomy pads, needles, and instruments, a few surgeons still consider a routine plain abdominal and pelvic radiograph standard procedure in the surgical suite when closure has been completed and before transfer to the postoperative recovery area.[8]

SUMMARY

Foreign bodies purposefully left behind should not be a problem. Those placed on a temporary basis should be removed within the anticipated prescribed time. Those left on a permanent basis must be removed if they become infected or are in other ways deleterious.

On the other hand, foreign bodies noted in an abdominal or pelvic location that were inadvertently left behind should be removed if they are deemed of concern. These include all items except a small portion of needle, which should be innocuous. Before and after removal of such items, careful explanation to the patient is mandatory.

REFERENCES

1. Cushing H: The control of bleeding in operations for brain tumors with the description of silver "clips" for the occlusion of vessels inaccessible to the ligature, Ann Surg 54:1, 1911.
2. Samuels PB and others: A new hemostatic clip: two year review of 1007 cases, Ann Surg 163:427, 1966.
3. Morgenstern L: Surgical shrapnel, Am J Surg 144:597, 1982.
4. Kokubo T and others: Retained surgical

sponges: CT and US appearance, Radiology 165:415, 1987.

5. Olnick HM and others: Radiologic diagnosis of retained surgical sponges, JAMA 159:1525, 1955.

6. Chau W, Lai K, and Lo K: Sonographic findings of intra-abdominal foreign bodies due to retained gauze, Gastrointest Radiol 9:61, 1984.

7. Morrison L and Homesley H: Carcinoma of the cervix complicated by a soup spoon, Obstet Gynecol 51(suppl 1):55, 1978.

8. Jones S: The foreign body problems after laparotomy, Am J Surg 122:785, 1972.

22

The Recurrent Small and Painful Vagina

Dionysios K. Veronikis

The vagina is a remarkably pliable and distensible organ and in the absence of pathology functions painlessly. When the vagina is used for surgical exposure during vaginal plastic surgery the goal is resolutely to reconstruct a functional, pain-free, pliable, distensible and well-supported structure. However, it is a given that following surgery the acquisition of scar tissue will locally reduce pliability as well as perhaps induce traction on healthy well-innervated neighboring tissue. Vaginal reconstructive surgery is similar to plastic surgery in that it involves the development of flaps. The anterior and posterior vaginal walls are mobilized by careful dissection, and the superfluous damaged areas are excised following the indicated reconstruction. The amount of vaginal wall that is removed, the reconstruction of the perineum and introital aperture, and the overall dimensions of the vaginal canal are many times guided by the indications for surgery, the type of operation performed, the status of the tissues, and the surgical judgment of the surgeon. As a general guide in gynecology, vaginal dimensions and judgment on adequacy of caliber, depth, and axis are dependent on the size of the individual surgeon's fingers. Second-guessing the effects of surgical healing and postoperative concerted conjugal function of the vagina following all types of reconstruction is perhaps the hallmark of the effective gynecologic surgeon. Therefore an unexpected finding that the patient's vagina is too small and/or painful postoperatively for coital comfort is not only annoying and distressful to the patient and disquieting to the surgeon, it also may require a reevaluation of surgical judgment.

There are no standards as to how small or large a vagina should be because a definition of an adequate vagina is one that admits and contains the woman's sexual partner with comfort. Thus tremendous variations exist, limiting conclusive statements on length and caliber except perhaps for one. If dyspareunia is present, then disproportion in female to male anatomy is a frequent cause of pain and discomfort, or an alteration in vaginal anatomic landmarks has resulted from surgical therapy. Yet surgery is not the only cause of dyspareunia; the etiology is highly varied, including congenital deformities such as agenesis of the vagina and uterus, absence of the lower half of the vagina, and transverse and longitudinal septa at any level, including imperforate hymen, as well as menopausal changes and psychosomatic factors.

In a general sense the mechanism of dyspareunia may be thought to be due to deficiency or a lack of tissue. Thus the goals of therapy are then directed at manipulating existing tissue hormonally and/or mechanically, depending on the patient's ability to participate, and/or surgically utilizing transfer of autologous tissue as indicated by the type of defect that exists.

History and Physical Examination

Dyspareunia is not a pathologic entity; it is a symptom complex referring to a patient's vaginal discomfort during coitus. It is a nonspecific term and requires further elucidation by careful and directed history. The history will help to establish the duration and severity and if apareunia has resulted. Specific questions such as the onset of pain in relation to the start of sexual activity and a description of the pain, measures that have been taken to relieve pain and whether they are helpful, whether coitus has ever been pain-free, whether it is painful every time attempted or just in certain circumstances, and a history of any sexual trauma or abuse that has been experienced. Characteristics of the pain described should further elucidate whether the pain perceived is superficial at or near the introitus upon intromission, if the pain is deep at the cervix or abdomen during thrusting, or whether the pain is constant throughout the entire vagina. All vaginal sites—introitus, middle and upper vagina—must be considered. Inquiries into previous treatments should include nonsurgical and surgical therapies and the results, as well as whether the dyspareunia is getting better, staying the same, or getting worse.

Following a complete history, a pelvic examination should be performed utilizing the information elicited in the interview to guide the examination. A suspicion of the anticipated defect and anatomic site and the expected physical findings should be formed before initiating the examination. Reassuring the patient that she is in control and that the pelvic examination will cease should it be uncomfortable and maintaining a continuous verbal dialogue with an explanation of the findings during the examination will relax the patient and allow her the opportunity to participate in identifying the site of her pain. The application of sufficient lidocaine jelly or ointment serves a dual purpose: lubrication in addition to short-term topical anesthesia. Guided by the history, inspection of the introitus, perineum, and vulva before palpation usually immediately offers much important information. Inspection is followed by and combined with a gentle single-digit examination of the introitus and the entire vaginal canal circumferentially, specifically palpating for ridges, levator muscle tone, and concurrently evaluating vaginal length, depth, axis, and caliber. A history of previous posterior colporrhaphy and/or perineorrhaphy would direct suspicion and examination at the introitus but not exclude the midvagina as a site for ridges and/or narrowing. An obstructed introitus from overzealous repair is readily identified by inspection. At times the external urethral meatus is visible only upon retraction of the labia. If questioned, such patients frequently also are troubled by postvoid urinary dribbling from the vagina acting as a pouch. A skin bridge above the fourchette will partially obstruct the lower introitus and, although it may permit intromission, will be a source of constant traction, abrasion, and trauma. A higher somewhat thicker skin bridge at times associated with tissue from lateral mobilization is referred to as a "dashboard" perineum. An office examination limited by pain from introital obstruction should warn the surgeon that perhaps midvaginal ridges or strictures are also present. If surgery is contemplated, a thorough examination under anesthesia will readily confirm and identify other sites requiring attention.

Postobstetric pain from a recent episiotomy may present with symptoms of an obstructed introitus or tenderness of the scar in the midline or mediolaterally. Occasionally crown sutures that reapproximate the pubococcygeal muscles in front of the rectum will produce a constant and unrelenting muscle spasm. A narrowed vaginal introitus in a patient with pliable tissues may not cause any other pain except transiently upon intromission. This most painful symptom may be due to intromission trauma of the external urethral meatus. Similarly, absence of a previous contributory surgical history with introital and/or urethral pain during intromission and recurrent cystitis related to coitus suggests a relative urethral hypospadias. A merging or lateral fusion of the hymen with the urethral meatus causes a pulling effect on the urethra into the vagina with intromission from the lateral attachments.

The midvagina is most commonly affected following posterior colporrhaphy. Painful ridges may sometimes be found beneath the midvaginal wall, usually the result of fibrosis from stitches that were placed into the belly of the levator muscle and tied across the midline (levator stitches). Similarly, overexcision of the posterior vaginal wall may result in an "hourglass" stricture.

Posthysterectomy dyspareunia may be caused by a foreshortened vagina, but this is usually due to fibrosis from infection, an upper vaginectomy, or more radical surgery. However, postoperative fixation of the ovary to the vaginal vault or prolapse of the fallopian tube will produce upper vaginal and/or abdominal discomfort. Some patients describe a transient postoperative pulling sensation when vaginal length is compromised.

A neovagina lined by a split-thickness skin graft will constrict in length and caliber if dilation or coitus is not continued for a long period of time. Similarly, patients with a bowel neovagina may present with introital stenosis at the perineal anastamotic site. Therefore, as a general guide, in a patient with a surgically constructed neovagina dyspareunia may be related to the type of neovagina constructed. Caliber and length requirements should be considered together since repair of an obstructed introitus that permits intromission postoperatively discloses a short vaginal canal causing pain.

If the vaginal wall retains some elasticity and the patient is optimistic and willing to participate in mechanically enlarging her own vagina, the use of the Ingram technique with the progressively longer or wider graduated vaginal dilators and/or coitus may restore the required dimensions without surgery.[1,2] The process is directed at first to achieving depth and then width as the dilators are progressively widened to increase width. The process requires from 3 to 9 months of sustained effort in which the dilator is generally worn for a total minimum of 2 hours per day. The time is usually divided between morning and evening. Supplemental vaginal estrogen, 1 to 2 grams at bedtime several times per week, especially if the vagina is inelastic, will restore elasticity and increase blood flow. In patients with a compromised vaginal length and/or width, vaginal appliances, such as dilators or obturators, become an integral part in the nonsurgical, preoperative, and/or postoperative treatment.

Basic Concepts of Tissue Manipulation in Reconstructive Surgery

Reconstructive surgical philosophy and surgical execution of procedures embrace techniques that are exacting and must meet the specific needs of a particular patient. The techniques and principles in plastic surgery are most often applied to skin and soft tissues. The fundamental surgical philosophy and the techniques from the inception of plastic and reconstructive surgery have been marked by preservation, transfer, and transplantation of tissues predominantly to relieve deficiency, which may be congenital, genetic, from surgical excision, or traumatic in origin.

The basic techniques include the use of skin grafts and flaps. Such reconstructive procedures should be part of the aramentarium of every surgical gynecologist. Myocutaneous grafts constitute more extensive and advanced procedures to repair considerable defects usually due to the surgical treatment of cancer. These procedures, although relevant, are beyond the scope of this chapter.

Perhaps a hallmark of vaginal surgery is the development of vaginal wall flaps, utilizing the avascular planes between organs to reduce blood loss, minimize tissue trauma, and gain access to potential pelvic spaces. This surgical attitude and exposure permits an entire array of therapy to the underlying structures and organs, as well as to the vagina, including excision of traumatized overdistended vaginal wall, excision of enterocele, repair of cystocele and rectocele, repositioning of the vagina over the levator plate, and reconstructing the perineum and introitus. It is this basic philosophy of exposure and flap generation that bridges plastic surgery with gynecologic reconstructive surgery. When the management of dyspareunia becomes surgical, it is imperative that a gynecologic reconstructive surgeon be versatile, able to apply several surgical techniques to remedy the same clinical situation to be able to choose the operation that best achieves the desired surgical goal for that particular patient. In planning an operation to correct a defect, our colleagues in plastic surgery are cognizant of the importance of the reconstructive ladder, escalating from simple to more complex techniques, all of which may ultimately achieve the desired surgical goal. From direct closure, the reconstructive ladder ascends to skin grafts, local flaps, and distant flaps. The most relevant to the gynecologic surgeon in the surgical treatment of the narrow and/or foreshortened vagina relate to split- and full-thickness skin grafts, Z-plasty, Y-V plasty, and random pattern skin flaps.

The success or failure of any operation is often determined prior to the incision. However, survival of a graft is determined by the surgical technique. The final functional result of a graft is directly related to intraoperative handling of tissues, the type of tissue, infection, and the patient's healing mechanisms. Skin and subcutaneous tissues that have been crushed and/or dried by prolonged exposure to air undergo different degrees of necrosis. Crushing, including the simple crushing effect of a forceps, may cause appreciable damage to both cells and vessels. The interstitial spaces fill with blood and lymph, providing a substance in which organisms can multiply, create infection, and compromise more tissue, which increases inflammation, reduces "take," and could result in more collagen deposition. Therefore the surgical philosophy of tissue handling is based on histopathology.

Tissue injury is incurred during surgery. However, atraumatic technique and appropriate instrumentation minimize tissue injury; sharp scissors and fine knife blades (no. 11 or 15), skin hooks, and sutures of proper size swaged on needles, all facilitate surgical technique and therapy. Electrocautery techniques probably provide the most rapid and effective hemostasis while not introducing foreign material into the wound. There is no evidence that wound healing is more impaired by prudent, focused electrical current than by use of suitable ligatures such as 5-0 polyglycolic acid sutures. Efficient coagulation and a decrease in trauma may be facilitated by bringing the active electrode in contact with a fine-tipped forceps that accurately grasps only the vessel. A fine-tipped needle electrode itself can also limit current spread and add precision. This method is especially helpful in obtaining nearly absolute hemostasis of the recipient bed prepared for a graft. Also, it is essential that the assistant blot the field, instead of wiping, the latter being an abrasive maneuver that may reopen coagulated vessels.

Epinephrine continues to be a reliable vasoconstrictor for surgical procedures, providing a "liquid tourniquet" that reduces blood loss and expedites surgery. Injection of a solution as dilute as 1:500,000 (1 ml ampule of 1:1000 epinephrine to 500 ml of 5% dextrose in water) will provide excellent hemostasis if the surgical team is able to wait approximately 7 minutes for initial pharmacologic effects.[3] Epinephrine solutions are commercially available in combination with local anesthetics such as 0.5% lidocaine and 1:200,000 adrenaline.

Autografts of skin are classified as a split-thickness (Thiersch's) graft or full-thickness (Wolfe's) graft. The split-thickness graft is further subclassified as thin, intermediate, and thick split-thickness, depending on the amount of dermis included in the graft. The setting of the dermatome, 10/1000 to 25/1000 inch, will determine the thickness and therefore the type of split-thickness skin graft that will be harvested. Translucency of the graft and bleeding pattern on the donor site are respective to the thickness, ranging from a translucent appearance and fine bleeding points to nearly opaque and large bleeding points.

The clinical importance of the graft thickness is that the thinner a skin graft, the more contraction will occur at the the recipient site during the months following transplantation. There is a constant interaction between the recipient site's relentless tendency to contract and the ability of the donor site tissue to resist. The contraction that results from a thick split-thickness skin graft is less than an intermediate, which in turn is less than a thin split-thickness skin graft. A full-thickness skin graft to recipient site interaction would result in the least amount of contraction.[4] However, a thin split-thickness skin graft may be more likely to survive and can await the growth of neovascularization longer because it does well during the plasmatic absorption phase, the first 48 hours after grafting.[5] The thin-graft recipient site does not have hair growing in the transplantation site even if the donor site was hirsute or from a hair-bearing area such as the suprapubic area of the anterior abdominal wall.[6] The thick-split thickness graft may contain some hair follicles that permit hair growth, which usually undergo atrophy. The donor site of a thin split-thickness skin graft reepithelializes more rapidly than a thick split-thickness graft and is usually more cosmetic.

A full-thickness skin graft contains epidermis and the entire dermis from the donor site. As a free graft, it is the most resistant to contraction. Before transplanting, all the subcutaneous fat should be removed because fat has fewer blood vessels than dermis and will impede the take. The fat is best removed by a sharp technique such as with a scissors.

An inherent principle of skin grafts and graft-recipient site interaction is contraction. Skin grafts undergo primary (graft elasticity) contraction and secondary (recipient bed) contraction. The elastic fibers of a skin graft cause it to shrink as soon as it is cut. Primary contraction is not the biologic phenomenon of contraction. Since elastic fibers are located in the dermis, thick grafts contract more than thin grafts at the time of harvest as a function of the amount of elastic fibers within the harvested graft. The lost surface area is easily recovered by stretching and tailoring the graft to fit the recipient bed as the graft is sutured in position. Full-thickness skin grafts primarily may lose 41% of their initial surface area, whereas a thin split-thickness graft may lose only 9%.[7] However, the biologic phenomenon of contraction that postoperatively plagues the patient and surgeon, as well as compromises surgical effectiveness, is the secondary, recipient bed contraction. The skin graft simply wrinkles on the steady, unrelenting, and continuous contraction of the recipient bed.[8] This phenomenon begins approximately on postoperative day 10 and continues for up to 6 months.[9,10,11] Postoperative splinting of the grafted site is the only means of preventing contraction. A complete take and using a full-thickness skin graft also decrease the degree of contracture. The most ideal interaction that will eliminate contraction is a full-thickness graft with complete take over a bony area.

Regardless of the graft type, good contact between the skin graft and its recipient bed is essential for vascularization of the graft and its survival. Graft movement is almost immediately eliminated by the thin fibrin network and serves as a glue to hold the surfaces together. The tension of the graft is also critical on the recipient site once sutured in place. Insufficient tension will result in wrinkles that do not become revascularized due to lack of contact with the recipient bed. Similarly, if there is too much tension, a stretched graft again results in a drumhead effect and prevents contact with the recipient bed.

Flaps can be classified according to blood flow, the anatomic region moved, whether the flap is local or distant, and whether it is a compound flap that combines skin with underlying attached muscle, cartilage, or bone. Perhaps the most applicable in reconstruction of the small vagina is the local or distant flap classification. Specifically, local flaps by definition lie adjacent to the recipient site and are manipulated in one of two ways: rotation or advancement. The rotational flaps, which include the transposition and interpolation flaps, have in common a pivot point and an arc through which the flap is rotated.

The transposition flap consists of donor tissue that is rotated to the immediate adjacent recipient site. The Z-plasty is an example of one such flap (Figure 22.1). Basically, two triangular skin flaps are rotated into the defect left by the other flap. The Z-plasty geometrically consists of a central member and two limbs that are usually parallel and extend outward in opposite directions from the central member. The limbs and the central member must always be of equal length, and the angle formed by each limb may be the same or may vary. The size of the angle created by the central member and each arm as well as the length of the central member are the only two variables. As the angle of each arm to Z-plasty is increased, there is a theoretical percentage gain in length.[12] However, the force required to transpose the flaps and pull them into their new position increases as the angle increases. Clinically the 60-degree Z-plasty facilitates transposition of the triangular flaps while obtaining maximal length. The angle of the limbs can vary from 30 to 90 degrees, and the angles need not be the same. However, each flap of donor triangle tissue will be used to graft the harvest site of the other and symmetry is clearly beneficial.

The greater the length of the central member, the greater the final length accomplished by the Z-plasty. The theoretical gain in length is the difference in length between the long diagonal *(CD)* and the short diagonal *(EF)* (Figure 22.1, *A*). The biomechanical properties of the skin may increase or decrease the theoretical gain.[13] At the completion of the Z-plasty, the original Z has been reversed and rotated 90 degrees on its axis and increased in length in the direction of the central member (Figure 22.1, *C*). Therefore the Z-plasty is an effective technique that may be used to increase the length of contracted skin by interrupting the scar tissue. A continuous circular contracture at the skin anastomotic site of a

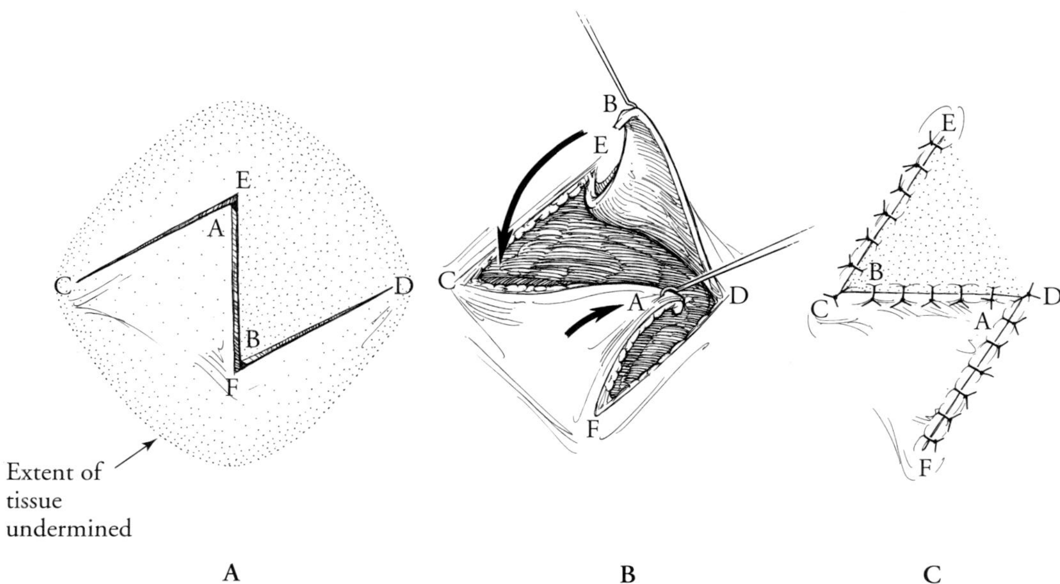

FIGURE 22.1 Sixty-degree Z-plasty. **A,** Components of the "Z" include the central member *EF,* and limbs *CE* and *FD.* The limbs must be equal to the central member. **B,** Triangular flaps *A* and *B* are rotated around each other by atraumatic technique. **C,** Completed Z-plasty with longer *EF* length. Note that the "Z" in **C** has been rotated 90 degrees and is reversed when compared to **A.**

bowel neovagina may be released by multiple Z-plasties interrupting the continuity of the circular scar and eliminating the annular band phenomenon.

The tissue of the interpolation flap is also rotated in an arc about a pivot point, as is the transposition flap. The difference between the two is that the donor site and the recipient site are not adjacent and the flap must be moved over intervening tissue (see Figure 22.7). It is essential that during the preoperative planning due consideration be given to the fact that these flaps are rotated only about the pivot point. Therefore reverse execution of the operative steps ensures the following: the flap created will be of adequate length, rotation can be accomplished without excessive buckling of the inside pivot tissue, and excessive tension on the outside pivot tissue and/or in the long axis of the flap is avoided. The initial minimal traction on the flap permits considerable stretching.[13] Continued traction will result in little additional length in the flap and may result in blanching on the skin surface, indicating vascular compromise. The success and surgical execution of the tissue transfer depends on the looseness of the skin. Clinically this is easily judged by approximating the donor site tissue between two fingers.

When the surface area of the donor site skin is not adequate for tissue transfer, the size of the donor tissue may be increased by an inflatable subcutaneous expander that will provide additional tissue for reconstruction (see Figure 22.7, *A, inset*). Tissue expansion requires the surgical implantation of an empty expander in the subcutaneous tissues of the donor site. Following initial healing, at 3- to 10-day intervals saline is used to fill and distend the expander through a buried or externalized injection port connector. Once the overlying tissue and skin are stretched sufficiently, the tissue expander is removed and the expanded tissue is used for reconstruction. Histopathology of expanded tissue has shown an increased thickness of the dermis, epidermis, and subcutaneous tissue compared with nonexpanded tissue with the patients serving as their own controls.[14] The increase in vascularity of the flap associated with tissue expansion can be noted clinically by an erythematous appearance of the skin overlying the expander. Thus tissue expansion is a technique that allows local host tissue to be increased in surface area, providing additional tissue for reconstruction, while also allowing primary closure of the donor site and stimulating angiogenesis prior to tissue transfer, facilitating flap survival.

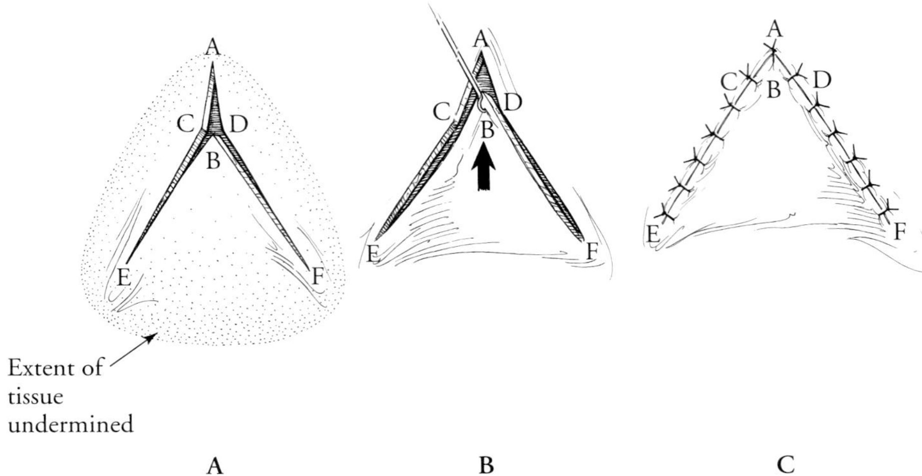

FIGURE 22.2 Y-V advancement flap. **A**, Length *AB* determines the advancement length, *CE* and *DF* correspond to the arms of the "Y." **B**, Triangular flap *B* is advanced to point *A* by gentle traction with a skin hook. **C**, The completed Y-V flap. Notice points *C* and *D* with intervening wedge of tissue. Initial "Y" incision has been closed as a "V."

The advancement flap technique, on the other hand, moves tissue directly forward into a defect without rotation or lateral movement. The Y-V advancement technique refers to the conversion of an initial Y incision to a final V-shaped closure (Figure 22.2). This is accomplished by advancing the wedge of donor tissue between the arms of the Y to the base of the Y. The Y-V advancement flap is effective in releasing and interrupting the continuity of contractures from scar tissue. The orientation of the advancing wedge of donor tissue is in a direction perpendicular to the axis of the contracture. A patient with a narrow and/or scarred introitus or a patient with a narrow introitus due to a skin bridge perineum provide ideal indications for the Y-V flap because it accomplishes interruption of the scar and opens the introitus by the diameter of the wedge of tissue, which may fortuitously be in excess. Usually advancement flaps are limited to the treatment of defects that require short length because excess tension will compromise blood flow in the flap. However, patients in older age groups have looser skin, which allows these types of flaps to be advanced further.

INTROITAL STRICTURE

A compromise of the introital perineum by a mechanical stricture may be surgically managed by a variety of techniques, which are influenced by the nature of the obstruction. Rarely, a stricture of the hymen requires incision or excision. Although hymenal ridges usually stretch with gentle examination and liberal use of a topical anesthetic followed by a short course of home dilation with an appropriate vaginal appliance, a thin persistent hymenal bridge can easily be excised using local anesthesia and sedation even in the office. However, a prominent and thickened hymen due to repeated trauma from intercourse or an almost complete occlusion of the introitus is best managed under general anesthesia. The hymen is incised in an "X" fashion, each of the four quadrants is excised, and size 3-0 polyglycolic acid sutures are placed around the introitus to approximate the mucosa and achieve hemostasis. Use of a topical anesthetic and a vaginal-introital appliance (obturator) or digital dilation postoperatively will gently stretch the hymenal remnants; warm sitz baths are started on the second postoperative day. Overzealous repair of obstetric lacerations and perineorrhaphy are common causes of a narrowed introitus. On the other hand, patients that have undergone vulvectomy and those patients with a neovagina constructed from bowel almost predictably will present with a narrowed introitus if long-term introital dilation by coitus or a suitable vaginal appliance is not continued. Although all surgeons attempt

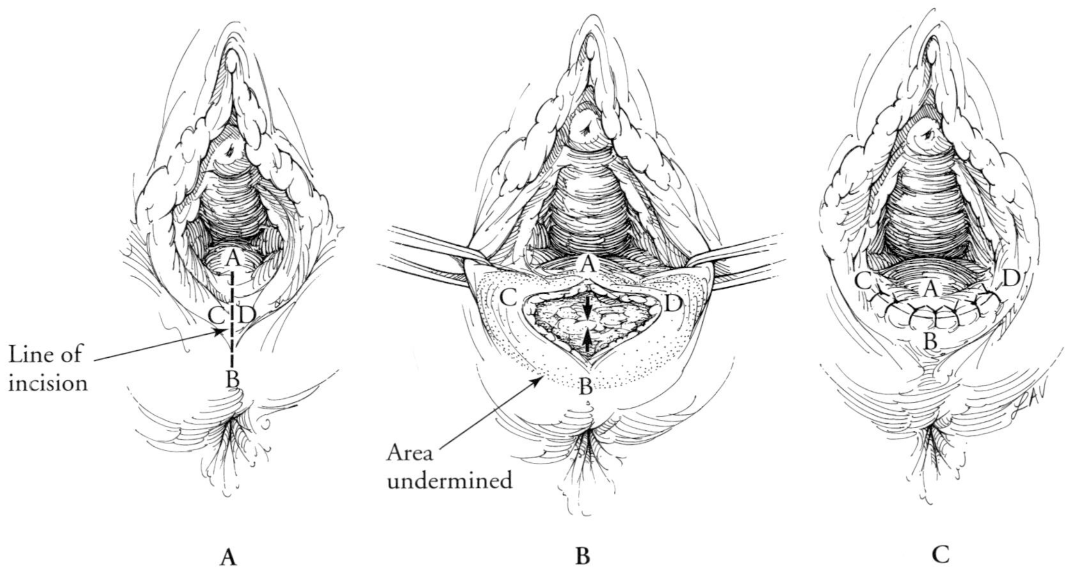

Figure 22.3 Midline perineotomy. **A**, Longitudinal incision *AB* through the contracted scar tissue. **B**, The skin and vaginal wall are released from the underlying scar. **C**, The mobilized vaginal mucosa and skin of the perineum are sutured without tension by interrupted absorbable sutures. Notice that vaginal point *A* and perineal point *B* are approximated.

to prevent such strictures at the time of initial operation, the perfect operative result may be transformed months to years later by aging, retraction of scar, diminished hormonal status, and decreased frequency of coitus to a functional narrowing.

A 5-year follow-up of patients after reconstructive surgery revealed that, of those with dyspareunia, 50% of cases were due to a mechanical obstruction of the introitus by a skin bridge.[15] A mechanical stricture of the perineum by a skin bridge or "dashboard" perineum secondary to surgery can be corrected by a vertical posterior midline introital incision with the vaginal mucosa closed transversely[16] (Figure 22.3). The skin flaps are undermined and mobilized, usually by scissors, and the incision is closed in a transverse direction with simple 2-0 polyglycolic acid suture or 2-0 nylon, which are removed on the postoperative day 7 to 10. A mechanical stricture of the introital perineum from narrowing may be treated in a similar fashion. The vaginal circumference in this operation is reconstructed with a compensation factor to allow for some postoperative contracture. The use of a vaginal appliance/obturator is an integral part of a satisfactory result.

When a midline perineotomy is closed transversely, one should consider that this will shorten the vagina by an amount equal to one half the length of the incision. Although this rarely leads to problems, the surgeon must be especially cautious in shortening a vagina with an already compromised length by previous surgery such as hysterectomy. From a functional point of view, the vaginal length required is relative to the patient's ability to contain her partner during coitus.

For the patient with an already shortened vagina the bilateral perineoplasty[17] is effective in releasing scar tissue and widening the introitus (Figure 22.4). When stenosis is present without a significant perineal body, such as congenital vulvar stenosis or postvulvectomy especially with superficial stenosis, a Z-plasty is very effective.[18,19] Z-plasty also may be useful in releasing a concentric scar contraction producing an annular ring phenomenon at the anastomotic site of a bowel neovagina (Figure 22.5). A useful combination is the bilateral perineoplasty with a concurrent bilateral Z-plasty when an adequate release is not obtained with either of these techniques individually. A Z-plasty can be performed at any point on the introitus.

The Y-V plasty interrupts an introital constriction specifically between the 4 and 8

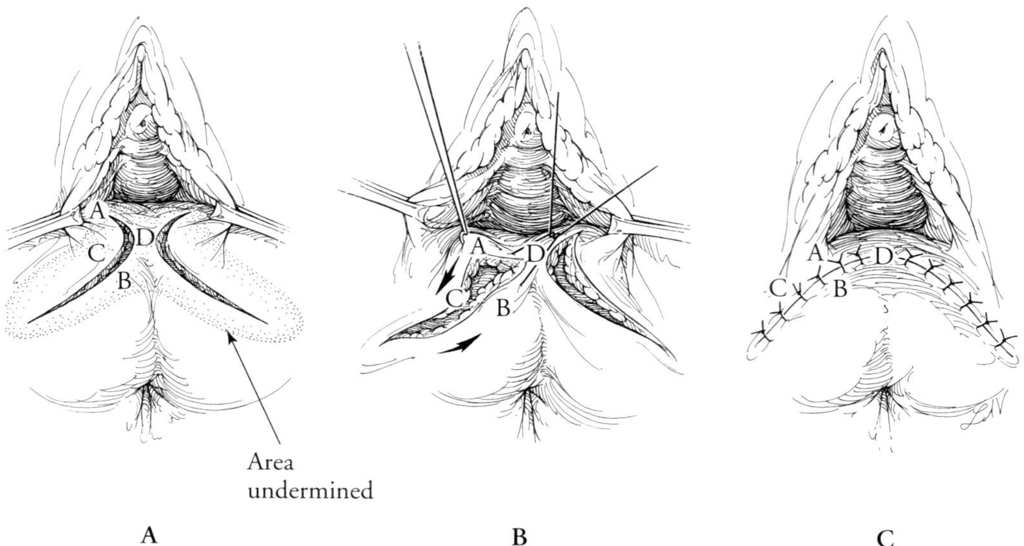

FIGURE 22.4 Bilateral episiotomy. **A,** Bilateral incisions with release of the contracted tissue and mobilization of vaginal mucosa and perineal skin. **B,** The incisions are closed by interrupted sutures. Point *D* is moved from a central position to the apex. **C,** In the end result, point *A* is adjacent to point *B*. Notice that points *A* and *C* have been mobilized laterally and inferiorly, enlarging the introitus.

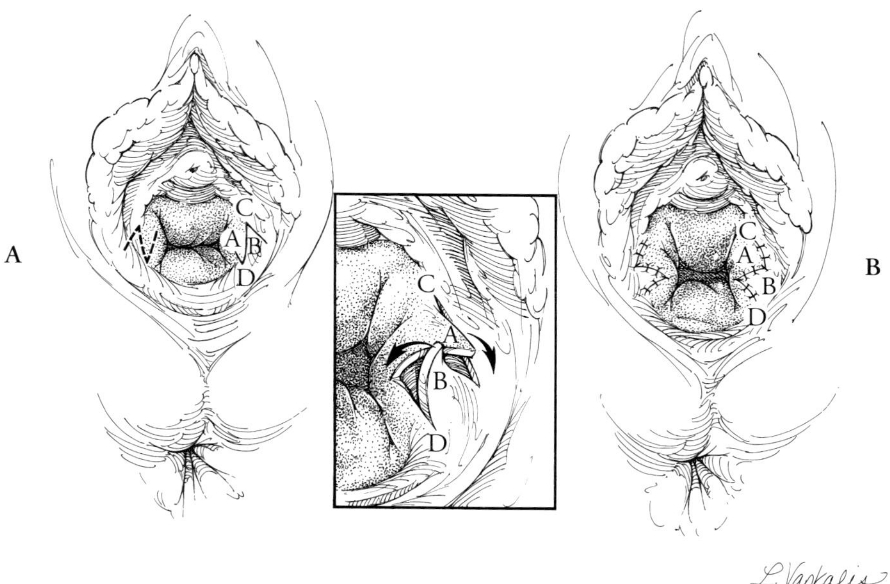

FIGURE 22.5 Bilateral Z-plasty for stenosed introitus by annular scar at the perineal anastomotic site of a bowel neovagina. **A,** Central member, *CD,* is placed over the anastomotic scar. *Inset,* Triangular flaps of mucosa *A* and skin *B* are mobilized and reversed. **B,** Final closure with interrupted sutures. Notice increased length of *CD* and interruption in the annular band phenomenon from the continuous scar.

o'clock positions. Fibrous tissue forming a partial constriction ring that palpates ridgelike may become shorter as the tissue becomes dense and contracts. The Y-V plasty interrupts the continuity of the scar, and the advancement of a triangular wedge of tissue releases the narrowing (Figure 22.6). Excision and release of scar tissue are also possible through this exposure.

The labial cutaneous transposition flap

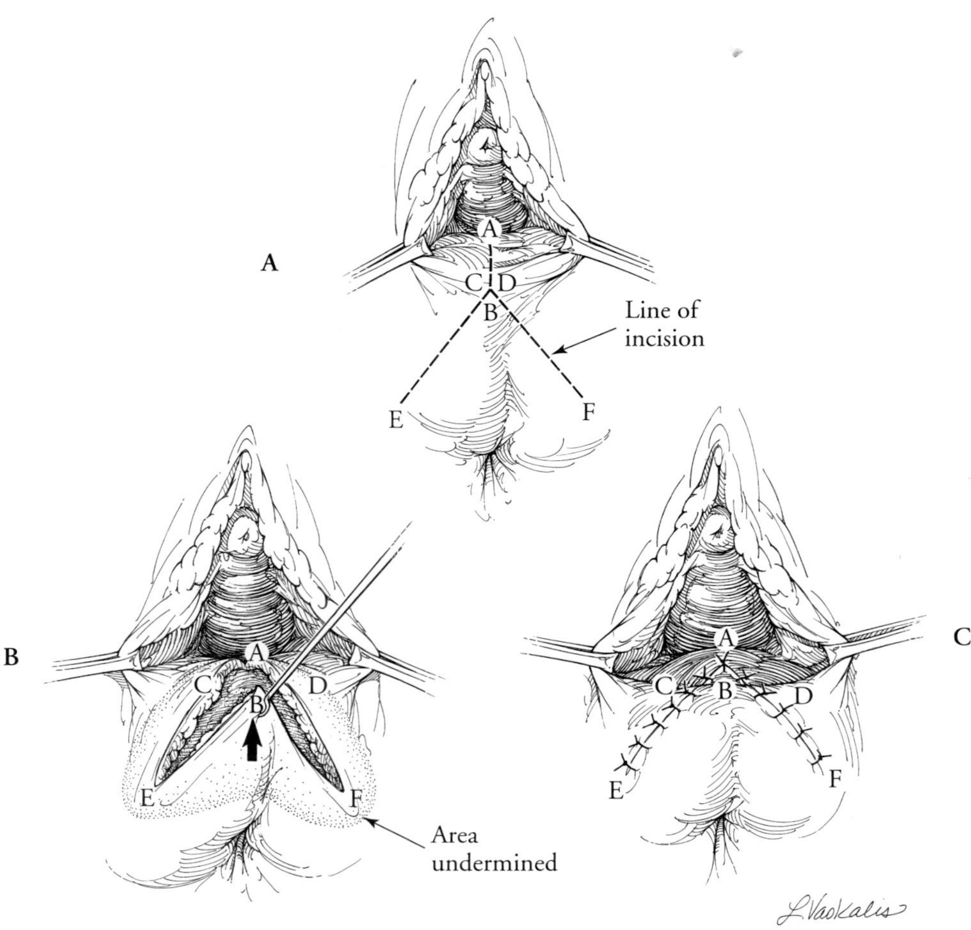

Figure 22.6 Y-V advancement flap. **A,** The initial incision *AB* releases the transverse scar. Incisions *CE* and *DF* form the flap. **B,** The angle of incisions *CE* and *DF* will determine the width of the flap and the subsequent introital aperture as flap *B* is approximated to point *A*. **C,** The triangular flap is secured into position with interrupted sutures. Notice points *C* and *D* in the lateral position.

(Figure 22.7) is useful when a bilateral perineoplasty and/or a Z-plasty and a Y-V plasty have been attempted or have been evaluated as not feasible. The tissue to be rotated and the graft site are marked with a surgical marking pen. Initially the subcutaneous tissue is thoroughly infiltrated with .5% lidocaine (Xylocaine) with epinephrine (Adrenalin) in a concentration of 1:200,000. This step also aids in obliterating the irregularities of the donor site and permitting the line of incision between the dermis and subcutaneous tissue to be visualized even more clearly. The full-thickness skin graft is cut with a no. 15 scalpel blade. Fine sutures can be inserted into the margins of the graft for traction and where identifying marks are located. Skin hooks also may be used for countertraction but Allis' and other crushing clamps should be avoided. Atraumatic technique is important to the success of these flaps, and traction by sutures and skin hooks is used for all handling, including rotating the flap to the new recipient site. Once in good position, initial simple interrupted sutures can be used for maintaining placement until final suturing is accomplished. The amount of fat left on the graft is not critical with this local transposition flap since there is a vascular pedicle at the base. This allows for a somewhat thicker flap and permits some padding. Although the flap may include the risk of containing some of the vulvar hair-bearing area from the labia majora, the risk of troublesome hair growth in the vagina is negligible as the hair follicles usually undergo subsequent atrophy. A labial cutaneous transposition flap may be performed bilat-

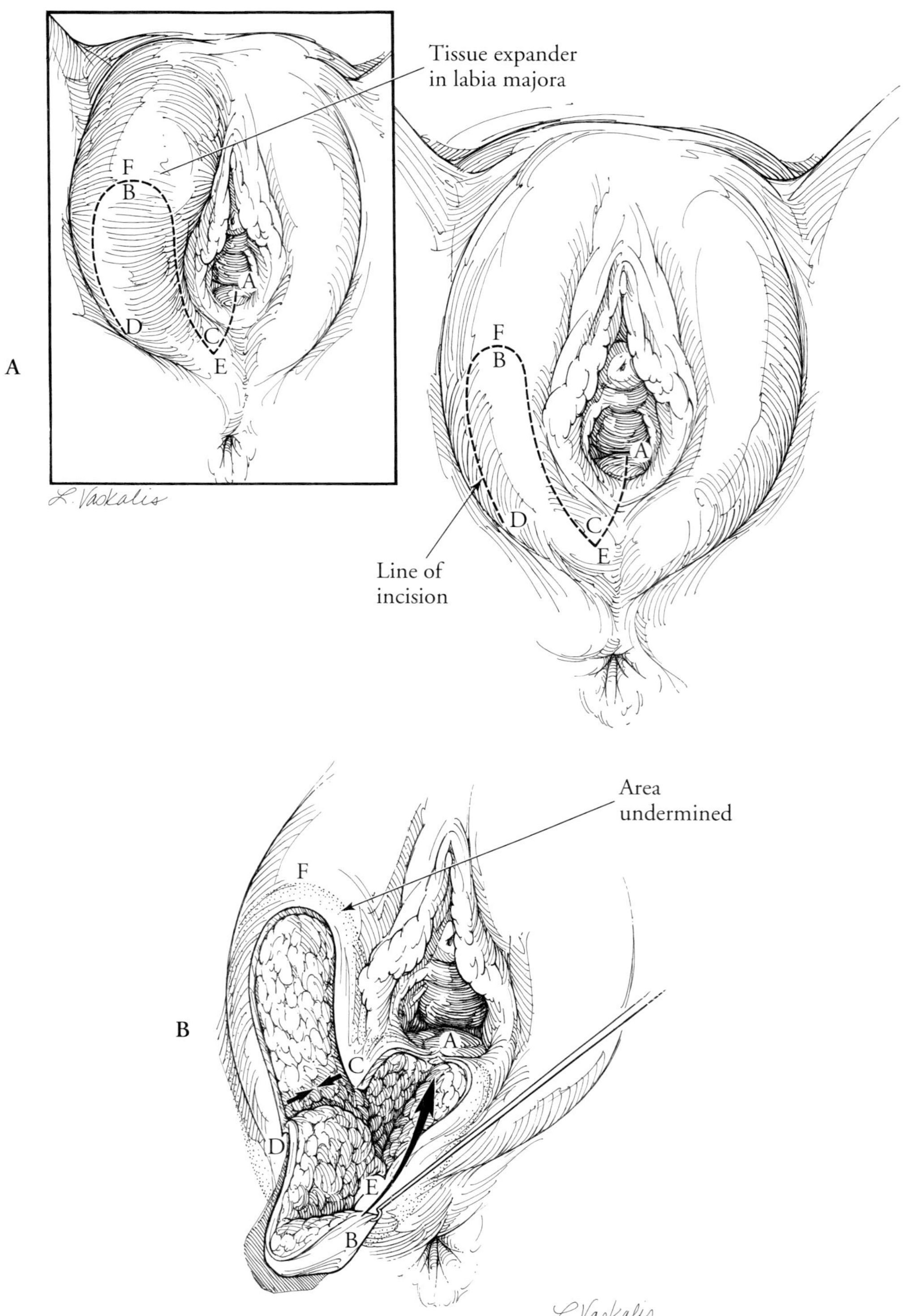

FIGURE 22.7 Labial cutaneous transposition flap. **A,** Execution of the surgical steps in reverse identifies the amount of tissue to be rotated. *Inset,* Same surgical procedure in a patient with a tissue expander. **B,** The flap *DBE* with some attached subcutaneous fat is created and rotated into the incision *AC* created past the introitus and in the vagina. Point *B* is gently brought to oppose point *A*.

Continued.

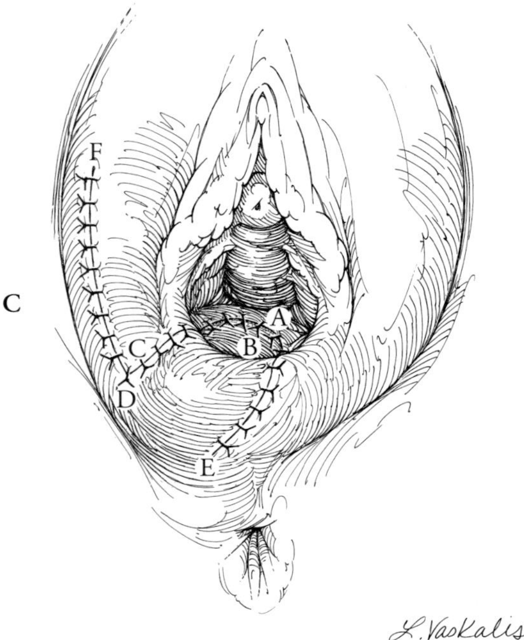

Figure 22.7, cont'd. C, The labial donor site defect and the flap are secured by interrupted sutures. Note the transposition flap *DBE* in new position. Introitus is enlarged by diameter of flap.

erally in a patient requiring still more vulvar space, or swinging of a gracilis cutaneous flap from the medial thigh may be useful. Alternatively, tissue expansion provides donor tissue for reconstruction by increasing the surface area of the skin.[20,21] One alternative approach when more tissue is required would be to use the tissue expansion techniques to create larger labial flaps. Depending on the size of the flaps needed, multiple expanders may be used. However, labial placement of more than one tissue expander may pose the problem of friction between the expanded skin, leading to chafing and erosion. This may be mitigated by the frequent application of lubrication and alteration in lifestyle during the expansion phase. The expansion may require a 6- to 10-week filling phase and to some extent depends on patient tolerance. A rapid-filling phase of 18 days was employed by Lilford, Sharpe, and Thomas[20] in a 14-year-old girl requiring a vaginoplasty. A 250-ml expander may provide a flap of 10 cm long by 8 cm wide. Tissue expanders are easily placed by creating a labial pocket from an inguinal incision to accommodate the expander. Care must be taken to place the expander flat without buckling in order to avoid extrusion during expansion. An expander with a remote injection port helps to prevent accidental trauma to the expander during filling, and a 25-gauge needle may be used to inject normal saline through the remote port. An added feature of tissue expansion is an increase in the vascularity associated with tissue expansion. Clinically the skin over the expander becomes reddened due to hyperemia.

An alternative is the vulvovaginal skin flap rotation, a modified Graves' operation, which is essentially a combination of the transposition and advancement flap techniques.[22] The Graves procedure was initially described as a method of treating vaginal agenesis.[23] When used for vaginal agenesis, four flaps, two from the medial thighs and two from the skin medial to the labia majora, are sewn together and inverted into the recipient site between the bladder and rectum. When an extensive midline stricture of the introitus and the lower half of the vagina is encountered that is more extensive than can be relieved by the above techniques, the two-flap modified Graves procedure provides a useful alternative approach (Figure 22.8). The modified Graves procedure creates two lateral flaps that are first rotated to the midline and sutured together to create a

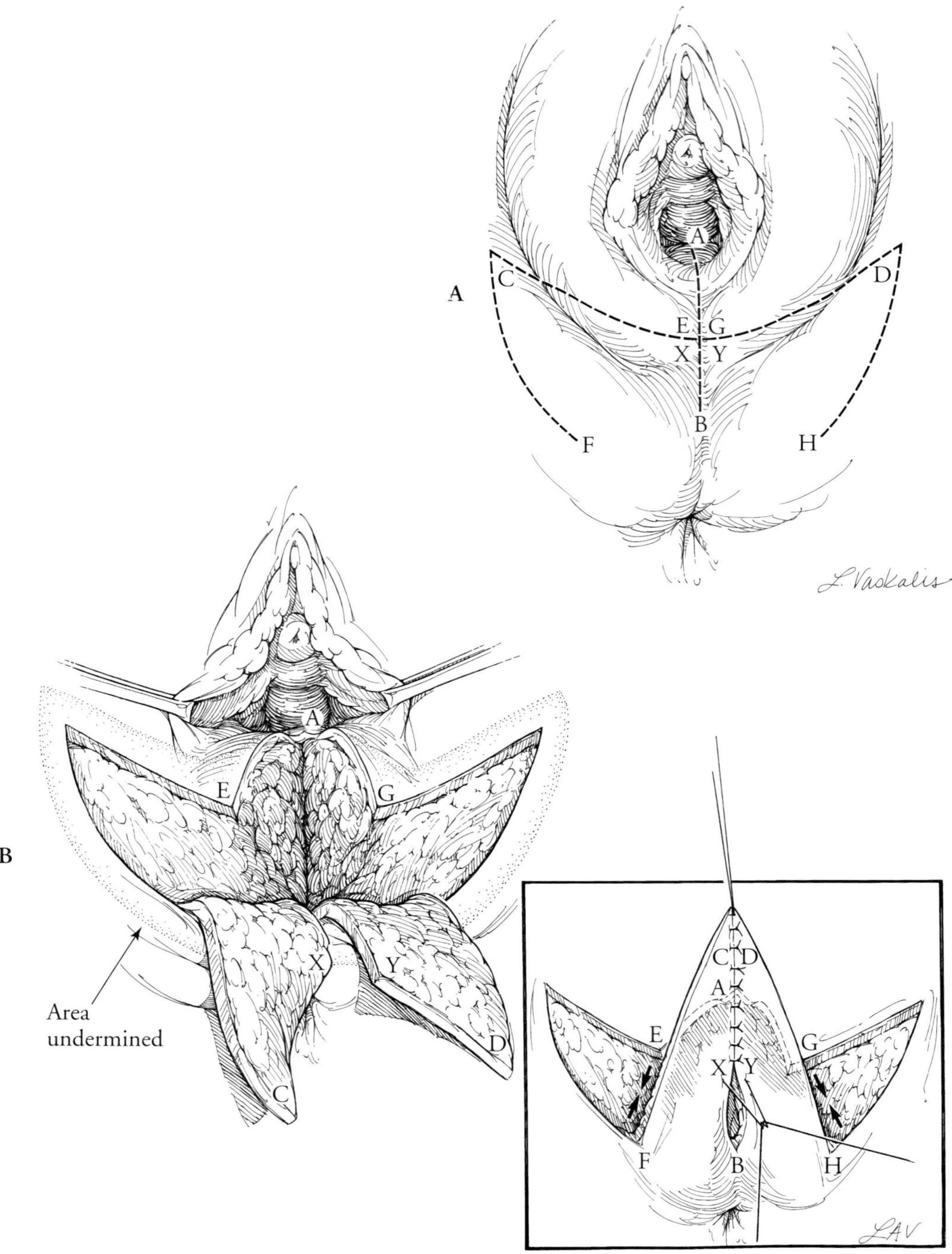

Figure 22.8 Modified Graves' operation. **A,** The flaps to be created are marked with a surgical marking pen. An initial midline incision is made from point *A* to *B.* This is followed by incising the demarcated skin, creating flaps *ECF* and *GDH.* **B,** Full-thickness skin flaps are developed; some subcutaneous tissue is allowed to remain. Surrounding skin is undermined as shown to facilitate mobilization. *Inset,* The medial margins of the flaps are sewn together in the midline. Notice points *CD* at the apex and *XY* at the midflap level. The newly united flap apex *CD* is mobilized by a traction stitch. Point *CD* is brought to point *A* in the vagina, and final flap position is tailored. Excess subcutaneous fat beneath the flap may be trimmed to eliminate contour defects.

Continued.

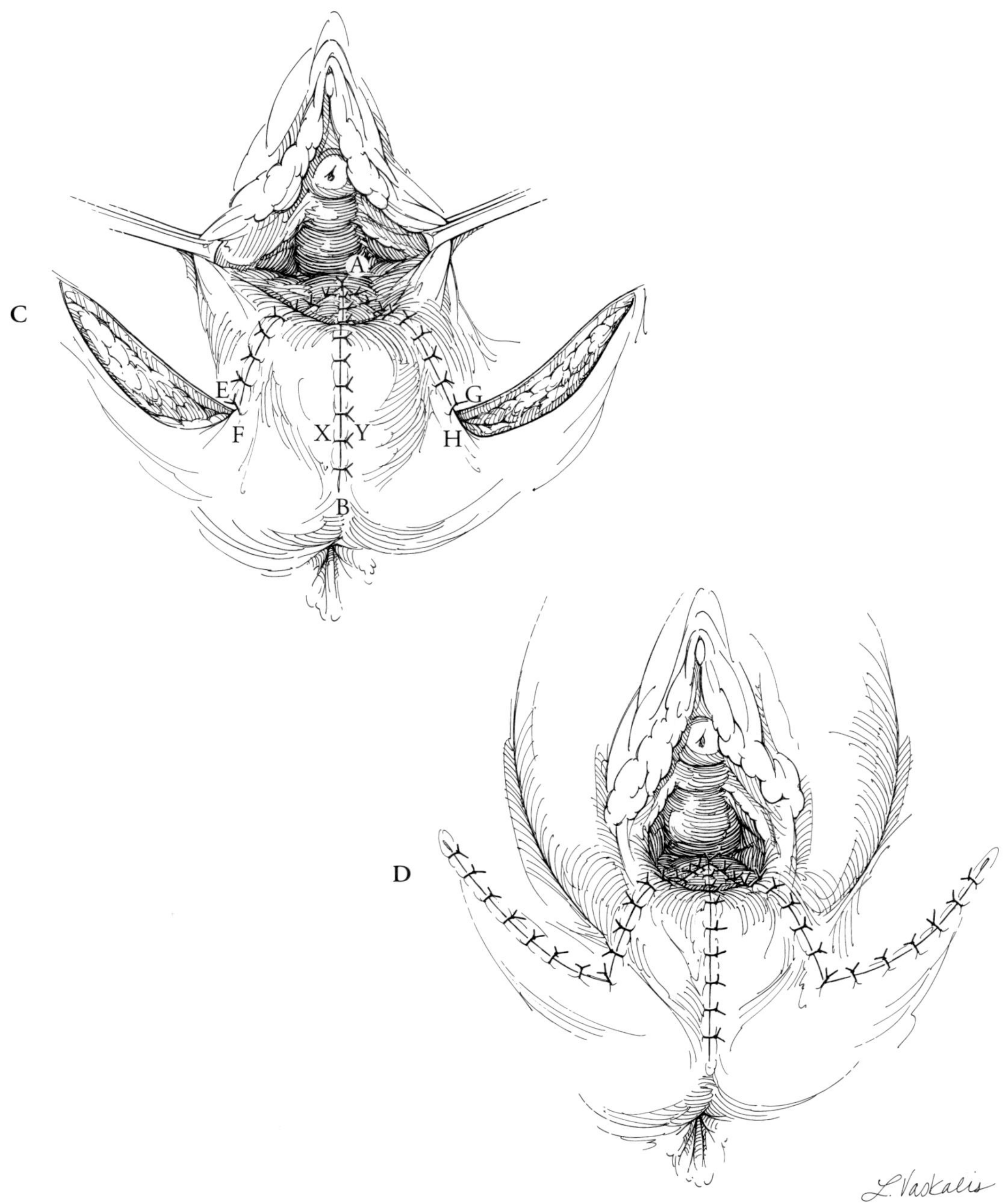

Figure 22.8, cont'd. **C,** Apex of new flap *CD* is secured to vaginal apex *A.* Lateral and distal points *F* and *H* of the flap are secured to points *E* and *G,* respectively. The flap is secured by interrupted sutures from points *CF* and *DH.* **D,** The remaining skin is closed with interrupted stitches. Closed suction drains may be placed beneath the skin flaps and brought out through a separate skin site. Final closed skin closure resembles a W. (Redrawn from Nichols DH and Randall CL: Vaginal surgery, ed 7, Baltimore, 1996, Williams & Wilkins.)

single inverted V-shaped flap. The second step is the advancement of the inverted V into the vagina. The incision lines required are a midline *(AB),* and two lateral V-shaped flaps, *(ECF)* and *(GDH).* Once the full-thickness flaps are raised, they are sutured together along their medial borders (*CX* and *DY*) to create a single inverted V-shaped flap *(FCDH).* When the flap is advanced past the introitus into the vagina, points *E* and *F* and points *G* and *H* will be approximated and sutured together. This is the maximum amount of advancement. The apex of the inverted V is gently pulled and sutured to point *A*.

MIDVAGINAL STRICTURE

Having an intrapelvic unbounded upper end, the vault of the vagina tends to be easily expandable. It is the midvagina that has limited expansion, and therefore defects appear as an hourglass deformity (Figure 22.9, *A*). Several intraoperative options exist when a midvaginal hourglass or full-length narrowing is observed at the completion of a reconstructive procedure or colporrhaphy due to excision of a little too much vagina. Palpable bands or ridges in the vagina that are localized at the conclusion of surgery may be adequately managed with simple lateral relaxing incisions[24] through the full thickness of the vaginal wall at the 3 and 9 o'clock positions (Figure 22.9, *B*). This is easily achieved with the scalpel blade. Palpation and repalpation will determine the extent of the incision and dissection. If the incision is rather large and the excised vaginal tissue is still available, an autograft may be placed to cover the defect.[24] Simply, a section of excised vagina is tailored to fit the elliptical defect. The full-thickness vaginal graft is then secured with interrupted 3-0 polyglycolic acid sutures (Figure 22.9, *C*). A grafted stricture release with full-thickness vagina or skin develops the least amount of contracture from scar tissue postoperatively. If vaginal tissue is not available, a donor site for a full-thickness skin harvest is an option.

A simple relaxing incision should be followed by the immediate use of a vaginal appliance and continued until complete healing has occurred to counteract the contraction effects of healing by secondary intention. A grafted stricture release will also require a vaginal appliance to ensure adequate vaginal caliber. However, the immediate use may be deferred until the initial postoperative edema has resolved and an office visit has confirmed good take of the graft. The duration of vaginal appliance therapy with relaxing incisions should be continued until healing by secondary intention is complete. A grafted stricture release with a full-thickness graft will require a shorter duration of intravaginal appliance therapy.

The management of a full-length decrease in caliber can be effectively addressed if the freshly excised vaginal tissue is still available. The excised vaginal wall from the anterior or posterior segments or both is evaluated for adequacy as well as "crush-spots," which ought to be excised if possible. After the posterior colporrhaphy is taken down, a free wedge of full-thickness vaginal wall autograft is placed between the posterior vaginal wall incisions. The graft is sewn with interrupted sutures of 3-0 polyglycolic acid sutures to each vaginal edge. If a single section of vaginal wall is not large enough to cover the defect, then two small sections will work nicely.

If identification of a stricture or narrowing should occur at some future postoperative time, the management may consist of relaxing incisions for small ridges and perhaps placement of an autograft of harvested free full-thickness skin from which the subcutaneous fat has been removed. The free skin graft may be placed laterally for hourglass strictures or along the full length of the posterior vaginal wall and perineum. Frequently, a narrowed introitus accompanies a full-length caliber decrease.

Alternatively, a lateral transposition flap is an option that allows some of the underlying fat to act as a cushion since a vascular pedicle exists at the base. This approach may also permit excision of a painful mediolateral episiotomy scar while providing added tissue to fill the gap and some subcutaneous fat to serve as padding. The use of a tissue expander broadens this approach to offer more tissue, allowing a longer and/or wider flap. Irrespective of the surgical procedure—a free full-thickness skin graft or a lateral transposition flap—infiltration at the site of harvest and at the site of vaginal incision or excision with 20 ml of .5% lidocaine with 1:200,000 epinephrine will produce a "liquid tourniquet" effect. Hemostasis must be optimal if a skin graft is to take. Bleeding points may be coagulated or ligated with fine suture. Needless to say, hematoma formation will prevent graft take by acting as a barrier and, if under tension, by decreasing blood flow, in addition to serving as a medium for infection.

The surgical construction or reconstruction of the vaginal caliber and/or length is best complemented with a vaginal appliance to optimize results. Relaxing incisions unsup-

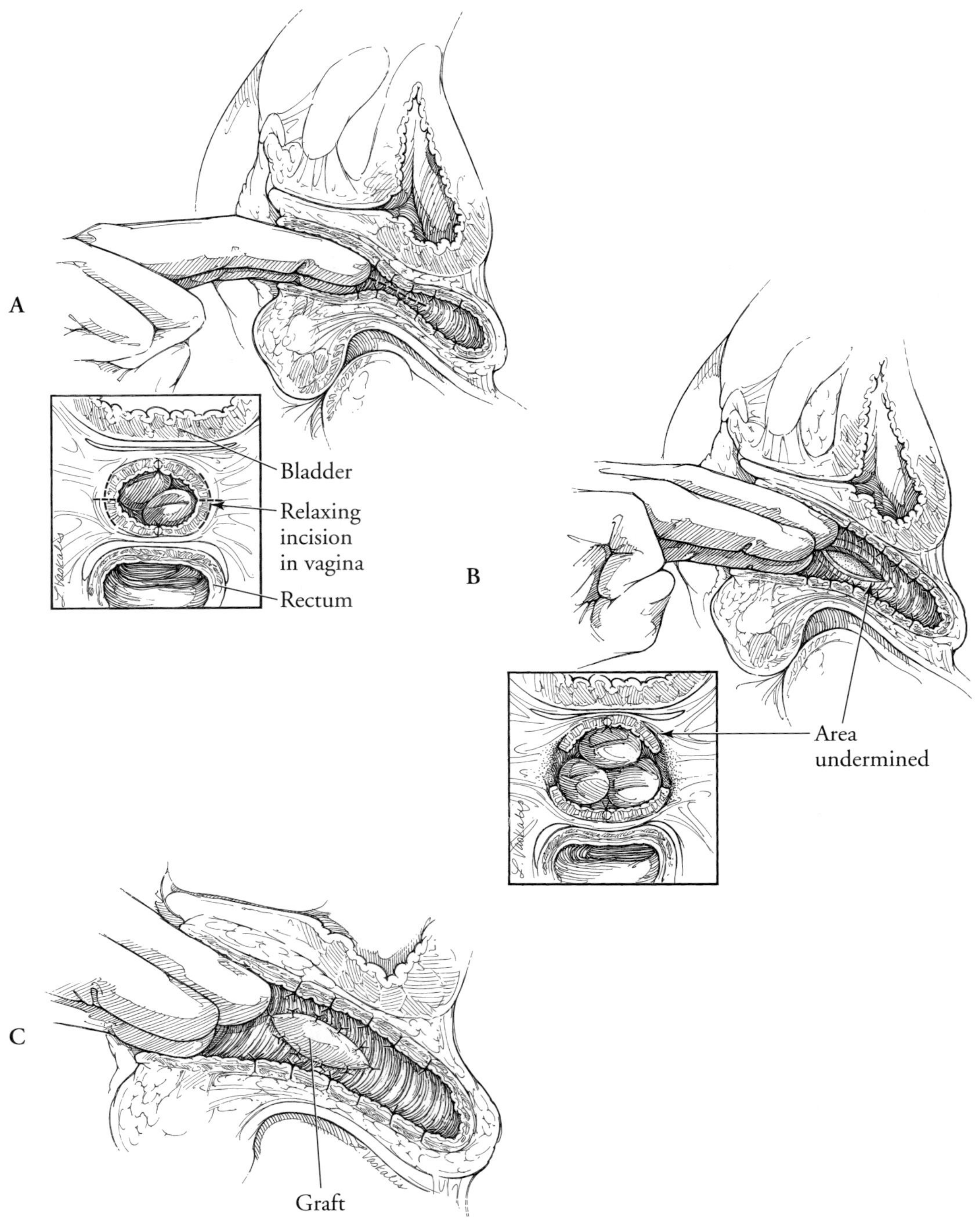

Figure 22.9 Midvaginal stricture. **A,** Digital examination discloses a midvaginal stricture in which the vagina has an hourglass configuration and will admit but two fingerwidths. *Insets,* The site of the lateral relaxing incision is indicated by the *dotted line.* The vaginal wall is also undermined for a centimeter in each direction perpendicular to the relaxing incision *(dotted lines)* in each direction, so that the vaginal caliber will admit three fingerwidths. **B,** The length and extent of the stricture is released by the full-thickness incision *(dotted line)* of the lateral vaginal wall at the 3 and usually 9 o'clock position. Note elliptical defect created during the dissection used to release the stricture. **C,** A full-thickness graft of the proper size may be fitted into the defect in the lateral vaginal wall created by the relaxing incisions. The graft may be from previously excised vagina if the stricture is identified at the time of a colporrhaphy, or a full-thickness skin graft at a later time. The graft is held in place by a few interrupted stitches. (Redrawn from Nichols DH and Randall CL: Vaginal surgery, ed 3, Baltimore, 1989, Williams & Wilkins.)

ported by grafting will heal very effectively by secondary intention but risk scar formation and contraction. Therefore such a patient should if possible be fitted at surgery with a vaginal appliance. Postoperative instructions may include a regimen of intermittent use, 20 to 30 minutes, several times during the day as well as continuous use during sleep for the first 2 or 3 weeks. This regimen during the initial several weeks of healing will avoid contraction by scar until a firm base of epithelialized granulation tissue has been established. Similarly, when grafts are utilized a short course of vaginal dilation started 7 to 10 days after grafting is beneficial. A plastic vaginal appliance of the required diameter that can be retained within the vagina for intermittent extended periods of time during the day and/or night is optimal. (The 2.5 and/or 3.5 cm in diameter graduated Lucite dilators, from 3 to 11 cm, developed by Ingram are manufactured by Faulkner Plastics, Inc, Tampa, Florida, and are available as sets within each of the diameters. Alternatively, individual dilators and a set of eight dilators with a fixed length of 15 cm and a variable diameter ranging from 1.0 to 4.5 cm are available from PM Designs, Inc, Boston, Massachusetts, as the Clarix vaginal dilator.) The Ingram and the Clarix appliances are cleaned with soap and water only between applications; they should not be boiled or autoclaved because high temperature will soften and glaze the Lucite. An office set permits preoperative assessment and can be gas sterilized. The selected vaginal appliance ideally would be just slightly wider than the required vaginal caliber at rest.

The patient may use as an appliance-obturator the barrel of a disposable plastic 60-cc conventional syringe or an Asepto syringe with the distal projecting tip removed, if a conventional acrylic or glass appliance is not available. Too often, however, the width of the barrel is not appropriate, or the barrel is too long, making extended postoperative therapy awkward, and the plastic edges may be painful if imprecisely trimmed. The appliance should be inserted as frequently as one's lifestyle and work permit for the initial 2 to 6 weeks. Lidocaine jelly in a 2%, 5%, or 20% concentration helps lubricate the appliance and provides some anesthesia. Intravaginal estrogen cream also may be used and is encouraged. Coitus after 2 weeks is not contraindicated and is best left to the patient's discretion.

VAGINAL LENGTH

When the vagina is of adequate diameter but is too short for coitus, depth may be added nonsurgically or surgically. Surgical length may be added at the vault or at the introitus with a Williams' vulvovaginoplasty. A coitally shallow vagina that has been shortened from previous vaginal surgery but maintained with adequate diameter can be managed nonsurgically as well as surgically. Candidates also include patients who have experienced partial vaginectomy, radical pelvic surgery, and post-McIndoe contraction. The nonsurgical treatment is an application of the Ingram bicycle seat technique, on which the patient sits at intervals each day using the wider 2.5 cm Ingram Lucite dilators. Duration of dilation will be shorter in simple posthysterectomy foreshortening and longer in patients treated by radical hysterectomy with radiation. McIndoe acknowledged that failures after inlay skin grafting resulted from improper management of the contractile phase.[11,25,26] This underscores that attempts to create a neovagina by any method should preferably be postponed until the patient is mature enough both physically and psychologically to cooperate. This is never more true than when the patient is responsible for the creation of her own vagina. A highly motivated mature patient will have the best chance of nonsurgical elongation of the vagina, though it may take up to a year. There is discomfort associated with this therapy, and lidocaine gel in a concentration from 2% to 20% is available and recommended to serve as both lubricant and anesthetic. Perhaps all patients with a shortened vaginal canal should be given a trial of conservative management while they await surgical therapy even if they insist on surgery. This is in part because all these patients will postoperatively require long-term management with a vaginal appliance (obturator) until they experience frequent coitus to ensure maintenance of length.

When the nonsurgical approach has been of limited benefit and further depth is required, construction of a new upper vagina may be accomplished by a partial split-thickness skin graft procedure. Although Abbe[27] and later McIndoe and Bannister[25] constructed a primary full-length neovagina using split-thickness skin grafts, the same principles apply to partial upper neovaginal construction. The reconstruction consists of incising the vaginal vault and creating an upper vascular recipient pocket (Figure 22.10, *A*). The skin graft donor site is chosen by the patient preoperatively. The buttock has the advantage of being more cosmetically acceptable, but a drawback is discomfort sitting until the donor site is healed. Other sites for consideration include the mons as well as the medial, lateral, posterior, and anterior thigh.

Removing a graft of split-thickness skin from its donor site is based on the principle that a sharp oscillating blade cuts into the skin at a predetermined thickness. This is usually controlled by a calibrated setting and chosen by the surgeon, usually 0.018 inches. The uniform thickness of a graft may also be checked as it is being cut by observing its translucency and the bleeding pattern of the donor's skin. The choice of instrument, knife, and drum-type, electrical, or air-driven dermatome usually depends on the surgeon's experience. Sterile mineral oil lubricates the donor site and reduces friction so the instrument can move forward smoothly. As the graft appears on the upper blade surface, an assistant lifts the graft to prevent blade bunching and ensures proper thickness. The flat graft is placed between moist layers of gauze.

After the split-thickness skin graft has been harvested, the donor site containing the hair follicles heals by epithialization. The donor site may be dressed with adaptic, xeroform, rayon cloth, or Opsite. The use of a semipermeable polyurethane membrane such as Opsite has been reported to be associated with almost complete absence of pain and discomfort as epithelialization continues[28]; with any method, the dressing comes away in about 14 days. When the site is completely exposed, it is lubricated with cocoa butter or lanolin.

If the harvested strip of split-thickness skin (usually 0.018 inch thick) is too narrow, it may be passed through a meshing device to expand and fenestrate the graft. This increases the surface area and allows for drainage. However, this is the exception rather than the rule as troublesome granulation tissue may develop at the site of each fenestration. The graft is usually tailored to conform to a soft stent and secured to itself by absorbable suture. The graft is held in constant opposition at the recipient site by a soft stent, which is removed between the seventh and tenth postoperative day. Following inspection, any extra graft tissue beyond the recipient site at the introitus may be easily trimmed at this time.

Long-term postoperative care and the success of a partial upper inlay-graft neovagina is very dependent on the patient's compliance with continued dilation of the new vaginal canal for at least 6 months. As recognized and emphasized by McIndoe, most failures of inlay skin grafting were the result of improper management of the contractile phase of the graft, as discussed previously in the section on basic concepts of tissue manipulation in reconstructive surgery. It is the secondary contraction of the recipient bed that plagues both the patient and the surgeon. The recipient bed contraction continues for up to 6 months, allowing and forcing the graft to wrinkle. The thin graft's inherent ability to inhibit and/or prevent contraction of the recipient bed is a dynamic process of contraction and countertraction between the recipient bed and graft, respectively. This dynamic process is altered as a function of graft thickness. A thicker skin graft will have less tendency to undergo secondary contraction because it contains sufficient dermis to afford resiliency and provides a stable interface to reduce and inhibit recipient bed contraction. A drawback of thick grafts is the necessity of split-thickness grafting of the donor site.

Horton has employed full-thickness skin grafts for construction of a neovagina in 50 patients with a 15-year follow-up.[29] The long-term advantages are virtually no shrinkage and the ability of the neovagina to grow with the patient.[29] Elliptical full-thickness skin grafts (14 × 6 cm) are obtained from the lateral hairless groin areas bilaterally.[30] The fat is removed from the undersurface of the skin and subsequently prepared in the same manner as a split-thickness graft. The donor sites are closed, primarily avoiding the healing phase required of a split-thickness donor site.

Similarly, a partial upper full-thickness skin graft vaginoplasty to treat a shallow vagina has

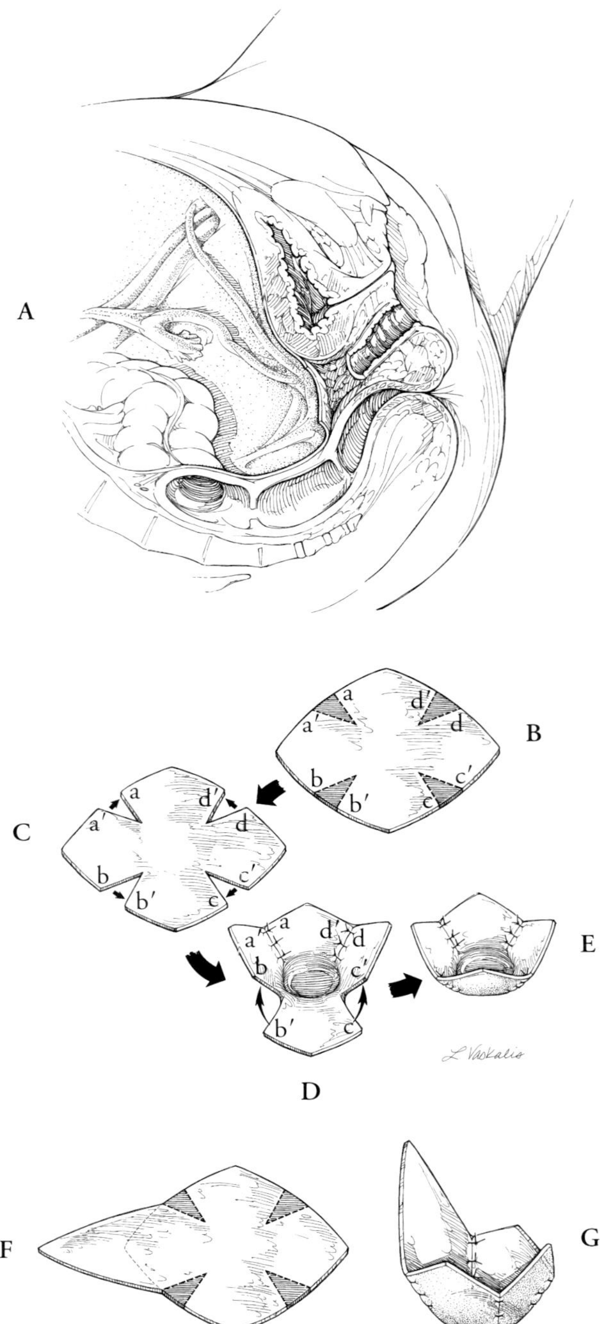

FIGURE 22.10 Vaginal elongation. **A,** The vaginal apex of the shortened vagina is opened, and a vaginal space is created up to the cul-de-sac peritoneum. Note that the peritoneum has been dissected off the posterior wall of the bladder and the anterior wall of the rectum. **B,** An elliptical full-thickness skin graft has been harvested and the subcutaneous fat removed. Four V-shaped wedges to be excised are marked by the dotted lines. **C** and **D,** Once the wedges have been excised, points *a, b, c,* and *d* are sutured to their respective counterpoint a^{I}, b^{I}, c^{I}, and d^{II}, by interrupted stitches. **E,** The folded tailored skin graft "cup" is ready for placement into the prepared recipient site. **F** and **G,** A variation of the full-thickness skin graft is a "cup" with a single extension that permits addition of vaginal length as well as concomitant restoration of caliber.

Continued.

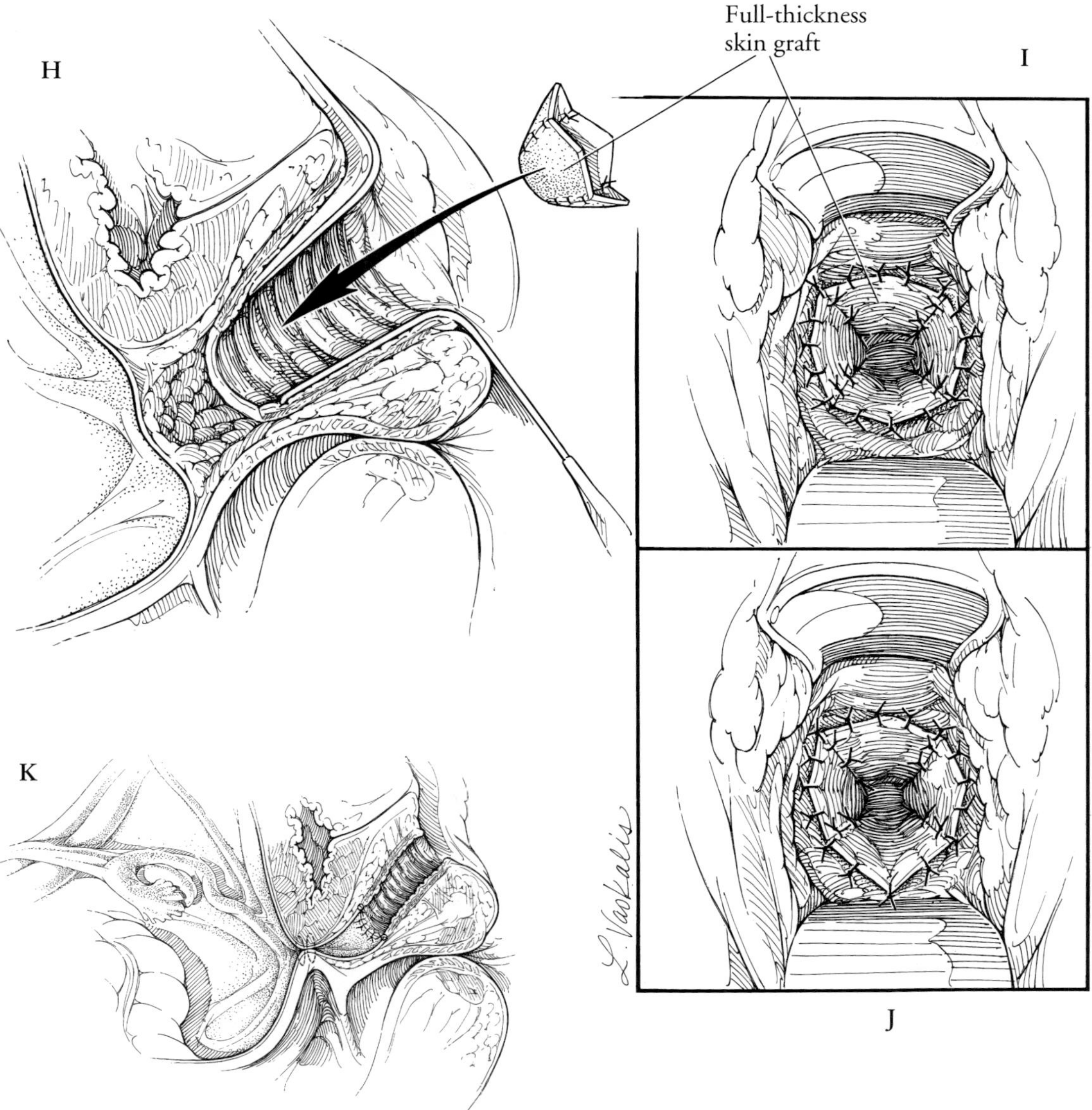

FIGURE 22.10, cont'd. H, The vaginal space having been created by mobilization of the peritoneum, the folded full-thickness skin graft "cup" is approximated to the recipient site. *Inset I,* The skin graft "cup" is sutured into position by interrupted stitches. *Inset J,* Skin graft "cup" with single posterior extension providing length and additional caliber is also secured by interrupted stitches. A split-thickness skin graft also may be used. **K,** An alternative to the full-thickness and split-thickness skin graft is the use of peritoneum as an advancement flap to cover the newly created upper vaginal space. The mobilized peritoneum from the bladder, rectum, and cul-de-sac is incised and pulled to the apex of the shortened vagina. The peritoneum is secured to the vagina by interrupted stitches. The new vaginal length is determined by the placement of the purse-string sutures into the peritoneum and subperitoneal retinaculum, which also establishes the new cul-de-sac.

been described by Morley and DeLancey.[31] An elliptical skin incision is made over the iliac crest, and a 10- by 3-cm section of full-thickness skin, which includes the dermis and epidermis, is harvested. The donor site is closed primarily. The full-thickness skin graft is easily tailored to fit the recipient site due to its elasticity. Sharp dissection should be used to clean the subcutaneous fat off the undersurface of all full-thickness skin grafts. Removal of the fat allows the take to occur between the dermis and the recipient bed. The graft is then sutured to the recipient bed by 3-0 polyglycologic acid sutures. Full-thickness grafts also may be placed at the time of partial vaginectomy to prevent postoperative shortening.[32] The placement of the graft or grafts may be achieved by several free grafts or by folding of the graft (Figure 22.10, *B* to *G*). Tailoring of the graft will provide the best fit into the recipient bed (Figure 22.10, *H*). Separate grafts allow for drainage, preventing the collection of fluid behind the graft. However, the nongrafted recipient bed will undergo contraction. Drainage also can be achieved by "piecrusting" a graft and creating areas of drainage.

Although a moulage can and should be created preoperatively with consideration to the donor site, the actual surface area will be determined after creating the upper vaginal recipient bed or at the time of vaginectomy. Intraoperatively sterile Telfa paper is invaluable in determining the precise amount of donor tissue required. This avoids complication due to inadequate or excess excision from the donor site and ensures enough tissue to cover the recipient bed, possibly from a single donor site. Depending on anticipated patient compliance, age, hormonal status, and/or coital partner with respect to the required length and tissue availability, a thoughtful consideration should be tolerance for anticipated shrinkage. However, this is more relevant to split-thickness grafts and must be performed with caution because considerable overcorrection and unnecessary exposure of the cul-de-sac of Douglas may lead to enterocele formation. On the other hand, as Amreich has pointed out, a short vagina that ends anterior to the levator plate will tend with time to become even shorter, as intraabdominal pressure may be transmitted in the axis of the vagina.[33]

A rather unique application of the transposition-flap principle is the Davydov peritoneal transplantation.[34,35,36] The procedure is a transposition of widely mobilized parietal peritoneum to line the cavity of the neovagina. The procedure may be performed concomitantly with radical hysterectomy while the abdomen is open or at the time of a vaginectomy. During the preparation of the recipient bed for a partial- or full-thickness skin graft, should the peritoneum be entered the surgeon then has the option of the Davydov peritoneal transposition (Figure 22.10, *I*). However, if the intent is to perform a Davydov and peritoneal entry becomes difficult due to scar tissue, the procedure also may be assisted by laparoscopy or in conjunction with laparoscopy being performed for another indication. Peritoneal entry also may be facilitated by instillation of indigo carmine solution in the bladder or by aspiration of peritoneal fluid by culdocentesis, as well as by digital palpation through the patient's rectum. Laparoscopically assisted mobilization of the peritoneum has the advantage of evaluating the pelvis, lysis of any adhesions, and directing mobilization before entering the cul-de-sac. Regardless of the surgical approach, the peritoneal dissection is continued circumferentially until a sufficient amount has been exposed to line the recipient vaginal bed. Once opened, the edge of the peritoneum is pulled to ensure adequate length and mobilization. The peritoneal edge is then sutured to the vaginal margin with interrupted 3-0 polyglycolic acid. The peritoneal cavity is then closed with several purse-string sutures, and the peritoneum is separately sutured to the wall of the bladder and rectum with 3-0 polyglycolic acid sutures to reduce distal tension. If a laparoscopy has been performed, inspection of the most cephalad purse-string suture will identify any peritoneal defect, which may be repaired by additional laparoscopic suturing. To prevent agglutination of the newly constructed partial upper vaginal peritoneal surfaces, a vaginal obturator is maintained for a minimum of 7 to 10 days. Coitus is permissible 2 weeks after surgery. The peritoneum is replaced by squamous epithelium from metaplastic transformation and/or growth from the vaginal edges. It assumes an acidic pH and undergoes cyclic changes.

Another versatile operation to create a neovagina was developed by Vecchietti as an abdominovaginal operation.[37] However, the operation also may be accomplished laparoscopically, which avoids the discomfort and disfigurement of a laparatomy scar.[32] In theory it is similar to the intermittent pressure technique of Frank and Ingram. The principal mechanism is a constant, round-the-clock traction requiring but 7 to 10 days to produce a vagina 9 to 10 cm in length. The pressure is delivered by a 1.5 cm acrylic "olive" attached to a suprapubic-mounted spring-traction device via the action of threads passed extraperitoneally. The constant upward traction to the olive is adjusted daily sufficient to advance the olive about 1 cm per day through the newly created invagination. Postoperatively the patient wears a vaginal dilator until intercourse is initiated. Although the invagination of Vecchietti was described for primary construction of a neovagina, it has been applied successfully to increase the depth of a foreshortened vagina (Figure 22.11). The above methods all add vaginal depth; an alternative is the Williams vulvovaginoplasty,[38] which adds length at the introitus.

The Williams procedure utilizes the full-thickness skin flaps of both labia majora, which are mobilized to the midline to produce an elongation of the vagina at the in-

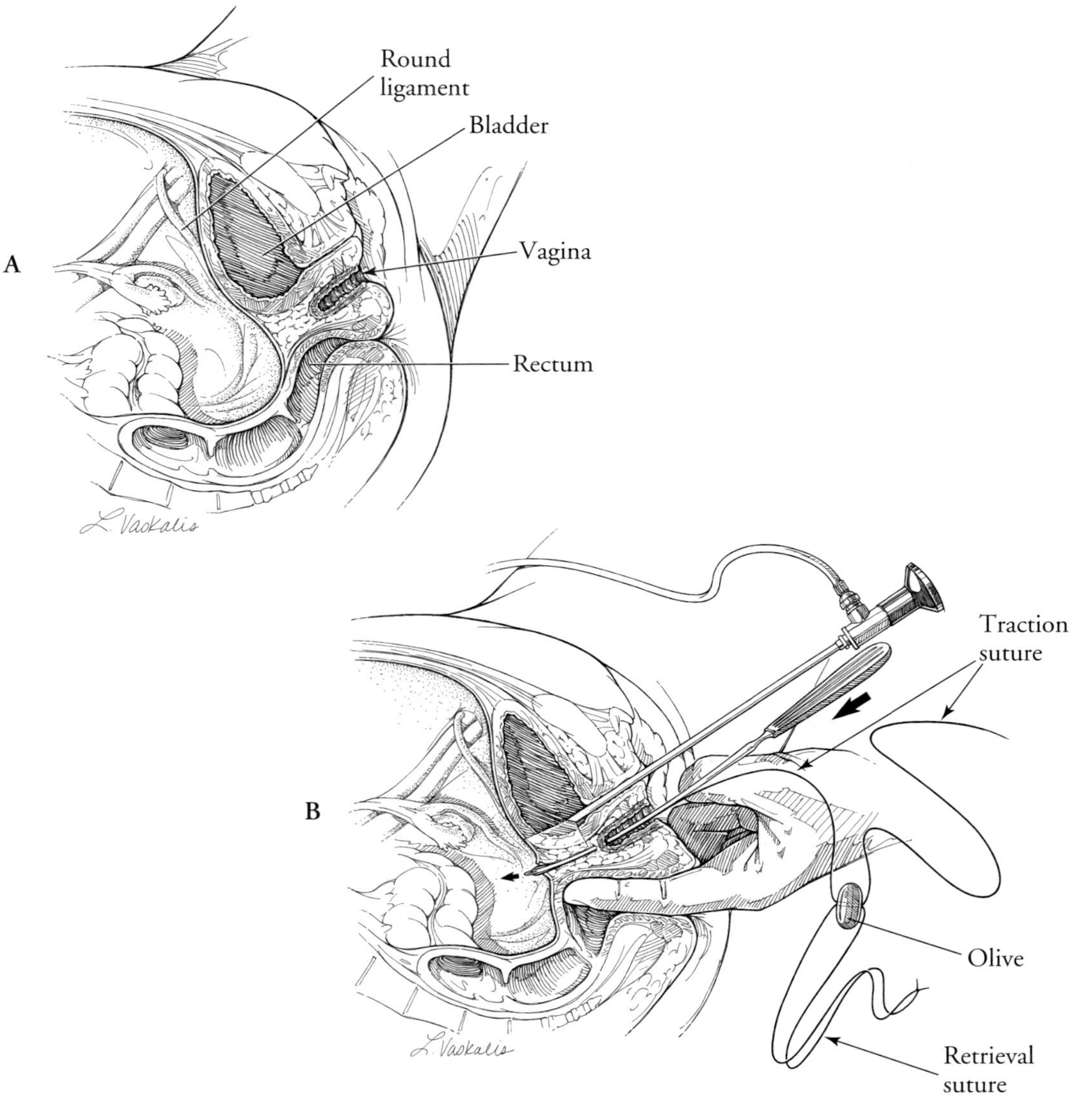

FIGURE 22.11 The Vecchietti operation. **A,** Anatomic relationships of cul-de-sac, bladder, rectum, and vault of short vagina. **B,** Under direct cystoscopic guidance and transrectal palpation, the straight Vecchietti ligature carrier is introduced through the cul-de-sac into the peritoneal cavity. Note one end of the traction suture is passed through the ligature carrier and "olive." A retrieval suture is also threaded into the "olive."

Continued.

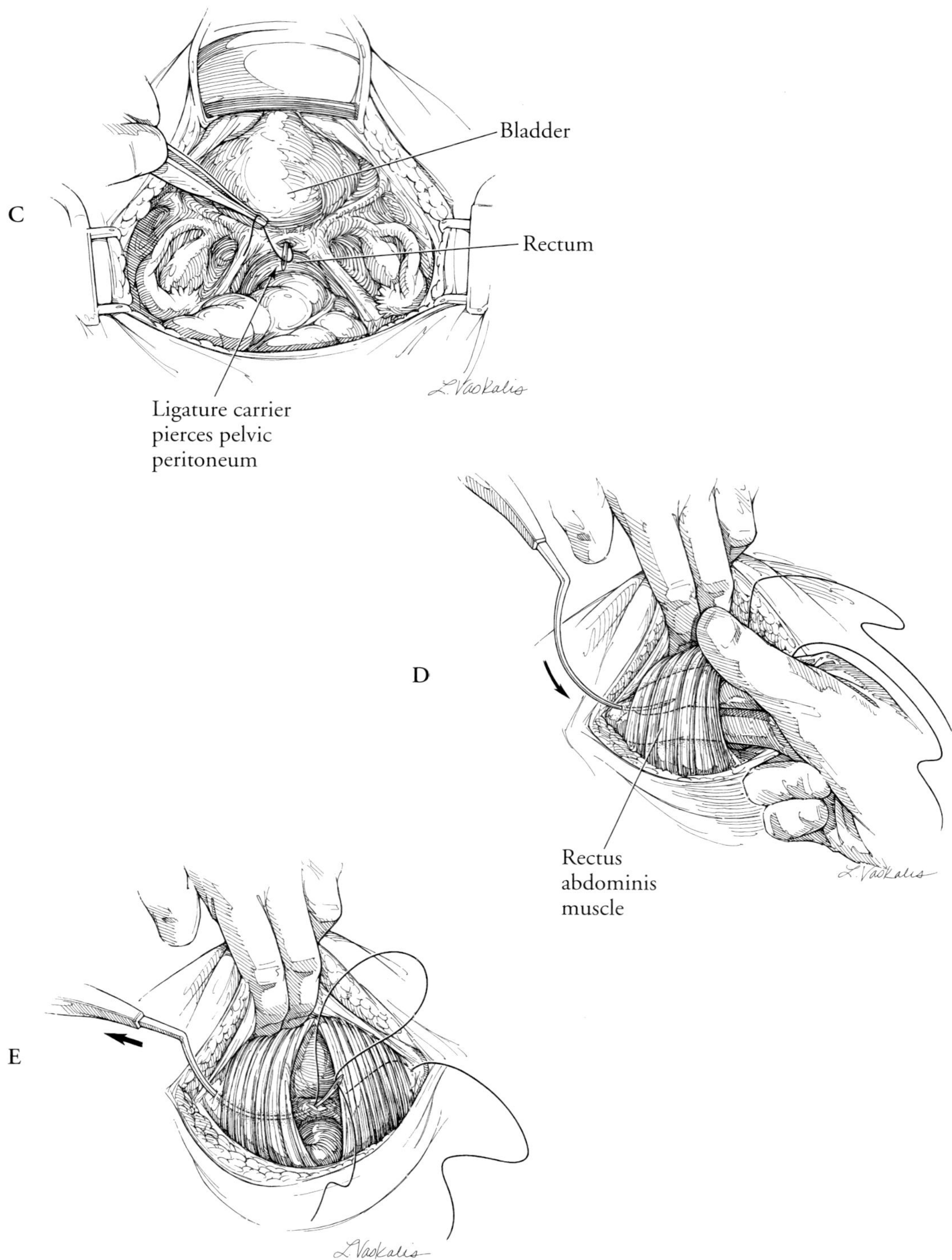

Figure 22.11, cont'd. **C,** Exposure through a laparotomy showing retrieval of the first end of the traction suture. A second pass will be required 1 cm apart to bring the other end of the traction suture into the pelvis. Alternatively, a single-pass technique would bring both sutures into the pelvis at the same point. **D,** The curved Vecchietti ligature carrier is passed lateral to the rectus muscles and under the peritoneum. **E,** The tip of the curved ligature carrier is brought through the initial opening in the cul-de-sac peritoneum created by the straight ligature carrier.

Continued.

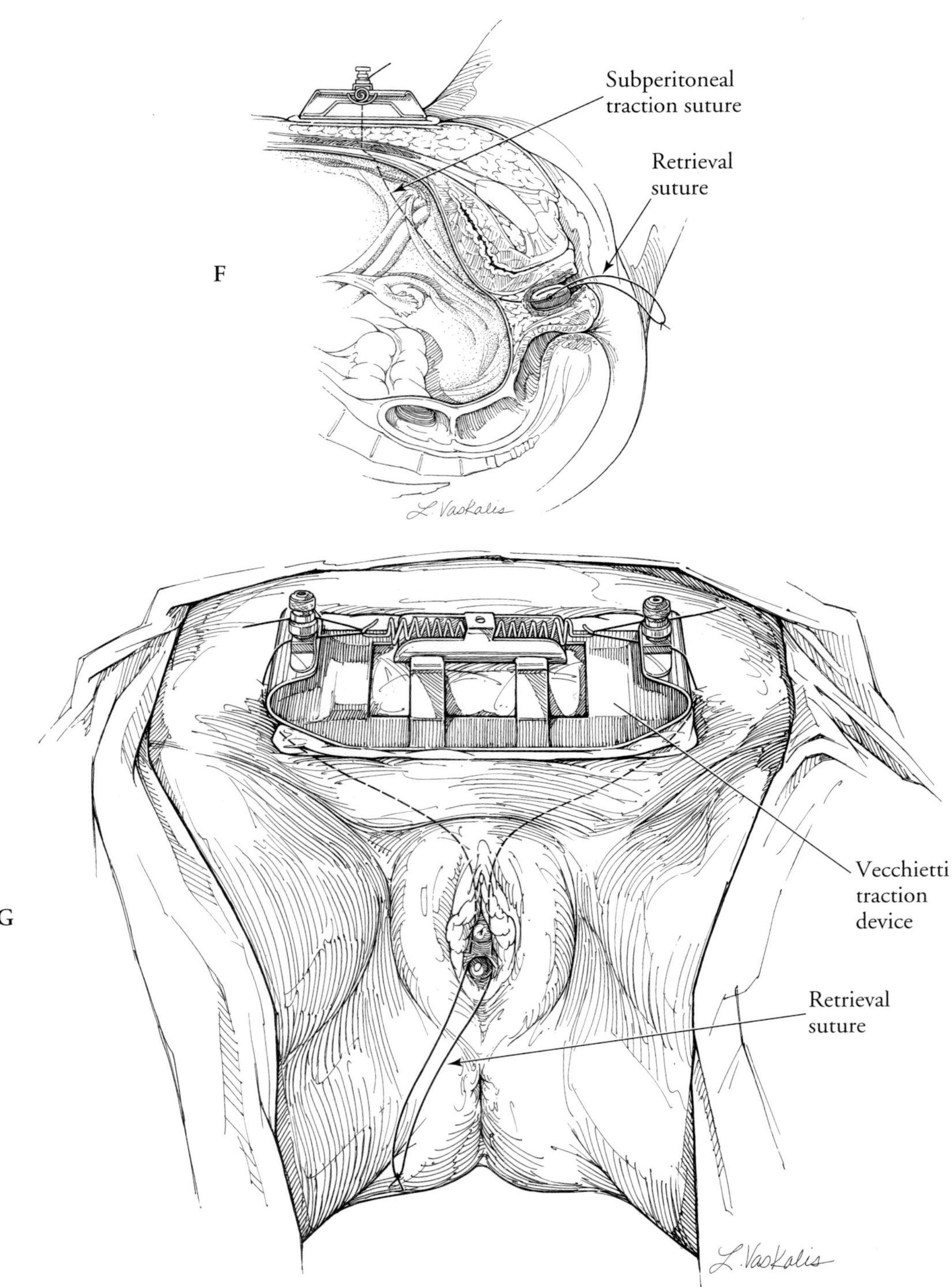

Figure 22.11, cont'd. **F**, Longitudinal view of "olive," traction sutures, and traction device in initial traction position. Note subperitoneal traction suture in the approximate path of the round ligament and over the iliac vessels. **G**, Suprapubic view of "olive," path of traction sutures, and traction device. (Redrawn from Nichols DH and Randall CL: Vaginal surgery, ed 4, Baltimore, 1996, Williams & Wilkins.)

troitus. A prerequisite is the availability of well-developed mobile labia majora. Although initially the vaginal axis is slightly more vertical, this has not proven to be a persistent impediment to coitus. With patience on the part of the patient and her partner, further depth may be added by wearing a progressively longer obturator and by frequent coitus. A gradual change to a more normal axis is achieved by a posterior rotation of the pouch, and with sustained use a normal vaginal depth and axis can be approximated.

The Williams vulvovaginoplasty is initiated by marking the most upper lateral edges of the U-shaped incision with a marking pen (Figure 22.12). These are located 4 cm lateral to the inferior portion of the urethra. The

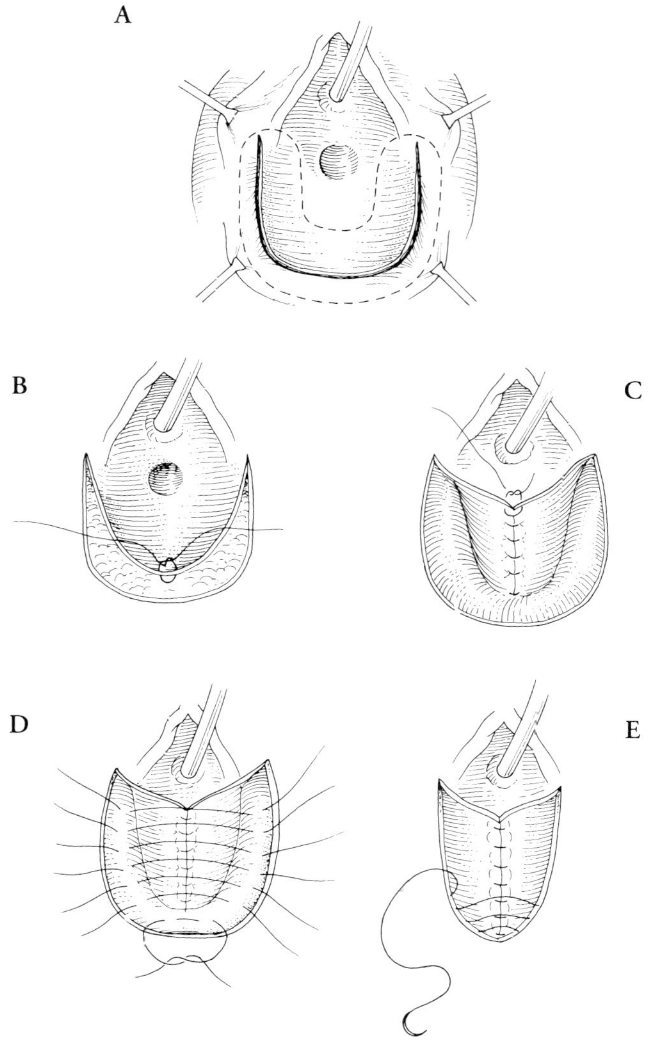

Figure 22.12 Williams vulvovaginoplasty. **A,** A U-shaped incision is created beginning approximately 4 cm lateral to the external urethral meatus *(dotted line).* **B,** The edges of the new vaginal pouch are undermined, creating flaps. The internal surface is approximated with interrupted stitches placed in such a fashion that the knots are within the vagina. **C,** This is continued until the level of the anterior hymenal site is reached. **D,** A perineorrhaphy may also be performed, and a second layer of interrupted sutures approximates the subepithelial tissue. **E,** The skin of the perineum is closed with a running subcuticular stitch. (From Nichols DH and Randall CL: Vaginal surgery, ed 4, Baltimore, 1996, Williams & Wilkins.)

tissue is then infiltrated with .5% lidocaine in 1:200,000 epinephrine, which serves as a "liquid tourniquet." The U-shaped incision is then made along the inner surface of the labia majora. The tissue surrounding the incision is undermined, creating a medial and lateral margin. The medial margin is then approximated using interrupted absorbable suture with the knots facing into the vaginal canal. A subcutaneous layer of interrupted stitches is placed from side to side. Usually the lateral margins are closed, resulting in a Y-shaped configuration, which may be closed with subcuticular or interrupted sutures or a combination. Occasionally a partial perineorrhaphy may be added between the medial and lateral margins, depending on individual anatomy. This may help add some distal length and support but must be done with caution.

On a rare occasion a patient will have a massively fibrosed and undilatable vagina. In this situation the entire vagina and scar tissue are excised by sharp dissection. A split-thickness skin graft is used to line the reconstructed vaginal recipient bed. Long-term use of a vaginal obturator is essential. It should be worn continuously for the first 6 months if possible, removed only during voiding and defecation. Subsequently it should be worn regularly at nighttime for several months and thereafter periodically to assure maintenance of a vagina of adequate size. Discomfort noted on insertion, signaling narrowing, or protrusion of extra obturator length that previously did not occur indicates the start of shortening, and the obturator should again be worn daily.

For the patient who returns with a short and narrow vagina after multiple procedures designed to maintain a functional neovagina or who is unable/unwilling to commit to long-term self-dilation therapy, an alternative surgical choice is the use of a segment of bowel to construct a neovagina.[39,40] This double operation requires a transabdominal bowel resection and anastomosis with all the inherent surgical risks. A two-team approach in this procedure will facilitate the operation. The patient must be counseled on the following possible developments: a postoperative mucoid discharge; introital stenosis, which may cause dyspareunia and require surgical treatment, and protrusion of the neovagina.[40]

OTHER CAUSES OF PAINFUL VAGINA

Vulvar vestibular syndrome may cause a patient to seek a second opinion or consultation following medical and/or surgical therapy. The syndrome should be recognized by the triad of introital dyspareunia, painful erythema at the hymenal sulcus, and point tenderness upon gentle palpation with a cotton applicator.[41] The characteristic historic features include a sudden onset of introital pain to coitus, touch, and insertion of tampons. The patient describes the tenderness to be within the vestibule. It is usually a severe pain that is reproducible by different examiners. Inspection is facilitated by gentle lateral reduction of the vulva, which initially may reveal typically normal-appearing tissues. Careful inspection, sometimes with the aid of a magnifying lens, may reveal faint punctate to several-millimeter erythematous lesions, superficial small ulcerations at the posterior fourchette, or, with long-standing vulvar vestibulitis, a transformation of the minor vestibular glands into vestibular clefts. Gentle palpation with a moist cotton-tipped applicator is effective in locating and mapping the tender areas precisely, which are usually concentrated at the 5 and 8 o'clock positions near the hymenal ring in the region where the minor vestibular glands are most abundant.

Nonspecific medical management includes topical lidocaine solution, topical corticosteroids, and intralesional as well as IM/Interferon. For those patients in whom conservative management is not curative, a surgical vulvar vestibulectomy and vestibuloplasty are required (Figure 22.13).

Two parallel U-shaped incisions are made cephalad and caudad to the posterior hymenal ring up to the 3 and 9 o'clock positions, and the tissue within the U is excised. The posterior vaginal wall is mobilized cranially for a distance of about 3 cm, and the vagina is sewn to the perineal skin with every attempt to keep the suture line out of the introitus.[42] If additional areas of vulvar vestibular syndrome develop in the future, the treatment can be repeated as necessary.

An occasional patient will demonstrate repetitive postcoital cystitis and frequently will

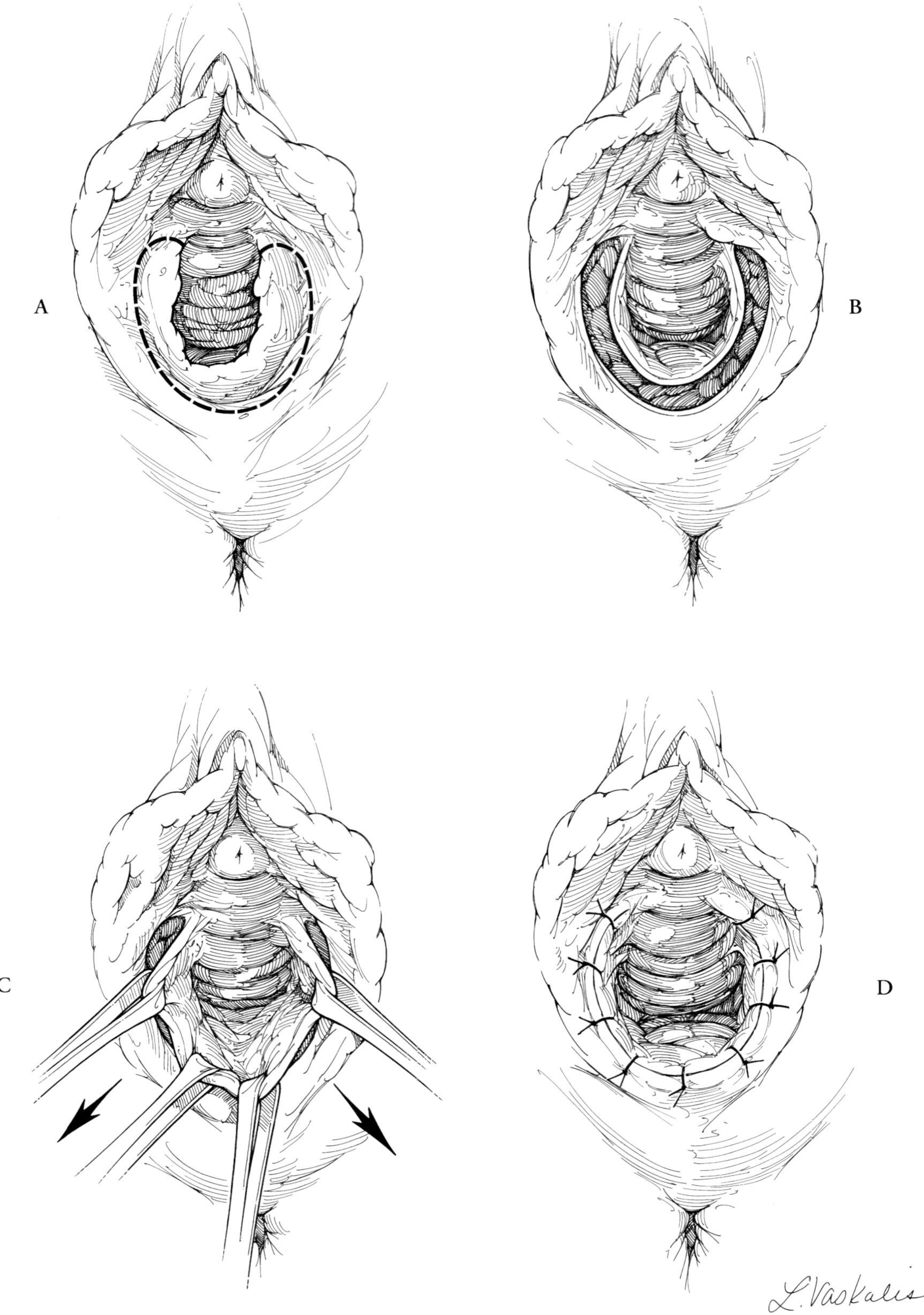

FIGURE 22.13 Vestibulectomy. **A,** The painful sites of the vestibular skin are identified preoperatively, and an inclusive incision is created. **B,** The full thickness of the skin and hymen is removed. **C,** The posterior vaginal wall is mobilized and advanced distally to cover the defect. **D,** The full thickness of the vagina is sewn to the skin of the vulva by two layers of interrupted synthetic sutures. Caution is used not to create a stricture lateral to the urethra. Areas may be left to heal by secondary intention. (From Nichols DH and Randall CL: Vaginal surgery, ed 4, Baltimore, 1996, Williams & Wilkins.)

complain of urethral discomfort with intromission. A rather consistent finding during digital examination or with a Lucite obturator is the observation that the external urethral meatus is drawn upward into the vagina. Paraurethral hymenotomy or hymenectomy is often a simple solution, which releases the urethral meatus from the vagina. Coincident perineotomy may be added if the introitus is too narrow and a trial of vaginal dilation has not been of benefit.

A palpable and painful neuroma may rarely develop beneath the posterior vaginal wall at the site of a previous episiotomy or posterior colporrhaphy. Its contribution to vaginal pain may be identified by the relief provided by anesthetic infiltration. Rarely, without any evidence of previous trauma, a most painful glomus tumor is the cause of severe introital dyspareunia.[43] The treatment for both is surgical excision.

Posthysterectomy dyspareunia without a compromise in vaginal length may occasionally be seen as a consequence of fixation of the ovary to the vaginal wall. When conservative management with suppression of ovarian function by oral contraceptives for a few months fails to provide relief, the ovaries must be freed from the vault of the vagina. Surgical intervention is directed at suspension to a higher position along the lateral pelvic side wall if they are still functional or removal if they are not.

Equestrian dyspareunia has been described in the literature. Examination reveals focal tenderness over the levator ani muscles. Interruption of riding, supplemented with prostaglandin inhibitors, has resulted in total cure after 1 month of therapy.[44]

An occasional patient will be the victim of a situation of psychosexual stress reflected as psychosomatic vaginal discomfort. Inability of the patient to identify a specific area during physical examination is reason to doubt the presence of an organic cause and perhaps consider a psychogenic component. If specifically questioned, the patient will usually divulge a long-standing history of abuse. Such patients may be reluctant to consider this cause, and consultation with a psychiatrist or psychologist, if accepted by the patient, will be beneficial.

Everted Shortened Vagina

The surgeon occasionally encounters the multioperated patient with total eversion of a shortened vagina. The vaginal depth may be too short to reach the sacrospinous ligament for colpopexy when repositioned into the pelvis. There are several treatment options that may allow for individualization. The Ingram dilators lubricated with estrogen cream may be used to lengthen the vagina[2] if the patient is willing to participate. Irrespective of the final vaginal length, several surgical alternatives exist. Sacrospinous colpopexy may be performed using a deliberate suture bridge of nonabsorbable synthetic mononfilament material, such as polybutester (Novafil) or polypropylene (Prolene, Surgilene).[32] Transabdominal sacrocolpopexy may be performed using an intermediate bridge of fascia lata or a synthetic material such as Mersilene mesh. Baden and Walker have suggested reattachment paravaginally on one or both sides as high as the vaginal length permits.[45] Additionally, if the labia are of sufficient size, a Williams' vulvovaginoplasty may be added as an additional procedure to provide a supplemental vaginal depth.

References

1. Ingram JM: The bicycle seat stool in the treatment of vaginal agenesis and stenosis: a preliminary report, Am J Obstet Gynecol 140:867, 1981.
2. Williams JK, Ingram JM, and Welden WS: Management of noncongenital vaginal stenosis and distortion by the bicycle seat stool technique, Am J Obstet Gynecol 150:166, 1984.
3. Miller SH and others: Alterations in the local blood flow and gas tension caused by epinephrine, Plast Reconstr Surg 73:797, 1984.
4. Rudolph R and Klein L: Healing process in skin grafts, Surg Gynecol Obstet 136:641, 1973.
5. Clemmesen T: The early circulation in split-skin grafts: restoration of blood supply to split-skin autografts, Acta Chir Scand 127:1, 1964.
6. Dudsinski MR and Rader JS: The mons pubis: an excellent graft donor site in gyneco-

logic surgery, Am J Obstet Gynecol 162:772, 1990.

7. Davis JS and Kitlowski EA: The immediate contraction of cutaneous grafts and its causes, Arch Surg 23:954, 1931.
8. Ragnell A: The secondary contracting tendency of the free skin grafts, Br J Plast Surg 5:6, 1952.
9. Billingham RE and Russell PS: Studies on wound healing, with special reference to the phenomenon of contracture in experimental rabbit skin, Ann Surg 44:961, 1956.
10. Corps BVM: The effect of graft thickness, donor site and graft bed shrinkage in the hooded rat, Br J Plast Surg 22:125, 1969.
11. McIndoe AH: The treatment of hypospadias, Am J Surg 38:176, 1937.
12. McGregor IA: Fundamental techniques of plastic surgery, ed 2, Edinburgh, 1962, Livingstone.
13. Gibson T and Renedi RM: Biochemical properties of skin, Surg Clin North Am 47:279, 1967.
14. Pasyk KA, Argenta LC, and Hasset C: Quantitative analysis of the thickness of human skin and subcutaneous tissue following controlled expansion with a silicone implant, Plast Reconstr Surg 81:516, 1988.
15. Simmons SC: Dyspareunia following repair—"the skin bridge"—and its prevention, Br J Obstet Gynaecol 70:476, 1963.
16. Huffman JW: Perineotomy, Surg Gynecol Obstet 92:355, 1951.
17. West JT, Ketcham AS, and Smith RR: Vaginal reconstruction following pelvic exenteration for cancer or postirradiation necrosis, Surg Gynecol Obstet 118:788, 1965.
18. Musset R: Traitment chirurgical des cloisons transversales du vagin d'origine congenitale par la plastie en Z, Gynec Obstet (Paris) 55:382, 1956.
19. Wilkinson EJ: Introital stenosis and Z-plasty, Obstet Gynecol 38:638, 1971.
20. Lilford RJ, Sharpe DT, and Thomas DFM: Use of tissue expansion techniques to create skin flaps for vaginoplasty: case report, Br J Obstet Gynaecol 95:402, 1988.
21. Patil U and Hixson FP: The role of tissue expanders in vaginoplasty for congenital malformation of the vagina, Br J Urol 70:554, 1992.
22. Nichols DH and Randall CL: Vaginal surgery, ed 2, Baltimore, 1983, Williams and Wilkins.
23. Graves WP: Operative treatment of atresia of the vagina, Boston Med Surg J 163:753, 1910.
24. Nichols DH and Randall CL: Vaginal surgery, ed 4, Baltimore, 1996, Williams & Wilkins.
25. McIndoe AH and Banister BJ: An operation for the cure of congenital absence of the vagina, Br J Obstet Gynaecol 45:490, 1938.
26. McIndoe AH: The treatment of congenital absence and obliterative conditions of the vagina, Br J Plast Surg 2:254, 1950.
27. Abbe R: New method of creating a vagina in a case of congenital absence, Med Rec 56:836, 1898.
28. Dinner MI, Peters CR, and Sherer J: Use of a semipermeable polyurethane membrane as a dressing for split skin graft donor site, Plast Reconstr Surg 64:112, 1979.
29. Horton CE: Personal communication, January, 1996.
30. Sadove RC and Horton CE: Utilizing full-thickness skin grafts for vaginal reconstruction, Clin Plast Surg 15:443, 1988.
31. Morley GW and DeLancey JOL: Full-thickness skin graft vaginoplasty for treatment of the stenotic or foreshortened vagina, Obstet Gynecol 77:485, 1991.
32. Nichols DH and Randall CL: Vaginal surgery, ed 4, Baltimore, 1996, Williams and Wilkins.
33. Amreich J: Aetiologie und Operation des Scheidenstumpfprolapses, Wien Klin Wochenschr 63:74, 1951.
34. Davydov SN: Modifisierte kolpoese aus peritoneum der excavatio rectouterina, Obstet Gynecol (Moscow) 12:55, 1969. Quoted in Kaser O and others: Atlas der gynakologischen Operationen, Stuttgart, 1983, Georg Thieme Verlag.
35. Rothman D: The use of peritoneum in the construction of a vagina, Obstet Gynecol 40:835, 1972.
36. Adamyan L: Additional international perspectives. In Nichols DH, editor: Gynecologic and obstetric surgery, St Louis, 1993, Mosby-Year Book, Inc.
37. Vecchietti G: Neovagina nella sindrome di Rokitansky-Kuster-Hauser, Attual Ost Gin 11:131, 1965.

38. Williams EA: Congenital absence of the vagina: a simple operation for its relief, Br J Obstet Gynaecol 71:511, 1964.

39. Pratt JH: Sigmoidovaginostomy: a new method of obtaining satisfactory vaginal depth, Am J Obstet Gynecol 81:535, 1961.

40. Turner-Warwick R and Kirby RS: The construction and reconstruction of the vagina with colocecum, Surg Gynecol Obstet 170:132, 1990.

41. Friedrich EG: Vulvar vestibulitis syndrome, J Reprod Med 32:110, 1987.

42. Marinoff SC and Turner MLC: Vulvar vestibulitis syndrome: an overview, Am J Obstet Gynecol 165:1228, 1991.

43. Kohorn EI, Merino MJ and Goldenhersch M: Vulvar pain and dyspareunia due to glomus tumor, Obstet Gynecol 67:41S, 1986.

44. Greiss FC: Equestrian dyspareunia, Am J Obstet Gynecol 150:168, 1984.

45. Baden WF and Walker T: Surgical repair of vaginal defects, Philadelphia, 1992, JB Lippincott Co.

23

Complications of Gynecologic Laparoscopy

JAMES H. DORSEY
HOWARD T. SHARP

Complications resulting from gynecologic laparoscopy are characteristically underreported and underestimated. This is in part due to the rapid evolution and performance of new and complicated surgical procedures that have not yet been adequately evaluated. Additionally, the lack of statistically adequate data that are traditionally associated with the descriptive reports of new surgical operations makes valid estimates of outcomes and complication rates impossible.

Clearly, the outcomes of a new laparoscopic procedure should not be assumed to be equal to those of a similar operation that has been performed for many years by traditional surgical techniques. Although the laparoscopic surgeon may feel that the endoscopic operation was performed in "exactly the same manner" as the traditional open one, this is seldom the case. Laparoscopy may provide a magnificent view of the surgical field, which is enlarged on a video monitor. However, the lack of ability to palpate tissue with an examining hand, the limitations of a relatively fixed angle of attack on tissue targets with long straight laparoscopic instruments inserted through trocar sleeves, and the differences in such simple maneuvers as knot tying are only a few of the easily recognized factors that place laparoscopic surgery in a separate domain.

One of the most recent examples of a new laparoscopic operation that has been adapted from the traditional one is the so-called laparoscopic Burch colposuspension procedure. In the open Burch procedure, the bladder neck is elevated by permanent-type sutures taken through Cooper's ligament and the pubovesical fascia. Over the years, a great deal of data have been acquired for both immediate and long-term outcomes of this operation. In one of the laparoscopic versions, a strip of mesh is fixed to Cooper's ligament and to the paravaginal fascia with a hernia stapling device. Obviously this technique differs greatly from the conventional approach to retropubic urethropexy, and no long-term results are as yet available for comparison. It seems premature to assume that laparoscopically fixed mesh produces the same outcome as an open Burch procedure in which carefully tied and accurately placed sutures are employed for the suspension. However, the method is currently being offered to patients with genuine SUI.

Despite the factors that make it difficult to gather valid outcome data and complication rates for new laparoscopic operations, the anecdotal reports, peer reviews, and medicolegal cases involving laparoscopic mishaps have often helped in understanding the etiology of laparoscopic surgical complications. Additionally, laboratory research on various divergent topics such as electrical capacitive coupling[1] and laparoscopic knot strength[2,3] have also given insight into laparoscopic mishaps and failures.[4]

The goal of laparoscopy is to provide a safer and less invasive surgical approach to accomplish an abdominal operation that would otherwise be performed through a laparotomy incision. Unfortunately, this goal is not always achieved. This chapter will focus on factors that often contribute to laparoscopic surgical complications, particularly those complications that require reoperation, and how to avoid the life-threatening dangers and additional surgical procedures that may accompany them.

Factors Contributing to Laparoscopic Complications

The majority of practicing gynecologic surgeons have not been trained in residency programs to perform advanced laparoscopic surgical procedures. It is clear that this situation has contributed to the emergence of a relatively large and definitely increasing number of laparoscopic surgical complications. This has led to governmental involvement in training and credentialing issues that were previously controlled by the medical profession.

After years of involvement with the peer review process and with the review of alleged laparoscopic malpractice cases, we have noted some constantly recurrent general causes of laparoscopic complications (Table 23.1).

Failure to Identify Important Anatomy

Because of the lack of ability to directly palpate intraabdominal organs, the laparoscopic surgeon often encounters difficulty in identifying important anatomic structures. This makes tissue dissection and lysis of adhesions challenging and at times hazardous, particularly if tissue planes are destroyed by the disease process. For example, endometriosis and resultant adhesions may obliterate the cul-de-sac, making separation of the anterior rectal wall from the posterior cervix and the vagina a dangerous task. The laparoscopic surgeon must therefore go to extra lengths to visually demonstrate the anatomy of the operative field.

Aggressive visual identification of anatomy may be accomplished in a number of ways. Certainly, proper positioning of the patient is necessary for adequate manipulation of the uterus during surgery. A uterine manipulator should be inserted well into the uterine cavity allowing for adequate motion of the uterus during the surgical procedure. The patient is placed in a modified lithotomy position with the buttocks well down on the edge of the operating table so that any instrument placed in the uterus, the bladder, the vagina, or the rectum may be depressed without hitting the bottom edge of the operating table. It should be possible to elevate the uterus to the anterior abdominal wall so that tension on surrounding adhesions, particularly those in the cul-de-sac, can be maintained. If the uterus is large or the adhesions thick, the various plastic intrauterine cannulas available for chromopertubation often do not suffice as manipulators since they may break whenever increased pressure is placed upon them. A metal rod or long cervical dilator taped to a Jacob's tenaculum or a Valchef manipulator should be used to ensure adequate motion and elevation of the uterus. When the uterus can be positioned and moved from below, it frees an abdominal instrument from this task, perhaps lessening the number of abdominal punctures necessary to achieve the operation.

Very often we perform cystoscopy, with or without ureteral catheterization, to ensure that injury has not occurred to the bladder or the ureters or to better delineate the anatomy of the urinary tract. Admittedly, ureteral catherization remains a controversial issue because some surgeons fear that problems such as ureteral spasm or renal infection may result. Wood, Maher, and Pelosi reported oliguria and anuria in 7 of 92 patients undergoing ureteric catheterization during laparoscopic hysterectomy.[5] Conversely, Quinlan, Townsend, and Johnson, in discussing a series of 317 women who had gynecologic surgeries in which there was high risk for ureteral injury, found catherization safe, simple, and of great benefit in ureteral identification.[6] In cases in which there are particularly dense pelvic adhesions, the stented ureter may still be difficult to see. However, we have routinely catheterized

Table 23.1 Common causes of laparoscopic complications

1. Failure to identify positively or to appreciate important surgical anatomy
2. Failure to understand completely the correct use of laparoscopic instrumentation and energy delivery systems, particularly when electricity is employed for dissection and coagulation
3. Inadequate training and experience of the surgeon in laparoscopic surgical techniques coupled with poor understanding of the effect that laparoscopic access has on the performance of these techniques
4. Failure to recognize when the laparoscopic approach is contraindicated or when it should be abandoned in favor of laparotomy

the ureters preoperatively in over 800 cases in which we anticipated difficulties identifying the ureters due to adhesions, endometriosis, or very large myomas and found it to be very helpful in the majority of instances. Although many patients have transient hematuria from ureteral catherization, we have not experienced any significant complications due to this practice. Obviously placement of the stent must be done carefully and trauma to the catheterized ureter avoided during the operative procedure. Also, to ensure that the catheter moves in the ureter, coiling of the catheter in the bladder should be avoided. The catheter should come straight from the ureteral orifice through the urethra and be taped to a Foley catheter. In most cases movement of the ureteral catheters will then give the surgeon a very good appreciation of ureteral position (Plate 1). This helps speed the operation and may make dissection of the ureter less difficult. We also firmly believe that this practice has helped us avoid ureteral injury at laparoscopic surgery. Certainly preoperative ureteral catherization helps identify ureteral injury. When a catheterized ureter has been stapled, clamped, burned, or otherwise damaged, such trauma is often evident on examination of the removed catheter (Plate 2).

The question of whether the gynecologist should be credentialed to perform cystoscopy often arises. In the early days of our specialty, it was expected that cystoscopy would often be performed by the gynecologist. Additionally, if a gynecologist is to perform urologic surgery for SUI, it seems quite illogical to assume that the same surgeon should not be able to inspect the bladder and perform indicated preoperative testing. It also seems inappropriate to deny the surgeon who performs pelvic reconstructive surgery the opportunity to check the bladder with a cystoscope for proper positioning or for damage. However, if a urologist must be called, arrangements should be made before initiating the surgery so that the ureteral stents may be placed quickly without interrupting the laparoscopic procedure. In our own OR, we always have a cystoscopy table ready for our use should the indication arise.

The use of a rigid sigmoidoscope is also of great benefit to the surgeon who is dissecting the cul-de-sac that is obliterated by adhesions. It is often impossible to tell exactly where rectum and vagina meet in these cases. A rigid sigmoidoscope passed to 15 or 20 cm can be easily visualized and palpated with laparoscopic instruments. In the obliterated cul-de-sac, where the rectum, the vagina, and the ureters may be pulled together, passage of the sigmoidoscope often speeds up our surgery and helps avoid rectal and low sigmoid damage.

Rectal probes also help define lower pelvic anatomy. One advantage of the rectal probe over the sigmoidoscope is that it is usually easier to keep it inserted in the rectum during the case. Often we use a rectal "sizer," an instrument designed to gauge rectal diameters during surgical resection with a stapling device, as a rectal probe. However, an additional advantage of the rigid sigmoidoscope is that it can be used to check for penetrating damage. As the scope is passed up into the sigmoid colon, air is pumped into the bowel through the scope in order to dilate and visualize its interior. If the laparoscopist fills the pelvis with irrigating fluid and watches for escaping gas, perforations in the wall of the colon can be readily identified. Since the gas ascends well up into the descending colon, the operator can be reassured that a significant portion of the colon is intact if no bubbles appear.

A vaginal probe is easily made by grasping a folded wet sponge with a sponge stick and inserting it into the vagina. Again, visualization and palpation of this instrument aids greatly in identification of the vaginal vault. One note of caution must accompany use of this probe. The vaginal fornices are usually so pliable and distensible that, if the probe is not directed to the middle of the cul-de-sac, the ureters may be displaced over the sponge and elevated by the vaginal probe, producing a distorted anatomic picture. It is helpful to first place an examining hand in the vagina and observe the anatomic location of the posterior fornix in the cul-de-sac by moving the fingers. Anatomic distortion produced by movement away from the midline is easily appreciated.

Aggressive identification of anatomy cannot be overemphasized as a great help in avoiding complications, and it is in the best interest of the patient for the laparoscopist to be able to perform cystoscopy and sigmoidoscopy intraoperatively. Certainly there is no substitute for thorough knowledge of anatomy. But in laparoscopy the surgeon should use every possible maneuver in order to avoid the complications associated with failure to appreciate laparoscopic anatomic landmarks.

Failure to Understand Laparoscopic Instruments and Energy Delivery Systems

Although many gynecologic surgeons may routinely use sophisticated instruments in open abdominal surgery, such as stapling devices and electrical forceps, these tools in laparoscopy are often put to very different use. For example, bipolar forceps in open surgery, if they are used at all, may be employed to cauterize small bleeders in skin and subcutaneous tissue. In laparoscopy, bipolar forceps are often used to coagulate the largest vessels that need to be secured when performing adnexectomy or hysterectomy, that is, the infundibulopelvic ligament and the uterine vessels. The excellent coagulation achieved by this instrument has helped make laparoscopic removal of these structures possible. However, there are inherent risks in the use of any energized instrument, and neither the unipolar nor the bipolar electrodes are exceptions.

Over the past 20 years there have been many technological advances in electrosurgery, such as the isolated circuit, return electrode monitoring, and the identification of capacitive coupling as a hazard in laparoscopic use of monopolar instruments. But to practice safe surgery and understand the hazards, the benefits, and the tissue effects of electrosurgical instrumentation, the surgeon should be formally educated in the principles of electrosurgery. Early attempts at laparoscopic sterilization involved the use of unipolar electricity to coagulate the fallopian tube. In a series of unipolar sterilizations performed at the Johns Hopkins Hospital during the early 1970s there were a surprising number of electrical bowel burns.[7] It was postulated that these injuries were most likely the result of one of several possible mechanisms, which included sparking or arcing. Although the exact electrical phenomena involved in those early burns remain unclear, the modern solid state electrosurgical generators have virtually eliminated the possibility of electrical burns occurring in the absence of direct tissue contact with the active electrode. Levy, Soderstrom, and Dail feel that microscopic examination of perforation sites can distinguish between electrical burns and intestinal punctures or mechanical rents.[8] Since bowel injury remains one of the most common of the major laparoscopic mishaps, this is an important distinction to make.

Most surgeons understand that breaks in the insulating material surrounding laparoscopic hand instruments may allow electricity to escape and cause inadvertent damage to tissue in contact with the faulty insulation points. If electricity is transferred to another instrument through a break in insulation, for example, from a pair of electrified scissors to the barrel of an operative laparoscope, the same type of mishap is possible if the scope inadvertently touches tissue. This transfer of electrical energy is referred to as the direct coupling of current from an active electrode to another conductor. Another type of current coupling may occur as a result of the electrical phenomenon of capacitance. Capacitive coupling of electrical energy from one perfectly insulated conductor into another metallic instrument is more difficult to understand and to detect. When electrical energy is passed through an insulated conductor that is itself surrounded by another metallic conductor, capacitance may allow up to 40% of the current flow to be induced or "coupled" to the surrounding metal. For example, an insulated unipolar needle that is passed through the channel of an operative laparoscope may transfer up to 40% of the current flowing through the needle to the laparoscope itself. At any given time, the laparoscopic surgeon may view only a relatively small area of the operative field. Recently Electroscope (Boulder, Colorado) developed a monitoring system, the Electroshield, that surrounds the active monopolar electrode and both identifies and then protects against capacitive and direct coupling.

Bipolar forceps were introduced in 1972 by J. Rioux because of the injuries that were felt to be due to unipolar electricity. The jaws of these forceps act as active and return electrodes so that the current passes only through the tissue located between the two. An undamped (cutting) wave form is used with bipolar forceps since this type of nonmodulated current produces the most profound coagulation. Various jaw configurations and sizes are available so that the volume of tissue coagulated at any one time may be determined by the surgeon. However, irrespective of jaw size, tissue coagulation always produces heat. Heat is conducted from the coagulation site and this lateral thermal spread may be difficult to predict and detect. In general, the larger the jaws of the instrument and the higher the power setting used, the more heat is produced and the greater the chance of adjacent tissue damage. During 1995 and 1996 we have reviewed four cases of severe injury secondary to the use of bipolar forceps. In one instance, the uterine vessels were coagulated during laparoscopic hysterectomy. The lateral spread of heat (not electricity) appears to have produced coagulation in adjacent tissue, including a segment of ureter. The patient developed urinary ascites and subsequently underwent emergency surgery for reimplantation of the ureter into the bladder. The other three cases involved rectal injuries and bipolar coagulation of endometriosis and adhesions. In these three cases, rectosigmoid perforation was delayed. In each case the surgeon believed that the forceps were not applied to the rectum. Nevertheless, the pathologic puncture was one of coagulation necrosis involving the rectal wall. One patient died from overwhelming sepsis, and the other two underwent successful resection and Hartmann's pouch procedures. All were critically ill. In no case was aggressive identification of anatomy initially carried out. It is possible that use of the rectal probe or sigmoidoscope and urethral catherization would have avoided these catastrophic injuries.

It is obvious that any instrument that produces heat may cause thermal damage during surgery. We have resected large bowel that was damaged when the coagulating device described by Semm (Endocoagulator, WISAP, Germany)[9] was applied to endometriosis on the rectosigmoid and a full thickness of bowel wall was damaged. Lasers have also produced serious injuries, but we have seen far fewer injuries with laser than with electricity. The question is unanswered as to whether this is because the laser is used less frequently by gynecologists than is electricity. Each laser wavelength produces a very predictable thermal injury. The surgeon does not have to worry about direct or capacitive coupling or current division and the path of least resistance.

It has been our impression that the stapling devices are both faster and safer for securing vascular pedicles at laparoscopy than is electricity. There were several early reports of ureters damaged by application of the stapling devices to the uterine vessels, and the implication was that the devices are inherently dangerous. However, it seems obvious that ureters are stapled by surgeons who do not appreciate the ureter's close proximity to the uterine artery just as ureters are burned by too close an application of the bipolar forceps. In all cases of which we are aware, injuries are the result of failure to recognize anatomy or failure to appreciate the physical characteristics of the instruments.

Inadequate Surgical Training for Laparoscopy

Many laparoscopic surgeons have not had an opportunity to spend the time necessary to acquire adequate knowledge and skills to perform complicated laparoscopic procedures.[10,11] Certainly the majority of gynecologic surgeons did not receive training in advanced laparoscopic surgical techniques during their residency program. Current residency programs in obstetrics and gynecology offer about 2 years of training (sometimes less) in the entire field of gynecologic surgery. This is not an adequate amount of time to properly prepare a surgeon to perform the many challenging operative procedures that are now a part of the gynecologic surgical armamentarium. Additionally, sound surgical judgment is an attribute that comes to the talented surgeon as a result of innate ability, excellent surgical training, and a significant amount of time spent in the practice of our specialty. In reviewing surgical mishaps that have resulted in malpractice actions, it is evident that incomplete training contributes to many. In 1996 we had the opportunity to operate on three women who had undergone laparoscopic Burch procedures in the recent past. All had major degrees of vaginal prolapse and persistent genuine SUI. Upon examination of all three patients, the only evidence that a surgical procedure had been carried out was the presence of scars from abdominal laparoscopic trocars. In one of these cases, the laparoscopic surgeon had never before performed an open retropubic urethropexy. In the other two, perusal of the operative reports showed that grossly inadequate suturing and knotting techniques had been employed for the suspension. All these women underwent major reoperation and pelvic repair. However, properly performed laparoscopic retropubic suspension may yield excellent results.[12]

In this country credentialing of the gynecologic surgeon is the prerogative of the hospital (usually a corporation) to which a gynecologist applies for privileges to practice the specialty. Specific privileges are usually granted after review of a "delineation of privileges" form by a committee of physicians who have been appointed to the credentialing committee. In many instances it appears that little effort is spent in ascertaining how much training or experience the physician actually has in the performance of a specific operative procedure. Unfortunately, not all surgeons are aware of the limitations of laparoscopic surgery or are able to predict when a surgical procedure exceeds those limitations.

Selecting Proper Indications for Laparoscopy or Abandoning the Laparoscopic Surgical Approach

Laparoscopy has received a great deal of publicity in the past decade. The laparoscopic surgeon is often placed under pressure by both patients and third-party payers to provide the "minimally invasive" and least expensive surgical service. Typically neither the patient nor the payer appreciates the complexity of the surgery. Vaginal hysterectomy has long been considered the preferable route for uterine removal since morbidity, cost, and recovery time are less than with abdominal hysterectomy.[13] Laparoscopically assisted vaginal hysterectomy (LAVH) is an operation that was designed to increase the number of hysterectomies that could be performed by the vaginal approach. However, several studies have shown that choice of hysterectomy route may be more influenced by the surgeon's "practice style" or personal preference than by adherence to accepted and standard indications.[14,15] One of the very valid criticisms of LAVH has been that some surgeons have performed this procedure on patients who could have been more properly treated by straightforward vaginal hysterectomy with reduction of morbidity and cost.[16]

Ovarian Malignancy Discovered at Laparoscopy

A more serious situation may arise when the laparoscopist encounters unexpected ovarian cancer in an adnexal mass. However, the disconcerting feeling of discovering ovarian cancer at laparoscopy pales in comparison to the surprise of the incidental listing of cancer on the pathology report. The possibility of malignancy always must be considered when performing laparoscopy for an adnexal mass. Although most of these masses encountered by the laparoscopist are benign if preoperative evaluation has been correctly performed, the role of laparoscopy in the evaluation and treatment of the adnexal mass remains controversial. In a survey of members of the Society of Gynecologic Oncologists, Maiman, Seltzer, and Boyce[17] reported on the laparoscopic management of ovarian tumors subsequently found to be malignant. In 42 cases of ovarian malignancy, complete excision was performed in only 12 (29%). Of these malignancies, 76% were less than 8 cm, 62% were cystic, 48% were unilocular, and 81% were unilateral. All four of these "benign" characteristics were found in 31% of the cases. Laparotomy was not performed at all in 12% cases, and the mean delay to laparotomy was 4.8 weeks. This survey emphasizes several potential dangers that may be associated with the laparoscopic management of the adnexal mass, including delay of treatment, incomplete staging, and the failure of preoperative testing to accurately predict malignancy. On the other hand, a 1991 survey conducted by the American Association of Gynecologic Laparoscopists reported only 53 cases of unsuspected cancer among 13,739 laparoscopies for ovarian cysts, for an incidence of 0.4% for incidental ovarian malignancy at laparoscopy. In considering laparoscopic management of adnexal masses, the following questions must be answered: (1) With what degree of certainty can ovarian malignancy be excluded preoperatively? (2) What routine steps should be taken at laparoscopy to avoid missing a cancer? (3) Are patients subjected to delayed treatment and a worse prognosis by performing a laparoscopic procedure?

Risk Factors for Ovarian Cancer. A family history of breast cancer and ovarian cancer are risk factors for ovarian cancer. Familial ovarian cancer, defined as having two or more first-degree relatives with ovarian cancer, may mean that the patient has up to a 50% chance of developing ovarian cancer, at an average of 20 years earlier than a control population.[18]

On physical examination, the presence of a fixed, solid, irregular mass or the presence of ascites should greatly increase the suspicion of malignancy.

Ultrasonographic estimation of ovarian size alone was studied retrospectively for pathologic correlation in postmenopausal women by Rulin and Preston.[19] Of 150 patients with ovarian masses, only 1 of 32 masses less than 5 cm in diameter was malignant. Six of 55 masses in the 5- to 10-cm range were malignant, and 40 of 63 in the 10-cm or greater group were malignant. When 180 patients of all ages were studied, only 1% of masses less than 5 cm and 11% of masses 5 to 10 cm were malignant. Other characteristics also may be evaluated ultrasonographically, such as ovarian shape and structure. Malignancy must be suspected when solid structures are seen within a cyst (including thick septa), bilateral ovarian abnormalities are seen, or in the presence of matted bowel or ascites. When these patterns were found on ultrasound scans, the positive predictive value was 73% (38/52 patients), and the negative predictive value was 95.7% (177/185).

Color flow Doppler imaging for detecting ovarian malignancy has not yet gained wide acceptance as a clinical modality. The initial reports were quite impressive, as one study reported a 96% positive predictive value and a 95% negative predictive value using a resistive index value of 0.4.[20,21,22] Unfortunately, other studies have produced mixed results. Wu and others[23] reported a sensitivity and specificity of 68.0% and 97.4%, respectively, for ovarian malignancy and a significantly high number of false negative rates for primary ovarian malignancies (30 of 79), malignancies with predominantly cystic elements (20 of 41), and malignancies with large diameters (27 of 63). The overall false negative rate was 32% (33 of 103).

CA-125 as a Tumor Marker. Approximately 89% of nonmucinous epithelial ovarian cancers are associated with an elevation of this tumor marker. However, several benign, common conditions also may cause an elevated CA-125 value (endometriosis, uterine leiomyomas, PID, adenomyosis, early pregnancy, and menstruation), resulting in limited utility and confusion in the premenopausal patient.

Malignancy in unilocular masses is much less common in the female of reproductive age. Halme calculated the absolute risk of malignancy in reproductive-aged females with a unilocular ovarian mass to be 0.25%, or 2.5:1000, based on the assumption that approximately 5% of all unilocular ovarian masses are neoplastic and that approximately 5% of these neoplasms are malignant.[24] This low risk of malignancy is cited by some as justification for the laparoscopic evaluation and treatment of adnexal masses.

In 1971 Barber and Graber wrote an editorial describing the postmenopausal palpable ovary as a pathologic state, based on three patients with ovarian cancer who had premenopausal-sized ovaries.[25] However, with improved noninvasive imaging techniques we are now able to manage adnexal masses based on more information than can be gained by palpation alone. Ultrasound studies have reported a 3% to 11% incidence of ovarian malignancy in postmenopausal ovaries less than 10 cm in size, opposed to a 63% to 71% incidence of malignancy in masses over 10 cm.[26]

Parker and Berek performed a pilot study of laparoscopic cyst aspiration and removal on 25 postmenopausal patients. Three patients required laparotomy, and all masses demonstrated benign pathology. In all cases, a preoperative CA-125 was obtained and was less than 35 units/ml, and strict preoperative ultrasonographic criteria were met.[27]

Tumor Spill and Prognosis. Intraoperative rupture of malignancy is one of the issues at the heart of the laparoscopic controversy because even the most thorough preoperative assessment cannot guarantee the absence of malignancy. In 1973 Webb and others reported a poorer prognosis after tumor spill.[28] However, with the use of multivariate analysis, newer data do not confirm this finding. Dembo and others studied 519 patients with stage I epithelial ovarian cancer and found that the only factors influencing relapse rate were tumor grade and the presence of dense adhesions and/or large volume ascites.[29] Intraoperative rupture was not found to have a negative prognostic effect. Similar findings were confirmed by Sevelda, Dittrich, and Salzer.[30] A recent study by Sainz de la Cuesta and others[31] reported a poorer prognosis in patients with intraoperative rupture but acknowledged that the difference in survival did not reach statistical significance.

Laparoscopy Versus Laparotomy for the Adnexal Mass. It is much easier to focus attention on cases that should not have been performed laparoscopically in the first place. An adequate preoperative evaluation, including physical examination, history, and ultrasonography, will help exclude patients who are at a high risk for cancer. If there are significant suspicions indicative of possible cancer, a laparotomy should be the initial procedure of choice. Routine laparoscopy for the complex adnexal mass in reproductive-aged women should be avoided. The two exceptions may be the dermoid cyst, because of its prevalence and relative ease of ultrasonographic diagnosis, and suspected endometrioma in the patient with known endometriosis and characteristic history and physical findings.

While a preoperative CA-125 determination is of limited utility in reproductive-aged women, it should be obtained in postmenopausal patients. Routine intraoperative steps should be taken prior to performing dissection, including obtaining peritoneal washings using 100 to 250 ml of saline. These washings may be discarded in cases of obvious benign tumors. Careful inspection of peritoneal surfaces, bowel, pelvis, and upper abdomen should be performed. Frozen sections should be performed on questionable lesions. Immediate staging laparotomy should be performed if cancer is found. Ovarian cysts should be removed rather than simply drained to make a histologic diagnosis.

Ultrasonographic criteria[32] for the laparoscopic management of postmenopausal masses should include: (1) simple cyst less than 10 cm with distinct borders; (2) no evidence of irregular solid parts or thick septa (> 2 mm); (3) no ascites; and (4) no matted bowel.

Abandoning the Laparoscopic Surgery. Any patient who is to undergo laparoscopic surgery must understand that it may become necessary to abandon the laparoscopic approach in favor of open abdominal surgery. Any surgeon who undertakes laparoscopic surgery must accept this fact and realistically inform the patient.

There are many examples of laparoscopic surgery that should have been converted to the traditional approach before the major complication occurred. Laparoscopic myomectomy is a procedure that has provided us with excellent illustrations of this point. On several occasions we have been called to the OR to deal with massive hemorrhage resulting from uncontrolled bleeding in a uterine myomectomy wound. In each of these cases, the surgeon failed to recognize the amount of blood loss, lacked the ability to control it, and, most seriously, failed to abandon the procedure in time to avoid blood loss that required very significant transfusion.

Laparoscopic surgery should be abandoned in the following situations: (1) when the difficulty of the surgery exceeds the ability of the surgeon; each surgeon must try to recognize the case or the time at which this occurs; (2) when it becomes obvious that the length of time required to perform the laparoscopic procedure so far exceeds the time required for open surgery that the benefits of laparoscopy are lost; and (3) whenever the surgeon's "comfort level" is seriously threatened by continuing the case. Quite obviously these are all very relative conditions that require surgical judgment and an honest evaluation by surgeons of their own laparoscopic surgical capability.

COMMON SITES OF LAPAROSCOPIC INJURY

The overwhelming majority of surgical complications reported in the literature or men-

TABLE 23.2 Most common laparoscopic injury sites in order of frequency

1. Anterior abdominal wall
2. Large and small bowel
3. Bladder
4. Great vessels
5. Ureters
6. Nerve

tioned in peer review and malpractice cases involve six different anatomic structures. These are listed in Table 23.2 in what seems to be the order of frequency in which injury is encountered. Although all six of these structures may be damaged in a number of different ways, gaining access to the abdominal cavity to perform laparoscopic surgery remains one of the most common mechanisms in the production of complications.

Access Injuries

Injuries resulting from gaining access to the peritoneal cavity by Veress needle and trocar placement include trauma to vessels in the anterior abdominal wall, the major abdominal and pelvic vessels, the bowel, and the bladder. We are aware of a case in which the bifurcation of the common iliac artery *and* the ureter were injured during umbilical trocar insertion. In addition to intraoperative injury, late postoperative complication may occur at the trocar sites, where omentum and small bowel may herniate through the fascial defect.

Anterior Abdominal Wall

Perhaps the most frequently encountered surgical injury in laparoscopy occurs when the lower quadrants of the anterior abdominal wall are penetrated for secondary trocar placement. It is in these locations that the superficial and deep epigastric vessels are most likely to be severed. Bleeding from the superficial epigastric vessels may be troublesome, but it is usually easy to deal with by conventional surgical techniques such as electrosurgical coagulation, clamping, and tying. On the other hand, the deep inferior epigastric artery is a larger vessel, arising from the external iliac artery just above the inguinal ligament. It runs cephalad in the properitoneal fat on top of the peritoneum approaching the rectus abdominis muscle laterally. At its origin, it has a mean diameter of 3.5 mm, and it branches often, entering the rectus abdominis in the middle third of that muscle.[33] When this vessel and its accompanying vein are severed, bleeding may be brisk with impressively rapid hematoma formation both properitoneally and intraperitoneally.[34]

A number of methods have been suggested for controlling the bleeding. These range from simple tamponade with large sutures passed through the entire thickness of the anterior abdominal wall and back out again to the use of special instruments designed to make suturing of the vessels under laparoscopic control an easier task. As with any vascular injury, speed is of primary importance in stopping the bleeding. In our hands, there have been two successful ways to quickly settle the problem. First, the wound is visualized laparoscopically, and finger pressure is exerted over the skin incision. The peritoneum just below the incision is grasped with a bipolar forceps that is passed either through another secondary insertion site or through an operative laparoscope, and the vessels are coagulated right through the peritoneum. If this maneuver is not successful after several attempts, the skin and fascial incisions are then enlarged to about 2 to 3 cm, the muscle fibers separated, and the vessels clamped and properly ligated. A trocar sleeve can then be placed into this incision. One fascial stitch will close the defect tightly enough to prevent escape of gas from around the sleeve. We have never had a patient complain about the slightly larger incision after the situation was explained.

Avoiding Access Injuries

Although Veress needle and initial trocar placement may be "blind," the surgeon must make every effort to appreciate the location of the important structures in and below the abdominal wall and to achieve a careful and controlled entry into the abdomen.

In initiating laparoscopy, several steps should be taken to lessen the possibility of vascular injury. When making the initial incision in the umbilicus, be it vertical or transverse, the knife blade should never be directed toward the aorta and should never penetrate the fascia. In the thin patient the aorta lies directly beneath the umbilicus, and at our own institution we have seen two aortic wounds made by a vertically directed no. 11 scalpel blade. Though it seems obvious that intraabdominal structures are endangered by an incision that is carried too deeply, we frequently have observed both residents and attending staff performing the "stab" type of incision dangerously close to the aorta. The initial umbilical incision should be made either transversely in the inferior curve of the umbilicus by directing the blade nearly parallel to the fascia or vertically by lifting the umbilicus between thumb and forefinger and incising the skin in a plane parallel with the long axis of the patient.

In order to understand the angle of Veress needle and trocar entry into the abdominal cavity, the surgeon should palpate the sacral promontory to locate the posterior boundary of the pelvic inlet. This structure lies just below the bifurcation of the aorta. It is therefore important that the surgeon make a very controlled needle and trocar penetration in the midline to avoid the common iliac vessels. The weight of the patient is a factor that must be taken into account. In a thin woman, safe entry usually dictates that needle and trocar be directed at a 45-degree angle from the horizontal in order to avoid the aorta, whereas in the obese patient with a thicker anterior abdominal wall a more vertical approach may be necessary. Hurd and others[35] studied the relationship of the aorta to the umbilicus in women of different weights and found the umbilicus in obese women to be well below the aortic bifurcation. We have found the use of the open Hasson technique for umbilical trocar insertion to be of great help in very obese patients. This technique allows the surgeon to palpate and incise the fascia of the anterior rectus sheath and to identify the rectus muscle and the posterior rectus sheath and peritoneum, offering a more controlled and familiar entry through the thick and difficult abdominal wall. In any event, if there is any suggestion of gastric distention, usually resulting from difficult intubation, a nasogastric tube should be inserted prior to the placement of a needle or trocar to avoid inadvertent injury to an overdistended stomach.

Instead of using a Veress needle to establish a pneumoperitoneum, direct trocar insertion is an alternative preferred by some surgeons. Dingfelder reported his series of 301 patients who underwent direct trocar insertion in 1978.[36] Subsequently several series of direct trocar insertions have been published.[37,38] The rationale for direct trocar insertion is that it avoids the possible complications associated with Veress needle placement, such as CO_2 embolus from inadvertent vascular insufflation and subcutaneous insufflation with failed pneumoperitoneum, possibly leading to failed laparoscopy. Copeland, Wing, and Hulka[39] reported only 3 complications occurring in over 2000 direct trocar insertions. They recommend the following: (1) obtaining adequate lower abdominal wall relaxation; (2) making an adequate incision; and (3) ensuring that only sharp pyramidal trocars be used. Due to the low incidence of Veress needle or trocar injury, a study with enough power to show a definitive safety advantage of the direct technique over the use of Veress needle insufflation will be difficult to perform. Injuries to the great vessels, bowel, and stomach have been reported using either technique, hence great caution should be used regardless of the surgeon's personal preference. Although it is generally felt that penetration of the bowel by a Veress needle seldom results in serious complications,[40] we have recently reviewed two cases in which this mishap appears to have produced two very serious cases of peritonitis, one of which resulted in the patient's death.

Other Methods of Insufflation. As previously mentioned, the use of Hasson open laparoscopic insufflation has been of assistance in the obese patient. However, this technique has not lowered the incidence of bowel injury at abdominal entry. We know of three unrecognized small-bowel injuries that occurred at the time of opening the umbilical incision. All three resulted in peritonitis, delayed diagnosis, and subsequent laparotomy with bowel resection. When the surgeon chooses this method of trocar placement, the incision should be large enough so that the anatomy of the anterior abdominal wall in this area is really visualized. Bowel that is adherent to the umbilical peritoneum is easily opened when the peritoneum is incised, particularly if this occurs through a tiny incision where anatomic landmarks may be difficult to identify.

Neely, McWilliams, and Makhlouf[41] have used the posterior vaginal fornix as an alternative insufflation site, and Morgan[42] described transfundal needle entry into the abdominal cavity for this purpose. Obviously if there are strong suspicions for anterior abdominal wall adhesions, there may be good reason to suspect cul-de-sac and other pelvic sites of adhesive disease. Vagina or fundus may offer *no safer* access than the umbilicus. Childers, Brzechffa, and Surwit[43] have successfully used the sixth intercostal space for Veress needle placement in patients at high risk for subumbilical adhesions, and we too have found this technique useful.

Secondary Trocar Sites. Even in patients undergoing diagnostic laparoscopy, additional trocar sites must be utilized so that the abdominal organs may be moved and inspected. Some surgeons employ a midline location and insert just one additional trocar for the manipulating instruments; however, this may be very limiting as far as proper exploration is concerned. Also great care must be exercised to avoid bladder injury. Foley catheter placement keeps the bladder empty but also may be used for inflating this organ with fluid to define its borders prior to trocar insertion. For any operation other than simple diagnostic laparoscopy or routine tubal sterilization, more than one laparoscopic surgical hand instrument is needed.

We prefer placing lateral trocars for better access to the adnexa and for moving bowel. Care must be taken during trocar insertion to avoid injury to the deep inferior epigastric vessels and the retroperitoneal great vessels. The deep inferior epigastric arteries should be visualized prior to trocar placement. These vessels are almost always seen pulsating just lateral to the umbilical ligament. Once the inferior epigastric vessels are appreciated, a 22-gauge needle may be placed through the abdominal wall at a safe location lateral to the vessels, allowing the surgeon to place the trocar along the same track as the needle to avoid the inferior epigastric vessels (Plate 3). We have found "transillumination" of the inferior epigastric vessels to be inadequate for identifying the inferior epigastric artery. We prefer to place lateral trocars using a two step motion. The first motion is made using gentle, straight downward force until the tip of the trocar is seen just piercing the peritoneum, away from the inferior epigastric vessels (Plate 4). Once the deep epigastric vessels are cleared, the angle of force is then changed and directed toward the midline, away from the great vessels, which often lie directly under or even medial to the trocar tip (Plate 5).

Trocar Removal and Subsequent Herniation. Trocar sheath removal should be performed under direct visualization to ensure that bleeding from an abdominal wall vessel has not been temporarily tamponaded by the trocar sheath. By leaving the laparoscope in the umbilical port during removal, the surgeon can make sure that bowel is not inadvertently suctioned through the umbilical incision. Kadar and others reported 6 cases of incisional hernias among 3560 operative laparoscopies (0.17%).[44] All occurred at extraumbilical sites involving 10- and 12-mm ports. However, other series reported a significant number of fascial defects at the umbilicus associated with the use of ports of 10 mm or greater diameter.[45,46] We have ourselves experienced three lower quadrant hernias in secondary 11.5-mm trocar sites. Consequently, closure of all fascial defects 10 mm or greater is highly recommended (Plates 6 and 7).

Bowel Injuries at Laparoscopy

Although access injury is still the most probable cause of bowel damage, particularly when small bowel loops are fixed to the abdominal wall by adhesions, we have seen a rapidly increasing number of malpractice cases that involve bowel injury sustained at the time of dissection and adhesiolysis. These injuries usually occur in one of three ways: (1) direct penetration of the bowel wall by the dissecting scissors or other instrument used to separate adhesions; (2) devitalization of the bowel wall secondary to traction, trauma, and damage to the blood supply; (3) direct or very close contact with an electrode, either unipolar or bipolar, or with some other energy source that produces heat.

Certainly a few bowel injuries are truly unavoidable. These are usually cases where there has been inadvertent access puncture or division of adhesions that are so dense that normal anatomy is impossible to identify. Previous abdominal surgery is not in itself an absolute contraindication for laparoscopy, and we have performed many successful laparoscopies on patients who have undergone major abdominal procedures. However, in many cases, observance of some commonsense surgical practices will greatly reduce the number of bowel injuries:

1. Always enter the peritoneal cavity carefully and maintain a high index of suspicion in patients who have undergone previous abdominal surgery, particularly if it involved a bowel resection or an incision extending around the umbilicus. Perform noninvasive visualization studies of the abdominal cavity in an attempt to identify adhesions and areas of danger. Preoperatively "bowel prep" the high-risk patient.
2. Treat tissue gently and avoid undue trauma when placing traction on adherent loops of bowel.
3. Use sharp *cold* dissection whenever gentle traction does not separate bowel that is densely adherent to other loops or other pelvic structures.
4. Be extremely careful whenever using electricity for adhesiolysis. Electrodes may damage delicate or distended thin bowel wall very quickly.
5. The surgeon always must understand the anatomy and know exactly where the patient's bowel, bladder, ureter, and great vessels are located.
6. Perform a laparotomy if the last condition cannot be fulfilled.

Inadvertent injury to the bowel usually does not in itself cause serious complications if the injury is recognized and immediately and properly repaired. The chances of severe sequellae are then minimized. Keeping a high index of suspicion for bowel injury is of paramount importance. If opening pressures are high at the time of Veress needle placement, bowel injury should be considered. After any laparoscopic operation the bowel should be carefully examined. Delay in the diagnosis of bowel injury does result in dire consequences. It must also be borne in mind that the bowel may have been injured in more than one location and very careful search must be made for other injured sites. Above all, the surgeon must listen to the postoperative complaints of the patient and immediately take action if any reasonable suspicion of bowel injury exists.

The repair of bowel injury may be carried out in several ways: (1) laparoscopically, if the surgeon is skilled at bowel surgery, laparoscopic suturing techniques, and if the type of injury is appropriate for laparoscopic repair; (2) through an enlargement of one of the trocar incisions if the injury area is relatively small and the surgeon knows that there are no other injuries; on several occasions we have successfully repaired small bowel through enlarged trocar incisions by simply delivering the loop of bowel out of the abdominal cavity and performing a routine type of suture or resection procedure; (3) at laparotomy after the abdomen has been opened through an appropriate incision; this is usually the most common and proper approach to injured bowel. In many cases the intended original operative procedure will have to be completed at laparotomy and thorough exploration with copious peritoneal lavage carried out. This latter step is extremely important, particularly in cases of large bowel injury where meticulous mechanical removal of contamination may be the difference between a smooth or complicated postoperative course. The usual postoperative management with antibiotics, nasogastric suction, and fluid and electrolyte replacement is carried out.

Bladder Injuries at Laparoscopy

Trocar injuries to the bladder most often occur as the result of placement of a secondary trocar in the lower abdomen near the midline. These injuries could be all but eliminated if the surgeon who uses this location for a secondary insertion would utilize a needle through the anterior abdominal wall to first localize the puncture site or insufflate the bladder with sterile water so as to identify its anatomic boundaries.

We are now seeing different types of bladder injury due to the more extensive and complicated types of surgery being performed laparoscopically. In our own institution we observed three laparoscopic bladder injuries during 1995 and 1996. One of these occurred during the resection of endometriosis over bladder peritoneum. The two others occurred when the bladder was inadvertently entered at the time of a laparoscopic Burch procedure. In each case the injury was immediately recognized.

After performing retropubic urethropexy, it is our custom to place a suprapubic catheter in the bladder. This is also done in any patient who sustains a penetrating bladder injury. In one of our cases, the bladder was entered as the space of Retzius was being developed. The opening simply was used for the placement of the suprapubic catheter and then closed more tightly with two laparoscopically placed purse-string sutures that drew the edges of the incision around the catheter. In the second case, the bladder was torn while being bluntly dissected away from the underlying pubovesical fascia. This was also repaired laparoscopically (Plate 8). Catheter drainage was maintained for 7 days before the suprapubic catheter was clamped and the patient allowed to void.

The diagnosis of bladder injury is usually quite straightforward. If there is any suspicion that the bladder has been inadvertently entered, the following procedures are carried out at the operating table. If a trocar has been placed in the bladder, it should be left temporarily in place as the diagnosis will be more easily clarified as the testing proceeds.

1. Fill the bladder through a Foley catheter with a dilute indigo-carmine blue solution. If the dye appears through the trocar site and not in the peritoneal cavity, the trocar has most obviously been placed through the suprapubic space into the bladder. If the dye appears in the peritoneal cavity, either there is a through-and-through trocar injury or the bladder has been entered surgically through the peritoneum.
2. Perform cystoscopy. This step will further clarify the situation anatomically.

Treatment of bladder injuries involve the following:

1. Repair of the defect. This may be performed laparoscopically if the surgeon is skilled at laparoscopic suturing and the defect is properly identified and easily closed. However, laparotomy is the conventional approach to repair and, if the defect is large or irregular, a multilayered closure is more appropriately accomplished with the abdomen open.
2. Drainage of the bladder must be established so that the bladder remains empty and properly decompressed during postoperative healing. This is preferably accomplished with a suprapubic catheter of adequate size. The suprapubic catheter is less likely to promote ascending UTI, and it may be clamped without removal when it is appropriate for the patient to attempt to void. Residual urine volume is easily measured after voiding by unclamping the catheter so that the patient need not undergo urethral catherization for this purpose.

Unrecognized bladder injury may result in a very ill patient. We know of an elderly patient who died of septicemia secondary to peritonitis and urinary ascites that went unrecognized for but 3 days. Immediate and proper surgical repair almost always results in a favorable outcome.

The postoperative patient with urinary ascites presents a diagnostic problem since the internal urinary leakage may stem from bladder or ureteral injury or both. Diagnosis is usually made by intravenous pyelography or by the enhanced CT scan. If the patient is allergic to the dye or if serum creatinine levels are elevated, cystoscopy and ureteral catherization may be performed. Ultrasonography may also help in localizing injury sites. Repairs should be carried out by a surgeon trained in competent urogynecologic surgery.

Injuries to the Great Vessels

The most immediate catastrophic event in laparoscopic surgery is a penetrating injury to the great abdominal or pelvic vessels. Trocar injuries have been the most frequent cause of significant vascular damage during laparoscopic surgery. Even massive hemorrhage from the great vessels may not be recognized immediately since retroperitoneal bleeding, particularly in the case of the aorta and vena cava, can go unnoticed by a surgeon who inserts the scope well past the injury site and then concentrates the view on the pelvis. Any significant drop in blood pressure should alert both anesthesiologist and surgeon of the possibility of hidden blood loss and an immediate search should be initiated for a possible bleeding site.

Postoperative signs of shock also must be immediately explained. We reviewed a case in which an unrecognized injury to the vena cava resulted in massive retroperitoneal hemorrhage. The patient maintained her vital signs at low normal levels for the first hour postoperatively but then experienced intermittent hypotensive episodes. It was not until she was in full-blown shock with dangerously low hypotension that a sonogram showed the hematoma.

Wheeler reviewed the literature on major vascular injury from the 1970s to the present and estimates that the overall risk is low, less than 1 per 1000 cases (0.1%).[47] He further postulates that this small risk statistically translates into a very high probability that the average gynecologic laparoscopist will experience such a major injury during his or her career.

Several laparoscopic operative procedures involve dissections around the great vessels: pelvic and para-aortic lymphadenectomy, sacral colpopexy, presacral neurectomy, and radical hysterectomy. We are aware of a laceration of the left external iliac artery that occurred during lymphadenectomy when the unipolar dissecting scissors inadvertently touched the vessel, producing almost instantaneously a defect in the wall of the vessel. We have also reviewed other cases of great vessel injury during adhesiolysis. It is probable that reports of great vessel damage will increase as more of these major laparoscopic surgical procedures are performed.

The diagnosis of major vessel injury is usually straightforward. These patients should undergo immediate laparotomy with repair of the vascular damage carried out, if possible by a competent vascular surgeon. This is no place for cautery or other ill-conceived and ineffective laparoscopic efforts for obtaining hemostasis. Delayed recognition of great vessel injury may result in death of the patient relatively quickly.[48] The majority of patients will need to be opened through a long lower midline incision in order for adequate exploration and repair to be carried out. This step plus open tamponade of the vascular injury should be carried out by the gynecologist if there is any significant delay in the arrival of a vascular surgeon.

Ureteral Injury

It seems safe to assume that if the surgeon were always aware of the exact location of the ureter of each patient, there would be very few ureteral injuries. Regardless of the instrumentation involved, the common denominator in ureteral injury is the surgeon's inability to properly identify the structure.

The ureter enters the pelvis at the bifurcation of the common iliac artery. It is in close proximity to the infundibulopelvic ligament just caudal to this point. It courses deeper into the pelvis just beneath the semitransparent pelvic wall peritoneum, very close to the hypogastric artery. In this position it is usually very easy to recognize. Stroking the peritoneum overlying the ureter with a laparoscopic instrument enhances visualization; however, this maneuver may prove less successful as laparoscopic surgery proceeds since the retroperitoneal structures may become somewhat edematous and the ureter less reactive. The right ureter may be much easier to visualize than the left since the sigmoid colon often overlies the bifurcation of the common iliac artery and may make visualization along the left pelvic wall very difficult, particularly in the obese patient with adhesive disease. The ureter passes beneath the uterine artery just lateral to the uterosacral ligament through a tunnel in the cardinal ligament (often referred to by the gynecologic oncologist as the "web"). As it passes through this condensation of endopelvic fascia, it is very difficult to identify unless it is dissected free of its covering.

Laparoscopically the ureter is most vulnerable to injury in four locations: (1) it may be damaged at the pelvic brim close to the infundibulopelvic ligament during efforts to secure the ovarian blood supply; (2) in the midpelvis where it is located just in or below the ovarian fossa as it courses beneath lateral parietal peritoneum, and efforts to free the ovary from dense lateral or inferior adhesions may cause injury; (3) it may suffer injury in the lower pelvis where it is close to the cervix and uterosacral ligament during operations involving the cul-de-sac or during laparoscopic hysterectomy; or (4) as it lies in the lateral borders of the presacral space just above the pelvic brim on either side of the sacral promontory, where it is subject to injury during procedures that involve dissections of this area. Recent reports of laparoscopic sacral colpopexy, presacral neurectomy, and para-aortic node dissections should make gynecologic surgeons aware of this anatomic ureteral location so that great care is taken to avoid injury to the ureter here, as well as injury to the great vessels.

In the vast majority of cases of ureteral injury that we have seen or reviewed, the damage was discovered postoperatively. Patients with ureteral obstruction occasionally have no symptoms. However, depending upon the type of injury and its location, most will have fever, rapid pulse, flank or abdominal pain, ileus, urinary ascities, or even fistula formation.

The postoperative identification of ureteral damage is usually straightforward. Renal sonography, intravenous pyelography if serum creatinine is not elevated, cystoscopy with ureteral catheterization, all help identify the problem rapidly.

We discussed ureteral catheterization earlier in this chapter, and to us the benefits of preoperative placement of these stents in patients undergoing complicated laparoscopic surgery far outweigh the disadvantages. The reports of unrecognized ureteral damage during laparoscopic surgery are certainly increasing.[49,50] Any operative step that helps avert this serious complication must be considered carefully.

Nerve Injury at Laparoscopy

Laparoscopy has introduced some new risks for nerve injury during pelvic surgery. The possibility of stretch and pressure injuries to the nerves of the lower extremities is inherent in the use of the modified lithotomy position so commonly employed for laparoscopic surgeries. This position often involves abduction, flexion, and lateral rotation of the hip as well as possible compression from stirrups or other holding devices for the lower leg and foot. Knowledge of the anatomic course of the nerves of the pelvis and lower extremities that could be involved may be helpful in avoiding this type of injury. Unfortunately, final positioning of the patient almost always occurs while she is under anesthesia, and the operator and other OR assistants must rely on judgment (sometimes on intuition) when deciding how much padding is needed or how much manipulation the anatomy can safely take. In addition to these passive-type injuries, actual nerve damage from direct surgical contact is also possible. Some of these injuries are avoidable if the surgeon has knowledge of the anatomic course of the nerves at risk. Other injuries are almost impossible to avoid even though the surgeon takes all possible precautions.

Femoral Neuropathy. The femoral nerve originates from the posterior divisions of the L2-L4 spinal nerves and traverses the psoas muscle until it courses the groove between the psoas muscle anteriorly and the iliac muscle posteriorly. As it exits the pelvis, it passes beneath the inguinal ligament and gives sensory branches to the anterior thigh and medial leg, and motor branches to the sartorius and quadriceps. In laparoscopy the most likely cause of femoral neuropathy is the use of lithotomy positioning where hyperabduction, flexion, or lateral rotation of the hips occurs.[51] Patients with femoral neuropathy commonly have difficulty with ambulation and numbness and paresthesias on the anterolateral aspect of the thigh. When the patient is examined, weakness is noted to varying degrees in the flexors, adductors, and external rotators of the hip, and upon knee extension. Quadriceps weakness is usually the most reliable sign. Decreased patellar reflex is the most common objective sign.

The Allen stirrups were designed to allow the patient to be placed in a relatively safe lithotomy position without excessive hip flexion or abduction. The patient's legs also may be elevated from a low to high stirrup position without repositioning the buttocks. This is most useful in performing procedures such as LAVH where the surgeon needs adequate access to the perineal area.

Obturator Neuropathy. The obturator nerve arises from the L2-L4 spinal nerves. Like the femoral nerve, it traverses the psoas muscle but, in contrast, passes lateral and superior to the hypogastric vessels (and ureter) in the obturator fossa until it reaches the obturator foramen. It then branches into its anterior and posterior divisions, which provide motor function to the leg adductors and sensory function to the hip, knee, and medial thigh. The affected patient may have presenting symptoms of sensory or motor deficits. Sensory deficits may result in reduced sensation over the medial aspect of the thigh or pain extending down to the medial thigh and into the knee.

The obturator nerve is most vulnerable to injury during procedures requiring retroperitoneal dissection such as colposuspension, paravaginal repair, and lymphadenectomy.[52] There is a reported case of partial fulguration of the obturator nerve during pelvic lymphadenectomy. Obturator nerve damage also has been reported to be associated with surgical resection of endometriosis. We are also aware of a case in which the obturator nerve was mistaken for the arcus tendineus pelvis and served as a suspension site during laparoscopic pelvic reconstruction.

Ilioinguinal and Genitofemoral Neuropathies. The ilioinguinal nerve is formed from the L1 spinal nerve and takes a retroperitoneal course that pierces the transversus abdominis muscle near the anterior iliac crest. It then courses through the transversus abdominis and internal oblique muscles to pass through the external inguinal ring. Patients with ilioinguinal nerve injury usually have presenting symptoms of hypoalgesia or hyperalgesia over the lower abdomen, radiating down the inner thigh into the labia majora. They may also demonstrate pain with extension of the thigh.

The genitofemoral nerve originates from the L1-L2 spinal nerves and descends dorsal to the parietal peritoneum on the surface of the psoas muscle. Patients with deficit typically have constant or intermittent pain over the inguinal region with radiation to the inner thigh and labia majora with point tenderness over the internal inguinal ring. These nerve injuries have been associated with laparoscopic herniorrhaphy using mesh and staples. Occasionally these nerves may be injured by secondary trocar punctures. This type of injury is extremely difficult to avoid since the location of secondary puncture sites is dictated by the disease process and the purpose of the laparoscopic surgery.

Peroneal and Sciatic Neuropathies. Peroneal neuropathy (footdrop) is usually associated with inadvertent and sometimes undetectable compression against the lateral aspect of the leg by stirrups or by OR assistants who inadvertently push against the leg. Patients may have presenting symptoms of footdrop or the inability to dorsiflex the foot. They may also display numbness over the dorsum of the foot. Every effort should be made to ensure that the patient's legs are well away from possible compression points and are well padded, as positions during laparoscopy may change both intentionally and unintentionally. If Allen-type stirrups are to be used, preoperative care should be taken to ensure proper padding and strapping of the legs. OR personnel should be instructed not to use the patient's leg as a hand rest. Fortunately, the vast majority of these injuries are transient, and complete recovery is to be expected. Sciatic neuropathy also has been reported at laparoscopy and attributed to lithotomy positioning.[53]

Conclusion

The incidence of laparoscopic complications appears to be rapidly increasing; however, the true incidence of surgical iatrogenic injury is unknown. Most of the estimates concerning these occurrences come from surveys of surgical professional organizations or from retrospective studies performed at active surgical centers. Hard conclusive data are not easily obtained. Not only is the numerator (number of complications) very possibly inaccurate, but the denominator (estimates of the total numbers of cases) in this equation may be even more misleading.

In this chapter we have discussed causes, injury sites, diagnosis, and the avoidance of laparoscopic complications. We have not addressed each specific laparoscopic procedure separately in the discussion of complications because almost any of the reported laparoscopic complications may occur with almost

TABLE 23.3 Recognition of complications

COMPLICATION	NUMBER	IMMEDIATE DIAGNOSIS	DELAYED DIAGNOSIS
Small bowel perforation	9	1	8
Large bowel perforation	7	0	7
Great vessel injury	3	2	1
Bladder perforation	4	2	2
Ureteral injury	1	0	1
Nerve injury	3	0	3
TOTAL	27	5	22

any laparoscopic operation. Unfortunately, every surgical procedure is associated with a set of inherent surgical risks. In laparoscopy the majority of these risks are associated with the majority of the advanced surgical procedures.

It is also clear that a majority of laparoscopic surgical complications, particularly those that may lead to lawsuits, are discovered postoperatively rather than intraoperatively. Laparoscopy is primarily an outpatient surgical exercise, and many of the operations that less than a decade ago were thought serious enough to require week-long postoperative hospitalization to ensure safe recuperation are now followed by discharge of the patient in under 8 hours. This practice reduces the cost of the surgical procedure only if the patient does not return to the hospital (sometimes desperately ill) to undergo another operation to correct a surgical complication. Table 23.3 summarizes the injuries sustained by 27 patients whose records were reviewed during 1996.

Of these patients, 14 underwent some type of adhesiolysis; 6 underwent LAVH; 4 had salpingo-oophorectomies; and 3 had diagnostic procedures. One of the nerve injuries was felt to be the result of positional compression. Only 4 of the 27 surgical injuries were discovered intraoperatively. Of the patients with vascular injury, 2 died, as did 1 with bowel injury and 1 with bladder injury. The message seems clear. Delay in the diagnosis of inadvertent intraoperative injury causes the patient pain and suffering and sometimes death, increases the cost of medical care tremendously, and often causes the surgeon emotional pain and suffering, plus a lawsuit.

Not all surgical complications are avoidable, but many undoubtedly are. The obvious duty of every surgeon is to take meticulous care to avoid surgical complications. Thorough abdominal exploration before the trocar sleeves are withdrawn, with particular attention paid to the common sites of inadvertent injury, is one of the most important mandatory steps at the conclusion of any laparoscopic operation.

REFERENCES

1. Odell RC: Biophysics of electrical energy. In Soderstrom RM, editor: Operative laparoscopy: the masters' techniques, New York, 1993, Raven Press.
2. Dorsey JH and others: Laparoscopic knot strength: a comparison with conventional knots, Obstet Gynecol 86:(4):536, 1995.
3. Sharp HT and others: A simple modification to add strength to the roeder knot, J Am Assoc Gynecol Lap 3(2):305, 1996.
4. Soderstrom RM and Levy BS: Bowel injuries during laparoscopy: causes and medicolegal questions, Contemp Ob/Gy 14:41, 1986.
5. Wood FC, Maher P, and Pelosi MA: Routine use of ureteric catheters at laparoscopic hysterectomy may cause unnecessary complications, J Am Assoc Gynecol Lap 3(3):393, 1996.
6. Quinlan DJ, Townsend DE, and Johnson GH: Are ureteral catheters in gynecologic surgery beneficial or hazardous? J Am Assoc Gynecol Lap 3(1):61, 1995.
7. Wheeless CR: Gastrointestinal injuries associated with laparoscopy. In Phillips JM, editor: Endoscopy in gynecology, Downey Calif, 1976, American Association of Gynecologic Laparoscopists.
8. Levy BS, Soderstrom RM, and Dail DH: Bowel injuries during laparoscopy: gross anatomy and histology, J Reprod Med 30:168, 1965.

9. Semm K: Endocoagulator: new possibilities for tubal surgery via pelviscopy, Excerpta Medica 370:242, 1974.
10. See WA, Cooper CS, and Fisher RJ: Predictors of laparoscopic complications after formal training in laparoscopic surgery, JAMA 270:2689, 1993.
11. Lipscomb GH, Stovall TG, and Ling FW: Basic laparoscopic knowledge among gynecologic laparoscopists, Am J Obstet Gynecol 171:1455, 1994.
12. Dorsey JH and Sharp HT: Laparoscopic sacral colpopexy and other reconstructive procedures for pelvic support defects. In Sutton C, editor: Baillieres Clin Obstet Gynaecol 9:749, 1995.
13. Thompson JD and Rock JA: Hysterectomy. In Thompson JD and Rock JA, editors: TeLinde's operative gynecology, ed 7, Philadelphia, 1992, JB Lippincott Co.
14. Dorsey JH, Steinberg EP, and Holtz PM. Clinical indications for hysterectomy route: patient characteristics or physician preference? Am J Obstet Gynecol 173(5):1452, 1995.
15. Kovac RS, Pignotti BJ, and Bindbeutel GA: Hysterectomy: a comparative statistical study of abdominal vs vaginal approaches, Mo Med 85:312, 1988.
16. Dorsey JH and others: Costs and charges associated with three alternative techniques of hysterectomy, N Engl J Med 335:476, 1996.
17. Maiman M, Seltzer V, and Boyce J: Laparoscopic excision of ovarian neoplasms subsequently found to be malignant, Obstet Gynecol 77:563, 1991.
18. Kock M, Gaedke H, and Jenkins H: Family history of ovarian cancer patients: a case control study, Int J Epidemiol 18:782, 1989.
19. Rulin M and Preston A: Adnexal masses in postmenopausal women, Obstet Gynecol 70:578, 1987.
20. Kurjak A and others: Transvaginal ultrasound, color flow, and Doppler waveform of the postmenopausal adnexal mass, Obstet Gynecol 80:917, 1992.
21. Fleischer AC and others: Color Doppler sonography of ovarian masses: a multiparameter analysis, J Ultrasound Med 12:41, 1993.
22. Lin PY and others: Color Doppler ultrasound in the assessment of ovarian neoplasms, J Ultrasound Med 1:172, 1993.
23. Wu C and others: Factors contributing to the accuracy in diagnosing ovarian malignancy by color Doppler ultrasound, Obstet Gynecol 84:605, 1994.
24. Halme JK: Laparoscopic management of persistent ovarian masses. In Hulka JF and Reich H, editors: Textbook of laparoscopy, ed 2, Philadelphia, 1994, WB Saunders Co.
25. Barber H and Graber E: The PMPO syndrome (postmenopausal palpable ovary syndrome), Obstet Gynecol 38:921, 1971.
26. Herrmann UJ, Locher GW, and Goldhirsch A: Sonographic patterns of ovarian tumors and the relation to the histologic diagnosis: prediction of malignancy, Obstet Gynecol 69:777, 1987.
27. Parker WH and Berek JS: Management of selected cystic adnexal masses in postmenopausal women by operative laparoscopy: a pilot study, Am J Obstet Gynecol 163:1574, 1990.
28. Webb MJ and others: Factors influencing survival in stage I ovarian cancer, Am J Obstet Gynecol 116:222, 1973.
29. Dembo A and others: Prognostic factors in patients with stage one epithelial ovarian cancer, Obstet Gynecol 75:263, 1990.
30. Sevelda P, Dittrich C, and Salzer H: Prognostic value of the rupture of the capsule in stage I epithelial ovarian carcinoma, Gynecol Oncol 35:321, 1989.
31. Sainz de la Cuesta R and others: Prognostic importance of intraoperative rupture of malignant ovarian epithelial neoplasms, Obstet Gynecol 84:1, 1994.
32. Granberg S, Wilkland M, and Jansson I: Macroscopic characteristics of ovarian tumors and the relationship to the histologic diagnosis: criteria to be used for ultrasound evaluation, Gynecol Oncol 35:139, 1989.
33. DeLancey JO and Hurd WW: Inability to insufflate the peritoneal cavity at the time of laparoscopy. In Nichols DH and DeLancey JO, editors: Clinical problems, injuries and complications of gynecologic and obstetric surgery, Baltimore, 1995, Williams & Wilkins.
34. Hurd WW and others: Laparoscopic injury of abdominal wall vessels: a report of three cases, Obstet Gynecol 82:673, 1993.
35. Hurd WW and others: The relationship of the umbilicus to the aortic bifurcation: impli-

cations for laparoscopic technique, Obstet Gynecol 80(1):48, 1992.

36. Dingfelder JR: Direct laparoscopic trocar insertion without prior pneumoperitoneum, J Reprod Med 21:45, 1978.

37. Byron JW, Fujiyoshi CA, and Miyazawa K: Evaluation of the direct trocar insertion technique at laparoscopy, Obstet Gynecol 74:423, 1989.

38. Byron JW, Markenson G, and Miyazawa K: A randomized comparison of Veress needle and direct trocar insertion for laparoscopy, Surg Gynecol Obstet 177:259, 1993.

39. Copeland C, Wing R, and Hulka JF: Direct trocar insertion at laparoscopy: an evaluation, Obstet Gynecol 62:655, 1983.

40. DeCherney AH: Laparoscopy with unexpected viscus penetration. In Nichols DH, and DeLancey JO, editors: Clinical problems, injuries and complications of gynecologic and obstetric surgery, Baltimore, 1988, Williams & Wilkins.

41. Neely MR, McWilliams R, and Makhlouf HA: Laparoscopy: routine pneumoperitoneum via the posterior fornix, Obstet Gynecol 45:459, 1975.

42. Morgan HR: Laparoscopy: induction of pneumoperitoneum via transfundal puncture, Obstet Gynecol 54:260, 1979.

43. Childers JM, Brzechffa PR, and Surwit EA: Laparoscopy using the left upper quadrant as the primary trocar site, Gynecol Oncol 50:221, 1993.

44. Kadar N and others: Incisional hernias after major laparoscopic gynecologic procedures, Am J Obstet Gynecol 168:1493, 1993.

45. Montz FJ, Holschneider CH, and Munro MG: Incisional hernia following laparoscopy: a survey of the American Association of Gynecologic Laparoscopists, Obstet Gynecol 84:881, 1994.

46. Plaus WJ: Laparoscopic trocar site hernias, J Laparoendosc Surg 3:567, 1993.

47. Wheeler JM: Major vascular injury at laparoscopy. In Corfman RS, Diamond MP, and DeCherney, editors: Complications of laparoscopy and hysteroscopy, Boston, 1993, Blackwell Scientific Publications, Inc.

48. Nordestgaard AG and others: Major vascular injuries during laparoscopic procedures, Am J Surg 169:543, 1995.

49. Assimos DG, Patterson LC, and Taylor CL: Changing incidence and etiology of introgenic ureteral injuries, J Urol 152:2240, 1994.

50. Senagore AJ and Luchtefeld M: An initial experience with lighted ureteral catheters during laparoscopic colectomy, J Laparoendoc Surg 4(6):399, 1994.

51. Hershlag A and others: Femoral neuropathy after laparoscopy: a case report, J Reprod Med 35:575, 1990.

52. Fishman JR, Moran ME, and Carey RW: Obturator neuropathy after laparoscopic lymphadenectomy, Urology 42:198, 1993.

53. Batres F and Barclay DL: Sciatic nerve injury during gynecologic procedures using the lithotomy position, Obstet Gynecol 62:925, 1983.

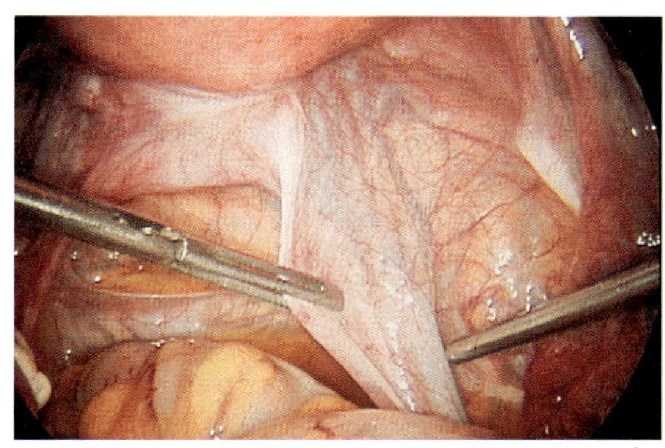

PLATE 1 Ureter has been catheterized, and when stent is moved, ureter is easily visualized. An instrument retracts the uterosacral ligament medially while the other forceps on the right points to the ureter. The ureter then passes through the web, where stent motion helps to identify it easily.

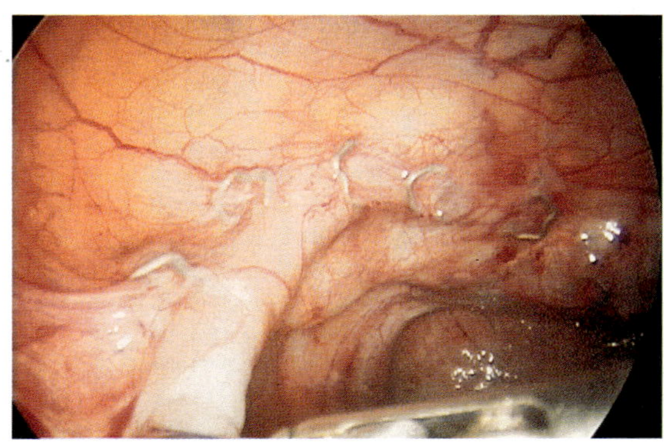

PLATE 2 This patient underwent LAVH 6 months previously. Apparently multiple hernia staples were used to close the parietal peritoneum, and one caused partial left ureteral obstruction. The ureter was catheterized, and the stent made removal of these staples and identification of the ureter quick and easy.

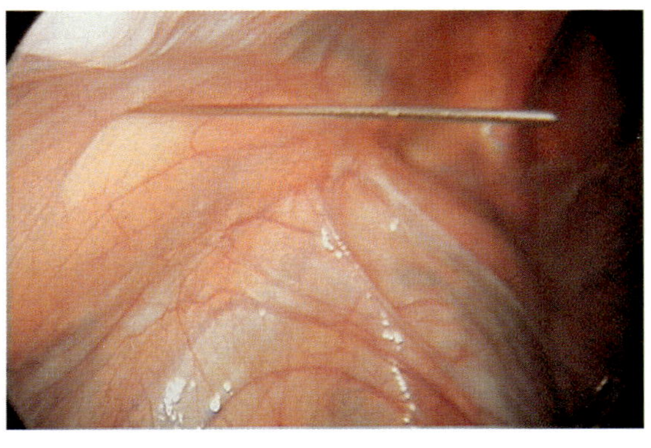

PLATE 3 Needle localizes trocar entry site. In this patient, the needle passes just lateral to the inferior epigastric vessels. Note how far lateral the path of the trocar is located. Iliac vessels are inferior and medial to the needle.

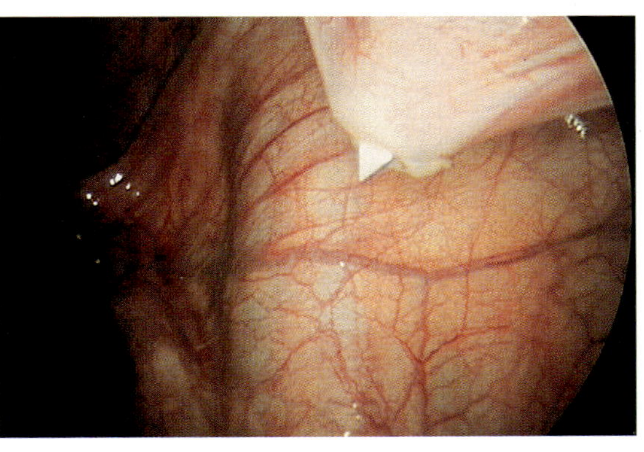

PLATE 4 Controlled entry means that the secondary trocars are carefully inserted through the anterior abdominal wall until the trocar tip is visualized. It is then directed away from possible injury sites.

Plate 5 Trocar sheath has been placed just lateral to inferior epigastric vessels and directly above external iliac vessels. Trocar sites are chosen to afford best approach to the operative site.

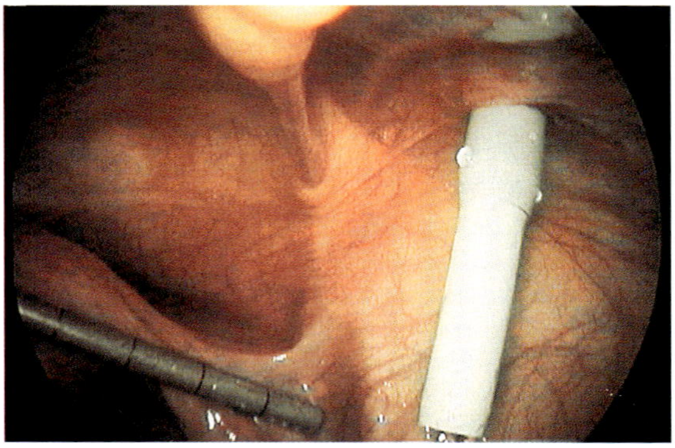

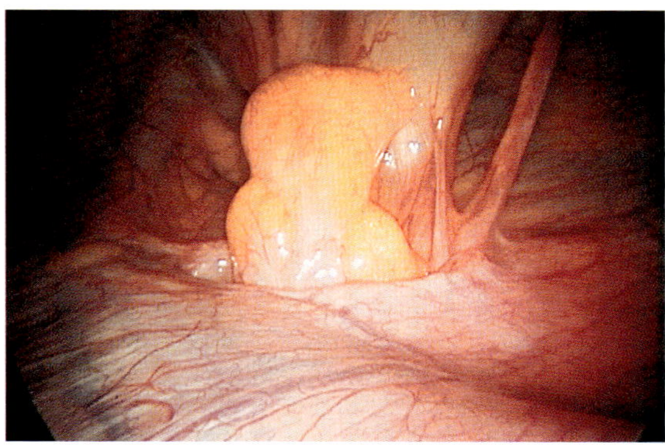

Plate 6 Omentum and bowel have herniated through the fascia at the site of an 11.5 mm trocar insertion. Fascia was improperly closed.

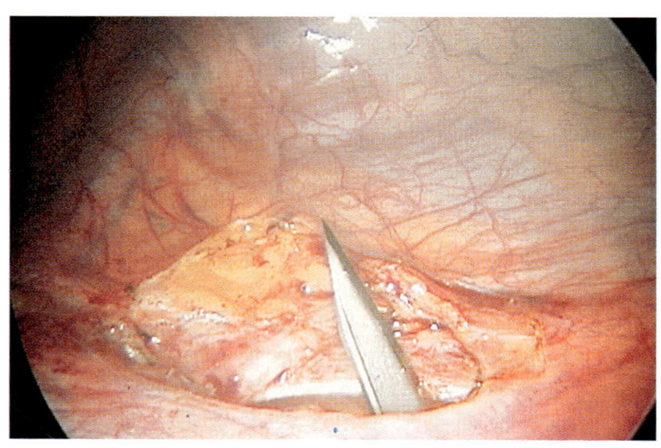

Plate 7 Bowel and omentum have been freed. Sac now is being excised, and broken closure of fascia will be accomplished. Note that the defect is much larger than original puncture site.

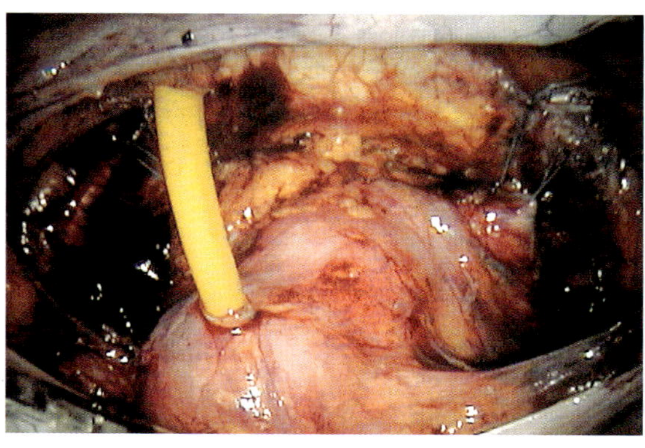

Plate 8 Space of Retzius has been opened and laparoscopic Burch procedure performed. Suspension sutures are seen in upper right-hand corner of photo. The bladder was entered when dissecting the vessel neck from the underlying pubovesical fascia. Two layered closure was performed and a suprapubic catheter left in place for 7 days. Recovery was uneventful.

24

Ovarian Remnant and Residual Ovary Syndromes

LOUISE LAPENSEE
KEITH B. ISAACSON

The ovarian remnant, the residual ovary, accessory ovary, and supernumerary ovary are all challenging benign ovarian syndromes that can result in the need for reoperation after previous gynecologic surgery. In this chapter, the ovarian remnant and the residual ovary syndromes will be discussed in detail, and the accessory ovary and supernumerary ovary, which are rare findings, will be reviewed briefly.

The residual ovary syndrome results when an ovarian pathologic condition (requiring surgical therapy) arises after hysterectomy in which an oophorectomy was not performed.[1] The ovarian remnant syndrome, on the other hand, refers to the presence of *functioning ovarian tissue* after an intended bilateral oophorectomy.

Confusion between the residual ovary and the ovarian remnant syndromes and between accessory and supernumerary ovaries occurs because of the similarity of the names. Supernumerary ovary, although it is an extremely rare gynecologic condition, deserves mention because it may be impossible to distinguish it from an ovarian remnant.[2] Also, it may present in a manner that mimics both the residual ovary syndrome and the ovarian remnant syndrome. A supernumerary ovary can be diagnosed when it becomes symptomatic or develops neoplasia when there has been no previous gynecologic disease. However, if the supernumerary ovary was not discovered at the time of hysterectomy, a subsequent ovarian problem will most likely be considered a residual ovary syndrome rather than a supernumerary ovary. Likewise, if a previous bilateral oophorectomy has been performed, subsequent evidence of ovarian function will lead to suspicion of an ovarian remnant syndrome rather than a supernumerary ovary.

Accessory ovary and supernumerary ovary both refer to congenital ectopic ovarian tissue. Accessory ovary is a portion of ovary in anatomic proximity to the main ovary, but it appears distinct.[1] It is usually attached to the broad ligament and is often connected to the normal ovary. In fact, the ectopic accessory ovary may actually have arisen when a small portion of ovarian tissue split off from the developing ovarian primordium.

A supernumerary ovary, on the other hand, is entirely separate from the normally placed ovary. It must also contain follicular ovarian tissue and arise from a separate primordium.[2,3] The clearest cases are those in which the supernumerary ovary lies in the retroperitoneal region.[4] The ectopic ovarian tissue has been found in the omentum, the mesentery of the bowel, and the lower pole of the kidney. It is thought to be either a result of arrested embryologic migration of germ cells en route from the yolk sac to the genital ridges or a result of detachment and transplant of a portion of the ovarian primordium from the genital ridge to the dorsal mesentary.[5] In either case, the supernumerary ovary has developed separately from the anlage of the normally placed ovary and has a separate blood supply. Since the supernumerary ovary has arisen as a result of developmental aberrancy, it is not surprising to find other associated genitourinary anomalies. Renal and ureteral abnormalities, bladder diverticulum, accessory fallopian tubes, and müllerian fusion defects such as unicornuate, bicornuate, or septate uterus, all have been found in association with a supernumerary ovary.[4]

Although the astute gynecologist should be attuned to the differences in the uncommon entities, occasional confusion is understandable. Indeed, in Wharton's classic discussion of the supernumerary ovary, the first case presented may likely be an example of ovarian remnant syndrome developing at the sites of two previously removed supernumerary ovaries.[4]

OVARIAN REMNANT SYNDROME CASE HISTORY

B.B.W. is a 42-year-old G1P1 woman who is status post–left salpingo-oophorectomy for an ovarian cyst and subsequent TAH and right salpingo-oophorectomy at the time of intraperitoneal hemorrhage from a ruptured right ovarian cyst. Her presenting symptom was right pelvic pain of several months' duration. The pain was constant but with periodic severe exacerbations. Severe dyspareunia made coitus extremely difficult. The patient also had a history of multiple episodes of PID, and at the time of hysterectomy, extensive pelvic adhesions.

Physical examination revealed a tender cystic mass in the right lower quadrant. Pelvic ultrasonography confirmed a 3- by 4-cm cystic mass in the right pelvis. Serum FSH level was 7.6 IU/L (postmenopausal normal level is 35 to 151 IU/L), serum luteinizing hormone (LH) level was 2.2 IU/L (postmenopausal normal level is 11 to 61 IU/L), and serum estradiol level was 186 pg/ml (postmenopausal normal level is 5 to 18 pg/ml).

At exploratory laparotomy, a 4- by 3-cm multicystic mass was found densely adherent to the right pelvic side wall and ureter. After lysis of extensive abdominal and pelvic adhesions, retroperitoneal dissection with removal of the peritoneum of the right pelvic side wall, including the mass and remnants of the round and broad ligaments, was accomplished. A similar dissection was carried out on the left side of the pelvis.

The pathologic examination of the cystic mass revealed ovarian tissue with a corpus luteum, multiple corpora albicantia, and ovarian stroma. Six weeks after surgery, the patient had an FSH level of 61.2 IU/L, an LH level of 19.7 IU/L, and an estradiol level of less than 10 pg/ml.

Etiology

The patient just described represents a case of ovarian remnant syndrome. The syndrome was first reported as a cause of ureteral obstruction by Kaufman in 1962[6] but probably dates into the last century. In 1875, prior to the common performance of hysterectomy, Goodman noted that women occasionally continued to menstruate following bilateral oophorectomy. The occurrence was attributed to "supplementary ovaries," but given the rarity of that gynecologic entity, the most likely explanation was an incomplete removal of ovarian tissue, as advanced by Malcolm in 1903.[4]

Confusion on the topic persisting to the present day is evidenced by the divergent views on the etiology of the ovarian remnant syndrome. The ovarian rest explanation, though it receives less support than the incomplete removal view, is based on the understanding of how the ovaries develop. In the human embryo, the primordial germ cells develop among the endodermal cells close to the allantois in the wall of the yolk sac. They then migrate along the wall of the hindgut and dorsal mesentery into the genital ridge, a distance of about 0.5 mm.[5,7]

Witschi,[4] in studying the migration of germ cells in the human embryo, found that occasionally there was a delay or failure of some of these cells to migrate. Although some of the cells that failed to reach the genital ridge degenerated, Witschi noted that others appeared normal. Should these germ cells induce the primitive mesenchyme of the mesentery or retroperitoneal area to undergo differentiation into ovarian stroma, functioning extragonadal ovarian tissue could result.

Although this explanation describes a probable etiology for supernumerary ovaries, it is a less likely explanation for the ovarian remnant syndrome than the incomplete removal theory. Support for the latter comes from the observation that ovarian remnant syndrome frequently arises in such settings as endometriosis or PID, where the initial dissection for removal of the ovaries was difficult.

The theoretical basis for this explanation is provided by data from animal studies. Parkes and Smith demonstrated the viability of homografts of ovarian tissue no bigger than 1 mm.[8,9] Shemwell and Weed[10] implanted ovarian cortex onto the peritoneum of four oophorectomized cats. Estrus was observed in two of the animals, while two had ovarian cysts at second laparotomy. Minke and others[11] showed that suturing devascularized ovarian tissue to intact or abraded peritoneum also resulted in the development of functioning ovarian tissue in rats. Payan and Gilbert[12] suggested that the pathogenesis of the disorder was related to the alteration of the soft tissue of the pelvis by inflammatory processes, tumors, or endometriosis, with vascular changes allowing ovarian remnants to function in ectopic locations. Consequently, in cases where extensive disease, adhesions, increased vascularity, or alteration of normal anatomy create the possibility of leaving behind even a tiny remnant of ovarian tissue, the cell may survive, reestablish a blood supply, and begin to function with the production of follicles, cysts, or corpora lutea. The functioning tissue is often retroperitoneal or encased in adhesions. This explains why pressure from an expanding cyst or bleeding from a corpus luteum frequently results in pain.

Obstruction of the distal ureter is occasionally encountered because of the propensity of the ovarian remnant to form cysts. Retroperitoneal reaction to the follicular fluid involved in ovulation can create local fibrosis and lead to cyclical ureteral obstruction.[13]

Diagnosis

Pelvic pain with or without a mass after hysterectomy and BSO is a diagnostic dilemma. The ovarian remnant syndrome is suspected when premenopausal levels of FSH and LH are present in a patient with documented bilateral oophorectomy. The diagnosis is confirmed by histologic demonstration of ovarian tissue at operation.[14] In addition to occurring after a hysterectomy and BSO, the syndrome also has been reported on the ipsilateral site of unilateral oophorectomy, although less commonly.[6,15,16] Obviously in these women, FSH and LH values in the premenopausal range would be expected. Ovarian remnant syndrome should be suspected in this case if there has been a history of surgery complicated by the presence of PID, endometriosis, diverticulitis, or severe adhesions. The symptoms can range from mild pelvic pressure, dull aches, dyspareunia, and constant or cyclic pelvic pain to an acute abdomen resulting from bowel and/or ureteral obstruction.

The symptoms from ovarian remnant syndrome usually occur within 5 years of the removal of both ovaries.[1,17] Postoperatively, patients can experience menopausal hot flashes that subsequently disappear. The symptoms of ovarian remnant syndrome are often delayed because some time must elapse before the lack of estrogen feedback to the central nervous system can induce a sufficient rise in FSH and LH levels to stimulate the development of the dormant ovarian remnant. Similarly, ovarian remnant syndrome is less likely to develop after unilateral oophorectomy as long as there is a functioning contralateral ovary. If a mass develops at the site where the previously removed ovary was located, neoplasia should be considered. However, Nezhat and Nezhat have reported three cases of ovarian remnant syndrome on the ipsilateral side of a previous unilateral oophorectomy in which pathology revealed only benign pathologic conditions (a corpus albicans, a follicular cyst, and a corpus luteum).[16] A pelvic mass that develops from an ovarian remnant in a postmenopausal woman must be considered malignant until proven otherwise by surgical removal. Any nonneoplastic ovarian tissue remaining in a postmenopausal woman after bilateral oophorectomy would be resistant to functional or dysfunctional stimulation by FSH or LH.

On physical examination, a tender pelvic mass is often found in women with ovarian remnant syndrome. In fact, up to 50% of patients with ovarian remnant syndrome have presenting symptoms of pelvic pain and a pelvic mass.[15] A transabdominal or transvaginal pelvic ultrasound examination is useful in delineating and evaluating a cystic mass. A CT scan and MRI are at this time of unproven value.

If GI complaints are present, barium enema, sigmoidoscopy, or both can be useful in demonstrating external compression from an ovarian remnant. Occasionally a patient will have flank pain or recurrent UTIs with a history of past bilateral oophorectomy. In this instance, an IV urogram should be done to eliminate an ovarian remnant obstructing a ureter.[1] Because ovarian remnants are frequently located near the ureter, an IV pyelogram is helpful to document the presence or absence of preexisting compromise of the urinary tract. Depending on the nature of any urinary tract symptoms, the gynecologist may wish to consider cystoscopy if the location of a mass or obstruction warrants ruling out a pathologic condition of the bladder.

Measurement of FSH, LH, and estradiol levels are definitely in order. Premenopausal levels in a patient with a history of bilateral oophorectomy indicate the presence of functioning ovarian tissue. Studies by Utian and others never recorded FSH levels less than 70 IU/L and LH levels less than 30 IU/L in postoophorectomy patients.[18] Even if a postoophorectomy patient has been on oral menopausal replacement therapy, levels of FSH have been reported to remain in the low postmenopausal range (50 to 75 IU/L) until levels of conjugated estrogens are given in doses as high as 2.5 mg per day.[18-20] On the other hand, estradiol, FSH, and LH levels in the menopausal range do not rule out an ovarian remnant. The amount of functioning ovarian tissue may be insufficient to suppress the gonadotropins.

Treatment

In the treatment of ovarian remnant syndrome, consideration may be given to three approaches: ablation, suppression, and removal. The advantages and disadvantages of each should be carefully weighed relative to the particular case under consideration.

Ablation. Ablation of the ovarian remnant by castration doses of deep radiation has the advantage of avoiding the technical difficulties and morbidity associated with a surgical treatment, as well as avoiding the possibility of recurrence. However, the dense pelvic adhesions that may make surgery difficult also pose significant risk of radiation enteritis or colitis to the immobilized bowel.[10] The dose of radiation required for castration of the premenopausal woman is usually about 2000 cGy. A smaller dose in the range of 500 to 700 cGy may be sufficient for a perimenopausal castration.[21] Small bowel injury occurs at a high incidence with dosages near 4000 cGy. These figures may make radiation appear to be a safe therapeutic regimen for the treatment of ovarian remnant syndrome, but the gynecologist must remember that radiation doses are usually reported as midline doses. Structures adherent to the anterior abdominal wall may, in fact, receive 15% to 20% more radiation than the intended area.[22]

A second caveat of castration by radiation is that an unexplored pelvic mass may represent a neoplasm. Shemwell and Weed have reported a case in which a woman presumed to have an ovarian remnant and treated with castration dosages of radiation subsequently died from adenocarcinoma that developed in an area of residual endometriosis.[10] Thus the decision to choose ablative radiation therapy for ovarian remnant syndrome must be accompanied by a reasonable certainty that a mass does not represent a neoplastic process. The patient must be followed carefully, and if the mass does not regress promptly, surgical exploration is mandatory.

Suppression. Suppressive therapy for an ovarian remnant may take several forms; the rationale behind each is to eliminate ovulatory surges of LH and/or to consistently suppress FSH. Again, an ovarian neoplasm should be ruled out and would not be expected to respond to suppressive therapy. In a woman with premenopausal levels of FSH, LH, and estradiol, however, an attempt at suppression is reasonable, especially if the surgical risk is high.

Gonadotropin suppression resulting in ovarian suppression has been reported with depot medroxyprogesterone acetate (Depo-Provera), danazol, GnRH agonist, estrogens, oral contraceptives, and a combination of these agents.[14,16,23,24] The number of cases in the literature varies from isolated case reports[23,24] to a limited series of 13 patients.[16] The results of suppressive therapy have been mixed, with approximately one half of the patients reporting pain relief.

Elimination of ovulatory surges can be accomplished with current oral contraceptive regimens until the perimenopausal years if there are no contraindications. Commonly used postmenopausal replacement regimens, on the other hand, do not completely suppress ovulatory function. The resolution of a pelvic mass and subsequent pain with the use of GnRH agonists is diagnostic as well as therapeutic by confirming the ovarian origin. There is concern, however, on the long-term consequences of the hypoestrogenic state induced by GnRH agonist treatment on calcium metabolism and trabecular bone strength. Therefore treatment should be limited to 6 months unless add-back therapy with an estrogen-progestin or bisphosphonate program is included. If an acceptable regimen is demonstrated to suppress ovulation function, some patients may be able to avoid surgical treatment.

Removal. To date, the most widely used treatment of ovarian remnant syndrome is surgical removal by laparotomy and more recently by operative laparoscopy. The important principle for the gynecologic surgeon to bear in mind is that not only should the identifiable mass be removed but all tissue in which an ovarian remnant could be located also must be removed. This principle becomes paramount on reviewing the operative histories of many of these patients. Patients who have been taken to surgery for the removal of a mass often come back again and again for removal of subsequent masses. The recurrence rate has been reported to be between 8% and 30%.[14] Removing all tissue in which a remnant could be located should take into consideration both of the proposed causes of the syndrome: the previous incomplete removal of ovarian tissue and stimulation of previously quiescent ovarian rests. The latter should remind the surgeon to search for the rare supernumerary ovary that can mimic ovarian remnant syndrome. Keeping this in mind, the bowel and its mesentary, the omentum, and the course of the ovarian vessels should be examined carefully. Adequate excision of the ovarian remnant and contiguous adherent tissue may require removal of bowel serosa and appendices epiploicae, the broad ligaments and underlying areolar and vascular tissues, and careful dissection to free an adherent ureter or pelvic vessel. The technical difficulty of the surgery in addition to frequent involvement of vital structures and the need for extensive dissection is often exacerbated by the distortions of anatomy from previous surgery and extensive adhesions, increasing the risk of vital organ injury. The complication rate is high, ranging from 16% to 30%.[14,25]

Occasionally an ovarian remnant syndrome is strongly suspected in a patient based on the history and steroid and gonadotropin hormone assays, but a mass cannot be identified. In the absence of a pelvic mass on pelvic examination and ultrasound examination, stimulation of any residual ovarian tissue with clomiphene citrate or gonadotropins before surgical intervention can aid in localization rather than proceeding with a retrograde dissection along both ureters. Kaminski and others[26] treated a patient with suspected ovarian remnant syndrome with a 10-day course of clomiphene citrate, 100 mg daily. Diagnosis was confirmed preoperatively by ultrasound examination, and the mass was easily localized at laparotomy and removed intact. Likewise, Kosasa and others[27] reported stimulation of ovarian remnant with human menopausal gonadotropins and human chorionic gonadotropin before surgery. Therefore a trial of ovarian stimulations with agents such as clomiphene citrate should be considered before surgery in any patient without an identifiable mass and with an FSH below 30 IU/L.

IV urograms and ureteral stents placed before the exploratory procedure can help identify the ureter during the dissection of an adherent mass. The ureteral catheters can be placed cystoscopically preoperatively or perioperatively. Another option is to perform an extraperitoneal cystostomy and catheterize the ureter if opening the peritoneum above the pathologic process and tracing the ureter inferiorly did not permit adequate visualization. Also, ureteroscopy[28] can facilitate the dissection, help rule out any intrinsic component of the obstruction, and assure adequate ureteral patency and integrity once the remnant has been removed. Undue manipulation of a ureter containing a semirigid catheter may otherwise add to the potential for ureteral injury. More recently, lighted ureteral catheters have been advocated for major laparoscopic pelvic surgery as a means of enhancing ureteral identification and decreasing the risk of ureteral injury.[29] The decision on whether or not to place ureteral catheters or perform a ureteroscopy is best made on an individual basis according to the adherent nature and location of the mass in relation to the course of the ureter.

Until recently surgery for ovarian remnant syndrome was traditionally done by laparotomy. Development of new laparoscopic instrumentation and techniques now allows access to and removal of the ovarian remnants even in the most complex cases associated with adhesions, endometriosis, and multiple previous laparotomies. Nezhat and Nezhat[16] used operative laparoscopy for the treatment of ovarian remnant syndrome in 13 patients. Nine patients reported complete pain relief, one had incomplete but satisfactory pain relief, two required bowel resection by laparotomy to obtain pain relief, and one, despite subsequent laparotomy, had persistent pain. There were no intraoperative or postoperative complications reported. All operations were performed on an outpatient basis, and the mean operating time was 130 minutes (range 90 to 230 minutes) with an average blood loss of less than 150 ml. Klutke et al.[28] reported a case in which an ovarian remnant following TAH and BSO resulted in unilateral ureteral obstruction. The obstructing tissue was successfully excised laparoscopically with simultaneous ureteroscopic monitoring without complications.

The American Society for Reproductive Medicine[30] recently published guidelines for attaining privileges in gynecologic operative endoscopy. If there is no extensive pelvic wall dissection, ureteral dissection, or bowel surgery required, laparoscopic surgery for ovarian remnant syndrome can be categorized as a level II procedure. However, most laparoscopic surgery for ovarian remnant syndrome is categorized as a level III procedure, requiring the surgeon to be skilled in advanced laparoscopic techniques.

When performed by an experienced surgeon, operative laparoscopy is preferable to laparotomy for surgically managing benign pelvic disease because patients have less blood loss, a shorter hospital stay, shorter recuperation period, less expense, and less fear of the procedure.[16]

Laparoscopy. The operative laparoscopy can be performed according to the following general outline. The patient is given an outpatient bowel preparation 1 day before surgery. After general endotracheal anesthesia is obtained, the patient is placed in the dorsal lithotomy position, in which the patient's lower legs are placed in Allen stirrups with the thighs flexed 10 to 20 degrees. This position allows access to the urethra, vagina, and rectum should intraoperative manipulation be needed (e.g., placement of ureteral stents via cystoscopy). A pelvic examination and bimanuel rectovaginal-abdominal palpation is performed, and the patient is then prepared and draped for laparoscopy. The patient's bladder is emptied, and a Foley catheter should be left in place to avoid recatheterization during a lengthy procedure, thereby decreasing the risk of bladder injury.

The surgery is performed using multipuncture operative laparoscopy. If the patient has undergone multiple previous laparotomies, the laparoscope can be inserted using an open laparoscopy technique or by a mapping technique in which the initial trocar is inserted in the left upper quadrant in an effort to decrease the risk of bowel injury.[16] After entry into the abdominal cavity, identification and restoration of normal anatomy often requires extensive lysis of adhesions. Any mass thought to represent an ovarian remnant should be evaluated in relation to the ureter, iliac vessels, bowel, bladder, and vaginal vault. In most cases, the ovarian remnant will be adherent to one or more of these vital structures. Therefore clear identification of these structures is necessary prior to adhesiolysis. Our preferred technique is to first identify the vital structures at a site distal to the mass where there is normal anatomy. The structure can then be traced to the adherent mass. This is done with the ureter at the level of the pelvic brim just as the ureter crosses over the iliac vessels (Figure 24.1). Once the ureter is identified, its course is traced down the pelvic side wall. If the ureter is not involved in the adhesive mass, a releasing incision is made in the peritoneum to allow the ureter to fall away from the area of dissection (Figure 24.2). If the ureter is involved in the adherent mass, then we pass a ureteral stent to allow for clear identification during adhesiolysis (Figure 24.3). This same exercise is done with the large and small bowel and the iliac vessels; they are located in an area free of adhesions and followed to the pelvic mass.

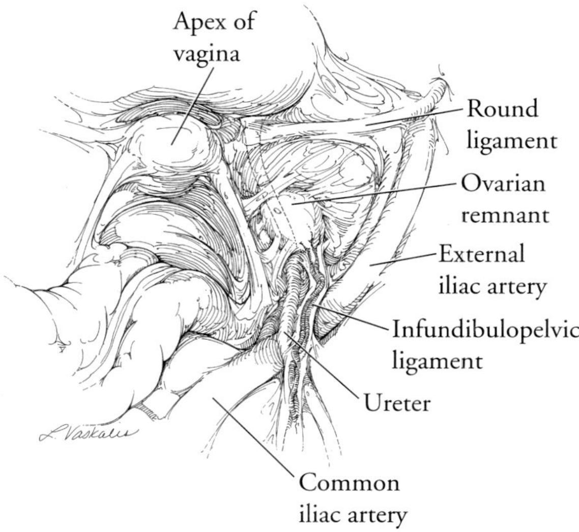

FIGURE 24.1 Identification of the vital structures (ureter, iliac vessels) distal to the ovarian remnant.

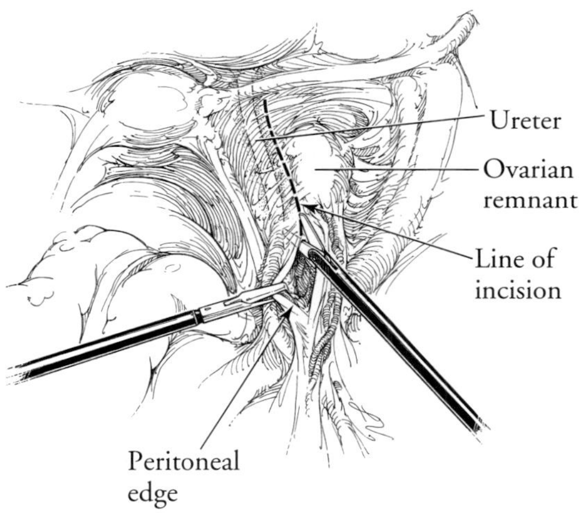

FIGURE 24.2 The course of the ureter has been traced down the pelvic side wall and is not involved in the adherent mass. Through a releasing incision, the ureter is allowed to fall away from the ovarian remnant.

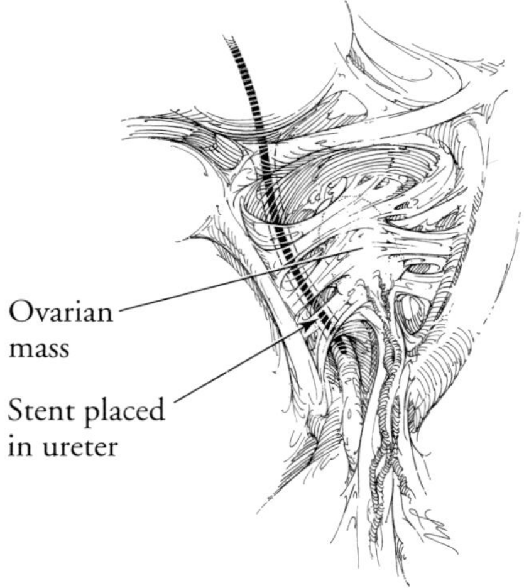

FIGURE 24.3 Placement of a ureteral stent is advised in any case where the ovarian remnant is involved with the ureter to permit adequate identification during adhesiolysis.

After these vital structures have been clearly identified, an effort is made to locate and ligate the ovarian vessels within the retroperitoneal space, again at a distance from the adherent ovarian mass (Figure 24.4). This is done to reduce the chance of hemorrhage during adhesiolysis.

Laparoscopic adhesiolysis and dissection of the ovarian remnant can be achieved as long as the surgeon is able to identify proper tissue planes. If at any time during dissection the tissue planes are lost due to dense adhesions, the procedure should be abandoned because the surgeon is likely to perforate a major vessel or bowel without warning. In this circumstance, the dissection should be performed via laparotomy to take advantage of the surgeon's own tactile feedback to avoid major vessel injury. Using traction and countertraction with minimally traumatic graspers and the magnification provided by the laparoscope, tissue planes should be adequately identified to allow for complete dissection in the majority of the cases.

Adhesiolysis is carried out using blunt and sharp dissection with the scissors or laser. It is best to use blunt dissection in avascular normal tissue planes and use either scissors or laser to lyse fibrous tissue (Figure 24.5). If the surgeon were to use only sharp dissection, then there would be an increased risk of injury to normal structures because of the lack of tactile feedback when using the laparoscope. In addition to having instruments available for cutting and hemostasis, an adequate suction-irrigating device is necessary to identify all sources of bleeding.

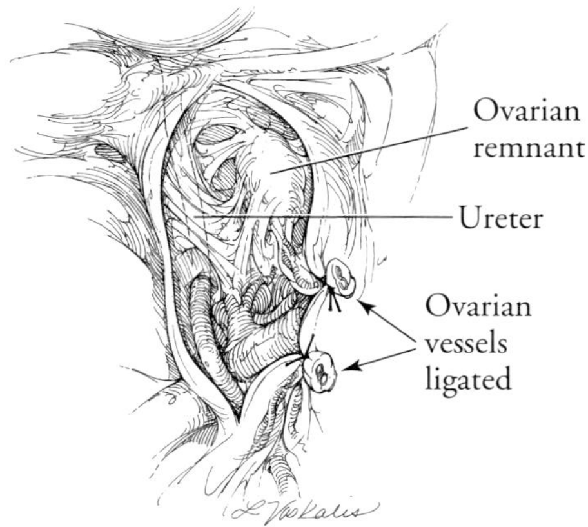

FIGURE 24.4 Identification and ligation of the ovarian vessels within the retroperitoneal space distal to the ovarian remnant.

The anatomy of the retroperitoneal space is identified in all cases in which an ovarian remnant is adherent to the lateral pelvic wall. As mentioned, the peritoneum is lifted in a nonadherent location and opened. The retroperitoneal space is then dissected to the infundibulopelvic ligament remnant for identification of the ovarian vessels while constantly viewing the course of the major pelvic blood vessels and the ureter. The ovarian blood supply is then interrupted via bipolar cautery, clips, or suture ligation. As long as proper tissue planes are identified, adhesions involving the bowel surface can be incised with the scissors or laser. Ovarian tissue imbedded in the muscularis of the bowel should be removed superficially with precaution not to enter the bowel lumen. If denuded, the serosa and muscularis layers of the bowel can be imbricated with one to three interrupted 4-0 polydioxanone extracorporal or intracorporal sutures. After freeing the ovarian tissue from its adhesions, the ovarian tissue is excised and submitted to the pathology department for histologic evaluation. If the ovarian mass is in a postmenopausal woman and carcinoma is suspected, the mass is placed in a plastic bag to prevent the spillage of cancer cells before removal through the abdominal wall.

It has been suggested that dissection of the contralateral ureter throughout its pelvic

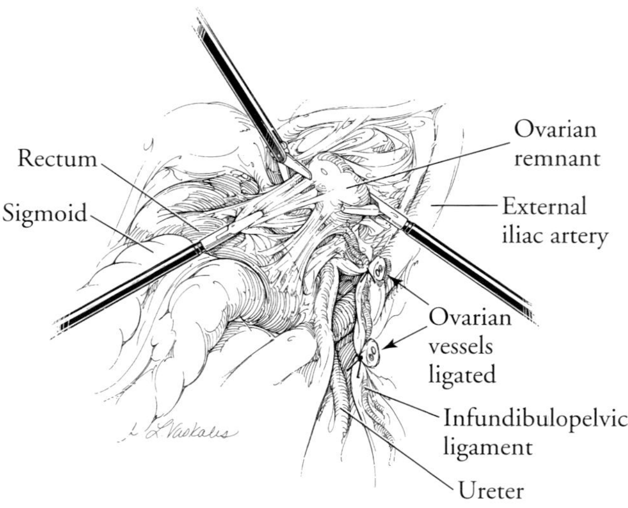

FIGURE 24.5 The adhesiolysis is carried out where tissue planes have been adequately identified. Using traction and countertraction with minimally traumatic graspers, fibrous tissue is lysed with scissors.

course as well as removal of surrounding tissues be performed on the opposite side of the ovarian remnant. This is to ensure that there is no "silent" remnant present that could lead to symptoms and repeat operation at a later date.[31] Considering the extensive dissection needed and the morbidity associated with the procedure, we recommend that the surgery be limited to the side where the ovarian remnant is located unless there is a strong suspicion that there are bilateral ovarian remnants, which is the exception rather than the rule.

Postoperatively, complications such as ileus or bowel obstruction, anemia, hematoma, lymphocyst formation, or urinary fistula can occur. The surgeon should be aware of persistent postoperative pain, nausea, vomiting, and/or fever, which can be an early warning sign of any of these complications.

In general, the advantage of operative laparoscopy over laparotomy is the reduced patient morbidity and rapid recovery of the patient when the procedure is performed by an experienced surgeon. The patient is usually discharged home the day of or the day after surgery.

Close follow-up of the patient is necessary for signs of recurrence. FSH, LH, or estradiol levels may be added to the pelvic examination to evaluate the effectiveness of treatment.[1] Adequate removal of a functioning ovarian remnant will usually result in a rise in FSH levels to more than 100 IU/L within 1 week of surgery, and in addition menopausal symptoms such as hot flashes may appear.[14]

Laparotomy. For most gynecologists, laparotomy and excision of the ovarian remnant remains the preferred approach for the treatment of ovarian remnant syndrome. The same general principles apply whether the surgery is performed by laparoscopy or laparotomy. The patient should be placed in the dorsal lithotomy position with the second assistant standing between the patient's legs in order to provide substantial retraction during the surgery. A Maylard incision should be considered for ideal exposure to the pelvic side walls. Careful lysis of adhesions to restore normal anatomy is performed. A retroperitoneal approach is usually needed for complete extirpation of the mass and adequate identification of ureter and vessels. Following complete dissection, reperitonization of the pelvis is often impossible and usually unnecessary. Occasionally a retroperitoneal space drain is needed to prevent lymphocyst formation if extensive dissection has been performed.

Prevention

The best way to prevent ovarian remnant syndrome is to remove all ovarian tissue at the initial operation. The same principles mentioned in removing an ovarian remnant apply when removing the ovaries at the first surgery. In the presence of endometriosis, PID, extensive adhesions, inflammatory bowel disease, or any other pathologic condition that alters normal pelvic anatomy, care must be taken to remove the entire ovary as well as the pelvic parietal peritoneum, which may be harboring ovarian cortical tissue. The ureters must be mobilized and retracted laterally as needed, allowing the excision of the cul-de-sac or pelvic side wall peritoneum if it is involved in periovarian adhesions.

With the advent of laparoscopic removal of ovaries, the same precautions are needed not to leave any ovarian tissue behind. Nezhat and Nezhat[16] reported two patients that presented with ovarian remnant syndrome following laparoscopic salpingo-oophorectomy using the endoloop technique. To prevent ovarian remnant syndrome, the infundibulopelvic ligament must be free of adhesions so that the endoloop ligature can be placed well below the ovarian tissue. Electrodesiccation and transsection of the infundibulopelvic ligament or application of surgical clips may be favored. When ovaries are densely adherent to the broad ligament, retroperitoneal dissection, meticulous adhesiolysis, and removal of peritoneum are essential before performing laparoscopic oophorectomy.

Also, because Minke and others[11] showed that devascularized ovarian tissue can reimplant on peritoneum in the rat, care must be taken when oophorectomy or cystectomy is performed by laparoscopy, because any specimens left in the abdominal cavity may result in persistent ovarian tissue. With these precautions, the patient's primary procedure hopefully will be curative, and she will be spared the trauma of reoperation for ovarian remnant syndrome.

RESIDUAL OVARY SYNDROME CASE HISTORY

D.M. is a 27-year-old G3P3 woman whose presenting symptom was crampy lower abdominal pain "about 12 days out of the month." Dyspareunia was so severe that following a recent attempt at coitus, she went to the emergency room because of incapacitating pain accompanied by nausea and vomiting. Her past surgical history included laparoscopic diagnosis of PID, subsequent bilateral salpingectomy, and later a vaginal hysterectomy for menometrorrhagia and uterine prolapse. On two occasions since hysterectomy, large ovarian cysts were noted at the time of laparoscopy for pelvic pain.

A markedly tender 4-cm cystic mass just posterior and caudal to the left vaginal fornix was found on pelvic examination. The pelvic ultrasound examination revealed a 4.8-cm left adnexal mass containing a 3.1-cm cyst. The patient was unable to tolerate attempted ovarian suppression with oral contraceptives, and pain was uncontrolled by nonsteroidal antiinflammatory agents.

Diagnosis

The residual ovary syndrome is characterized by symptoms of lower abdominal and back pain, deep dyspareunia, and occasional disturbance of the urinary tract in women in whom one or both ovaries were preserved at the time of hysterectomy.[32] In most cases, a fixed tender mass near the vaginal cuff is found on pelvic examination. It is estimated that 1% to 3%[33] of posthysterectomy patients will eventually present with the residual ovary syndrome, and up to 10% of patients[33-35] with preserved ovaries will need a second operation for ovarian disease. Reoperation occurs within 5 years of hysterectomy in one half of these cases.[33] The pain that is found in 77% of patients with residual ovary syndrome may be continuous or intermittent and varies in intensity from a bothersome ache to incapacitating cramps. Radiation of the pain to the legs, back, or both can occur, and some patients report vasomotor symptoms, nausea, and vomiting.

Disturbance of the urinary tract can be manifested as frequency, urgency, dysuria, and recurrent UTIs. Interestingly, 30% to 50% of patients have had a pelvic surgical procedure before their hysterectomy. The most common indications that led to hysterectomy are dysfunctional uterine bleeding, leiomyomas, pelvic pain, and pelvic floor relaxation.

A mass is found in more than one half of the patients with residual ovary syndrome. Whether or not a mass is present, the ovary is usually located close to the vaginal cuff, contributing to the dyspareunia.[32,33]

Transabdominal or transvaginal pelvic ultrasonography, CT scan, or MRI, all may be useful in locating the ovaries before surgery. Adhesions and perioophoritis, as well as retroperitoneal location of the ovary, may prevent follicular rupture into the peritoneal cavity and give rise to an expanding polycystic mass. The ultrasound examination may show solid and cystic areas, making it difficult to distinguish the residual ovary from neoplasia.[36] A barium enema is appropriate if neoplasia is a strong consideration or if GI complaints are present.

If the mass is suspicious for malignancy, appropriate tumor markers should be obtained prior to the surgery. Just as mentioned for the ovarian remnant syndrome, an IV pyelogram is often appropriate to document the presence or absence of preexisting compromise of the urinary tract. If urinary tract symptoms are present, a cystoscopy should be performed to rule out a pathologic condition of the bladder.

At the time of surgery, periadnexal adhesions to the vaginal cuff, pelvic side wall, and bowel are almost universally found. If the ovary is retroperitoneal, the ureter and other retroperitoneal structures may be encased by the process. The ovary is cystic in more than one half of the cases, and most of those cysts are functional. In up to 10.3% of patients, the cause of the cyst is endometriosis.[37] Benign neoplasia of the ovary is present in up to 13.7% of patients with residual ovaries, and the incidence of malignant neoplasia ranges from 0.5% to 8.2%.[37-40]

Treatment

The management of residual ovary syndrome is similar to the management of the ovarian remnant syndrome (see previous section). If a pelvic mass is present, it should be managed as a pelvic mass would be in any other woman of comparable age with the application of the usual criteria for surgical exploration. If there is no mass or if a mass is thought very unlikely to represent a neoplastic process, a trial of ovarian suppression with medroxyprogesterone acetate, a combination estrogen-progestin regimen, or GnRH analogs may be considered. Ablation of the ovaries by castrating doses of radiation has very little place in the current management of residual ovary syndrome. In most cases, surgery by a laparoscopic approach or by laparotomy will be performed with the treatment options being oophoropexy or unilateral or bilateral oophorectomy.

Oophoropexy rather than oophorectomy may be performed in young women in whom preservation of ovarian function is important. Microsurgical technique should be applied to free the ovary from surrounding adhesions, and the ovaries are then suspended out of the pelvis by suturing or clipping them intraperitoneally to the psoas muscle (Figure 24.6). They should be marked by radiopaque surgical clips for subsequent identification should that ever prove necessary. Extreme care should be exercised to avoid torsion of the infundibulopelvic ligament. If there is a question of compromise to the ovarian blood supply, the viable ovary will demonstrate a timely greenish fluorescence under Wood's light after rapid IV injection of 3 to 4 ml of a 20% solution of fluorescein dye. Oophoropexy can also be performed by laparoscopy. The ovaries are sutured to the psoas muscle using intracorporal or extracorporal sutures. They can then be marked with staples using a hemoclip applier.[41]

In most cases of residual ovarian syndrome, unilateral or bilateral salpingo-oophorectomy is the procedure of choice. Because of previous surgery and the frequency of perioophoritis and adhesions, an approach similar to that used in the ovarian remnant syndrome may be helpful (see previous description). A laparoscopic approach should be favored in most cases because of the advantages cited previously. Laparoscopic surgery for the residual ovary syndrome is considered a level II procedure requiring advanced laparoscopic techniques.[30] In most cases, the surgery will be uneventful, requiring less pelvic side wall dissection, bowel surgery, and ureteral dissection than surgery for ovarian remnant syndrome, rendering the laparoscopic procedure the preferred approach for most gynecologists. Consideration may be given to preoperative bowel preparation and to the placement of ureteral catheters with the same indications previously mentioned.

The surgery for residual ovary syndrome is performed using multipuncture operative lap-

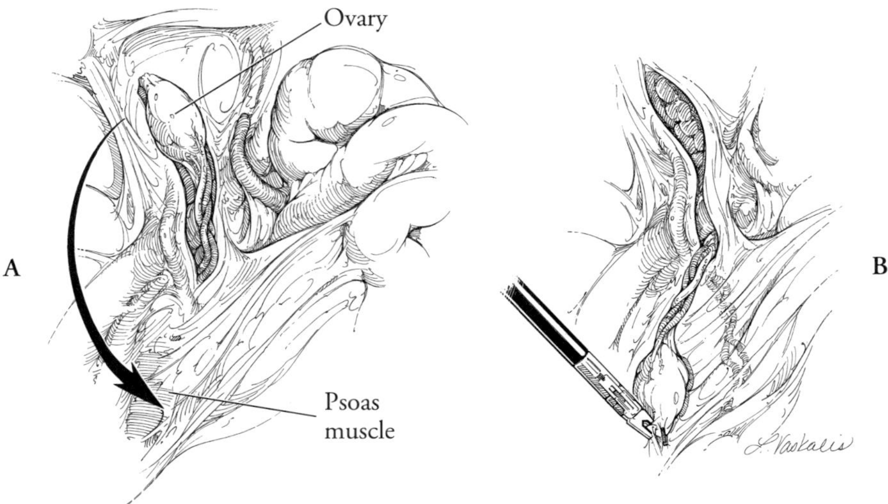

Figure 24.6 **A,** Oophoropexy is favored in young women with a residual ovary to preserve ovarian function. The ovary is freed from surrounding adhesions and suspended out of the pelvis to the psoas muscle. **B,** Clipping of the ovary intraperitoneally to the psoas muscle.

aroscopy. Lysis of adhesions will probably be necessary to restore the landmarks of pelvic anatomy. A retroperitoneal approach will often be helpful and necessary if the ovarian mass is itself retroperitoneal and encasing the ureter or other retroperitoneal structures. To enter the retroperitoneal space, the round ligament is identified, cauterized, and transsected. The incision in the peritoneum is then extended cephalad along the pelvic side wall parallel to the infundibulopelvic ligament. The retroperitoneal space is developed using blunt and sharp dissection, and adhesions are lysed until the ureter and the course of the major blood vessels can be traced. With the ureter under direct visualization (see Figure 24.2), the ovarian vessels can then be isolated, electrodesiccated and transsected, or the surgeon may choose to apply surgical clips. Proceeding caudally, blunt and sharp dissection can be used to free the adnexa from the pelvic side wall, from remaining portions of the broad ligament, from the bladder, and from the vaginal cuff (see Figure 24.5). If the ovary is densely adherent to other pelvic structures, an attempt to remove the serosal layer of these organs along with the ovary should be undertaken to prevent subsequent development of the ovarian remnant syndrome. If the surgeon elects to remove the ovary with an endoloop ligature, care must be taken to remove all adhesions from the infundibulopelvic ligament so that the ligature can be placed well below the ovarian tissue. The peritoneal defect does not have to be closed.

Prevention

The residual ovary syndrome is one of a number of considerations in the continuing debate over ovarian conservation at the time of hysterectomy. An awareness of the essential metabolic functions of the ovaries persuades most gynecologists not to perform oophorectomy at the time of hysterectomy in premenopausal women unless otherwise indicated. If the initial procedure is being performed abdominally, the operative morbidity for TAH versus TAH with BSO is the same in most cases. Proponents of prophylactic oophorectomy look mainly toward prevention of ovarian cancer and less toward prevention of residual ovary syndrome. On the other hand, it is estimated that to save one woman from ovarian cancer, prophylactic oophorectomy must be routinely performed in 700 to 3300 women at the time of hysterectomy.[42,43]

The decision of whether to perform prophylactic oophorectomy must be individualized, and dogmatic recommendations regarding management are best avoided. Careful and considerate information regarding the advantages and disadvantages of retaining the ovaries should be given to each patient. The impact of menopausal symptoms, the risk of osteoporosis and cardiovascular disease, psychologic changes, age, parity, menstrual status, family history, personal history, postoperative follow-up, cultural factors, and the patient's preference, all should be thoroughly discussed prior to performing a prophylactic oophorectomy. Age and proximity to natural menopause are two of the most important considerations, because the incidence of ovarian cancer increases significantly after age 40 and peaks at age 80.[44,45] Moreover, not all patients can take HRT, and the degree to which pills, pellets, and patches can mimic the complex endocrinologic function of the human ovary is debatable.

Although an in-depth discussion of the pros and cons of ovarian conservation is beyond the scope of the present chapter, consideration of some of the possible causes of the residual ovary syndrome have a bearing on the decision to retain or remove the ovaries in an individual patient. Since nearly all ovaries requiring removal in the residual ovary syndrome are found to have perioophoritis and adhesions, ovaries found to be so involved at the time of hysterectomy might be viewed with greater suspicion, particularly if the patient has significant pelvic pain. If a decision is made to retain these ovaries, adhesions should be lysed as much as possible using microsurgical techniques, and the placement of adhesion barriers should be considered at the conclusion of the surgery.

In addition to pelvic adhesive disease at the time of hysterectomy, Grogan has suggested two additional high-risk groups for developing residual ovary syndrome: patients who have experienced conservative pelvic surgery before their hysterectomy and patients coming to hysterectomy with the diagnosis of dysfunctional uterine bleeding.[37] The first group is of concern because 35% to 50% of patients with residual ovary syndrome give such a history. The second group is of concern because the uterus being removed is merely the target organ. The dysfunction lies further upstream in the hypothalamic-pituitary-ovarian axis and can reside in the ovary itself. Women who had a unilateral oophorectomy at the time of hysterectomy are also at higher risk for the residual ovary syndrome. Plöckinger and Kölbl retrospectively studied 1265 women status posthysterectomy for benign conditions with at least one ovary saved. The risk of having secondary ovarian pathologic findings was significantly higher in women who had only one ovary saved (7.6%) compared with those who had both ovaries saved (3.4%).[38]

An ovary cannot function properly if its blood supply is compromised. Variation in ovarian blood supply[21] ranges from sole dependence on the ovarian artery to sole dependence on the uterine artery. Generally the medial half of the ovary and the medial two thirds of the fallopian tube are supplied by the uterine artery; the remaining lateral portions are supplied by the ovarian artery. If the ovaries are to be retained at the time of hysterectomy, the clamps containing the utero-ovarian ligaments should be placed as close to the uterus as possible. Even this maneuver will not spare the occasional ovary that derives essentially its entire blood supply from the uterine artery. If the surgeon has any doubt regarding ovarian blood supply, it may be tested with fluorescein dye as described previously, or the surgeon may listen for arterial pulsations with a sterile Doppler probe.

Unless diseased, the tube should be retained with the ovary in order to prevent the interruption of the arcade of vessels running through the mesosalpinx and mesovarium. Likewise, care should be taken not to twist or stretch the ovarian vessels during reperitonization if it is performed.

The pedicles containing the ligated utero-ovarian ligaments should not be tied together in the midline of the pelvis, especially in the premenopausal woman. The resulting adhesions to the vaginal vault may cause dyspareunia. At abdominal hysterectomy, consideration may even be given to elevating and suspending the ovaries out of the pelvis. Surgical clips on the utero-ovarian ligaments will identify their location on subsequent radiographic studies. Finally, if a decision has been made to remove the ovaries, care should be taken that they be removed in their entirety to prevent the development of the ovarian remnant syndrome and thus merely substituting the risk of one reoperative benign ovarian syndrome for another.

References

1. Price FV, Edwards R, and Buchsbaum J: Ovarian remnant syndrome: difficulties in diagnosis and management, Obstet Gynecol Surv 45(3):151, 1990.
2. Cruikshank SH and Van Drie DM: Supernumerary ovaries: update and review, Obstet Gynecol 60:126, 1982.
3. Harlass F, Magelssen D, and Solsson AP: Supernumerary ovary: a case report, J Reprod Med 32:459, 1987.
4. Wharton LR: Two cases of supernumerary ovary and one of accessory ovary, with an analysis of previously reported cases, Am J Obstet Gynecol 78:1101, 1959.
5. Printz JL and others: The embryology of supernumerary ovaries, Obstet Gynecol 41:246, 1973.
6. Kaufman JJ: Unusual causes of extrinsic ureteral obstruction, part 1. J Urol 87:319, 1962.
7. Sadler TW: Urogenital system. In Langman: Medical embryology, Baltimore, 1985, Williams & Wilkins.
8. Parkes AS and Smith AU: Proc R Soc Lond 140:455, 1953.
9. Smith AU and Parkes AS: Preservation and transplantation of normal tissues, Ciba Foundation Symposium, New York, 1954, Churchill Livingstone.
10. Shemwell RE and Weed JC: Ovarian remnant syndrome, Obstet Gynecol 36:299, 1970.
11. Minke T and others: Ovarian remnant syndrome: study in laboratory rats, Am J Obstet Gynecol 171:1440, 1994.
12. Payan HM and Gilbert EF: Mesenteric cyst–ovarian implant syndrome, Arch Pathol Lab Med 111:282, 1987.
13. Horowitz MI and Elguezabel A: Obstruction of the ureter by recent corpus luteum lo-

cated in the retroperitoneum: report of two cases, J Urol 95:706, 1966.

14. Steege JF: Ovarian remnant syndrome, Obstet Gynecol 70:64, 1987.
15. Symmonds RE and Pettit PDM: Ovarian remnant syndrome, Obstet Gynecol 54:174, 1979.
16. Nezhat F and Nezhat C: Operative laparoscopy for the treatment of ovarian remnant syndrome, Fertil Steril 57(5):1003, 1992.
17. Lee RA: Ovarian remnant syndrome. In Nichols DH and DeLancey JOL, editors: Clinical problems, injuries and complications of gynecologic and obstetric surgery, ed 3, Baltimore, 1995, Williams & Wilkins.
18. Utian WH and others: Effect of premenopausal castration and incremental dosages of conjugated equine estrogens on plasma follicule-stimulating hormone, luteinizing hormone, and estradiol, Am J Obstet Gynecol 132:297, 1978.
19. Schiff I and others: Oral medroxyprogesterone in the treatment of menopausal symptoms, JAMA 244:1443, 1980.
20. Simon JA and diZerega GS: Physiologic estradiol replacement following oophorectomy: failure to maintain precastration gonadotropin levels, Obstet Gynecol 59:511, 1982.
21. Mattingly RF and Thompson JD: Leiomyomata uteri and abdominal hysterectomy for benign disease. In TeLinde's operative gynecology, ed 6, Philadelphia, 1985, JB Lippincott Co.
22. Brown CB and Go RT: Diagnostic radiographic techniques in gynecologic oncology. In Sciarra JJ, editor: Gynecology and obstetrics, Philadelphia, 1985, Harper & Row, Publishers.
23. Nelson DC and Avant GR: Ovarian remnant syndrome, South Med J 75:757, 1982.
24. Koch MO, Coussens D, and Burnett L: The ovarian remnant syndrome and ureteral obstruction: medical management, J Urol 152:158, 1994.
25. Pettit PD and Lee RA: Ovarian remnant syndrome: diagnostic dilemma and surgical challenge, Obstet Gynecol 71:580, 1988.
26. Kaminski PF and others: Clomiphene citrate stimulation as an adjunct in locating ovarian tissue in ovarian remnant syndrome, Obstet Gynecol 76:924, 1990.
27. Kosasa TS and others: Diagnosis of a supernumerary ovary with human chorionic gonadotropin, Obstet Gynecol 47:236, 1976.
28. Klutke J and others: Laparoscopic treatment of ureteral obstruction secondary to ovarian remnant syndrome, J Urol 149:827, 1993.
29. Senagore AJ and Luchtefeld M: An initial experience with lighted ureteral catheters during laparoscopic colectomy, J Laparoendosc Surg 4(6):399, 1994.
30. Society for Reproductive Surgeons, The American Fertility Society: Guidelines for attaining privileges in gynecologic operative endoscopy, Fertil Steril 62(6):1118, 1994.
31. Lee RA: Residual ovarian disease after hysterectomy. In Stovall TG, editor: Hysterectomy, New York, 1993, Elsevier Science Publishing Co.
32. Bukovsky I and others: Ovarian residual syndrome, Surg Gynecol Obstet 167:132, 1988.
33. Christ JE and Lotze EC: The residual ovary syndrome, Obstet Gynecol 46:551, 1975.
34. Hajj SN and Mercer LJ: Retrograde dissection of the adnexa in residual ovary syndrome, Surg Gynecol Obstet 165:451, 1987.
35. Ranney B and Abu-Ghazaleh S: The future function and fortune of ovarian tissue which is retained in vivo during hysterectomy, Am J Obstet Gynecol 128(6):626, 1977.
36. Gray R and others: Postoperative residual ovary syndrome: an uncommon cause of pelvic mass, J Can Assoc Radiol 34:56, 1983.
37. Grogan RH: Reappraisal of residual ovaries, Am J Obstet Gynecol 97:124, 1967.
38. Plöckinger B and Kölbl H: Development of ovarian pathology after hysterectomy without oophorectomy, J Am Coll Surg 178:581, 1994.
39. Reycraft JL: Discussion of Counsellor, Am J Obstet Gynecol 69:543, 1955.
40. Grundsell H and others: Some aspects of prophylactic oophorectomy and ovarian carcinoma, Ann Chir Gynaecol 70:36, 1981.
41. Williams RS and Mendenhall N: Laparoscopic oophoropexy for preservation of ovarian function before pelvic node irradiation, Obstet Gynecol 80(3):541, 1992.
42. Schweppe KW and Beller FK: Prophylactic oophorectomy, Geburtshilfe Frauenheilkd, 39(12):1024, 1979.

43. DeNeef JC and Hollenbeck ZJR: The fate of ovaries preserved at the time of hysterectomy, Am J Obstet Gynecol 96:1088, 1966.

44. Prophylactic oophorectomy, ACOG Technical Bulletin No. 111, 1987.

45. Barber HRK: Ovarian cancer, Cancer 36(3):149, 1986.

Bibliography

Berek JS and others: Avoiding ureteral damage in pelvic surgery for ovarian remnant syndrome, Am J Obstet Gynecol 133:221, 1979.

Dmowski WP, Radwanska E, and Rana N: Recurrent endometriosis following hysterectomy and oophorectomy: the role of residual ovarian fragments, Int J Gynaecol Obstet 26:93, 1988.

Major FJ: Retained ovarian remnant causing ureteral obstruction, report of two cases, Obstet Gynecol 32:748, 1968.

Parker GA: Ovarian remnant and residual ovary syndromes. In Nichols DH, editor: Reoperative gynecologic surgery, St Louis, 1991, Mosby.

Phillips HE and McGahan JP: Ovarian remnant syndrome, Radiology 142:487, 1982.

Randall CL, Hall DW, and Armenia CS: Pathology in the preserved ovary after unilateral oophorectomy, Am J Obstet Gynecol 84:1233, 1962.

25

Repair of Chronic Third- and Fourth-Degree Obstetric Lacerations

John O.L. DeLancey
Marc R. Toglia

Third- and fourth-degree obstetric lacerations are an uncommon but serious complication of vaginal delivery. It is becoming increasingly apparent that obstetric trauma to the anal sphincter complex can be associated with significant dysfunction of the anal continence mechanism and is far more common than previously recognized.[1-5] Rectovaginal fistulas and chronic third- and fourth-degree perineal lacerations are probably the most commonly recognized cause of anal incontinence seen in an obstetrician/gynecologist's practice. This chapter will discuss the diagnosis and management of the last two conditions. Since accurate therapy requires a thorough understanding of the anal continence mechanism, the pathophysiology of these conditions will be reviewed as well.

Prevention Considerations

The prevention of third- and fourth-degree lacerations has received appropriate consideration recently. Oftentimes, leaving the perineum intact rather than cutting a median episiotomy can accomplish this. Recognized risk factors for obstetric lacerations that involve the anal sphincter include nulliparity, instrumental delivery, infant weight greater than 4 kg, persistent occiput posterior position, and a prolonged second stage.[4] The value of a midline episiotomy in protecting against sphincter injury is questionable, and several studies have suggested that episiotomy itself increases the risk of anal sphincter rupture.[2,6,7,8]

Avoidance of episiotomy in an attempt to minimize the likelihood of sphincter injury is not without consequences. Clear evidence exists that a prolonged second stage of labor is associated with increased degrees of denervational pelvic floor nerve injury and can predispose to future development of urinary incontinence and pelvic organ prolapse. The obstetrician is therefore constantly faced with the dilemma of attempting to protect the pelvic floor from acute muscular injury or avoiding neurologic injury from prolonged impact of the fetal head against the pelvic floor.

Once a third- or fourth-degree laceration has occurred, it must be recognized as a significant problem. No less attention should be paid to correcting this defect in the delivery room than to correcting it in the gynecologic OR. The basic tenets of repair surgery mandate the following: adequate exposure and lighting, good visualization of the anatomic structures involved, adequate anesthesia, and the proper instruments and assistance. This may involve moving the patient from the labor/delivery room to the delivery/operating room, placing a pudendal nerve block, or calling upon the anesthesiologist to redose the epidural anesthetic. All of these efforts will pay off in preventing a third- or fourth-degree laceration from becoming more than a transient problem for the patient.

Anatomy and Physiology

Chronic third- or fourth-degree lacerations are part of a spectrum of pelvic floor defects involving the perineal body, rectovaginal septum, and anorectum. Clinical management of these conditions requires a thorough understanding of the normal anatomy (Figure 25.1) and physiology of this area. Anal continence is a complex physiologic mechanism that requires both intact anatomic structures and appropriate neuromuscular control.

External Anal Sphincter

The external anal sphincter is a teardrop-shaped body of striated muscle that encircles the lower part of the anal canal before attaching to the coccyx posteriorly through the anococcygeal raphe. Unlike most other striated muscles, the external anal sphincter, along with the puborectalis muscle, maintains a constant resting tone that contributes to the closure of the anal canal at rest. During sudden distention of the rectum with a fecal bolus, the external anal sphincter contracts reflexively to preserve continence and to allow us to defer defecation to an appropriate time.

Internal Anal Sphincter

The internal anal sphincter is the thickened, downward continuation of the circular smooth muscle layer of the colon, lying between the anal mucosa and the external anal sphincter. Together with the external anal sphincter, it forms a cylindrical muscular complex that, measured in the midline, is 18.3 mm thick and 28.0 mm long.[9] It is important for clinicians to recognize that 54% of the anterior thickness of this sphincter complex is attributable to the internal anal sphincter and that physiologic studies have shown that the internal anal sphincter is responsible for 75% to 85% of the resting tone of the anal canal.[10,11] Unlike the external anal sphincter, this structure is not under voluntary control, and its function is mediated by reflex arcs at the spinal cord level. As intestinal contents fill the rectal

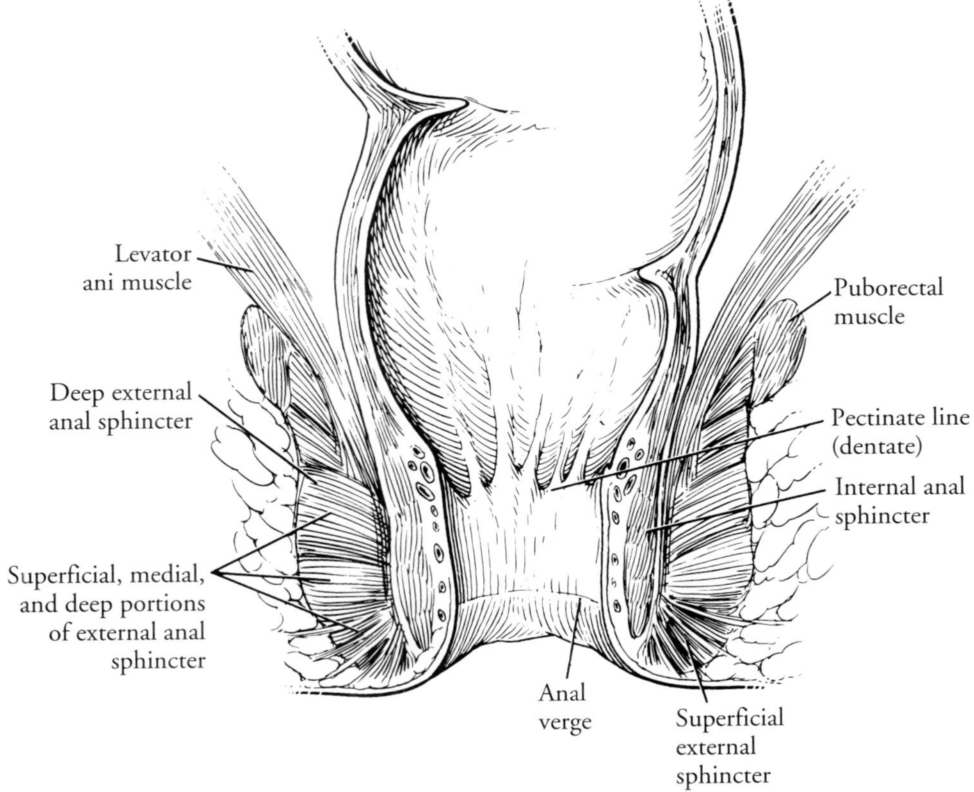

Figure 25.1 Anatomy of the anal continence mechanism. (From Lee RA: Atlas of gynecologic surgery, Philadelphia, 1992, WB Saunders Co.)

ampulla, the internal anal sphincter temporarily relaxes to allow the sensory rich upper anal canal to "sample" the contents and to determine whether this bolus represents solid, liquid, or gas. Once sampled, the internal anal sphincter contracts again to augment anal closure and preserve continence.

Puborectalis Muscle

Although the puborectalis muscle is not found within the perineal body and is therefore not involved in chronic third- and fourth-degree lacerations, it plays a critical role in anal continence and should be considered in any discussion regarding fecal control. The puborectalis muscle is a portion of the levator ani that originates on the inner surface of the pubic bones and passes behind the anorectal junction to form a U-shaped sling that "kinks" the rectum towards the pubic bone. Like the external anal sphincter, this striated muscle maintains a constant resting activity that creates an approximately 90-degree angle between the anal and rectal canals.[12,13] Continence of solid stool is maintained primarily by the action of the puborectalis, which is the reason why many patients with chronic fourth-degree lacerations remain continent of solid stool.

SYMPTOMS

Symptoms arising from injury to the anal continence mechanism can be understood by examining the physiologic role that each component of the continence mechanism plays in maintaining fecal control. The external anal sphincter is critical for providing immediate temporary augmentation of canal closure during times of sudden rectal filling with gas or liquid stool. Therefore injury to the external anal sphincter is associated with fecal urgency and urge-related incontinence of liquid or loose stool and flatus. Solid stool is maintained high in the pelvis by the action of the puborectalis muscle and the low compliance and generous capacity of the rectum and lower sigmoid colon. Damage to the puborectalis is associated with a flattening of the anorectal angle and difficulty in maintaining continence of solid stool. The internal anal sphincter is chiefly responsible for maintaining continence at rest, and also plays an important role in maintaining continence of liquid stool and flatus. Contraction of both the external and internal anal sphincters at the conclusion of a bowel movement help empty the anal canal by forcing stool either back up into the rectal ampulla or out through the anal orifice. Injury to these structures can therefore be associated with postdefecation seepage or fecal staining.

Normal continence requires an extraordinary sensorimotor coordination in order to allow the sphincteric complex to first distinguish between solid, liquid, and gaseous forms of intestinal contents and to allow gas to pass while remaining continent to the other two forms of feces. Much of this ability lies within the highly accurate sensation of the upper anal canal as well as sensory receptors within the levator ani.[14,15] Faulty continence can occur not only from pudendal nerve injury, which denervates the external anal sphincter and puborectalis, but also from damage to the sensory receptors that provide feedback.

DIAGNOSTIC EVALUATION

It is essential that the clinician determine the pathophysiology for the patient's complaints before initiating therapy. In the majority of cases, attentive history taking and focused physical examination can sufficiently diagnose most problems without needing to resort to sophisticated diagnostic studies.[16,17] States of increased GI motility, decreases in the normally compliant rectal reservoir, and central nervous system lesions, all can give rise to faulty anal continence. These conditions have been summarized elsewhere and are beyond the scope of this chapter.[17] It is important to recognize that patients with a chronic third- or fourth-degree laceration may have additional alterations of the anorectum that significantly contribute to their symptoms. This is especially true with both irritable bowel syndrome and inflammatory bowel disease. In one large series of women with both Crohn's disease and rectovaginal fistulas, 67% of subjects thought their symptoms related to their intestinal disease were more important than those attributed to their fistula.[18]

Clinical evaluation of the anal continence

mechanism is easy for the clinician who is adept at pelvic examinations and who possesses a clear understanding of the relevant anatomy and physiology. The following steps in this evaluation should prove useful in the management of patients with chronic third- and fourth-degree lacerations.

Inspection of the Perineum

Clinical evaluation begins with careful inspection of the vaginal introitus, perineum, and anal verge. Chronic fourth-degree lacerations are characterized by a disruption in the external anal sphincter anteriorly, loss of the perineal body, and attenuation of the rectovaginal septum[19] (Figure 25.2). When the external anal sphincter is disrupted anteriorly, there is typically dimpling of the perianal skin at 2 and 10 o'clock, which becomes more prominent when this muscle contracts. Subcutaneous separation of the sphincter can be present in a third-degree laceration and is associated with loss of the radial creases of the anal verge between these locations, which has been called the dovestail sign[16] (Figure 25.3).

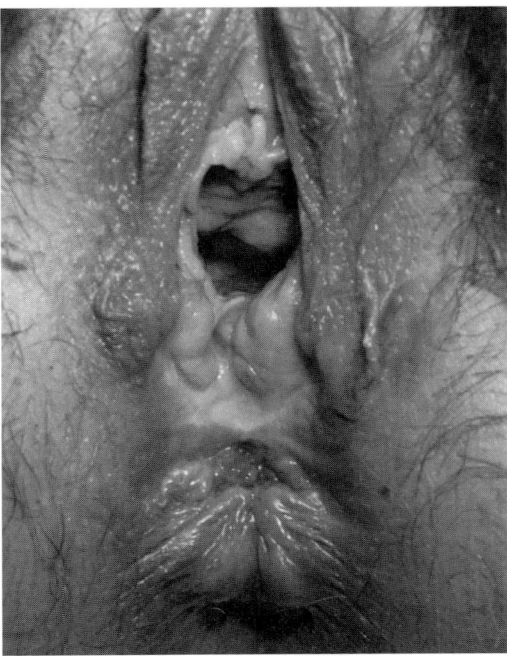

Figure 25.2 Chronic fourth-degree laceration. Note the absence of any perineal body and the posteriorly contracted separated sphincter muscle.

Determination of whether the external anal sphincter is intact or not is the most critical part of an evaluation for a chronic third- or fourth-degree laceration. Probably the most common error made in the evaluation of anal incontinence following a vaginal delivery is to assume that the external anal sphincter is intact when there is simply a taut band of perineal tissue bridging the anal and vaginal canals. Anal endosonography has demonstrated that persistent defects in this structure are surprisingly common following the primary repair of third- and fourth-degree obstetrical lacerations.[4,5]

The distal vagina must be carefully inspected to rule out small pinpoint fistulae that often accompany chronic fourth-degree lacerations. These typically appear as a small dimpling in the vaginal mucosa with the velvety red appearance of the underlying tissue

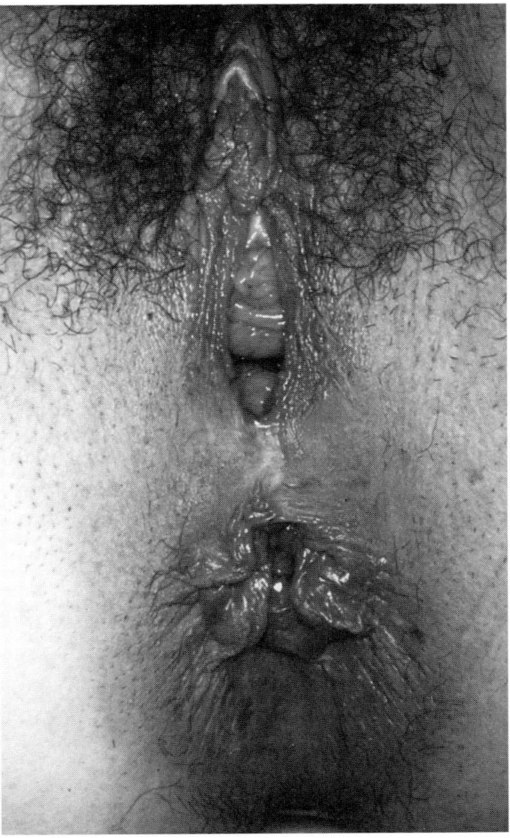

Figure 25.3 Chronic third-degree laceration. The perineal body is intact, but the sphincter is separated as indicated by the anterior loss of the perianal skin folds.

exposed. Such defects should be probed with fine silver wire probes to see if there is any communication with the anus. If the patient's symptoms suggest a fistula and none is evident, methylene blue dye mixed with surgical jelly can be instilled into the rectum using a catheter tip syringe. The colored jelly can be massaged into the rectovaginal septum with a gloved finger. The appearance of dye within the vaginal vault with either technique is highly suggestive of a fistulous tract.

Palpation

The integrity of the external anal sphincter and puborectalis can be evaluated by observation of the anal verge during voluntary muscular contraction and by digital palpation. The external anal sphincter should contract concentrically, and the actions of the puborectalis muscle pull the anus inward and toward the symphysis. Mechanical defects in the external anal sphincter are often apparent as a loss of the palpable muscular ring anteriorly on rectovaginal examination. The torn ends of the sphincter muscle can be located by inserting an index finger into the anal canal and palpating the substance of the external anal sphincter muscle at the 8 o'clock position between the finger and thumb. The muscle can then be followed anteriorly until its substance is lost and the end of the sphincter identified. Once the defect has been delineated, the remainder of the perineal body and rectovaginal septum can be evaluated to determine the integrity of these structures. Chronic third-degree lacerations represent an incompletely healed episiotomy in which the perineal skin is often intact but the underlying structures, including the anal sphincter complex, remain separated. In patients with a chronic fourth-degree laceration the perineal body is nonexistent and the rectovaginal septum is attenuated. Typically the vaginal mucosa and rectal mucosa appear fused and are devoid of the intervening connective tissue layer.

Neurosensory Examination

A focused neurosensory examination is essential prior to recommending surgical repair. Sphincter separation is often associated with denervation to this structure.[20] Although EMG studies or motor nerve conduction studies can objectively document injury to the sphincter complex, physical examination is oftentimes sufficient to direct therapy. A separated sphincter that exhibits brisk and strong voluntary contraction of the intact segment indicates that the muscle has retained a significant portion of its innervation. On the other hand, the absence of contraction or dimpling of the perianal skin with voluntary contraction suggests that there has been significant denervation of this structure. Although surgical intervention may be warranted in some of these individuals, they should be counseled preoperatively that the procedure may not restore complete continence.

DIAGNOSTIC TESTING

Many sophisticated diagnostic tests have been devised for evaluating the anal continence mechanism. These techniques have added to our understanding of how the continence mechanism works. We find, however, that they are rarely necessary for the evaluation of straightforward separated sphincters. The most frequently used studies include EMG, motor nerve conduction studies, anal manometry, and anal imaging studies. They will be briefly described to provide the reader with an understanding of their role in managing difficult cases.

EMG has been used to evaluate the integrity of external anal sphincter innervation following traumatic injury. EMG is a study of the electrical activity produced by the depolarization of muscle membranes. Nerve injury is characterized by reinnervation of the affected motor unit and a subsequent increase in "fiber density." EMG studies provide indirect evidence of neurologic injury by measuring the amount of reinnervation or increase in fiber density. Motor nerve conduction studies also have been used to study pelvic nerve damage. These studies are performed by stimulating the axon of the nerve and measuring the speed with which the action potential reaches the muscle innervated by that nerve. This time delay is called the nerve latency. A noninvasive technique for measuring the pudendal nerve terminal motor latency (PNTML) was developed by Snooks and Swash to evaluate pelvic floor neurophysiology following vaginal birth. Prolongation of the PNTML is indicative of injury to the pudendal nerve.

Anal manometry can be used to evaluate the sphincteric muscles under simulated physiologic conditions. Anorectal pressures are measured at different parts of the anorectum during both rest and voluntary contraction. Resting anal pressure is an indirect measure of the resting tone of the internal anal sphincter, whereas pressures measured during voluntary contractile effort reflect the functioning of the external anal sphincter.

Anal endosonography is a recently introduced technique for imaging both the internal and external anal sphincters.[21] This technique is ideally suited for evaluating sphincter function following vaginal delivery and has provided much insight into both the investigation and management of anal incontinence in these patients. Although originally described using a special probe inserted within the anal canal, similar results can be obtained using a probe placed against the perineal body and directed perpendicular to the axis of the anus. This procedure helps confirm mechanical disruption to both the internal and external anal sphincters. We have found it to be especially helpful in demonstrating defects in the internal anal sphincter that are impossible to determine clinically. Although sonographic studies are not absolutely essential, they do lend a degree of precision and objectivity that can be helpful in optimizing the results of surgical reconstruction.

MRI is capable of demonstrating highly detailed anatomy of the anorectum.[22] As such it is probably the most revealing anatomic study in terms of delineating sphincter defects. However, the great expense of these studies has limited their use as a research tool at the present time.

Surgical Repair Techniques

Reconstructive surgery for obstetric trauma involving the anorectum aims to restore the continuity of both the external and internal anal sphincters. In addition, attention should be directed at reestablishing a normal perineal body and rectovaginal septum, as the muscular support between the vagina and rectum is extremely limited. The ultimate goal of such a repair should be to reconstruct a sphincter complex that is at least 2 cm thick and at least 3 to 4 cm long. The results of such meticulous technique will also lengthen the anal canal and restore the functional high pressure zone within the anal canal.

Primary Repair of Third- and Fourth-Degree Lacerations at Delivery

Recent studies suggest that the primary repair of obstetric sphincter lacerations yield imperfect results.[4,5] It is our belief that these acute lacerations should be treated as thoroughly and meticulously as we would approach a chronic third- or fourth-degree laceration. First and foremost, the obstetrician should be satisfied that the basic tenets of reconstructive surgery have been satisfied: good exposure and lighting, adequate anesthesia, and the proper tools and assistance. The goal of this multilayer repair should be the reconstruction of a muscular cylinder that is at least 2 cm thick and 3 cm long, to reestablish the normal anatomic length of the anal canal and to reconstitute the perineal body. The uterus should be well contracted so that there is minimal bleeding from this area, and consideration should be given to placing a vaginal pack to prevent postpartum uterine bleeding from obscuring the operative field. A self-retaining vaginal retractor, such as a Gelpi retractor, can be quite effective in providing adequate exposure.

The steps involved in repairing a third- or fourth-degree laceration are illustrated in Figures 25.4 to 25.6. In the case of a fourth-degree laceration, the first layer of the repair should approximate the submucosa of the anorectum. We prefer to use a running suture of either 3-0 or 4-0 delayed absorption material such as polyglactin to create a watertight seal. In order to accomplish this, the suture should be started at least 5 mm above the defect in the anal mucosa and carried down to the anal verge. The second layer consists of a reapproximation of the disrupted fibers of the internal anal sphincter using a similar running 3-0 delayed absorbable suture.

Repair of the external anal sphincter should accomplish an end-to-end anastomosis of the disrupted sphincter capsule and its contained

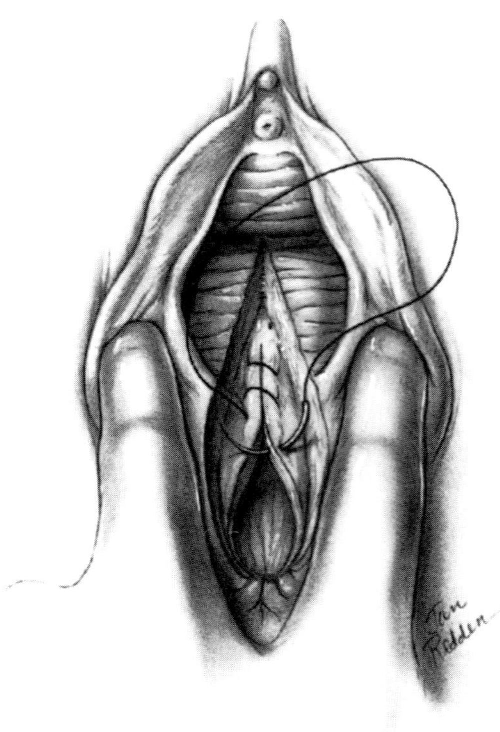

FIGURE 25.4 Closure of the bowel with a running suture anchored in the submucosa and muscularis of the anorectum. (From Hankins GDV and others: Operative obstetrics, Norwalk, Conn, 1995, Appleton & Lange.)

sphincter muscle. This can be accomplished by placing four to five interrupted sutures widely through the capsule and muscle. Visualization of the sphincter muscle itself is important to make sure that all areas are approximated. We are currently using a 2-0 delayed absorbable suture for this layer. Next, the intervening rectovaginal fascia and perineal body are approximated over these layers using interrupted sutures. Lastly, the vaginal mucosa and the remainder of the perineal body and skin are approximated.

Early Repair of Episiotomy Breakdown

Episiotomy infection and breakdown are an uncommon but important postpartum complication. In a retrospective review of more than 7,000 deliveries in which a median episiotomy was performed, Harris reported an 11% rate of third- or fourth-degree extension that resulted in a 0.1% incidence of rectovaginal fistulae and a 0.1% incidence of episiotomy infection.[23] Traditional teaching has held that the secondary repair of episiotomy dehiscence should be delayed for a minimum of 2 to 3 months to allow for revascularization and formation of scar tissue around the ends of the external anal sphincter. Unfortunately, this approach commits the woman to an extended period of physical, social, and sexual disability and is without scientific foundation.

There has been considerable discussion recently concerning the early repair of episiotomy dehiscence, and this cumulative experience has been summarized.[24] Hankins and others have reported their experience with early repair of episiotomy dehiscence in 31 patients, including 12 with clinical evidence of infection.[25] In all patients, aggressive wound debridement was performed on an inpatient unit, and antibiotics were administered to patients with clinical evidence of infection. Surgical repair was delayed until the wound was free from exudate. Satisfactory results were obtained in 94%. Others have reported similar experiences.[26,27,28]

A protocol for early repair of episiotomy breakdown has recently been proposed.[24] Once the diagnosis has been made, the wound should be carefully inspected and thoroughly debrided using IV analgesia or regional anesthesia if necessary. Suture fragments should be removed at this time. Subsequent wound care should consist of twice daily cleansing with a povidone-iodine impregnated scrub brush to remove any exudate. A single broad-spectrum antibiotic can be administered at the clinician's discretion. Secondary repair is then performed when the wound surfaces are free from exudate and covered by pink granulation tissue.

There are several advantages to these early repairs. Prolonged incontinence and loss of sexual function are avoided, and it allows the patient to return to her normal activities sooner. One disadvantage of this approach includes committing the patient to an extended hospital stay during the early postpartum period, which may interfere with breastfeeding and maternal-child bonding. Another is that some early attempts at repair may still fail, and there may be need for additional surgical procedures.

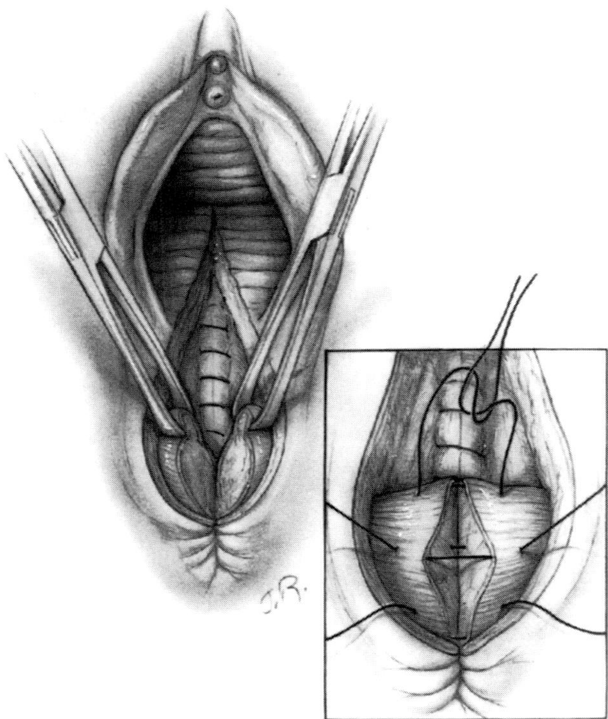

FIGURE 25.5 Approximation of the external anal sphincter muscle and its capsule. (From Hankins GDV and others: Operative obstetrics, Norwalk, Conn, 1995, Appleton & Lange.)

Repair of Chronic Third-Degree Lacerations

In repairing a chronic third-degree laceration we use an arch-shaped incision beginning over one end of the sphincter and extending to the other side. The first goal of repair is to dissect and identify the separated sphincter muscle (see Figure 25.3). The ends are typically located between the 2 and 3 o'clock position and the 9 and 10 o'clock position within the perineal body. The ends of the sphincter should be grasped with Allis' clamps and sharply mobilized with Metzenbaum's scissors. Locating these ends can be difficult, especially if there has been extensive scarring. Palpation of the intact portion of the external anal sphincter posteriorly while tugging on the tissue grasped within the Allis' clamps can help the surgeon to determine the location of these torn ends. In addition, we prefer to use a muscle stimulator to cause the muscle to contract, aiding in its identification. Once properly identified, both ends of the sphincter should be widely mobilized in order to obtain a tension-free anastomosis. The remainder of the perineal body should be reconstructed and the skin closed in whatever direction (transverse or vertical) the edges most naturally approximate.

Repair of Chronic Fourth-Degree Lacerations

When a fourth-degree laceration breaks down, the vaginal mucosa becomes attached to the rectal wall (Figure 25.7). The easiest way to excise the scarred tissue and enter the proper perineal planes is to excise the midline scar by grasping the lateral margins with Allis' clamps and cutting transversely with Mayo's scissors (Figure 25.8). This allows the surgeon to enter the rectovaginal space (Figure 25.9). The rectal wall should be mobilized from the rectovaginal septum and vaginal mucosa. Surgical dissection should be carried out to reach normal tissue. The location of normal tissue planes can be anticipated by palpating the rectovaginal septum before surgery to delineate the lateral extent of the central irregular scarred tissue and its junction with the pliable resilient normal tissue. Wide mobilization at each tissue plane

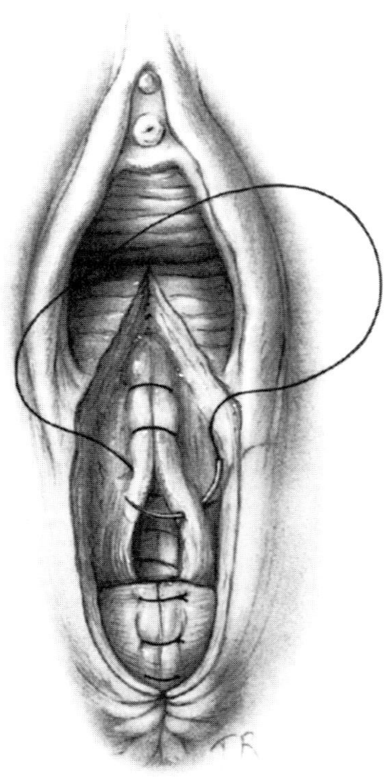

FIGURE 25.6 Closure of the internal anal sphincter muscle shown here after approximation of the external sphincter repair. We prefer to approximate this layer prior to repair of the external sphincter. (From Hankins GDV and others: Operative obstetrics, Norwalk, Conn, 1995, Appleton & Lange.)

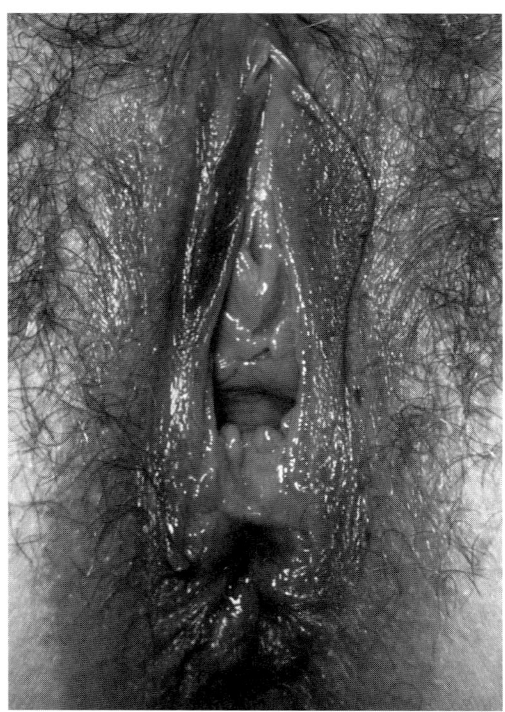

FIGURE 25.7 Chronic fourth-degree laceration. Note how the vaginal wall and rectal wall have become fused without intervening perineal body or anal sphincters.

to reach normal tissue will allow for tension-free approximation. Lateral dissection will reveal the retracted ends of the internal anal sphincter, which can be grasped with clamps and pulled toward the midline. The internal sphincter has usually fused with the external sphincter and can most easily be found extending cephalad from the sphincter until the intact bowel wall is found (Figure 25.10).

Once the tissues have been mobilized, repair is begun at the upper margin of the anal defect. We prefer a running suture of either 3-0 or 4-0 delayed absorption material that is begun above the defect and continued down to the anal verge. This suture should firmly grasp the submucosal layer of the bowel (Figure 25.11). This initial layer pulls the torn ends of the internal anal sphincter medially into the operative field. If necessary, additional dissection should be performed at this time to mobilize the internal anal sphincter in all

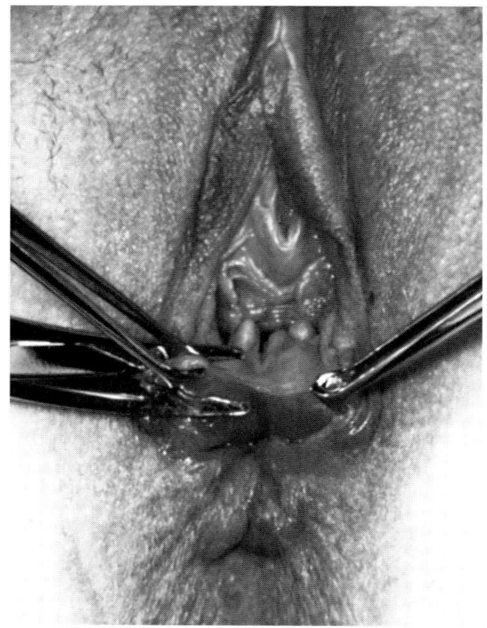

FIGURE 25.8 Excision of the scar in preparation for entering the rectovaginal space. An Allis' clamp is placed at each end of the scar, and Mayo scissors are used to remove the cicatrix.

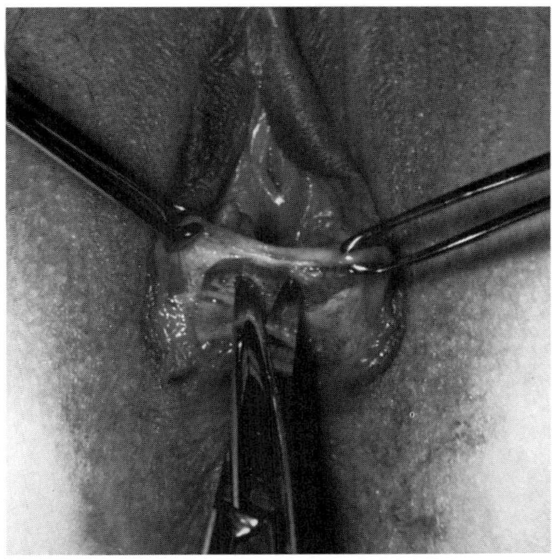

Figure 25.9 Anterior traction on the vaginal wall facilitates entry into the rectovaginal space.

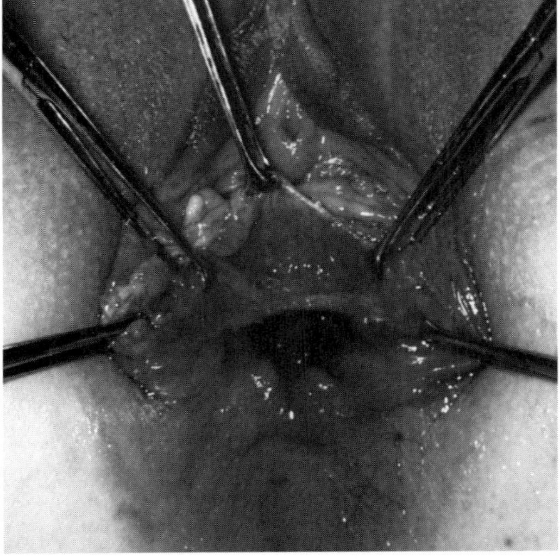

Figure 25.10 Completed dissection prior to closure. The most posterior pair of Allis' clamps are on the external anal sphincter. The adjacent pair of clamps are on the separated edges of the internal sphincter, with the middle Allis' clamps marking the upper margin of the internal sphincter defect. The bowel wall can be seen immediately ventral to the anal canal.

directions. Closure is accomplished with a running 2-0 delayed absorbable suture in a fashion similar to the first layer (Figures 25.11 and 25.12). Care must be taken to make sure that this suture is pulled tightly to get adequate approximation.

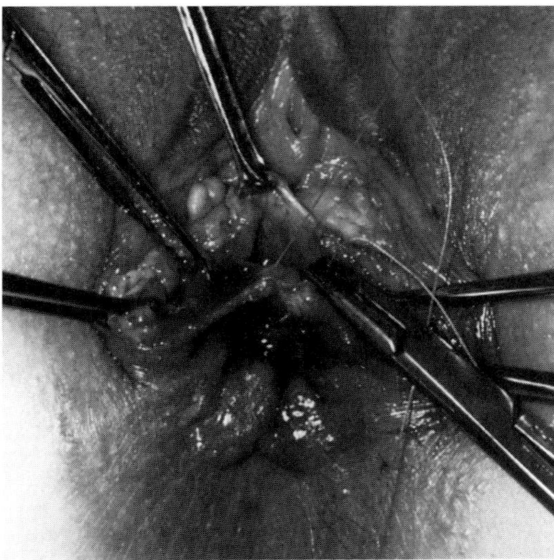

Figure 25.11 Closure of the anorectal wall.

Repair of the upper portions of the rectovaginal septum should be accomplished next. Interrupted 2-0 delayed absorbable suture can be used to bring the tissues cephalad to the external sphincter together. We find it easier to accomplish this before attempting the repair of the external anal sphincter because the tissues are more accessible prior to sphincter closure. Since the lateral margins of the perineal body fuse with the inner surfaces of the levator ani muscle, this repair brings the levators in close approximation, adding bulk to the rectovaginal septum and perineal body and reinforcing the repair in this area.

The divided ends of the external anal sphincter should then be united in the midline with a series of interrupted delayed absorbable or permanent suture (Figure 25.13). A 2-0 suture should provide adequate tensile strength while minimizing the knot size. Currently we prefer to perform an end-to-end anastomosis, although others have preferred an overlapping sphincteroplasty. The most cephalad and inferior suture should be placed first, and at least four to five sutures should be used to reunite the ends of the external anal sphincter.

Further support of the repair can be accomplished by careful reapproximation of the subcutaneous tissues of the vagina and perineal body. Finally, the vaginal mucosa and perineal skin should be approximated with a running,

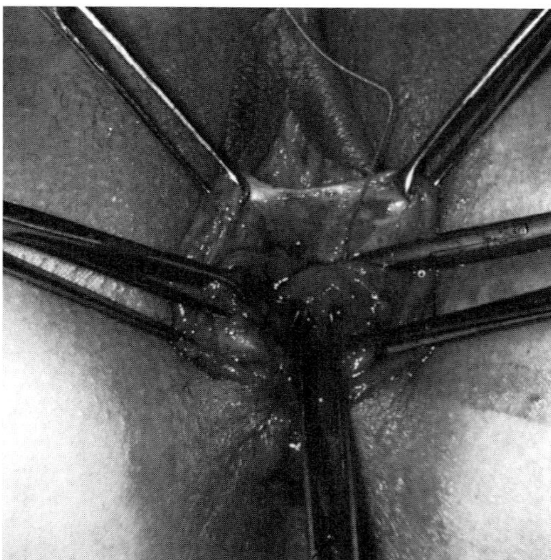

Figure 25.12 Closure of the internal sphincter.

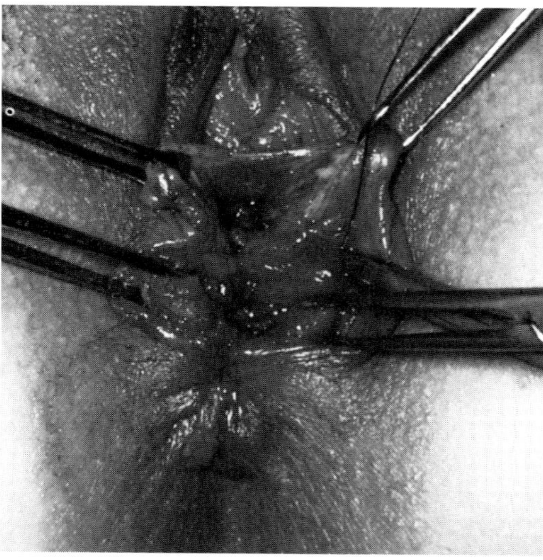

Figure 25.13 Closure of the external sphincter.

nonlocking 3-0 delayed absorbable suture (Figure 25.14).

The end result of this repair should be the reconstruction of a cylindrical sphincteric complex that is approximately 2 cm thick and 3 cm long. The perineal body and rectovaginal septum should be of sufficient thickness and length to restore the normally supportive roles of these structures. The anus should easily admit one finger following the repair.

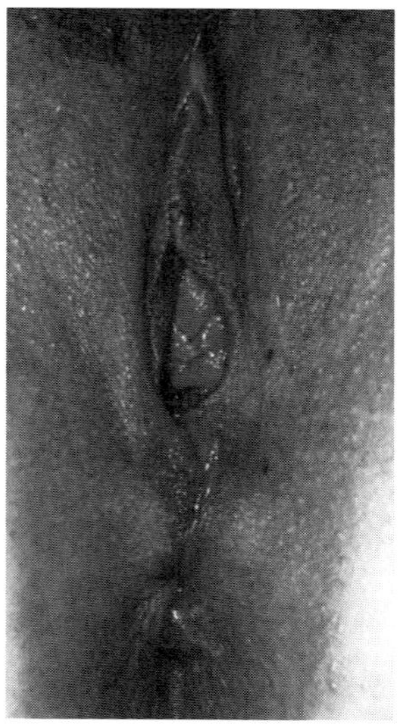

Figure 25.14 Completed repair.

Preoperative Considerations

The approach to the preparation and management of the lower GI tract both preoperatively and postoperatively varies considerably. Optimal success depends on several basic factors: the tissues involved must be free from infection; nutritional deficits should be corrected; and the lower GI tract must be adequately prepared and emptied prior to the procedure.

It is often helpful to institute a low-residue diet several weeks prior to the procedure. This will result in a decrease in stool volume, which will also become small and hard in consistency. This may decrease the continuous seeding of the disrupted tissue with liquid stool just prior to the surgical procedure. A clear liquid diet is instituted in the last 48 to 72 hours prior to the surgical repair.

Modern methods of cleansing the large bowel most commonly involve using an oral lavage agent such as GoLYTELY. We prefer to give these agents on preoperative day 2 instead of on the day before surgery, in order to decrease the chance that a thin fecal effluent will be present at the time of the repair. More extensive preparation of the colon and rectum is typically unnecessary and should be avoided to prevent significant metabolic and electrolyte disturbances. Tap water or Fleet enemas should be given the evening before surgery to complete the emptying of the lower colon and rectum.

Preoperative oral antibiotics such as erythromycin base and neomycin may be administered on the day before surgery but must be administered after the completion of the antegrade bowel preparation so that these agents remain with the lumen of the bowel. A single dose of a broad-spectrum parenteral antibiotic such as cefoxitin or cefotetan should be given within 30 minutes of the surgical incision. The prolonged use of IV antibiotics is best avoided in these patients since it is not possible to completely sterilize either the gut or the vagina, and the antibiotics can serve only to select out more resistant bacteria.

Postoperative Considerations

There are many different philosophies and practices in the management of these patients during the postoperative period. Some surgeons prefer to institute a high-fiber diet during the postoperative period to keep the stool soft and loose. Others prefer the opposite approach and utilize a low-residue diet to decrease the size and number of bowel movements. Our personal preference is to place the patient on a clear liquid diet for the first 2 to 3 days postoperatively and then to advance them to a low-residue diet plus a stool softener or a tablespoon of a mineral oil emulsion twice a day. On around the fifth postoperative day, the patient can be given a mild laxative such as Milk of Magnesia, cascara, or castor oil to promote a loose stool. The patient can then be switched to either a regular or high-fiber diet to keep the stool soft. Enemas are best avoided as a means of stimulating a bowel movement in the postoperative period.

Patients should be instructed in proper wound care prior to leaving the hospital. Sitz baths contribute to proper hygiene and often improve patient comfort. Sitz baths should be limited to 10 to 15 minutes, 2 to 3 times a day, because longer periods of time can lead to tissue maceration. Following the sitz bath the patient should be instructed to dry the area thoroughly using a dry towel. A heating lamp or a blow dryer used on a low setting can also be used to keep the area dry. Patients also should be instructed to cleanse themselves after each bowel movement with soft toilet tissue. The use of Tucks pads often may be soothing.

Postoperative infections are uncommon but can have a devastating effect on the repair. We prefer to reexamine these patients on a weekly basis during the early postoperative period in an attempt to identify early signs of infection so that they can be treated conservatively before a wound breakdown occurs.

The Future

Technical advancements over the last few decades in antibiotics, suture material, and wound care have greatly improved our ability to successfully treat women with chronic third- and fourth-degree obstetric lacerations. Although the results of sphincter repair during the first 6 weeks are usually quite satisfying to the surgeon and patient alike, attenuation of the perineal body may occur over time. This observation was recorded by Miller and Brown in the 1930s when they introduced the idea of performing a paradoxical incision posteriorly in the sphincter in order to relieve the tension on the anterior anastomosis.[29] Although this procedure is more often discussed than performed in modern times, it should continue to focus our attention on the inherent difficulties involved in reconstructive surgery involving the anal sphincter. It is possible that there is a role for longer-acting monofilament or permanent sutures in these repairs.

References

1. Haadem K, Ohrlander S, and Lingman G: Long-term ailments due to anal sphincter rupture caused by delivery: a hidden problem, Eur J Obstet Gynecol Reprod Biol 27:27, 1988.
2. Sorensen M and others: Sphincter rupture in childbirth, Br J Surg 80:392, 1993.
3. Sorensen SM and others: Perineal rupture following vaginal delivery: long term consequences, Acta Obstet Gynecol Scand 67:315, 1988.
4. Sultan AH and others: Third degree obsteric and sphincter tears: risk factors and outcome of primary repair, BMJ 308:887, 1994.
5. Sultan AH and others: Anal sphincter disruption during vaginal delivery, N Engl J Med 329:1905, 1993.

6. Borgatta L, Piening SL, and Cohen WR: Association of episiotomy and delivery position with deep perineal laceration during spontaneous delivery in nulliparous women, Am J Obstet Gynecol 160:294, 1989.
7. Green JR and Soohoo SL: Factors associated with rectal injury in spontaneous deliveries, Obstet Gynecol 73:732, 1989.
8. Henriksen TB and others: Episiotomy and perineal lesions in spontaneous vaginal deliveries, Br J Obstet Gynaecol 99:950, 1992.
9. Aronson MP, Lee RA, and Berquist TH: Anatomy of anal sphincters and related structures in continent women studied with magnetic resonance imaging, Obstet Gynecol 76:846, 1990.
10. Sweiger M: Method for determining individual contributions of voluntary and involuntary anal sphincters to resting tone, Dis Colon Rectum 22:415, 1979.
11. Frenckner B and Euler CV: Influence of pudendal block on the function of the anal sphincters, Gut 16:482, 1975.
12. Parks AG, Porter NH, and Hardcastle J: The syndrome of the descending perineum, Proc R Soc Med 59:477, 1966.
13. Parks AG: Anorectal incontinence, Proc R Soc Med 68:681, 1975.
14. Duthie HL and Gairns FW: Sensory nerves and sensation in the anal region in man, Br J Surg 47:585, 1960.
15. Taverner D and Smiddy FG: An electromyographic study of the normal function of the external anal sphincter and pelvic diaphragm, Dis Col Rec 2:153, 1959.
16. Toglia MR and DeLancey JOL: Anal incontinence and the obstetrician-gynecologist, Obstet Gynecol 84:731, 1994.
17. Madoff RD, Williams JG, and Caushaj PF: Fecal incontinence, N Engl J Med 326:1002, 1992.
18. Radcliffe AG and others: Anovaginal and rectovaginal fistulas in Crohn's disease, Dis Colon Rectum 31:94, 1988.
19. Stricker JW and others: Surgical correction of anal incontinence, Dis Colon Rectum 31:533, 1988.
20. Snooks SJ, Henry MM, and Swash M: Faecal incontinence due to external sphincter division in childbirth is associated with damage to the innervation of the pelvic floor musculature: a double pathology, Br J Obstet Gynaecol 92:824, 1985.
21. Law PJ, Kamm MA, and Bartram CI: Anal endosonography in the investigation of faecal incontinence, Br J Surg 78:312, 1991.
22. Aronson MP, Lee RA, and Berquist TH: Anatomy of anal sphincters and related structures in continent women studied with magnetic resonance imaging, Obstet Gynecol 76:846, 1990.
23. Harris RE: An evaluation of median episiotomy, Am J Obstet Gynecol 106:660, 1970.
24. Ramin SM and Gilstrap LC: Episiotomy and early repair of dehiscence, Clin Obstet Gynecol 37(4):816, 1994.
25. Hankins GD and others: Early repair of episiotomy dehiscence, Obstet Gynecol 75:48, 1990.
26. Hauth JC and others: Early repair of an external sphincter ani muscle and rectal mucosal dehiscence, Obstet Gynecol 67:806, 1986.
27. Monberg J and Hammen S: Ruptured episiotomia resutured primarily, Acta Genecol Scand 66:163, 1987.
28. Ramin SM and others: Early repair of episiotomy dehiscence associated with infection, Am J Obstet Gynecol 167:1104, 1992.
29. Miller NF and Brown W: The surgical treatment of complete perineal tears in the female, Am J Obstet Gynecol 34:196, 1937.

26

Postpartum Hysterectomy

David L. Barclay
Paul J. Wendel

Postpartum hysterectomy, by definition, is an unplanned operation dictated by circumstances encountered after a cesarean section or a vaginal delivery. The majority of the operations are performed immediately after delivery or within the next 24 hours. Rarely, however, delayed postpartum hemorrhage or a refractory pelvic infection may necessitate removal of the uterus.

The first hysterectomy at the time of cesarean section was performed in 1868 by Horatio Robinson Storer.[1] The patient had a large abdominal tumor obstructing the birth canal and prohibiting vaginal delivery, even with craniotomy. A subtotal hysterectomy and BSO were performed. The cervical stump was exteriorized after a metallic cord had been firmly tied around the lower uterine segment. The patient died from sepsis. The first successful operation was performed in 1876 by Edoardo Porro of Pavia, Italy, after a very carefully planned and executed cesarean section on a 25-year-old primigravid dwarf who had a skeletal deformity from rickets, resulting in absolute disproportion.[1] The Porro operation was defined as a subtotal hysterectomy and BSO.

The Porro operation was necessitated by the fact that after cesarean section the uterine incision remained open, draining purulent lochia into the peritoneal cavity. Maternal mortality after cesarean section was essentially 100% prior to the introduction of the Porro operation. In about 1882, Max Sänger, a German surgeon, introduced the use of a large number of sutures deep and superficial to secure perfect closure of the uterine wound and prevent spillage of blood and lochia into the peritoneal cavity.[2] The Sänger operation was called the conservation cesarean section, whereas the Porro operation was called the radical cesarean operation. Cesarean hysterectomy became relegated to emergency situations such as infection after prolonged labor and hemorrhage.

For the purposes of this review, postpartum hysterectomy will be limited to gestations beyond 24 weeks; therefore bleeding and infection associated with ectopic pregnancy, postabortal infections, and gestational trophoblastic disease will not be considered.

Excessive bleeding and severe infection are the most frequent indications for an unplanned peripartal hysterectomy. Evaluation of blood loss at delivery has always been imprecise. By tradition, blood loss of 500 ml or more at vaginal delivery has been defined as postpartum hemorrhage.[3] Quantitative evaluation of blood loss, however, has suggested an average blood loss of 500 ml with vaginal delivery, 1000 ml with cesarean section, and 1400 ml for elective cesarean hysterectomy.[4] Gahres, Albert, and Dodek reviewed 19 studies of postpartum blood loss and found an average loss of 450 ml after vaginal delivery.[5] Combs, Murphy, and Laros suggested that a decrease in hematocrit of 10% or the necessity for blood transfusion would be a satisfactory definition for postpartum hemorrhage.[6] Mee has estimated that postpartum hemorrhage occurs after approximately 2% to 4% of vaginal deliveries and 6% of cesarean sections.[7]

The causes of postpartum hemorrhage fall roughly into four categories: uterine atony, placental disorders, ruptured uterus, and uterine or lower genital tract lacerations. These causes are essentially the same after either cesarean or vaginal delivery with the exception of extension of the uterine incision into the uterine vessels, parametrium, or vagina. A consumption coagulopathy, most often associated with abruptio placentae and a Couvelaire uterus, is a rare occurrence in modern-day obstetrics. Modern antimicrobial drugs have reduced the need for removal of the uterus for a severe uterine infection.

The obstetric surgeon must decide when uterine hemorrhage or infection cannot be controlled without removal of the uterus. Hysterectomy can be a very effective and immediate solution to the emergent situation, but that decision must be tempered by the experience and skills of the surgeon and the desires of the patient. Less definitive measures to control uterine hemorrhage may result in significant blood loss, incurring the risks of multiple transfusions and perhaps the inability to completely control hemorrhage. Modern antimicrobial agents may effectively control uterine and pelvic infections, but are the risks of intensive (conservative?) therapy greater than that of the expeditious removal of the uterus at the time of cesarean section?

Management of Postpartum Hemorrhage

Identification of the cause of obstetric hemorrhage is the key to management. Typically the placenta separates within 5 to 15 minutes of delivery. The uterus becomes firm and rises somewhat in the abdomen, and the placenta advances into the vagina and can be removed by gentle traction on the umbilical cord. The placenta is inspected for complete removal and for evidence of a succenturiate lobe. If there is not prompt separation of the placenta with descent into the vagina, manual exploration of the uterine cavity may be necessary. Some have recommended routine manual exploration of the uterine cavity and removal of the placenta. In general, however, this is not a routine procedure, and manual exploration is reserved for those cases in which the placenta does not promptly separate and descend. The uterus is stabilized with the abdominal hand, and the dominant hand is placed through the tightening internal os of the cervix for exploration of the cavity. The placenta can be peeled from the uterine wall by gentle manipulation with the palm beneath the surface of the placenta. The placental site is somewhat difficult to evaluate considering that it has a very irregular configuration. A sponge may be placed across the examining fingers to wipe away residual membranes and perhaps placental tissue in the cavity. The corpus can then be massaged until it is firm.

If hemorrhage occurs after separation of the placenta, the birth canal should be carefully inspected for vaginal or cervical lacerations. The lower uterine segment can be explored for laceration or separation of a prior scar from cesarean section. Constriction of the interlacing fibers of the uterine wall constricts the blood vessels of the placental site, resulting in adequate hemostasis. In the absence of adequate uterine contractility, uterine atony may result in excessive bleeding from the placental bed. Contractility may be augmented by infusing a dilute solution of 20 units of oxytocin in 1000 ml of crystalloid, which can be infused rapidly. Pitocin should not be given in a concentrated IV solution as this may cause further hypotension. IM or direct myometrial injection of prostaglandin may assist in uterine contractility but may cause bronchospasm in women with asthma. Methylergonovine in doses of 0.2 mg IM has been used in the past but is contraindicated in patients who are hypertensive. Repeated attempts at bimanual massage of the uterine fundus and administration of pharmacologic agents may be necessary for sufficient control of postpartum hemorrhage from uterine atony. Care must be taken that there is not excessive, unreplaced blood loss resulting in a rapidly deteriorating condition of the patient. The next step is laparotomy for surgical control of hemorrhage.

If there is uterine contractility but excessive blood loss, the vagina, cervix, and lower uterine segment should be examined for laceration. Vaginal and cervical lacerations can be repaired through the vagina; however, if there is extension into the base of the broad ligament or lower uterine segment, laparotomy is ordinarily necessary. If implantation of the removed placenta had occurred in the lower uterine segment, there may well be bleeding from the placental site in the noncontractile lower uterine segment. Under these circumstances, it is very difficult to be certain that there is not an element of placenta accreta.

At this point, a tube of blood should be observed for clot retraction and clot lysis, providing clinical evidence of sufficient clotting factors. Studies to detect a coagulopathy may be submitted. However, results rarely return in a timely manner to aid in the decision-making process in acute hemorrhage.

If laparotomy is mandated, the purpose is to identify the cause of hemorrhage, if possible, and secure hemostasis by arterial ligation or ultimately by hysterectomy if hemorrhage cannot be controlled. Hysterectomy can be performed quickly and is effective in control of bleeding, but that decision must be tempered by the experience of the surgeon and the desires of the patient for subsequent fertility. This decision-making process should not be so time consuming that there is an inordinate blood loss prior to surgery. A large component of the excessive blood loss in the treatment of uterine atony is secondary to the decision-making process rather than the operation itself.

Uterine Atony

Clark and others reported in 1984 that 43% of emergency hysterectomies in their series were performed for uterine atony.[8] This is somewhat less than the 67% incidence reported by O'Leary and Steer.[9] In the Tulane series, extending from 1938 to 1967, 31.6% of operations were performed for that indication.[10] In the early years of the Tulane study, the Couvelaire uterus associated with abruptio placentae and a consumption coagulopathy was a common indication (Figure 26.1).[11] This is a rather dramatic undertaking and is an infrequent occurrence. Clark and others found that hysterectomy for atony has a statistically significant association with amnionitis, oxytocin augmentation of labor, cesarean section for labor arrest, preoperative magnesium sulfate infusion, and increased fetal weight.[8] In 23% of their patients, there was no identifiable risk factor causing the atony. Rarely, uterine fibroids may interfere with uterine contractility and/or closure of the uterine incision, causing hemorrhage (Figure 26.2).

Immediate treatment consists of venous access for infusion of crystalloid, bimanual fundal compression, and rapid infusion of a dilute solution of 20 units of oxytocin. In the absence of prompt response or in the presence of excessive bleeding, consideration should be given to operative intervention for arterial ligation or hysterectomy, depending upon the experience of the surgeon and the desires of the patient.

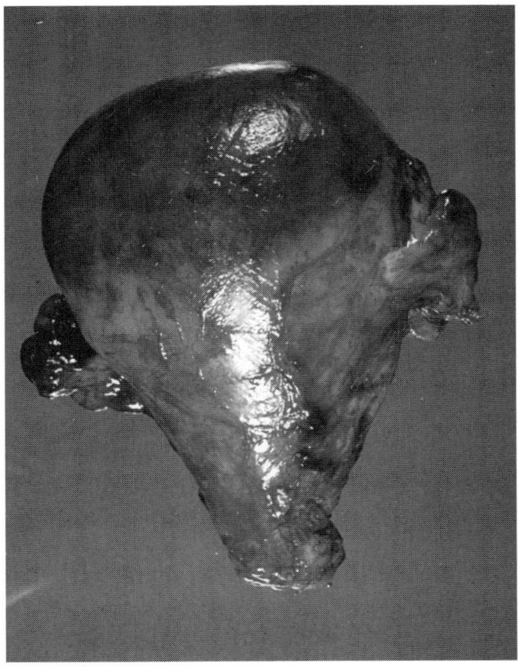

Figure 26.1 Couvelaire uterus removed for postpartum hemorrhage.

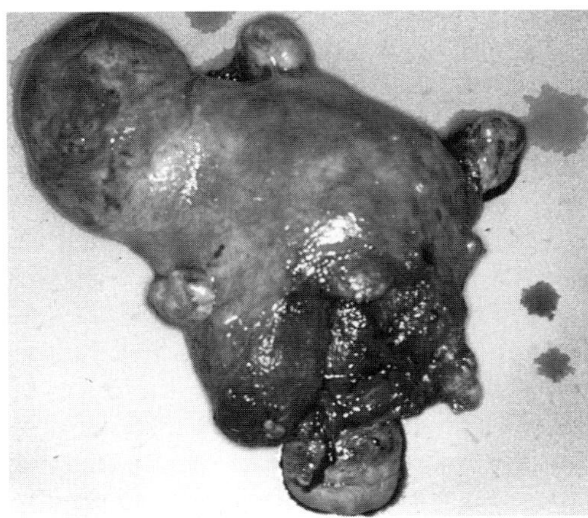

Figure 26.2 Myomatous uterus removed because of inability to close the incision and to control bleeding.

Abnormal Placentation

During the last decade the abnormally adherent placenta has become the most common indication for peripartal hysterectomy. This is particularly true in the patient who has undergone one or more prior cesarean sections. The emerging significance of placenta previa accreta in a patient who has had one or more cesarean sections was documented by Read, Cotton, and Miller in 1980[12] and Clark, Koonings, and Phelan[13] in 1985. This was further confirmed by Stanco and others[14] in 1993 and Zelop and others in 1993.[15] In the latter study, the risk of hysterectomy with placenta previa was markedly increased with parity and a history of prior cesarean section. The incidence by parity increased from 1 in 143 deliveries in nulliparous women with placenta previa to 1 in 4 deliveries in multiparous women with 4 or more deliveries. Four or more deliveries, prior cesarean sections, and repeat cesarean birth for placenta previa resulted in 1 in 14 chance of hysterectomy for hemorrhage. Stanco and others[14] reported 123 cases of emergency peripartum hysterectomy, of which 61 were performed for hemorrhage from placenta accreta; 41 of these patients (67.2%) had undergone a prior cesarean section.

Bleeding from the placental implantation site usually involves a noncontractile lower uterine segment in a patient who has undergone a cesarean section for placenta previa. The lower segment is less resistant to penetration by the placenta, causing placenta accreta, increta, or percreta; the last may result in laceration of the uterine vessels when the placenta is removed. The placenta may penetrate through a previous low-segment incision and into the base of the bladder. Finberg and Williams[16] reported that the antenatal diagnosis of placental invasion into the myometrium may be possible by ultrasonography in women with prior cesarean sections with anterior placenta at the level of the bladder. He described three sonographic criteria that may aid in the diagnosis of an accreta in this scenario: (1) the loss of the normal hypoechoic retroplacental myometrial zone, (2) thinning or disruption of the hyperechoic uterine serosa–bladder interface, and (3) presence of focal exophytic masses beyond the uterine serosa. The incidence of placenta previa is about 2%, and the chance of a patient having had a prior cesarean section is about 15%; the combination of the two risk factors has significantly increased the necessity for an emergency unplanned hysterectomy at the time of cesarean section.

The diagnosis of an abnormally adherent placenta is based on clinical examination and exploration of the uterine cavity after either abdominal or vaginal delivery. The placental site in the corpus is difficult to evaluate by manual palpation, and therapeutic decisions are made strictly on the basis of hemorrhage. After removal of the uterus, the pathologist may not confirm the clinical diagnosis of an abnormally adherent placenta; however, a need for hysterectomy is based on the necessity to control hemorrhage. It is suggested that, on occasion and under some circumstances, local excision and repair by oversewing of the implantation site may negate the necessity for hysterectomy. However, Zelop and others,[15] found the procedure unsuccessful in 27 patients in whom they attempted to oversew the placental bed; hysterectomy was necessary. Conservative management should be considered, however, as recorded by Cho and others[17] in 1991. Their patients were treated by placing a series of deep interrupted through-and-through sutures in a circular pattern surrounding the bleeding implantation site; however, with deep invasion into the uterine wall (placenta increta or percreta), this is not possible. Invasion anteriorly into the base of the bladder or laterally into the uterine vessels complicated the operation.

In the series reported by Zelop and others,[15] 75 patients underwent hysterectomy for abnormal placentation; 25% of those patients underwent a subtotal hysterectomy. Three of the patients underwent reexploration for persistent bleeding within the lower uterine segment and cervix. The authors recommended, and we agree, that a subtotal operation may not be effective in the treatment of a placenta accreta located in the lower uterine segment because the cervical branch of the uterine artery may well be intact and cause continued hemorrhage. In the series recorded by Stanco and others,[14] 25 of the 55 patients undergoing hysterectomy for placental accreta underwent a subtotal hysterectomy. Fortunately, only 1 of those patients required secondary surgery for removal of the cervix and placement of a pelvic pack.

Obstetric Uterine Rupture

Although rupture of the pregnant uterus can be a catastrophic event, many reported cases are simply separation of previous low-segment uterine scars, although classified as uterine rupture. The occurrence may be asymptomatic and result in no adverse outcome. The literature is somewhat confusing because there are confounding variables regarding the outcomes for patients who had simple asymptomatic dehiscence.

In 1984 Plauché and others[18] reported an incidence of catastrophic life-threatening rupture of 1 in 2174 deliveries on the Louisiana State Charity Hospital Service. This was somewhat more than the incidence derived from a survey of the English literature. Their estimate was that major catastrophic uterine rupture would occur in approximately 1 in 2200 deliveries. The principal cause of rupture of the pregnant uterus is the existence of a uterine scar, usually resulting from a previous cesarean section. Catastrophic rupture implies complete separation of the uterine incision and rupture of the fetal membranes. The vertical incision extending into the muscle of the corpus, or particularly a "T" incision, is especially liable to rupture, which may occur spontaneously before the onset of labor.

It is not surprising that the prior cesarean section scar healing in the involuting uterus may be defective. Although prior hysterotomies and myomectomies in the nonpregnant patient have been related to uterine rupture, in general the healing is much better. Severe postpartum uterine infection after cesarean section on occasion may result in complete dehiscence of the incision, particularly if there has been extension of a vertical incision into the muscular corpus. This is particularly true if a cesarean section is performed prior to development of a satisfactory lower uterine segment. Complete dehiscence may result in spillage of infected lochia into the abdominal cavity, prompting a hysterectomy. If the corpus adheres to the abdominal wall, the area of dehiscence may be walled off; however, on occasion there may be drainage through the incision in the abdominal wall, resulting in a uterocutaneous fistula. If secondary healing occurs prior to epithelialization of the tract, spontaneous closure is the rule. However, these incisions are quite vulnerable with a subsequent pregnancy. An interval hysterosalpingogram, after a low transverse cesarean section, may demonstrate extravasation of dye (Figure 26.3). Silent dehiscence of this variety

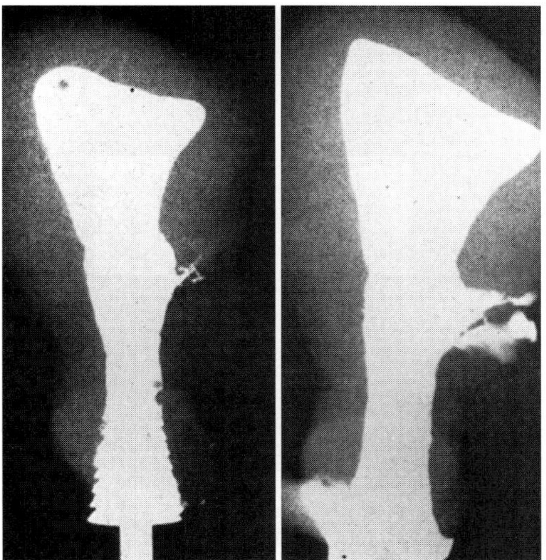

Figure 26.3 Hysterosalpingogram demonstrating defect in an old low cervical cesarean section scar.

was a major reason for cesarean hysterectomy in the original series reported from the Charity Hospital of New Orleans, Tulane Service.[10] In fact, Dyer, Nix, and Weed,[19] from that institute, in the era of "once a section, always a section," felt that the uterus ultimately reached a "section saturation point." This was a suitable indication for hysterectomy at the time of cesarean section.

Forceps delivery is the most common cause of uterine rupture in the absence of a prior cesarean section. Classical application of the Kielland forceps can lacerate the lower uterine segment beneath the bladder flap or otherwise cause a tear of the cervix, extending into the lower uterine segment.

Spontaneous rupture may occur from extension of a prior cervical and vaginal laceration into the lower uterine segment and possibly uterine vessels (Figure 26.4). A low transverse cervical excision may extend into the uterine vessels, parametrial tissues, or lower uterine segment and vaginal fornix. If arterial ligation is unsuccessful and hysterectomy is performed, it is necessary to perform a total removal of the uterus and cervix and suture of any extension into the vaginal fornix.

Coagulopathies Causing Postpartum Hemorrhage

The classic cause of a postpartum consumption coagulopathy is a concealed severe abrup-

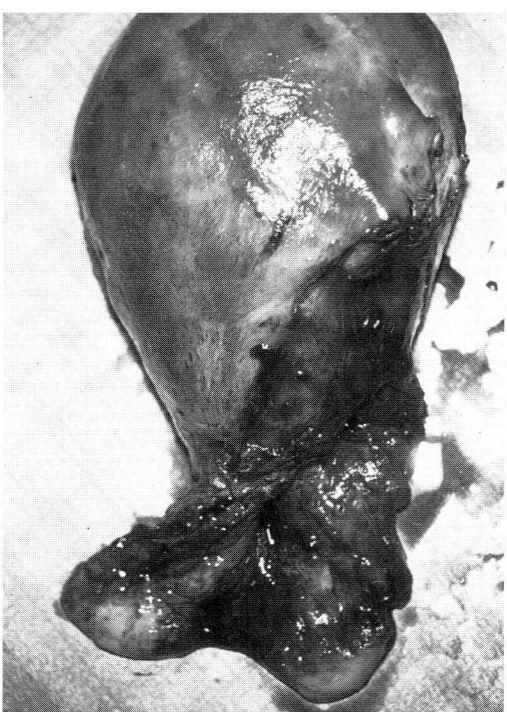

FIGURE 26.4 Laceration extending from the vaginal fornix into the lower uterine segment.

tio placentae with or without an associated Couvelaire uterus. This was the most common cause for postpartum emergency hysterectomy in the early Tulane series. Amniotic fluid embolism can also cause a profound coagulopathy and postpartum hemorrhage. Massive hemorrhage may lead to a coagulopathy over time, not from consumption, but from loss of critical levels of clotting factors. Medical management is the treatment of choice if the causative agent can be identified before embarking on an emergency hysterectomy for hemorrhage.

INDICATIONS FOR LAPAROTOMY

After vaginal delivery, indications for laparotomy are uncontrolled hemorrhage from uterine atony, placental site bleeding, or extension of a vaginal and cervical laceration into the base of the cardinal ligament. For immediate control of hemorrhage the obstetrician should consider manual compression of the aorta and specific ligation of the bleeding point if possible. Ligation of the anterior division of the hypogastric arteries has been considered to be the next step, although Burchell[20] demonstrated in 1968 that even after ligation of the hypogastric artery there is continued blood flow in the uterine artery with a decreased pulse pressure. Therefore that procedure may be helpful in decreasing the amount of bleeding but is not the total answer.

An alternative, suggested by O'Leary,[21] is ligation of the uterine vessels at the level of the internal os. He reported a 95% success rate in 200 patients who sustained post–cesarean section hemorrhage. The uterus is placed on tension and elevated out of the pelvis. An absorbable suture on a large needle is then placed through the lower uterine segment medial to the ascending branches of the uterine vessels and back through the avascular portion of the broad ligament, after which the ligature is secured. This is performed bilaterally. If there is not sufficient control of bleeding, a second pair of sutures may be placed in a similar manner just beneath the junction of the utero-ovarian ligament and the corpus uteri. With a fundal implantation of the placenta there may be significant flow through the ovarian vessels anastomosing with the ipsilateral uterine vessels. Pregnancies subsequent to uterine artery ligation have not been compromised.

Internal iliac (hypogastric) artery ligation is a procedure that has been most commonly used in control of pelvic hemorrhage from uterine or rectal carcinoma or after pelvic trauma or obstetric hemorrhage. There is an extensive literature on the subject, and it is apparent that the proper procedure is not always successful in controlling excessive bleeding when it is used prophylactically before a cesarean hysterectomy or in the treatment of postpartum hemorrhage. There is significant variability in the anatomy of the hypogastric artery and its branches. It was illustrated by Lipschütz[22] in 1918 that there is extensive collateral circulation after ligation of the entire hypogastric artery in contrast to ligation of the anterior division, which gives rise to the uterine and vaginal arteries. Ligation serves to decrease the pulse pressure as described by Burchell and perhaps increases the possibility for clotting.

The technique of hypogastric arterial ligation has been illustrated in many publications and may be a significant surgical challenge for the obstetrician who is unfamiliar with dissection of the pelvic sidewall and development of the perivesical and perirectal spaces. Incision of the peritoneum over the common and external iliac vessels allows entry into the retroperitoneal space. If the round ligament is clamped and cut, there is increased exposure in the retroperitoneal space, and the perivesical space can be developed without difficulty. The hypogastric artery can then be identified and traced into the pelvis. Although some have advocated ligation of the common internal iliac artery, it is probably ineffective in controlling hemorrhage and places the hypogastric vein, which is intimately adherent to the undersurface of the artery, at significant risk when a right angle clamp is placed beneath the artery for placement of a ligature. The vein has a very thin wall and can easily be torn in this procedure. An alternative is to identify the anterior division, which becomes the obliterated hypogastric or superior vesical artery, which can be identified and grasped with a Babcock's clamp. The uterine artery can be secured safely and rather quickly with hemoclips. The final clip can be placed on the anterior division of the hypogastric artery at its point of origin from the common trunk. While the obstetrician pursues this course of action, it must be remembered that there is continuous blood loss. Although preservation of the uterus may be a high priority, the obstetrician cannot allow the patient to become sufficiently blood-volume depleted to slip into shock prior to commencement of the definitive operation consisting of hysterectomy.

Hemorrhage during or immediately after cesarean section is usually caused by uterine atony; abnormal placentation; extension of a transverse incision into the uterine vessels, cardinal ligament, and perhaps even the fornix of the vagina; or extension of a low vertical incision into the anterior wall of the vagina. If immediate surgical repair with or without arterial ligation does not control hemorrhage, then the obstetrician has no alternative but to perform a hysterectomy. Perhaps a subtotal hysterectomy may be adequate for control of hemorrhage from uterine atony. However, it may not control hemorrhage associated with placenta previa or extension of a cervical laceration or cesarean section incision into the uterine vessels and cardinal ligament.

Operative Technique

Removal of the uterus immediately after cesarean section or during the first 24 hours after vaginal delivery is an infrequent operation that is distinctly different from hysterectomy in the nonpregnant patient. In the face of impending shock from blood loss, the obstetrician is faced with an operation that reportedly is associated with excessive blood loss and significant risk to the urinary tract.[23] Several basic surgical principles facilitate the operation:

1. The abdomen is opened through a low vertical incision.
2. The corpus is placed on constant tension by the first assistant. This is somewhat more difficult in the absence of a uterine incision but is an absolute necessity to maintain anatomic relationships.
3. Sharp dissection is used throughout, particularly when skeletonizing the uterine vascular pedicles.
4. All vascular pedicles down to the the uterine arteries on both sides are secured before ligation is performed.
5. Low ligation of the uterine vessels requires that the ureters be identified by palpation.
6. Compression of the lower uterine segment between the thumb and forefinger allows identification of the dilated and soft cervix, and clamps can be placed on the vagina.

If a cesarean section had been performed, the incision can be left open or, if bleeding, closed with a running suture or secured with towel clamps, and the corpus is delivered through the incision. If the ovaries are to be preserved, the operation is begun by placing a clamp on the round ligament, which is cut, and the anterior leaf of the broad ligament is incised to the bladder flap incision. The avascular portion of the broad ligament is penetrated, and the utero-ovarian ligament and fallopian tube are doubly clamped and cut, with a third clamp securing the proximal pedicle to prevent back-bleeding. With constant tension on the corpus, the broad ligament is incised sharply with the scissors and the uterine vessels skeletonized. This dissection is performed quite easily, and the veins can be protected if the corpus is on constant tension; however, there is a tendency to "wander" laterally as the vessels are dissected. Therefore the ureters, which are quite easily palpated in the cardinal tunnel, should be identified prior to placing a clamp on the uterine vessels quite low. If all of these pedicles on both sides are secured prior to attempting suture ligature, there should be a significant decrease in uterine hemorrhage, after which each pedicle can be secured with a suture. Utero-ovarian vessels are usually tied with a free tie followed by a suture ligature. If the pedicle is entirely too large, the utero-ovarian ligament can be secured separately. During this entire procedure of vascular pedicle ligation the corpus is maintained on constant tension, which decreases back-bleeding. Additional pedicles can then be taken on the uterosacral ligaments and on the base of each cardinal ligament. Compression of the lower uterine segment and cervix between the thumb and forefinger allows identification of the lower limits of the cervix and application of a clamp on the vagina on either side. The vagina can then be entered anteriorly or posteriorly, the cervix circumscribed, and the specimen removed. We ordinarily close the vagina with angle and interrupted figure-of-eight sutures. Whether or not a drain is left in the pelvis is the surgeon's option. Ordinarily the peritoneum is not closed either in the pelvis or during closure of the abdominal wall. The pelvis is thoroughly irrigated and the abdominal cavity explored to ensure removal of all laparotomy pads. The abdominal wall is usually closed in one layer with the exception of skin with a continuous far-and-near absorbable suture.

SUMMARY

Removal of the uterus in the immediate postpartum period is an uncommon and anxiety-producing event, usually precipitated by life-threatening hemorrhage. The problem must be recognized promptly and decisions made quickly. The patient should be examined in an orderly manner as described in the text. When to perform a laparotomy is the most difficult decision. After entering the peritoneal cavity, one must progress in an orderly manner from arterial ligation to hysterectomy if absolutely necessary.

It must be recognized that hysterectomy under these circumstances is quite different from hysterectomy in the nonpregnant patient. The approach to the operative procedure as described in outline fashion is very important. Constant tissue tension on the uterus, for instance, is essential for maintenance of anatomic relationships. If one can confidently identify the course of the ureter and reflect the bladder from the vagina and lower uterine segment, only one pedicle may be necessary below the uterine vessels. Clamping of all vascular pedicles before placing a suture ligature gives immediate control of hemorrhage.

The surgeon who has had the opportunity to perform several hysterectomies after cesarean section in the absence of emergency circumstances can appreciate the details and relative simplicity of the operation.

REFERENCES

1. Speert H: Edoardo Porro and cesarean hysterectomy, Surg Gynecol Obstet 106:245, 1958.
2. Durfee RB: Evolution of cesarean hysterectomy, Clin Obstet Gynecol 144:841, 1982.
3. Cunningham FG and others: Williams obstetrics, ed 19, Norwalk, CT, 1993, Appleton & Lange.
4. Pritchard JA and others: Blood volume changes in pregnancy and the perum II. Red blood cell loss and changes in apparent blood volume during and following vaginal delivery, cesarean section and cesarean section plus total hysterectomy, Am J Obstet Gynecol 84:1271, 1962.
5. Gahres EE, Albert SH, and Dodek SM: Intrapartum blood loss measured with Cr^{51}-tagged erythrocytes, Obstet Gynecol 19:455, 1962.
6. Combs CA, Murphy EL, and Laros RKL Jr: Factors associated with postpartum hemorrhage with vaginal birth, Obstet Gynecol 77A:69, 1991.
7. Mee HK: Blood transfusion in contemporary obstetric practice, Obstet Gynecol 75:940, 1990.

8. Clark SL and others: Emergency hysterectomy for obstetric hemorrhage, Obstet Gynecol 64:376, 1984.
9. O'Leary JA and Steer CE: A 10 year review of cesarean hysterectomy, Am J Obstet Gynecol 90:227, 1964.
10. Barclay DL: Cesarean hysterectomy: thirty years experience, Obstet Gynecol 35:120, 1970.
11. Barclay DL: Cesarean hysterectomy at the Charity Hospital of New Orleans: 1,000 consecutive operations, Clin Obstet Gynecol 12:635, 1969.
12. Read JA, Cotton DB, and Miller FC: Placenta accreta: changing clinical aspects and outcome, Obstet Gynecol 56:31, 1980.
13. Clark SL, Koonings PP, and Phelan JP: Placenta previa/accreta and prior cesarean section, Obstet Gynecol 66:89, 1985.
14. Stanco LM and others: Emergency peripartum hysterectomy and associated risk factors, Am J Obstet Gynecol 168:879, 1993.
15. Zelop CM and others: Emergency peripartum hysterectomy, Am J Obstet Gynecol 168:1443, 1993.
16. Finberg HJ and Williams JW: Placenta accreta: prospective sonographic diagnosis in patients with placenta previa and prior cesarean section, J Ultrasound Med 11:333, 1992.
17. Cho JY and others: Interrupted circular suture: bleeding control during cesarean delivery in placenta previa accreta, Obstet Gynecol 78:876, 1991.
18. Plauché WC and others: Cesarean hysterectomy at Louisiana State University, 1975 through 1981, South Med J 76:1261, 1983.
19. Dyer I, Nix FG, and Weed JC: Total cesarean hysterectomy at cesarean section and in the immediate puerperal period, Obstet Gynecol 65:517, 1953.
20. Burchell CR. Physiology of internal iliac artery ligation, J Obstet Gynaecol Brit Cwlth 75:642, 1968.
21. O'Leary JA: Stop of hemorrhage with uterine artery ligation, Contemp Ob/Gyn 28:13, 1986.
22. Lipschütz B: A composite study of the hypogastric artery and its branches, Am J Surg 67: 584, 1918.
23. Nichols DH, editor: Gynecologic and obstetric surgery, St Louis, 1993, Mosby.

27

Obstetric Genital Tract Fistulas

THOMAS E. ELKINS

The obstetric genital tract fistula is a surgical condition that remains far too common in our world. This is true even though it is seen almost solely in the underdeveloped countries, where there may be only 1 doctor for every 200,000 persons (as in parts of northern Nigeria), and that doctor may not be able to perform a cesarean section. Most estimate that 1 to 2 women develop obstetric genital fistulas for every 1000 births. Because of the scarce number of surgeons available to repair these fistulas, it is estimated that somewhere over 20,000 severely debilitated women in west Africa are currently awaiting repair of some form of obstetric fistula.[1]

The effects of this situation are tragic. Some aspects of this total social disaster have been documented in recent years by Tahzib[2] and others. It occurs most commonly in primigravid adolescents with no prenatal care. Over 90% of these young persons are illiterate. The intended child in the pregnancy dies in over 95% of cases.[3] The mothers are then usually divorced by their husbands as being unfit wives once they have survived prolonged obstructed labor only to develop a genital tract fistula. They often become outcasts and beggars. Some remain hidden in shame from society, along with the stench of urine and feces about them, until repair can be achieved.[4]

The causes of this ancient problem are many and varied. The lack of obstetric service availability is at the top of the list, but other factors are also important. Socioreligious traditions often create a scenario that is conducive to neglected, obstructed labor in young women. For example, many remote Moslem and Coptic tribes of sub-Saharan Africa practice early selling of young girls as wives to older men desiring children. As soon as menses occur, pregnancy is attempted, even though the female's pelvis may be far from fully developed. Many of these same tribes require that no male (i.e., most physicians) touch their wives or that no wife be allowed to visit a modern hospital facility (especially if money is required) without the husband's direct authorization, which may not be given.

At times vaginal outlet obstruction can be the result of scar formation secondary to female circumcision. This remains a tragic and senseless custom among remote tribes in parts of west Africa. The amount of tissue removed, and thus the scar formation that occurs, differs widely. For example, in northern Ghana, only clitoridectomy is practiced; while in the Sudan and Somalia, large amounts of labial tissues are damaged as well.[5] This creates a more serious problem at delivery on occasion. This is a notable factor in up to 5% of fistulas in some areas, such as the Sudan.[6]

Another local practice that often leads to suburethral and urethral fistula formation after delivery are the "gishiri" cuts made by many traditional birth attendants, especially in northern Nigeria. This is an anterior episiotomy that attempts to create room for the delivering fetus through a tight introital outlet. It is made with a long "gishiri," or sickle-shaped knife. In parts of Nigeria, this is implicated in up to 13% of fistula cases.[6]

The development of the bony pelvis also has direct implications for the rate of obstructed labor and fistula occurrence. The classic west African pelvis is android or anthropoid in shape. This gives a small, very narrow opening through which childbirth must occur. Nutritional deficiencies such as rickets are not uncommon in developing countries. This also contributes to the high incidence of bony pelvic structures that are poorly formed for childbirth in endemic fistula areas such as sub-Saharan Africa.

As Waaldijk has described, the "obstruction" in obstructed labor goes far beyond the medical and physical problems encountered by the young woman of the Third World.[1] It is usually thought to take 48 hours of intense pressure on the pelvic floor by the fetus in active, obstructed labor for a fistula to form. The "obstruction" includes the illiteracy that prevents her from knowing about prenatal care or safe delivery methods. It includes the lack of roads, transportation, and modern communication. These are some of the reasons why Harrison states that only universal education can reverse the maternal mortality and morbidity rates seen in west Africa.[7] It is notable that in the large fistula series from the Mayo Clinic in 1988 of Lee, Symmonds, and Williams, obstetric trauma was the cause of urogenital fistulas in only 8% of 300 patients, and none of that "trauma" was "obstructed labor."[8] Most were due to cesarean sections when an obstetric cause was considered. Gynecologic surgery accounted for over 80% of the 300 total cases.

One last major concern that is only now beginning to be addressed is the focus of major international funding agencies toward the problems of maternal mortality and maternal morbidity in developing countries. During the past 25 years enormous amounts of funds were allocated worldwide for maternal and child health. Most, however, went to the development of children's health programs, which have been remarkably successful.[9] Village-level, low-cost intervention with such programs as immunization and oral rehydration have saved many lives worldwide. Similar low-cost efforts have been the focus of maternal health efforts as well. For the past 20 years, U.S. agencies have focused almost solely on family planning programs (contraception, sterilization, abortion, etc.), to the exclusion of any other initiatives. This has failed to make any appreciable difference in maternal mortality rates. Maternal death ratios of 6 to 10 women per every 1000 deliveries are common in major teaching centers across west Africa, while even higher rural numbers are beginning to be reported.[10] Only recently have funding agencies seen the wisdom in developing professional services to specifically address maternal health problems. This stems in part from the realization that maternal mortality can be reduced only by the active use of prenatal clinics and regionalization of services to provide reasonable access to IV fluids, blood, antibiotics, and operative obstetrics.[11]

In terms of the obstetric fistula problem—the most prominent form of maternal morbidity in west Africa—major factors in the magnitude of the problem include a lack not only of obstetric professionals but also of surgically trained physicians who can repair the growing number of patients. Less than 200 physicians are thought to be able to repair anything beyond the minimally difficult fistula across sub-Saharan Africa.[12] This is further complicated by the fact that the majority of patients are found in the remote, northern portions of west African countries, whereas most surgeons are located in the major cities far to the south near the coastline.

The problem of the obstetric fistula is one of massive proportion in the poorly developed countries outside the industrialized nations. It is widely known as the vesicovaginal fistula (VVF), the term applied to this problem in Africa. It is a problem with an ancient history but hopefully a limited future as the international health community becomes more concerned and active.

It is interesting to note that I have seen obstetric fistulas from tissue necrosis secondary to obstructed labor on four separate occasions. In each situation, the second stage was beyond 2 hours (usually beyond 4 hours), and leakage did not begin for 48 to 72 hours after delivery. As prolonged second stages with epidural anesthesia become more common, VVF may become more familiar in the United States.

The History of Obstetric Fistula Repair: A History of Gynecologic Surgery

Obstetric genitourinary fistulas have been known since the beginning of history. One of the mummified wives of an eleventh dynasty Egyptian king was found to have a large midvaginal VVF. Avicenna of Persia was the first to describe a fistula as being the cause of urine leakage after difficult vaginal delivery.[6,13]

Many have attempted repairs of these large defects over the centuries. Fatio of France described a technique of mobilizing the vagina away from the bladder and closing the two separately. However, no evidence shows that he was ever successful.[14] de Lamballe had some success in France in the early 1800s.[15] Diffenbach, the master plastic surgeon of Germany, was quoted as saying "the lucky cure of a VVF is the rarest of occurrences." He described full wards of miserable, leaking women with little hope of recovery.[6] Mettauer was the first American to record a cure of an obstetric fistula in Virginia in 1840.[16]

J. Marion Sims did much to change all of this and became known as the father of modern gynecologic surgery for his efforts.[17] He began his work in Montgomery, Alabama, where he published his classic paper on repair methods. He and Dr. Thomas Emmet then founded the first fistula hospital in New York City in the late 1800s. Sims successfully repaired 200 of 270 patients.

The Sims technique involved simply denuding the fistula tract edges and then mobilizing the vagina minimally away from the bladder before closure with interrupted wire sutures.

Shortly after the report of Sims' successes, Maurice Henry Collis of Ireland developed the split-flap technique for wide mobilization of large fistula tracts, followed by tension-free layered closure in 1861.[18] This technique was later defined more extensively by Halban of Germany.[19] It is notable that in this technique the fistula tract is NOT excised. This preserves all tissue possible for use in reapproximation. It also prevents intravesical bleeding postoperatively, which can result in catheter obstruction from blood clots, bladder distention, disruption of suture lines, and repair failure. In the late 1800s two urologic surgeons, Von Dittel and Trendelenburg, popularized transabdominal approaches to obstetric fistulas, a route preferred by most urologists even today.[20]

Many expert surgeons added their contributions to the obstetric fistula repair story. The Mayo brothers encouraged overlapping layers sewn in opposite directions, to close defects without compromising blood supply.[21] Norman Miller of Michigan spoke against purse-string suturing of small defects and described placing the patient in the prone position postoperatively for 48 hours to allow bladder mucosal healing without gravitational pressure from the transurethral catheter.[22] Halban of Germany emphasized wide mobilization of tissues to facilitate VVF repairs.[19] Lawson later emphasized the prone, jackknife position for suburethral VVF repair, which was challenged by Miller of Michigan and others.[23]

A number of surgeons began to look for ways to bring new tissue and new blood supply into the area. Heinrich Martius of Germany described the bulbocavernosus graft in the early 1930s before later modifying this approach to include the fibrofatty tissue beneath the labia majora[24,25] (Figure 27.1). Ingelman-Sundberg made extensive use of gracilis muscle grafts in attempts to repair large VVFs.[26] This method was first attributed to Garlock in the 1920s[27] (Figure 27.2). Wein, Mallory, and Greenberg[28] and Orford and Theron[29] and others utilized omental J-flaps extensively to interpose tissue between the vagina and the bladder in transabdominal repairs (Figure 27.3). Today the modified Martius graft is used most commonly with obstetric fistula repairs.[30] It has an extensive blood supply that allows it to be detached either superiorly or inferiorly and still maintain its usefulness in providing neovascularity, tissue bulk, and separation of suture lines. Detaching the graft at the level of the clitoris leaves the pudendal artery supply intact. Detaching the graft at the level of the introitus leaves the inferior epigastric blood supply intact (Figure 27.4). Many different tissues have been used in adjunctive repair methods to assist in closure of these difficult-to-manage defects. However, none has consistently taken the place of primary bladder closure.

Outstanding surgeons continued to dedicate much of their career focus to the successful repair of the obstetric fistula. The 1950s and 1960s were times when Professors Mahfouz, Moir, and Lawson wrote extensively from their experience in north and west Africa.[23,31,32] They were successful in raising the fistula repair rate overall to beyond 65%, with higher rates being seen for suburethral types.

The 1970s through the 1990s have seen the development of fistula repair centers across north and west Africa. Sister Ann Ward, M.D., a missionary obstetrician in

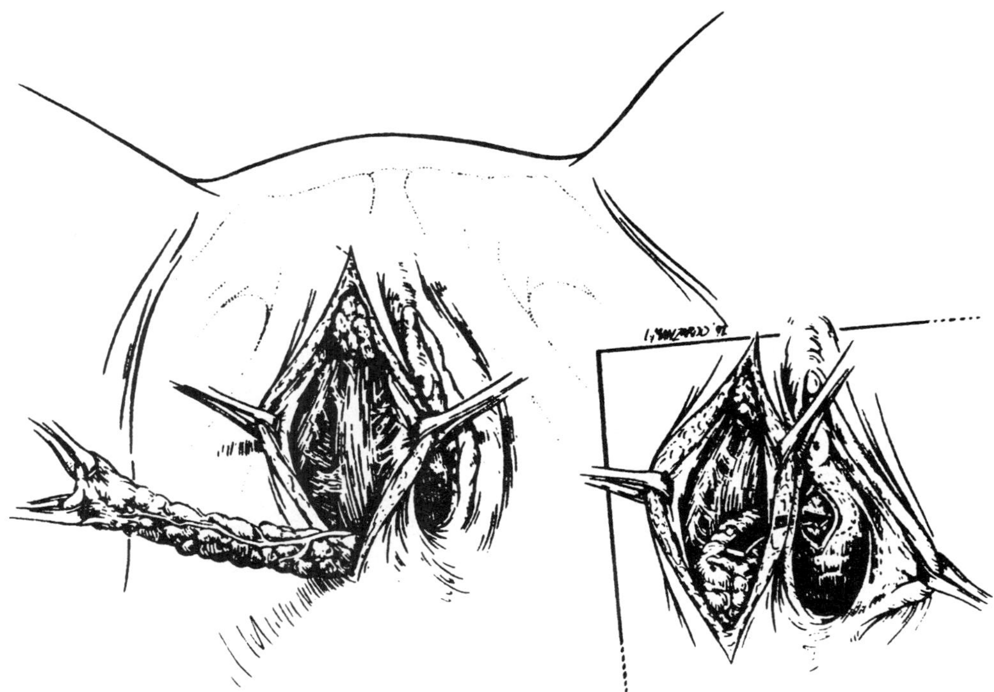

Figure 27.1 The modified Martius graft involves fibrofatty tissue from the labium majus, where the round ligament originates. (From Fitzpatrick C and Elkins TE: Int Urogynecol J 4:287, 1993.)

Anua-Uyo, Nigeria, has reported on over 2500 VVF repairs.[33] Dr. Kees Waaldijk has established centers at Kano and Katsina, Nigeria, and repairs approximately 1000 VVFs per year.[34] Professor Henry Ojengbede has established a fistula ward at the University College Hospital in Ibadan, Nigeria, where he has done over 1000 repairs.[35] A similar service has been established at Korle Bu Teaching Hospital in Accra, Ghana, under Dr. T.S. Ghosh, and at the Komfo Anokye Teaching Hospital in Kumasi, Ghana, under Professor J.O. Martey.[36] Dr. J. Abbo in Khartoum, Sudan, has a similar vast experience and operates a VVF hospital that bulges with patients.[37]

The premier fistula hospital was established by Drs. Catherine and Reginald Hamlin in Addis Ababa, Ethiopia, in the 1960s.[38] Over 15,000 patients have been surgically cured at the hospital, run by Dr. Catherine Hamlin with recent help from Dr. Steve Arrowsmith, Professor John Kelley, and excellent Ethiopian physicians and staff.[39,40] The center provides psychosocial support and rehabilitation services for patients, as well as surgical expertise.

After centuries of struggling simply to close obstetric fistulas, all of these contemporary surgeons are performing large numbers of repairs, with excellent successful closure rates of 80% to 95% generally. The focus of attention has therefore centered upon several "fistula issues":

1. Programs in maternal health, prenatal care, and obstetric care aimed at prevention of further VVFs
2. New repair methods to close the most difficult fistulas (those needing urethras, the combined VVF-rectovaginal fistula [RVF], etc.)
3. New repair methods to reduce the 60% complication rate (gynatresia, SUI, small bladder syndrome, etc.) that accompanies even successful repairs
4. The training of more surgeons in endemic areas to help with fistula repairs

Types of Obstetric Fistulas

Classification

Most classifications in the past have been anatomic in origin. For example, Moir and Lawson used the following anatomic categories:

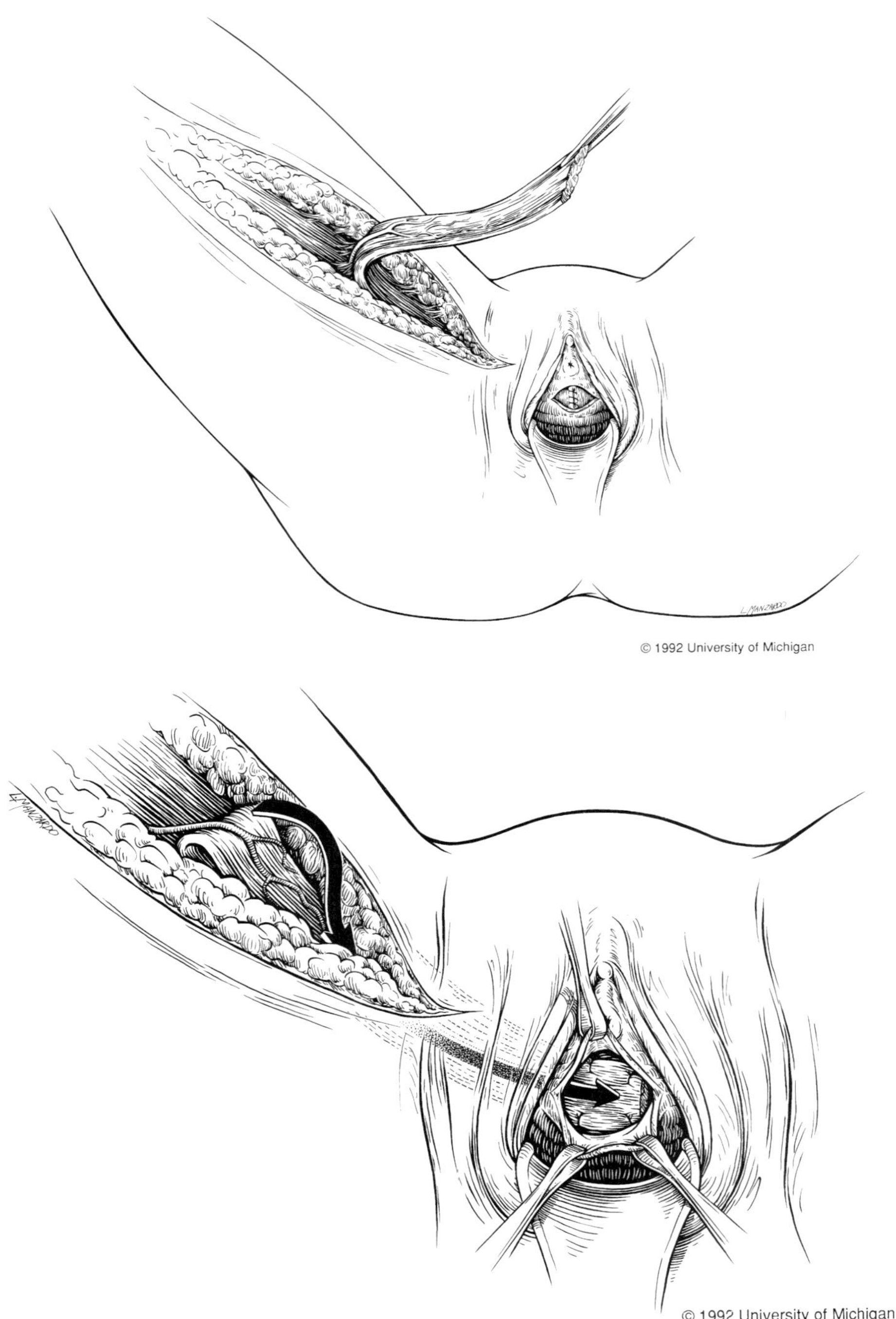

FIGURE 27.2 The gracilis muscle graft requires extensive leg dissection and muscle mobilization. (From Fitzpatrick C and Elkins TE: Int Urogynecol J 4:287, 1993.)

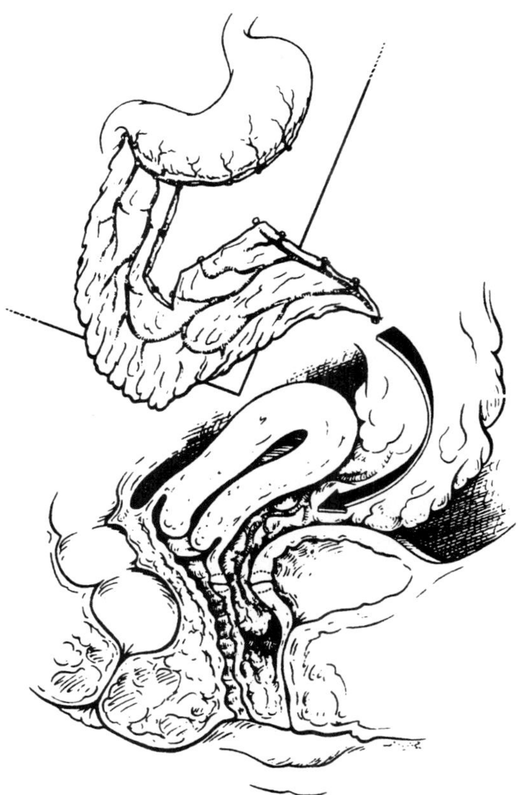

Figure 27.3 The omental J-flap mobilizes readily into the pelvis. (From Fitzpatrick C and Elkins TE: Int Urogynecol J 4:287, 1993.)

suburethral fistula, total urethral loss, midvaginal fistula, juxtacervical fistula, and uterovesical fistula[32,23] (Figure 27.5). Less common fistulas in this classification would include combined vesicovaginal and rectovaginal fistulas, the ureterovaginal fistula, and the colonovesical fistula. Waaldjik has recently submitted a further classification, basing his categories on the degree of operative difficulty in repairing each fistula type and the amount of complications to be expected from even the successful closure of each fistula type.[41] In this system, for example, those fistulas involving the functional closing mechanism for urinary output need special consideration. In this chapter, the anatomic classification will be used (Figure 27.5).

Suburethral Vesicovaginal Fistulas

These represent the most common type of obstetric fistulas. They represent prolonged tissue trauma right at the base of the pubic bone, which involves the urethrovesical neck and lower proximal urethra (Figure 27.6). The standard split-flap technique described previously is sufficient for closure in 95% to 97% of these lesions. However, because of the wide disruption of periurethral fascia caused by this dissection, 10% to 25% of patients will have significant type II (hypermobility-related) SUI despite successful closure.[42] Therefore most surgeons prefer to elevate the vesical neck at the time of repair with vaginally placed sutures that resemble Marshall-Marchetti-Kranz sutures in the United States.

Midvaginal Vesicovaginal Fistulas

These fistulas are thought to develop from prolonged midpelvic obstruction in labor. They are often quite large, measuring 4 to 6 cm in diameter (Figure 27.7). It is not uncommon to see the ureteral orifices clearly present on the lower, lateral edges of the fistula (Figure 27.8). Prolapse of the bladder wall through the fistula is also common with this type of fistula (Figure 27.9).

Wide dissection with the split-flap method is used to mobilize the bladder enough to reapproximate its edges in layers. Ureteral catheters are usually placed to help the surgeon avoid the ureters.

Many surgeons still prefer 2-0 or 3-0 chromic catgut for inner bladder layers, since it dissolves quickly, and stone formation would be uncommon. 2-0 or 3-0 Vicryl on a CT-2 needle is preferred for outer bladder layers because of its prolonged tensile strength.

One of the major problems in repairing these larger VVFs is the loss of vaginal tissue that occurs if reapproximation of fistula edges is attempted, and the small bladder syndrome that may result from bladder closure over large defects. The problem of postoperative vaginal atresia (and thus dyspareunia or sexual nonfunction) has been addressed in part by using full-thickness, modified Martius grafts[43] (Figures 27.10 and 27.11). The Hamlins and Dr. Steve Arrowsmith have long used vaginal–labia minora grafts to close such defects.

The small bladder syndrome results when a functional capacity of less than 20 to 25 ml is all that remains after closure of a large midvaginal VVF. This causes constant sensations

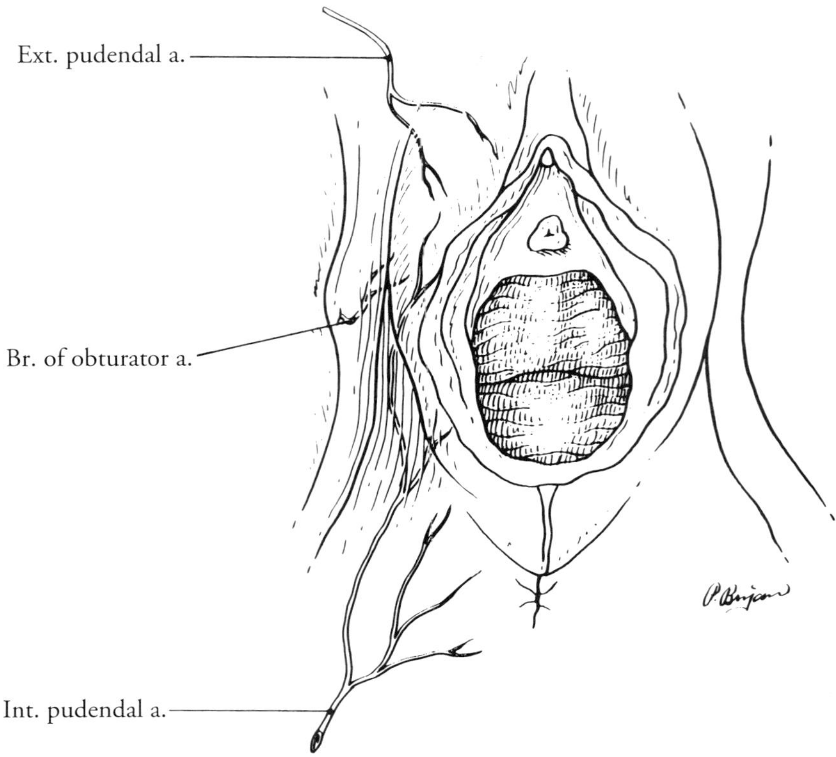

FIGURE 27.4 The extensive blood supply of the labium majus is the main reason for the Martius graft's usefulness, since it brings neovascularity into the region of the surgery.

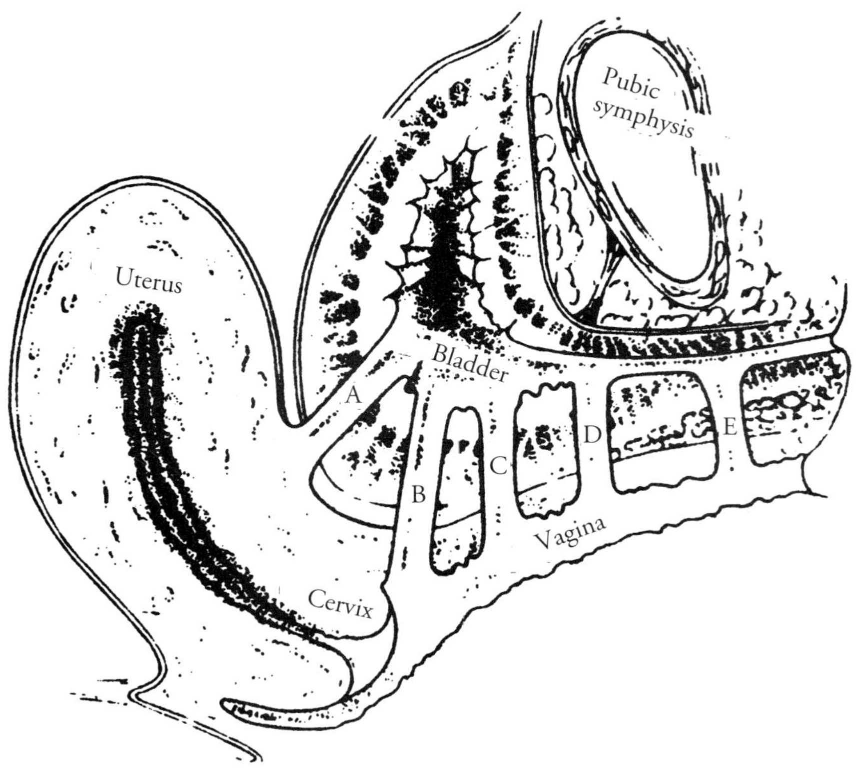

FIGURE 27.5 The different types of obstetric fistulas. **A**, Vesicocervical fistula. **B**, Juxtacervical fistula. **C**, Midvaginal fistula. **D**, Suburethral fistula. **E**, Total urethral loss. (From Elkins TE: Am J Obstet Gynecol 170:1108, 1994.)

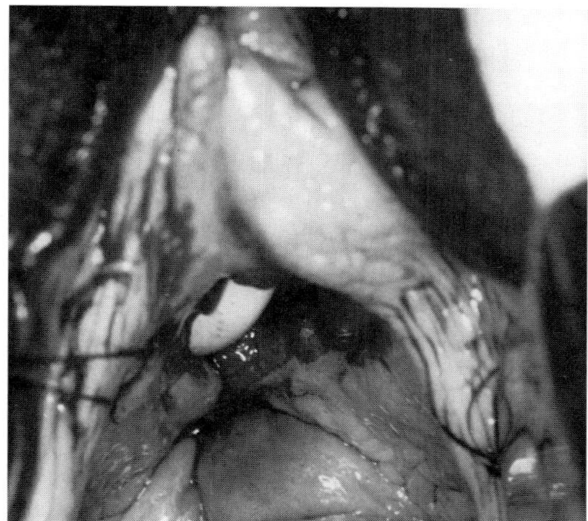

Figure 27.6 A typical suburethral obstetric fistula, the most common obstetric fistula. (From Elkins TE: Am J Obstet Gynecol 170:1108, 1994.)

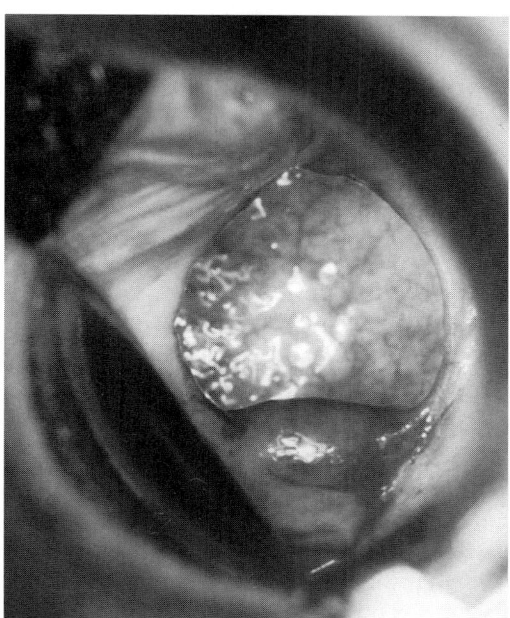

Figure 27.7 A midvaginal, large, cavernous fistula. (Reprinted with permission from The American College of Obstetricians and Gynecologists. Elkins TE: Obstet Gynecol 72:307, 1988.)

of urgency and frequency, as well as bladder spasms. Standard bowel augmentation cystoplasty techniques have been troublesome because of the build-up of obstructive mucus and bladder obstruction. Autoaugmentation holds some promise for these patients and is now being attempted.

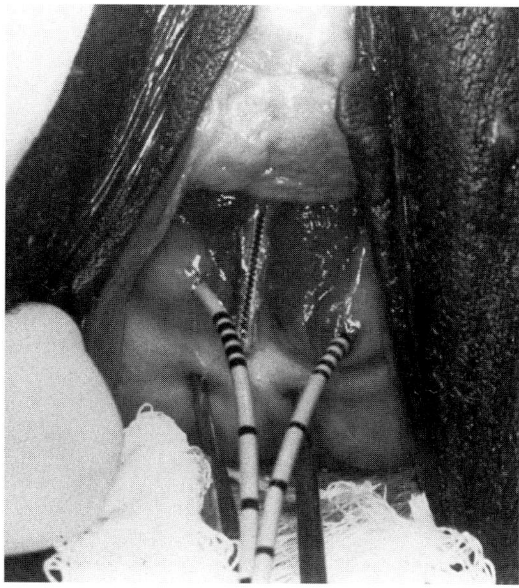

Figure 27.8 A midvaginal fistula with ureteral catheters at the fistula edges. (Reprinted with permission from The American College of Obstetricians and Gynecologists. Elkins TE: Obstet Gynecol 72:307, 1988.)

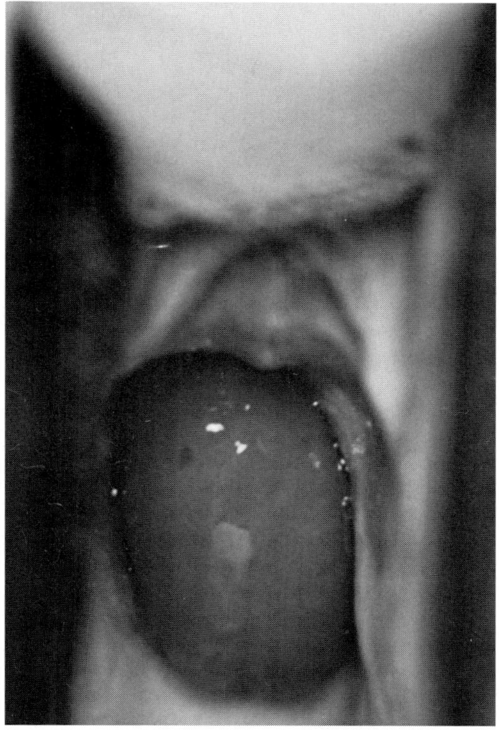

Figure 27.9 A midvaginal fistula with prolapsing bladder. (From Elkins TE: Am J Obstet Gynecol 170:1108, 1994.)

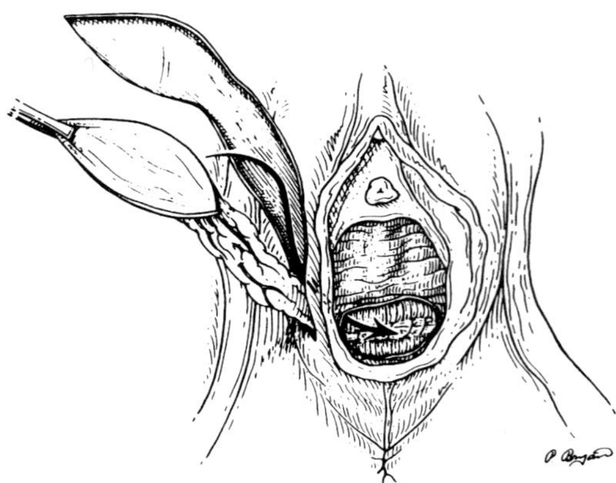

FIGURE 27.10 A full-thickness modified Martius graft to preserve vaginal depth.

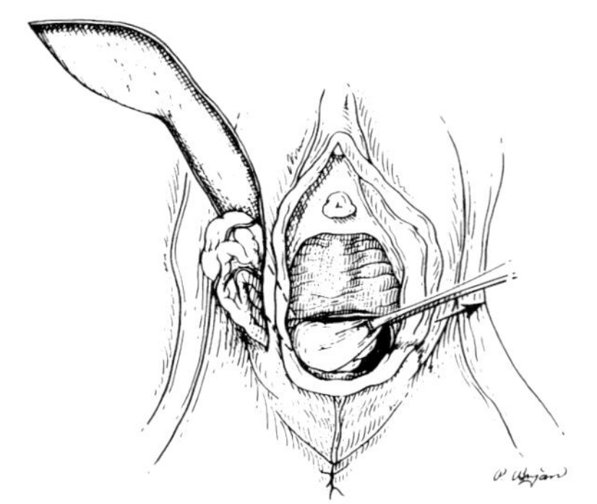

FIGURE 27.11 Pulling the full-thickness graft through the Martius tunnel.

Approaching the Large Vesicovaginal Fistula

On many occasions the large VVF can be one of the simplest dissections if all edges are visible and the urethra is still connected to the bladder.

When the fistula is first visualized and palpated, an attempt is made to pass a Foley catheter into the bladder. If it goes easily, a simpler repair awaits. If the urethra has formed a stricture and is no longer connected to the bladder, then a more difficult repair involving retropubic anterior bladder wall mobilization lies ahead. In this instance, the strictured urethra is manually opened by a uterine sound forced into the bladder cavity. This is followed by urethral dilators and finally a 16-French Foley catheter.

The best place to enter the space of Retzius vaginally when faced with a large VVF (which has sloughed a portion of the urethra, or not) is the same place used to do this for a Pereyra, Raz, or Stamey procedure. The technique of achieving a retroperitoneal position should be the same. An incision is made at the urethrovesical junction, or just beneath the pubic bone, through whatever vaginal epithelium is available. This incision is carried laterally along the fistula edge on both sides. Sharp and blunt dissection allows lateral and superior exposure of the bladder (and the lower urethra if it is intact), just as in a dissection for a Kelly's plication. The index finger of the left hand is then placed directly on the pubic bone (still hidden by endopelvic fascia) to the left of the patient's urethra, or remnant thereof. Metzenbaum's scissors are then pushed upward through the endopelvic fascia at a 45-degree angle away from the urethra, by placing the scissors between finger and bone, with tips toward the pubic bone. This usually is successful in mobilizing even the badly scarred bladder away from the pubic bone. The same procedure is then carried out on the patient's right side.

These maneuvers should allow the surgeon to feel the pubic tubercle and even Cooper's ligament without tissue covering these structures.

The incision through the vaginal epithelium should then be extended to encircle the large fistula tract, staying approximately 2 to 5 mm away from the red, friable bladder mucosal edge.

Placing a finger into the space of Retzius through the holes created above in the endopelvic fascia allows gentle blunt and sharp dissection of the bladder wall away from the vaginal epithelium. The surgeon gently sweeps his or her finger inferiorly and posteriorly, following the incision made above. Constant use of Metzenbaum's scissors to pierce and spread tissues is also helpful at this stage. Care must be taken to be superficial to the puborectalis and bulbocavernosus muscles attached to the lateral pubic rami, or excessive hemorrhage may occur.

When the surgeon has successfully mobilized the bladder in this fashion on both sides, it is clear that the space of Retzius has been entered anteriorly, and the paravaginal space is clearly palpable and visible laterally.

The inferior portion of the large midvaginal fistula is usually easily dissected by spreading with Metzenbaum's scissors to elevate vaginal epithelium away from the bladder and ureters. During this posterior dissection, ureteral orifices are usually identified and cannulated with ureteral stents or small pediatric feeding tubes. These may be removed at the end of the repair, or in several days if any question of ureteral entrapment or compromise is present.

If the large (4 to 6 cm in diameter) VVF is truly midvaginal only and the urethra is intact, then wide mobilization, followed by layered closures, and placement of a Martius graft yields a high success rate. (This was the situation in the ACOG video I produced in 1988.)

If the entire urethra, or almost all of the urethra, is missing, a Tanagho type of anterior bladder wall flap may be created to add urethral length or to serve as an entirely new urethra. This is described in detail elsewhere.[46]

Even when most or all of the urethra is intact, one of the most difficult parts of the repair when urethral stricture (and nonconnection with the bladder) has been present is the closure of the lateral, superior angle at the urethrovesical junction on both sides. Even with aggressive anterior bladder wall mobilization, this small angle may be almost retropubic in location and very prone to leak. Patients who have lateral, recurrent failures have even learned where the defect is and often announce on return to the clinic: "Lunga, lunga" (small-hole leak).

A one- or two-layer bladder closure is usually reinforced with a Martius graft.[24] The large, raw surface area is then best closed by creating a lateral side-wall vaginal pedicle graft of epithelium. Or a full-thickness Martius graft, as described by Margolis and others, prevents vaginal atresia and strictures.[43]

Juxtacervical Vesicovaginal Fistulas

Obstruction at the pelvic inlet is thought to result in a juxtacervical VVF. In this fistula the lower edge is often visible vaginally (Figure 27.12). The upper edge of the fistula may be visible or may be high on the cervix. Often a combined transvaginal and transabdominal mobilization is required to free the fistula edges circumferentially from the vagina and

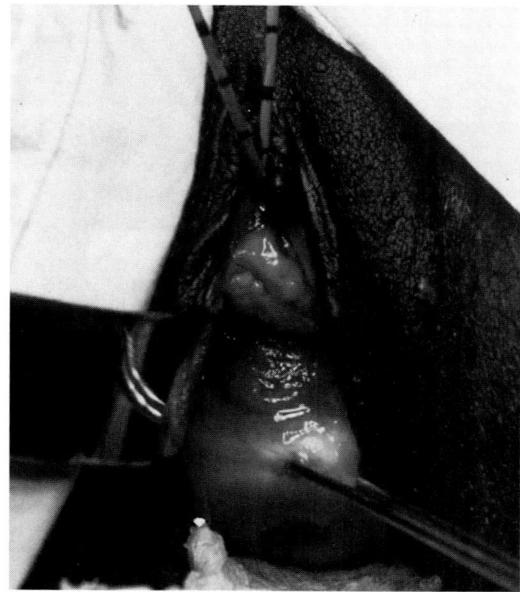

Figure 27.12 Typical juxtacervical obstetric fistula. (From Elkins TE: Am J Obstet Gynecol 170:1108, 1994.)

cervix. The transperitoneal approach involves dissecting the entire bladder away from the lower uterine segment, cervix, and upper vagina. A multilayered fistula closure is then possible. An omental J-flap is a helpful adjunctive procedure in these cases. It is interposed between the bladder and vagina, which are each closed separately.[28]

The juxtacervical fistula and the uterovesical fistula are often approached through an extraperitoneal, transvesical approach. This is a simple approach that requires opening the dome of the bladder and then dissecting the vagina (or the cervix or the uterus) away from the bladder through the fistula tract itself.[44]

Success rates for all of these methods approach 90% to 95% in multiple series.

Total Urethral Loss

Loss of the urethra is thought to be caused in most instances by prolonged obstruction at the pelvic outlet (Figure 27.13). This did represent one of the most difficult to repair fistula types. Even if urethral tissue was successfully fashioned from nearby labial tissue, the development of type III SUI (due to the lack of intrinsic sphincteric function) was extremely

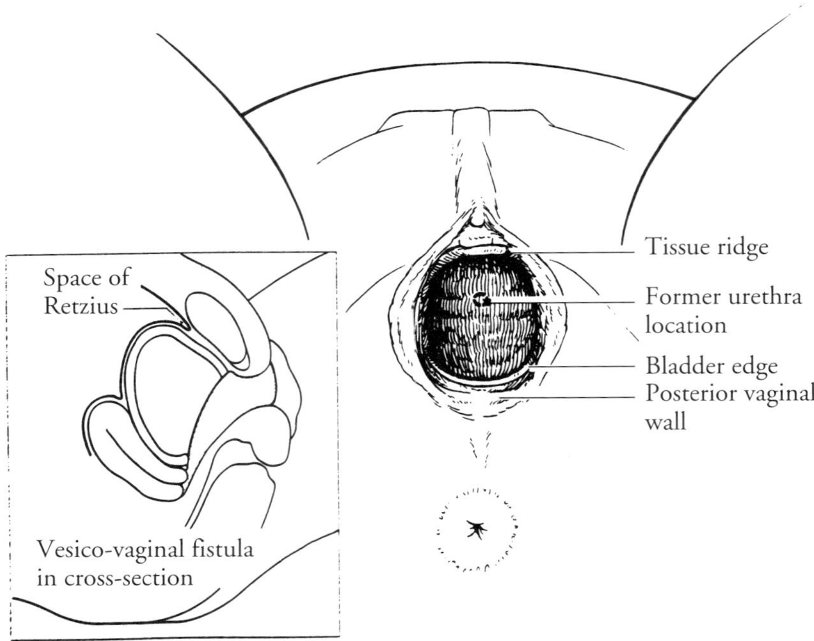

FIGURE 27.13 Schematic view of total urethral loss. (Reprinted with permission from The American College of Obstetricians and Gynecologists. Elkins TE and others: Obstet Gynecol 79:455, 1992.)

common. Techniques to utilize anterior bladder wall tissue in forming a neourethra had been developed by Tanagho with a transabdominal approach.[45] This has now been modified to be used with a transvaginal approach and has resulted in successful urethral formation in up to 90% of patients. A sling procedure, following placement of a Martius graft, has become a standard component of this operation[46] (Figure 27.14).

Older techniques, followed by sling placement, must still be used if the large VVF is below the urethral loss. Using the anterior bladder wall for a new urethra in this setting simply leaves too little bladder capacity behind, and a small bladder syndrome results.

Injuries to the urethra caused by the "gishiri cut" are readily repaired by mobilizing remaining urethral tissue laterally and accomplishing a midline closure. This is possible because of the incision-like injury to the urethra, rather than the crushing loss of usable tissue caused by prolonged obstruction.[6]

Combined VVF-RVF

Combined VVF-RVF cases have the lowest total closure rate in most recent series (Figure 27.15). Only 60% to 65% are both closed initially, and high rates of gynatresia or vaginal stenosis follow most successful repairs.[47]

Most contemporary surgeons favor a more liberal use of diverting colostomy in these patients, with broader use of full-thickness grafts that replace vaginal tissue, rather than utilize what little of it remains to close defects.

The RVF resulting from obstetric trauma is generally unlike that seen after full episiotomy breakdown or buttonhole formation due to poor episiotomy healing, which are common in the United States. The RVFs secondary to tissue necrosis from obstructed labor are larger, often off-center, and usually much higher in the vaginal canal than the usual postpartum RVF seen in the United States. Mobilization often involves literally peeling the rectosigmoid and fistula tract away from the lower portions of the pubic rami.

Ureterovaginal Fistulas

Ureterovaginal fistulas also are seen after long obstructed labor. However, they are most commonly seen after cesarean section or cesarean hysterectomy. In developing countries not all operative obstetrics is performed by obste-

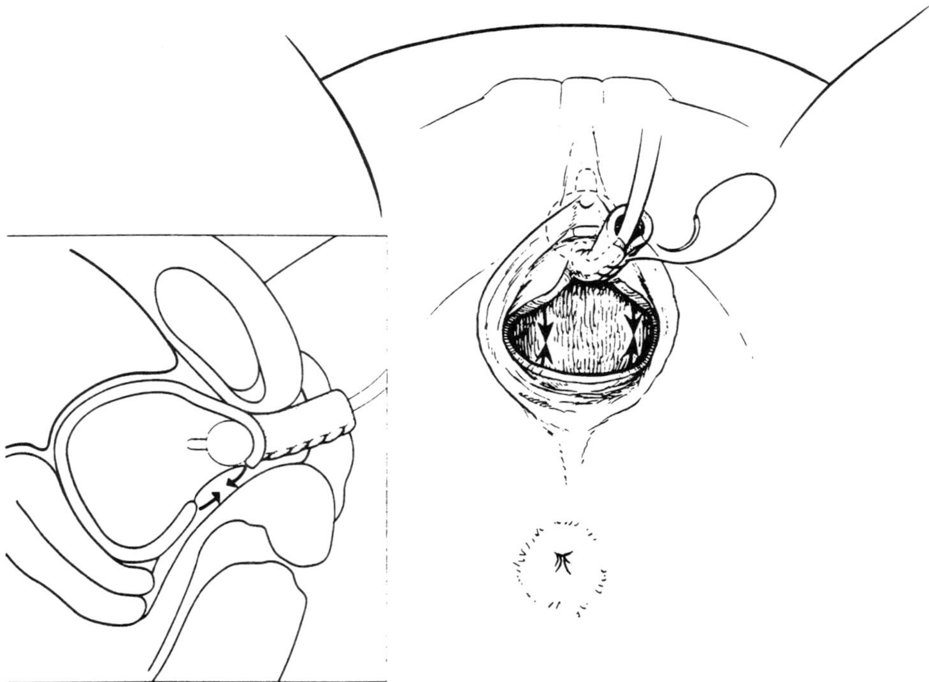

Figure 27.14 Neourethra formation from the mobilized anterior bladder wall. (Reprinted with permission from The American College of Obstetricians and Gynecologists. Elkins TE and others: Obstet Gynecol 79:455, 1992.)

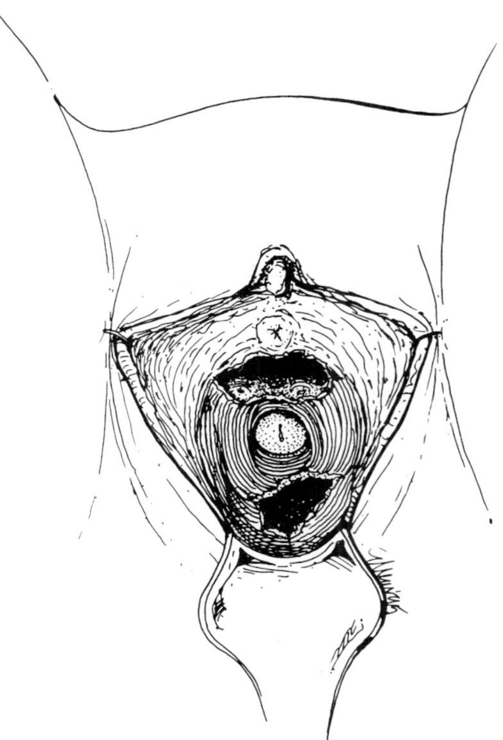

Figure 27.15 The most difficult to repair obstetric fistula: the compound VVF-RVF.

tricians. Inadequately trained surgeons may be ill prepared to manage the challenges presented to them by the extensive tissue necrosis and sepsis associated with prolonged, obstructed labor. Ureters may easily be damaged in such settings.

Techniques of ureteral reimplantation, reanastomosis, and reinsertion into the bladder using Boari flaps, etc., are beyond the scope of this chapter. It simply should suffice to say that all these procedures may become useful in achieving dryness for the patient who has a urogenital fistula after obstetric trauma.

Small High Vaginal Vault Fistulas

Small high vaginal vault fistulas usually follow cesarean hysterectomy and resemble the kind of VVFs seen most frequently in the United States. These are commonly repaired by the Latzko technique.[48] By this method, vaginal epithelium is excised in a wide circle around the tiny fistula tract, which is usually excised. A layered closure is done, which produces a partial colpocleisis. Recent series show this method to be 95% successful in gynecologic fistulas in the United States.[49]

Special Considerations

Diagnosis of the Obstetric Fistula

Most patients begin to experience urine leakage in 1 to 7 days after delivery, with leakage around day 3 to 7 being most common. In most instances the lesion is very palpable and visible on examination. If not, methylene blue may be inserted via a Foley catheter into the bladder.[50] Original insertion of this catheter should be done as soon as possible after prolonged labor. Six weeks of drainage may prevent fistula occurrence, or at least limit the size of the tissue damage. Blue staining of vaginal pads implies the presence of a VVF, which may be confirmed with cystoscopy. If no leakage occurs, one ampule of indigo carmine may be injected IV with fluid hydration. Within 5 to 12 minutes, vaginal pads should be stained blue, identifying a ureterovaginal fistula. This may then be confirmed by a retrograde IV pyelogram, if available. Leakage through the cervical os implies a vesicouterine fistula.

Timing of the Repair

Obstetric fistulas, because of the extensive tissue necrosis seen with them, were always thought to need maximal delay between the time of delivery and the time of repair before surgery could be accomplished successfully. Three-to-four month delays were considered standard. However, Waaldjik recently discussed a large series of patients in which he immediately began excision of dead tissue and attempted complete repair as soon as all fistula edges appeared viable. His success rates were comparable to (or slightly less than) those achieved by waiting much longer before attempting repairs.[51]

Immediate transurethral catheter drainage of the bladder following prolonged labor is thought by Kelly to be effective in preventing VVFs.[50] He further notes that small obstetric VVFs may completely resolve with 3 to 4 weeks of catheter drainage of the bladder. Performing these procedures, while providing nutritional support, is highly recommended before attempting surgery.

Postoperative Bladder Drainage

Many have stated in the United States that the Foley catheter can be removed after only 1 to 3 days of drainage if the urine is clear of microscopic hematuria. In the large obstetric fistulas, a more conservative approach is usually recommended. Transurethral catheter drainage for 14 to 21 days is the standard. In the immediate postoperative period (24 to 48 hours postoperatively), patients are encouraged to drink profusely until their urine appears to be similar in color to water. This reduces the problem of catheter tip obstruction from tissue debris or blood clots.

Some surgeons (Ghosh, in Accra, for example) prefer suprapubic catheter drainage to avoid any catheter pressure on suture lines.

Nonoperative Complications Associated with Obstetric Fistulas

Between 5% and 65% of patients who develop obstetric fistulas from prolonged obstructed labor have some degree of peroneal nerve palsy, or footdrop. The injury tends to be transient in most instances and does seem to respond in part to physical therapy.[52]

Secondary amenorrhea occurs in 10% to 20% of fistula patients, as well. This is thought to be due to one of four mechanisms: (1) Asherman's syndrome (intrauterine synechiae) resulting from untreated postpartum endometritis; (2) Sheehan's syndrome (from excessive hemorrhage at the time of delivery, causing pituitary necrosis); (3) extensive uterine tissue necrosis in labor that results in minimal remaining endometrial tissue, and (4) pituitary and ovarian dysfunction secondary to the severe debilitation and malnutrition of these patients. Initial studies by Ojengbede have shown that Asherman's syndrome is probably the most common cause, but severe debilitation and malnutrition is surely a factor as well.[35,53]

Training Surgeons to Perform Fistula Surgery

There is a massive need to train surgeons of all types to repair vesicovaginal and other obstetric fistulas. Waaldjik (Nigeria) is a perfect example of the capacity of someone other than a gynecologist or urologist to repair obstetric fistulas, since he was first an orthopedic surgeon and then a plastic surgeon before going to Nigeria.[54] Several pilot studies have been done to identify fistulas that are at high risk for repair failure, so that these may be transferred to major VVF centers. Other pilot projects have looked at the minimal time necessary to train someone knowledgeable in pelvic surgery to do fistula repairs. Two to four weeks seems sufficient for such persons to then achieve 90% to 95% success rates in a significant number of repairs. "First World" assistance in developing "Third World" expertise is sorely needed to reduce the number of patients now suffering from obstetric fistulas in west and north Africa alone. This, combined with the steady growth of programs to improve women's health care and diminish the alarming rate at which new fistula patients are being seen, holds the key to solving one of the world's greatest tragedies of the 1990s.

References

1. Waaldijk K and Armuja YD: Obstetric fistula in northern Nigeria: a major health problem, Int Urogynecol J 4:126, 1993.
2. Tahzib F: An initiative on vesicovaginal fistula, Lancet 2:1316, 1989.
3. Harrison K: Child-bearing, health, and social priorities: a survey of 22,774 consecutive births in Zaria, northern Nigeria, Br J Obstet Gynaecol 92(suppl 5):1, 1985.
4. Murphy M: Social consequences of vesicovaginal fistula in northern Nigeria, J Biosoc Sci 13:139, 1981.
5. Brody S and Elkins TE: Female circumcisions in northern Ghana, Int J Gynecol Obstet (in press).
6. Zacharin R: Obstetric fistula, New York, 1988, Springer-Verlag.
7. Harrison KA: Maternal mortality in developing countries, Br J Obstet Gynaecol 96:1, 1989.
8. Lee RL, Symmonds RE, and Williams TJ: Current status of genitourinary fistula, Obstet Gynecol 72:313, 1988.
9. Rosenfield A: Maternal mortality in developing countries: an ongoing but neglected epidemic, JAMA 262:376, 1989.
10. Elkins TE: Maternal mortality and morbidity in the developing world: personal reflections and a profession's commitment, Women's Health Issues 2:146, 1992.
11. Sciarra JJ: Reproductive health: a global perspective, Am J Obstet Gynecol 168(6):1649, 1993.
12. Elkins TE and others: Recognition and management of patients with high risk vesicovaginal fistula: implications for teaching and research, Int Urogynecol J 5:183, 1994.
13. Derry DE: Note on five pelves of women of the eleventh dynasty in Egypt, J Obstet Gynaecol Br Emp 42:490, 1935.
14. Fatio J: Helvetisch-vemunstige wehemuner, Basel, 1752.
15. Jobert de Lamballe AJ: Traite des fistules vesico-uterines, Paris, 1852, Balliere et Fils.
16. Mettauer JP: Vesico-vaginal fistula, Boston Med Surg J 22:154, 1840.
17. Sims JM: On the treatment of vesicovaginal fistula, Am J Med Sci 23:59, 1852.
18. Collis MH: Further remarks upon a new and successful mode for treatment of vesicovaginal fistulas, Ir J Med Sci 31:302, 1861.
19. Halban J: Operative technique of vesicovaginal fistulas, Am J Obstet Gynecol 33:1073, 1937.
20. Trendelenburg F: Uber blasenschneidanfistaloperationem und uber backehochlagerung bei operationen, Samml Klin Vortr 355(109):3373, 1890.
21. Mayo CH and Walters W: The operative treatment of vesicovaginal fistulas, Surg Clin North Am 4:399, 1924.
22. Miller NF: The surgical treatment and postoperative care of vesicovaginal fistula, Am J Obstet Gynecol 44:873, 1942.
23. Lawson JB: Tropical obstetrics and gynaecology: vesicovaginal fistula—a tropical disease, Trans R Soc Trop Med Hyg 83:454, 1989.
24. Martius H: Uber die behandlung von blasensheidenfistela, insbesondere mit hilfe emir lappenplastik, Geburtsh Gynäkol 103:22, 1932.
25. Elkins TE, DeLancey JOL, and McGuire EJ: The use of modified Martius graft as an adjunctive technique in vesicovaginal and rectovaginal fistulas repair, Obstet Gynecol 75:727, 1990.
26. Ingelman-Sundberg A: Pathogenesis and operative treatment of urinary fistulas in irradiated tissue. In Youssef AF, editor: Gynecologic surgery, Springfield, Ill, 1960, Charles C. Thomas, Publisher.
27. Garlock JH: The cure of an intractable vesi-

covaginal fistula by use of a pedicaled muscle graft, Surg Gynecol Obstet 255:255, 1928.

28. Wein AJ, Mallory TR, and Greenberg SH: Omental transportation as an aid in genitourinary reconstructive procedures, J Trauma 20:473, 1980.
29. Orford HJL and Theron JLL: The repair of vesicovaginal fistulas with omentum: a review of 59 cases, S Afr Med J 67:143, 1985.
30. Betson JR: The bulbocavernosus fat pad transplant for severe stress incontinence and vesicovaginal fistula, Am J Surg 271:129, 1961.
31. Mahfouz N: Urinary fistulae in women, Obstet Gynecol 64:23, 1957.
32. Moir JC: Personal experiences in the treatment of vesicovaginal fistulas, Am J Obstet Gynecol 71:476, 1956.
33. Ward A: VVF repairs: personal series. Invited panel at the American Urogynecology Society meeting, Orlando, Fla, November 1, 1989.
34. Waaldijk K: The surgical management of bladder fistula in 775 women in northern Nigeria, Nijmegen, 1989, Benda.
35. Ojengbede OHA: VVF repairs: personal series. Invited panel at the American Urogynecology Society meeting, Orlando, Fla, November 1, 1989.
36. Martey JO: VVF repairs: personal series. Invited panel at the American Urogynecology Society meeting, Orlando, Fla, November 1, 1989.
37. Abbo AH and Mukhtar M: New trends in the operative management of urinary fistulae, Sudan Med J 13:126, 1975.
38. Hamlin RHJ and Nicholson EC: Reconstruction of urethra totally destroyed in labor, Br Med J 2:147, 1969.
39. Arrowsmith SD: Genitourinary reconstruction in obstetric fistulas, J Urol 152:403, 1994.
40. Kelly J: Vesicovaginal and rectovaginal fistulae, R Soc Med 85:258, 1992.
41. Waaldijk K: A classification of obstetric fistulas, Int J Gynaecol Obstet (in press).
42. Schleicher D, Ojengbede OHA, and Elkins TE: Urologic evaluation after closure of vesicovaginal fistulas, Int Urogynecol J 4:262, 1993.
43. Margolis T and others: Use of a full thickness Martius graft to restore vagina depth in patients with large vesicovaginal fistulas, Obstet Gynecol 84:148, 1994.
44. Mack WF: Urologic complications of pelvic surgery, Br J Urol 41:641, 1969.
45. Tanagho EA: Neourethra: rationale, surgical technique, and indications. In Stanton S and Tanagho EA, editors: Surgery for female incontinence, Berlin, 1980, Springer-Verlag.
46. Elkins TE and others: Transvaginal mobilization and utilization of the anterior bladder wall to repair vesicovaginal fistulas involving the urethra, Obstet Gynecol 79:455, 1992.
47. Elkins TE: Surgery for the obstetric vesicovaginal fistula: a review of 100 operations in 82 patients, Am J Obstet Gynecol 170:1108, 1994.
48. Latzko W: Postoperative vesicovaginal fistulas: genesis and therapy, Am J Surg 58:211, 1942.
49. Tancer ML: Observations on prevention and management of vesicovaginal fistula after total hysterectomy, Surg Gynecol Obstet 175:501, 1992.
50. Kelly J: Vesicovaginal fistulae. In Studd J, editor: Progress in obstetrics and gynaecology, London, 1983, Churchill-Livingstone.
51. Waaldijk K: The immediate surgical management of fresh obstetric fistulas with catheter and/or early closure, Int J Gynaecol Obstet 45:11, 1994.
52. Waaldijk K and Elkins TE: The obstetric fistula and peroneal nerve injury: an analysis of 947 consecutive patients, Int Urogynecol J 5:12, 1994.
53. Bieler EU and Schnabel T: Pituitary and ovarian function in women with vesicovaginal fistulae after obstructed and prolonged labor, S Afr Med J 50:257, 1976.
54. Thornton JG: Should vesicovaginal fistulae be treated only by specialists? Trop Doct 16:7, 1986.

28

Medical/Legal Implications

Saul Lerner

A disproportionately larger number of lawsuits are filed following a second operation than following the initial operation. Gynecologists must keep this in mind when they have to reoperate. The question they should ask themselves is, "Is this procedure now that much more difficult that it should be done by a gynecologist who is much more experienced in this type of problem?" One of the major causes leading to a poor outcome on a secondary operation is the failure of surgeons to recognize that this procedure has been so infrequent in their practice that they may not be the best person to undertake this second attempt. There are gynecologists in most areas who seem to have referred to them these more unusual and difficult cases. Both for the patient's interest and for legal protection, gynecologists would do well to recognize their limitations and refer their patients appropriately. On occasion this same advice might apply to the original surgery. There are operations that are rarely but necessarily done, and since the gynecologist may not have much experience performing such surgery, it would be best for everyone if such a case were referred to a regional center experienced in managing this problem.

Any time that an operation has to be repeated for the same problem, there is a natural assumption on the part of the nonmedical public that the surgeon who performed the first operation did it improperly. Given the present malpractice climate wherein some opportunistic lawyers vigorously advertise free consultation for anyone who believes he or she may have been the victim of such less than perfectly performed surgery, it is inevitable that many of these cases will progress to a lawsuit. What can be done to minimize risk in such an atmosphere? If surgeons are to survive in an unfavorable environment, they must accept the fact that the nature of the playing field has changed and mount a defensive strategy to meet the new challenge.

It is impossible to guarantee a perfect result in each case. There are too many extraneous factors beyond the surgeon's control that influence the final result, such as poor tissue in an individual patient or lack of compliance on the patient's part. Thus it is probably inevitable that if gynecologists are busy enough, they will probably be the victim of lawsuits.

Many surgeons, having informed the patient that surgery will have to be performed to deal with the patient's problem, recognize the patient's apprehensive reaction as inordinate and may tend to overdo it in trying to alleviate that apprehension. In so doing, they may leave the patient with the feeling that nothing can go wrong and the result inevitably will be perfect. We all know that we cannot give guarantees of a perfect result. Yet the fact is that many plaintiffs claim that the surgeon guaranteed their problem would be solved by the surgery. Surgeons must go out of their way when explaining the operation to the patient to make sure that no guarantee is being offered. The surgeon must honestly explain the possibility of failure and even give honest statistics on failure rates. Certain operations have a higher degree of failure to permanently solve the patient's problem, such as repair operations as opposed to ablation of an organ, and recognizing that possibility, the surgeon, in obtaining consent for surgery, must inform the patient of the possibilities for failure so that consent will be *informed consent.* But, as a defensive strategy, that would not be enough. Surgeons must take the time to document in the office record that they explained the possibility of failure or eventual recurrence of the problem. Most gynecologists are busy and are frequently behind schedule in the office, but if they are unwilling to take the time to provide such documentation, they must accept the idea that they are ignoring the reality of the playing field and leaving themselves vulnerable if sued.

Surgery performed to correct such problems as SUI, prolapse of the uterus, fistulas, cystocele, rectocele, or enterocele will generally be successful for a period of time, but there is a definite eventual recurrence rate for each of these. I am not going to discuss each of these separately but will discuss the problem of pregnancy following sterilization (which is generally followed by repeat sterilizing procedure) more in depth since the same principles apply to almost all the other problems.

It is generally accepted that 2 or 3 sterilization procedures in every 1000 will fail, and the woman will eventually find herself pregnant. It is also generally assumed that in most of the failures the procedure was performed properly. The healing process in the human is unpredictable; fistulous tracts that allow sperm or egg to bypass the manufactured barrier can develop, and the patient becomes pregnant—a true natural accident. However, the first reaction of a layperson (i.e., either a patient or a member of a jury) is that the operation was improperly done. Many lawyers know that the resultant pregnancy was not the result of a surgical error, but they are aware of the public perception. Thus the basis for most lawsuits in this category is not that the operation was improperly done but that the patient was not informed that the operation carries with it a chance of failure. The best defense against the charge that the operation was not properly done is an operative note clearly stating that each tube was traced out to its distal end, the fimbria were seen, and thus the tube was clearly identified before the tubal occlusion was accomplished. Too often the surgeon who is being sued rushes to review the operative note only to find that the resident who dictated the note simply said, "A Fallope ring was applied to each tube." At that point, the surgeon can only wish that he or she had taken the time to read the note before signing it.

Sometimes it is impossible during laparoscopic sterilization or minilaparotomy to trace the tube completely to its fimbriated end, but the surgeon is confident that the grasped structure is, indeed, the tube because the round ligament can be traced as a separate structure. What to do? Good medical practice (even if there were no malpractice threat) requires that the patient be informed that there was some uncertainty that the divided structure was tube and that she must not have unprotected intercourse until a hysterogram can be performed 3 months later. Most important, when the operative note is dictated, the plan of management should be clearly stated, and the surgeon should document in the record that he or she so instructed the patient.

Informed Consent

Now, let us return to the problem of informed consent. I am repeatedly amazed at how often there is a signed consent form in the medical record, yet the plaintiff claims a lack of informed consent. The general claim is that a clerk thrust a paper at the patient and demanded that it be signed. A good lawyer will note that when a car is taken in for repair, the driver must sign a long complicated document before leaving (without having read the document). The only practical precautionary defense against lack of informed consent is proper documentation, reinforced by the surgeon taking the time from an admittedly busy office to explain the nature of the operation, its side effects, its permanence, and its unavoidable inherent failure rate to the patient. Informed consent requires that the patient understand the nature of the act: in the example of tubal sterilization, that it is not a method of birth control but of terminating the childbearing period. I tell patients that they must not think of the procedure as something that can be reversed if they decide to have another baby since the reversability success rate is only 70%. Since subsequent pregnancy is the cause of most lawsuits in this category, it must be explained to the patient that no matter which technique is used, and, in spite of the fact that the operation is properly performed, about 2 or 3 women in 1000 will become pregnant because of the body's remarkable capacity to repair itself. Naturally such explanations must be given in such a manner that the surgeon is sure the patient understands what is being said. Survival tactics demand that surgeons record in their notes that they explained all of this to the patient. As a further defensive move, I recommend that surgeons give the patient a booklet on sterilization (e.g., ACOG's booklet) that mentions the inherent failure rate and record in their notes that such a booklet was given to the patient. The inevitable claim that is heard in court is "He told me that after this operation I would never be able to get pregnant." Although most hospitals have each patient sign a consent form before surgery, for sterilization procedures, the surgeon should have the patient sign a witnessed form in the office. Such a consent form must explicitly include information about the permanence of the procedure and the lack of guarantee.

Informed Refusal

The recent concept of informed refusal has coincidentally evolved with the law of informed consent, in which a patient participates with the physician in a process of decision making about proposed plans and surgical procedures offered as a remedy to the problem.[1] The patient also has the right to refuse any recommended treatment or procedure, and this is known as informed refusal.[2] When fiscal reimbursement for a procedure has been denied to the patient by the health insurance carrier, or the patient expresses a religious conviction that is in contrast to the surgeon's recommendation or declines treatment because of personal preference, these circumstances and the reasons given for the decision should be documented by the surgeon in the patient's clinical record, noting that the risks and benefits of the proposed procedure were discussed with the patient, who then refused the treatment. If the proposed treatment is refused for economic reasons, this should be stated, further noting the surgeon's efforts on behalf of the patient to convince the managed care provider that coverage should be provided, and also noting that the surgeon informed the patient of the likely consequences if surgery or treatment is not given.

Additional Considerations

Another reason for returning the patient to the OR for a second procedure is the discovery of a retained sponge or abdominal pad inadvertently left in the peritoneal cavity during the first operation (see Chapter 21).

This is a puzzling phenomenon since in each case it will be found that the sponge and pad count are noted in the record as having been correct. Yet it does happen occasionally in good hospitals involving good surgeons. All surgeons feel this is the fault of the circulating and scrub nurse, and therefore they are not guilty of negligence. Yet the courts, for the most part, do not agree. They still hold to the "captain of the ship" theory that the surgeon is responsible for all that happens in the OR. Too often a spirited defense is futile. The best way to deal with this problem is to recognize that it does indeed occur and take measures designed to reduce the possibility of it happening.

The most commonly employed tactic is to receive all sponges in sponge sticks and establish a procedure that when replacement sponges are required the scrub nurse refuses to provide one until she receives the soiled one back. Pads inserted into the abdomen should always have a Kelly's clamp affixed to the tail of the pad so that the clamp lies outside the wound. Occasions will arise when the surgeon must use a free sponge or pad in such a way that it cannot be clamped. This frequently happens in the course of a vaginal approach to the peritoneal cavity. In such cases, the surgeon, realizing that an unattached sponge has been left in the peritoneal cavity, can attach the Kelly clamp to the front of his or her surgical gown, seizing the underlying shirt in the process. The clamp on the surgical gown is removed when the free sponge has been removed. Thus, at the completion of the surgery, should the gown clamp be discovered as the gown is taken off, the surgeon will be reminded that there still is a sponge in the patient. If there is any question of the status of the sponge or pad count, x-rays seeking out a radiopaque marker must be performed in the OR before the patient is allowed to leave the room.

Not all second operations are done because of recurrence of the original problem. On occasion a patient will require a second operation very soon after the first operation to deal with an unexpected complication such as postoperative hemorrhage, intestinal obstruction, or evisceration. Once again the nonmedically trained person suspects that the original operation was not properly done, and such a situation lends itself to exploitation by an opportunistic lawyer. It is most important to have careful documentation of the surgeon's preoperative assessment of the case. Keep in mind that the claim frequently made in the ensuing lawsuit is that the diagnosis of the complication should have been made earlier in the course of events, and this would have prevented the serious sequelae that followed. When the patient is not doing as well as should have been expected postoperatively, that is the time for the surgeon to seek consultation—not a corridor consultation but an official one documented in the record. Granted that such consultation may not be necessary for management of the patient's problem, it is of great help in mounting a defense in a subsequent lawsuit (or, better still, in discouraging a stalking lawyer).

Frequently, when such emergency surgery has to be performed, the patient may not be alert and in command of all of her senses. Under such circumstances, the husband or parent should be asked to substitute for the patient and grant consent for the surgery. Again, it must be informed consent. Sometimes the husband or other close relative is not immediately available and the situation is urgent, requiring haste in getting the patient to the OR. In that case, a surgical colleague (or even a medical one) should be asked for a consultation to agree that the surgery is both necessary and urgent.

Many times the lawsuit, when filed, is also directed against the hospital. It would be wise under certain circumstances when it is reasonable to anticipate such a possibility to alert the administrator on call so that he or she can set in motion such risk management moves as are indicated.

All surgeons have had the experience of being in the midst of an operation and making an unanticipated discovery requiring removal of another organ or doing something other than what was told to the patient before surgery. Even though the surgeon is fully competent to handle this new development, he or she should seek supportive consultation with a colleague as an extension of the consent process. Naturally the existence of such a consultation should be recorded in the surgeon's operative note, but also the consultation report should be written separately in the record, signed by the consultant.

The most common malpractice claim against gynecologists concerns failure to diagnose breast cancer early enough, but that is beyond the scope of this book on repeat gynecologic operations and will not be discussed.

The next most common problems concern alleged failure to sterilize properly and ectopic pregnancy. Most suits related to ectopic pregnancy involve delayed diagnosis, but a certain number involve repeat ectopic pregnancy in the same tube. Most gynecologists prefer to conserve organs whenever possible, and many operations are done in which the pregnancy is removed from the tube by one means or another and the tube reconstructed. There is some disagreement on the wisdom of this approach, since it leaves a scar in the tube that could trap a subsequent fertilized egg on its journey through the tube to the uterus, setting up another ectopic pregnancy. I will not discuss the merits of the different surgical techniques employed to reduce the possibility, but I will point out that this possibility should be properly disclosed to the patient before surgery.

Although there still are some true emergencies with ruptured ectopic pregnancy requiring rapid course of action to deal with hemorrhage threatening the patient's life, most ectopic pregnancies are diagnosed early using a combination of quantitative human chorionic gonadotropins, ultrasonography, and/or laparoscopy, leaving plenty of time for discussion of her problem with the patient. The various approaches to her problem, with their advantages and disadvantages, should be explained to the patient. The possibility of repeat ectopic pregnancy should be presented to the patient fairly, and she should be allowed to select the procedure of her choice, conservation of the tube or excision. The gynecologist can certainly recommend his or her choice to the patient as long as it is done fairly. Consent to surgery must be informed consent. This means explaining alternatives, side effects, possible complications, and possible failure rates to the patient. The wise surgeon not only explains all of these, but also documents in the chart that each of them has been explained.

REFERENCES

1. American College of Obstetricians and Gynecologists: Ethical dimensions of informed consent, ACOG Committee Opinion No. 108, Washington, DC, 1992.
2. American College of Obstetricians and Gynecologists: Informed refusal, ACOG Committee Opinion No. 166, Washington, DC, 1995.

Index